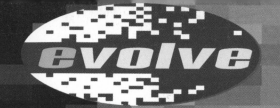

The Latest *Evolution* in Learning.

Evolve provides online access to free learning resources and activities designed specifically for the textbook you are using in your class. The resources will provide you with information that enhances the material covered in the book and much more.

Visit the Web address listed below to start your learning evolution today!

▶▶ *LOGIN: http://evolve.elsevier.com/Chabner/language/*

Evolve Learning Resources for Chabner's, *The Language of Medicine*, 7th Edition offers the following features:

- **Course Management System**

  The Evolve Course Management System (CMS) is a customizable course environment that provides powerful online instructor and student tools and any free learning resources available.

- **Learning Resources**

  The Evolve Learning Resources are free resources designed specifically for students and instructors using the corresponding textbook.

- **Weblinks**

  Hundreds of active websites keyed specifically to the content of the book. The Weblinks are continually updated, with new ones added as they develop.

Think outside the book... *evolve*.

The Language of Medicine

The Language of Medicine

Davi-Ellen Chabner, B.A., M.A.T.

A Write-in Text Explaining Medical Terms

7th edition

SAUNDERS

An Imprint of Elsevier

SAUNDERS

An Imprint of Elsevier

11830 Westline Industrial Drive
St. Louis, Missouri 63146

THE LANGUAGE OF MEDICINE   0-7216-9757-7

NOTICE

Medicine is an ever-changing field. Standard safety precautions must be followed, but as new research and clinical experience broaden our knowledge, changes in treatment and drug therapy may become necessary or appropriate. Readers are advised to check the most current product information provided by the manufacturer of each drug to be administered to verify the recommended dose, the method and duration of administration, and contraindications. It is the responsibility of the licensed prescriber, relying on experience and knowledge of the patient, to determine dosages and the best treatment for each individual patient. Neither the publisher nor the editor assumes any liability for any injury and/or damage to persons or property arising from this publication.

International Standard Book Number 0-7216-9757-7.

Acquisitions Editor: Jeanne Wilke
Developmental Editor: Becky Swisher
Publishing Services Manager: Pat Joiner
Project Manager: Sarah E. Fike
Designer: Ellen Zanolle

Printed in Chile.

9   8   7   6   5   4   3   2   1

For my mother, Estelle Rosenzweig

With love and gratitude for your confidence,
support, and encouragement

And, especially, for the time that we spend together
now

Preface

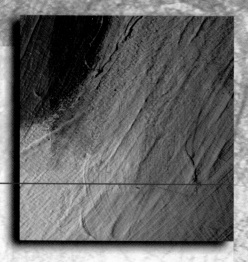

Welcome to the 7th edition of *The Language of Medicine*! This edition is about continuity. It has been twenty-eight years since the first edition was published, and I continue to find satisfaction in teaching and writing about medical terminology. You, as students and teachers, continue to motivate me with your valuable suggestions and comments. Because of the ease of communication via email, you have made a big difference in this edition. Thank you for writing to me and contributing to the success of this book throughout the years.

More than ever, this new edition reflects your continuing interest in the clinical relevance of medical terminology. Thus, I have added more case scenarios to illustrate how medical terms are used in sentences and up-to-date information about disease processes and new procedures. Plus, you will find additional full color illustrations and photographs that enhance your ability to see medical terms in action. Clearly, the best way to study medical terms is to understand them in their proper context, which is the anatomy, physiology, and pathology of the human body.

In addition to valuable reviews and continual feedback from instructors, medical reviewers have provided insight and advice about relevant and important medical terminology. My daughter, Elizabeth Chabner Thompson, MD, MPH, also contributed medical vignettes to each chapter and meticulously examined each chapter for clarity, simplicity, and practicality. Throughout, *The Language of Medicine* emphasizes explaining terminology rather than rote memorization of terms.*

---

*Continuing in this edition is the omission of the possessive form of all eponyms (e.g. Down syndrome, Tourette syndrome, Alzheimer disease). While the possessive form remains acceptable, this text is responding to a growing trend in promoting consistency and clarity. This decision is supported by The American Association for Medical Transcription in their Manual of Style (2002) and the American Medical Association in their Manual of Style, 10th edition (Williams and Wilkins), as well as by major medical dictionaries.

The fundamental features you have come to trust in learning and teaching medical terminology remain unchanged in this new 7th edition. These are:

- Simple, nontechnical explanations of medical terms.
- Workbook format with ample spaces to write answers.
- Explanations of clinical procedures, laboratory tests, and abbreviations related to each body system.
- Pronunciation of terms with phonetic spellings and spaces to write meanings of terms.
- Practical Applications sections with case reports, operative and diagnostic tests, and laboratory and x-ray reports.
- Exercises that test your understanding of terminology as you work through the text step-by-step (answers are included).
- Review sheets that pull together terminology to help you study.
- Comprehensive glossaries and appendices for reference in class and on the job. NEW to this edition is a Drug Appendix that alphabetically lists drugs and their uses.

The CD-ROM included with this new edition is packed with additional information, images, and video clips to test and expand your understanding. Chapter by chapter, I have added more case studies, examples of medical records, and a wealth of new images to illustrate terminology. Additionally, on the CD-ROM, you can hear me pronounce the relevant terms on the pronunciation of terms section in every chapter (more than 3,000 terms in all!). A useful CD-ROM glossary helps you analyze and divide terms into their individual word parts.

My *Medical Language Instant Translator* (for sale separately) is a uniquely useful resource for all allied health professionals and students of medical terminology and has been updated for this new edition. It is a pocket-sized medical terminology reference with convenient information at your fingertips! Included are:

- Explanations of common office and hospital procedures and laboratory tests.
- Abbreviations, acronyms, and symbols.
- Frequently prescribed drugs and their uses.
- Glossaries to help you decipher medical terms without consulting a dictionary.
- Medical terms that are commonly confused.
- Full-color illustrations of body systems.
- Surgical terminology, including instrumentation and procedures.

The Language of Medicine Instructor's Curriculum Resource (including an instructor's manual, CD-ROM with test bank, and image collection) is available with even more new quizzes, teaching suggestions, crossword puzzles, medical reports, and reference material. The image collection contains all figures and photos from this new 7th edition.

My continued goal in writing *The Language of Medicine* is to help students learn and to help instructors teach. Using an interactive, logical, interesting, and easy-to-follow method, you will find that medical terminology comes "alive" and stays with you. Undeniably, the study of this language requires commitment and hard work, but the benefits are great. The knowledge that you gain will jump start your career in the medical workplace and help you for years to come.

Each student and teacher who selects *The Language of Medicine* becomes my partner in the exciting adventure of learning medical terms. Continuity is crucial. Continue to communicate with me through email (*MedDavi@aol.com*) with your suggestions and comments so that further printings and editions may benefit. A website connected to *The Language of Medicine* and dedicated to helping students and teachers is located at *http://evolve.elsevier.com/Chabner/language*. I hope you will tell me what you would like to see on that website so that we can make it a useful part of the learning process. You should know that I still experience the thrill and joy of teaching new students. I love being in a classroom and feel privileged to continue to write this text. I hope that my enthusiasm and passion for the medical language is transmitted to you through these pages. Work hard, but have fun with *The Language of Medicine*!

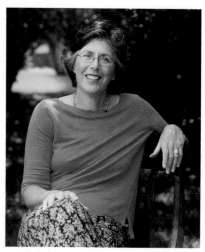

Davi-Ellen Chabner

Acknowledgment

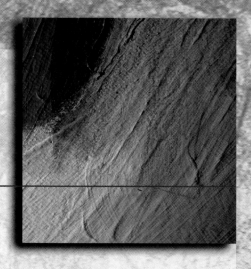

Once again, my indispensable editor, Maureen Pfeifer, has shepherded this edition to completion. My gratitude goes deep for her brilliant and effective guidance on every aspect of the work. She has uncanny good sense and is willing to trouble-shoot, tackle, and solve whatever problems arise. I trust her keen intelligence, excellent judgment, and loyalty and know that any success of this edition (or other editions that she has collaborated on with me) is, in large part, because of her tireless (even with two babies in tow) efforts on its behalf. Maureen, thanks for your continuing friendship and confidence in *The Language of Medicine*.

I am grateful to my devoted daughter, Elizabeth Chabner Thompson, M.D., M.P.H., who besides making valuable and extensive editorial contributions, sustained me with her boundless energy, enthusiasm, ideas, and support. She did all this while incubating her fourth child!

To the medical reviewers (listed on a separate page), and foremost to my husband, Bruce Allan Chabner, M.D., I owe much thanks. These experts took time from busy schedules to provide essential advice and information on chapters related to their specialties. I appreciate their outstanding assistance and interest in the text.

I am also indebted to the instructors (listed on a separate page) who extensively reviewed this book and gave me their feedback. Many experienced instructors personally communicated with me to offer comments and suggestions that are reflected in this new text. Since they are "on the front lines" with *The Language of Medicine*, I especially value their guidance. Special thank you to Judy Aronow, Chris Palpias, Nancy Kotyk, Charlotte Bowers, Alice Noblin, Barbara Barranco, Alan Rosenberg, Leslie Jebson, Michelle Green, Susan Webb, Julie Lopez, Efram Miranda, Brandy Ziesemer, Lola McGourty, Karen Lockyer, Gino Gentile, R.N., Jeannetta Blackmun, Colleen Closser, Linda Alford, Helen Horiuchi, and Terri Stroh, and Joyce Y. Nakana. I am also grateful to the many students who have shared their ideas and comments, including Judy Hensley, Julie Kahler, Debbi Segreti, Michelle Cordeiro, Jean Fox, Pauline Fletcher, Fran Grohman, Pamela LaCuran, and Mary Peterson. I listen to each of you!

Jim Perkins, Assistant Professor of Medical Illustration, Rochester Institute of Technology, once again did excellent work on the artwork. I appreciated his superb illustrations and careful attention to detail, clarity, and accuracy in every image.

Many people at Elsevier were integral to the completion of this edition. In particular, I want to thank Ellen B. Zanolle, Senior Book Designer, Art/Design, who not only designed the cover and interior of this new edition, but also supervised the complicated layout and composition of the text. Ellen, you were a life-saver and essential! Becky Swisher, Developmental Editor, Health Professions II, and Sarah Fike, Project Manager, Book Production, were crucial to the completion and coordination of various aspects of production. Special thanks to Becky for her work on the CD-ROM and *Medical Language Instant Translator* and for bolstering my flagging spirits along the way! Thank you, Sarah for picking up the project midstream and doing such a good job.

My gratitude also to Andrew Allen, Publishing Director, Health Professions II Editorial, and Jeanne Wilke, Executive Editor, Health Professions II Editorial, for their unwavering, strong support. Thanks to Katherine Tomber, Editorial Assistant, Health Professions II Editorial; Pat Joiner, Publishing Services Manager, Book Production; Kim Hamby, Product Manager, Marketing; Jaleen Nowell, Multimedia Producer, Multimedia Production; Sharon Salomon, Creative Director, Creative Services; and Peggy Fagan, Director of Publishing Services, Book Production; for their hard work and countless hours devoted to this new edition.

With utmost pleasure, I thank my grandchildren, Bebe, Solomon, Ben, and Gus, for helping their "Mimi" relax with precious hours of fun and enjoyment. My devoted family and close friends also gave much sustaining encouragement and understanding (especially long-suffering Bruce) while I was spending so much time on my work. Special thanks to Juliana Carmo, who cheerfully helped with so many aspects of my life during the writing of this edition.

Davi-Ellen Chabner

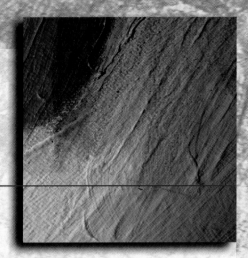

Reviewers

Medical Reviewers

Elizabeth Chabner Thompson, M.D., M.P.H.
Scarsdale, New York

Bruce A. Chabner, M.D.
Clinical Director, Massachusetts General Hospital
  Cancer Center
Professor of Medicine
Harvard Medical School
Boston, Massachusetts

Barry S. Coller, M.D.
David Rockefeller Professor of Medicine
Rockefeller University
New York, New York

Michael J. Curtin, M.D.
InterMountain Orthopedics
Boise, Idaho

Carlos Jamis-Dow, M.D.
Department of Radiology
Georgetown University Hospital
Washington, DC

Fred H. Hochberg, M.D.
Neurology Department
Massachusetts General Hospital
Boston, Massachusetts

Richard T. Penson, M.R.C.P., M.D.
Clinical Director
Medical Gynecologic Oncology
Massachusetts General Hospital
Boston, Massachusetts

Henry E. Schniewind, M.D.
Instructor in Psychiatry
Harvard Medical School
Boston, Massachusetts

Amy Simon, M.D.
Assistant Professor of Medicine
Director, Asthma Center
Tufts University School of Medicine
Boston, Massachusetts

Daniel I. Simon, M.D., F.A.C.C., F.A.H.A.
Associate Director, Interventional Cardiology
Brigham and Women's Hospital
Associate Professor of Medicine
Harvard Medical School
Boston, Massachusetts

Norman Simon, M.D.
Professor of Medicine
Northwestern University
Feinberg School of Medicine
Chicago, Illinois

Jill A. Smith, M.D.
Associate Chief of Ophthalmology
Newton-Wellesley Hospital
Newton, Massachusetts

Arthur Sober, M.D.
Associate Chief of Dermatology
Massachusetts General Hospital
Professor of Dermatology
Harvard Medical School
Boston, Massachusetts

Instructor Reviewers

Richard R. Espinsoa, R.Ph., PharmD.
Department Chair for Allied Health Sciences
Associate Professor, Registered Pharmacist
Austin Community College
Austin, Texas

Karen Jackson, A.S., N.R.-C.M.A.
Remington College
Department Chair, Medical Assisting Program
Garland, Texas

Patricia McLane, B.S., M.A., R.H.I.A.
Instructor, Health Careers
Henry Ford Community College
Dearborn, Michigan

Tammy Miller, R.N.
Medical Coordinator
Douglas Education Center
Monessen, Pennsylvania

Bonnie Petterson, R.H.I.A., B.S., M.S.
Department Chair, Health Information Technology
Phoenix College
Phoenix, Arizona

Kay Shepherd, R.N., B.S.N.
Secondary School Nurse
High School Health Academy Instructor
Washington High School
Vinton, Iowa

Ann Haber Stanton, B.A., C.M.T.
Medical Transcription QA Specialist
Medical Terminology Instructor
Career Learning Center of the Black Hills
Rapid City Regional Hospital
Rapid City, South Dakota

Lisa Teasley
President
Med Scripts
Wetumpka, Alabama

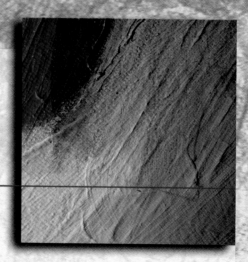

Contents

Chapter 3

Suffixes   75

Chapter 4

Prefixes   109

Chapter 5

Digestive System   139

Chapter 6

Additional Suffixes and Digestive System Terminology   185

Chapter **7**

Urinary System   213

Chapter **8**

Female Reproductive System   253

Chapter 9

Male Reproductive System   305

Chapter 10

Nervous System   333

Chapter 11

Cardiovascular System   383

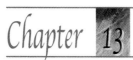

Chapter **12**

Respiratory System   441

Chapter **13**

Blood System   487

Chapter 14

Chapter 15

Chapter 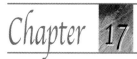 16

Skin 629

Chapter 17

Sense Organs: The Eye and the Ear 669

Chapter 18

Endocrine System 719

Chapter 19

Cancer Medicine (Oncology) 769

Chapter **20**

Radiology and Nuclear Medicine 817

Chapter **21**

Pharmacology 849

Chapter **22**

Psychiatry 887

chapter 1

Basic Word Structure

This chapter is divided into the following sections

In this chapter you will

- Learn basic objectives to guide your study of the medical language.
- Divide medical words into their component parts.
- Find the meaning of basic combining forms, prefixes, and suffixes of the medical language.
- Use these combining forms, prefixes, and suffixes to build medical words.

I. Objectives in Studying the Medical Language

There are three objectives to keep in mind as you study medical terminology:

1. **Analyze words by dividing them into component parts.** Your goal is to learn the *tools* of word analysis that will make understanding complex terminology easier. Do not simply memorize terms; think about dividing terms into component parts. This text will show you how to separate both complicated and simple terms into understandable word elements. Medical terms are very much like individual jigsaw

puzzles. They are constructed of small pieces that make each word unique, but the pieces can be used in different combinations in other words as well. As you become familiar with word parts and learn what each means, you will be able to recognize those word parts in totally new combinations in other terms.

2. **Relate the medical terms to the structure and function of the human body.** Memorization of terms, although essential to retention of the language, should not become the primary objective of your study. A major focus of this text is to *explain* terms in the context of how the body works in health and disease. Medical terms explained in their proper context will also be easier to remember. Thus, the term **hepatitis,** meaning inflammation **(-itis)** of the liver **(hepat),** is better understood when you know where the liver is and how it functions. No previous knowledge of biology, anatomy, or physiology is needed for this study. Explanations in the text are straightforward and basic.

3. **Be aware of spelling and pronunciation problems.** Some medical terms are pronounced alike but are spelled differently, which accounts for their different meanings. For example, **ilium** and **ileum** have identical pronunciations, but the first term, **ilium,** means a part of the pelvis (hip bone), whereas the second term, **ileum,** means a part of the small intestine. Even when terms are spelled correctly, they can be misunderstood because of incorrect pronunciation. For example, the **urethra** (ū-RĒ-thrăh) is the tube leading from the urinary bladder to the outside of the body, whereas a **ureter** (ŪR-ĕ-tĕr) is one of two tubes each leading from a single kidney and inserting into the urinary bladder. Figure 1–1 illustrates the difference between the urethra and the ureters.

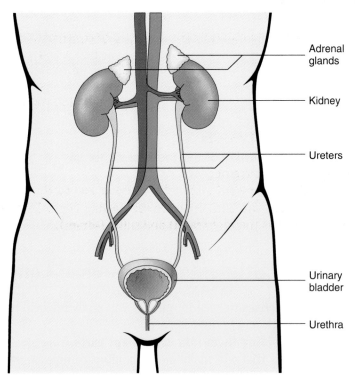

Adrenal glands

Kidney

Ureters

Urinary bladder

Urethra

Figure 1–1
_____

Urinary system.

II. Word Analysis

Studying medical terminology is very similar to learning a new language. At first, the words sound strange and complicated, although they may stand for commonly known English terms. For example, the term **otalgia** means "ear ache," and an **ophthalmologist** is an "eye doctor."

Your first job in learning the language is to understand how to divide words into their component parts. Logically, most terms, whether complex or simple, can be broken down into basic parts and then understood. For example, consider the following term:

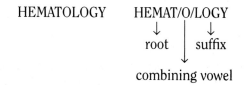

The **root** is the *foundation of the word*. All medical terms have one or more roots. For example, the root **hemat** means **blood**.

The **suffix** is the *word ending*. All medical terms have a suffix. The suffix **-logy** means **study of.**

The **combining vowel** (usually o) *links the root to the suffix or the root to another root*. A combining vowel has no meaning of its own; it only joins one word part to another.

It is useful to read the meaning of medical terms *starting from the suffix and moving back to the beginning of the term*. Thus, the term **hematology** means **study of blood.**

Here is another familiar medical term:

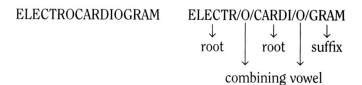

The root **electr** means **electricity.**
The root **cardi** means **heart.**
The suffix **-gram** means **record.**
The entire word means **record of the electricity in the heart.**

Notice that there are two combining vowels in this term. They link the two roots (**electr** and **cardi**) as well as the root (**cardi**) and suffix (**-gram**).

Try another term:

GASTRITIS   GASTR/ITIS
                ↓   ↓
              root suffix

The root **gastr** means **stomach.**
The suffix **-itis** means **inflammation.**
The entire word, reading from the end of the term (suffix) to the beginning, means **inflammation of the stomach.**

Note that the combining vowel, o, is missing in this term. This is because the suffix, **-itis,** begins with a vowel. The combining vowel is dropped before a suffix that begins with a vowel. It is retained, however, between two roots, even if the second root begins with a vowel. Consider the following term:

GASTROENTEROLOGY   GASTR/O/ENTER/O/LOGY
                        ↓   ↓   ↓
                       root   root   suffix
                               ↓
                        combining vowel

The root **gastr** means **stomach.**
The root **enter** means **intestines.**
The suffix **-logy** means **study of.**
The entire term means **study of the stomach and intestines.**

Notice that the combining vowel is used between **gastr** and **enter,** even though the second root, **enter,** begins with a vowel. When a term contains two or more roots related to parts of the body, anatomical position often determines which root goes before the other. For example, the stomach receives food first, before the small intestine, thus **gastroenteritis,** not enterogastritis.

In summary, remember three general rules:
1. Read the meaning of medical terms from the suffix back to the beginning of the term and across.
2. Drop the combining vowel (usually o) before a suffix beginning with a vowel: **gastritis** *not* **gastroitis.**
3. Keep the combining vowel between two roots: **gastroenterology** *not* **gastrenterology.**

In addition to the root, suffix, and combining vowel, two other word parts are commonly found in medical terms. These are the **combining form** and **prefix.** The combining form is simply the root plus the combining vowel. For example, you are already familiar with the following combining forms and their meanings:

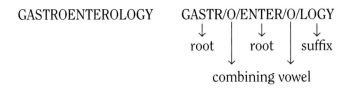

HEMAT/O   means   **blood**
  ↗   ↗
root + combining vowel = COMBINING FORM

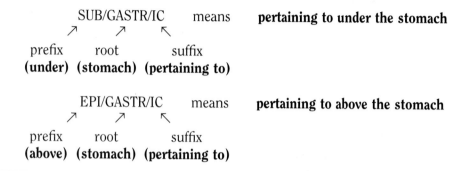

GASTR/O   means   **stomach**

root + combining vowel = COMBINING FORM

CARDI/O   means   **heart**

root + combining vowel = COMBINING FORM

Combining forms are used with many different suffixes. Remembering the exact meaning of a combining form will help you understand different medical terms.

The **prefix** is a small part that is attached to the *beginning of a term*. Not all medical terms contain prefixes, but the prefix can have an important influence on meaning. Consider the following examples:

SUB/GASTR/IC   means   **pertaining to under the stomach**

prefix   root   suffix
(under) (stomach) (pertaining to)

EPI/GASTR/IC   means   **pertaining to above the stomach**

prefix   root   suffix
(above) (stomach) (pertaining to)

In summary, the important elements of medical terms are the following:
1. **Root:** foundation of the term
2. **Suffix:** word ending
3. **Prefix:** word beginning
4. **Combining vowel:** vowel (usually o) that links the root to the suffix or the root to another root
5. **Combining form:** combination of the root and the combining vowel

---

III. Combining Forms, Suffixes, and Prefixes

In previous examples you have been introduced to the combining forms **gastr/o** (stomach), **hemat/o** (blood), and **cardi/o** (heart). The following list contains new combining forms, suffixes, and prefixes with examples of medical words using those word parts. Your job is to write the *meaning* of the medical term in the space provided. As you do this, you may wish to divide the term into its component parts by using slashes (e.g., **aden/oma**).

If you have a question about the correct pronunciation of a term, consult the Pronunciation of Terms section at the end of each chapter. In addition, the CD-ROM that accompanies this text contains the pronunciations of most terms on the Pronunciation of Terms lists. Although most medical terms can be divided into component parts and understood, others defy simple explanation. This text provides additional information when those terms are introduced, but you may wish to consult a medical dictionary as well.

To test your understanding of word parts and terminology in this chapter, complete the exercises on pages 14 to 22 and check your answers on pages 23 to 25. Then, as a final review, give the meanings for the combining forms, suffixes, and prefixes on the Review Sheet, pages 29 and 30.

Write the meanings of the medical terms that follow in the spaces provided. The notes in italics below the terms will help you define them. Simple definitions are best. The first one has been filled in as an example.

Combining Forms

Combining Form	Meaning	Terminology	Meaning
aden/o	gland	adenoma	*tumor of a gland*

The suffix -oma means tumor or mass.

adenitis _____

The suffix -itis means inflammation.

arthr/o	joint	arthritis _____	
bi/o	life	biology _____	

biopsy _____

The suffix -opsy means process of viewing. Living tissue is removed from the body and viewed under a microscope.

carcin/o	cancerous, cancer	carcinoma _____	

A carcinoma is a cancerous tumor. Carcinomas grow from epithelial (surface or skin) cells that cover the outside of the body and line organs, cavities, and tubes within the body.

cardi/o	heart	cardiology _____	
cephal/o	head	cephalic _____	

(sĕ-FAL-ĭk) The suffix -ic means pertaining to. If an infant is born with its head delivered first, it is a cephalic presentation.

cerebr/o	cerebrum (largest part of the brain)	cerebral _____	

The suffix -al means pertaining to. A cerebrovascular accident (CVA) occurs when damage to blood vessels (vascul/o means blood vessels) in the cerebrum causes injury to nerve cells of the brain. This condition is also called a stroke.

cis/o	to cut	incision _____	

The prefix in- means into and the suffix -ion means process.

excision _____

The prefix ex- means out.

crin/o   secrete (to form and give off)   endocrine glands _____

The prefix endo- means within; endocrine glands (e.g., thyroid, pituitary, and adrenal glands) secrete hormones directly within (into) the bloodstream. Other glands, called exocrine glands, secrete chemicals (e.g., saliva, sweat, tears) through tubes (ducts) to the outside of the body.

cyst/o   urinary bladder; a sac or a cyst (sac containing fluid)   cystoscopy _____

(sĭs-TŎS-kō-pē) The suffix -scopy means process of visual examination.

cyt/o   cell   cytology _____

derm/o
dermat/o   skin   dermatitis _____

hypodermic _____

The prefix hypo- means under, below.

electr/o   electricity   electrocardiogram _____

The suffix -gram means record. Abbreviations are ECG or EKG.

encephal/o   brain   electroencephalogram _____

Also called an EEG.

enter/o   intestines (usually the small intestine)   enteritis _____

The small intestine is narrower but much longer than the large intestine (colon).

erythr/o   red   erythrocyte _____

The suffix -cyte means cell. Erythrocytes carry oxygen in the blood.

gastr/o   stomach   gastrectomy _____

The suffix -ectomy means excision or removal.

gastrotomy _____

The suffix -tomy means incision or cutting into.

gnos/o   knowledge   diagnosis _____

The prefix dia- means complete. The suffix -sis means state of. A diagnosis is made after sufficient information has been obtained about the patient's condition. Literally, it is a "state of complete knowledge."

prognosis _____

The prefix pro- means before. Literally, "knowledge before," a prognosis is a prediction about the outcome of an illness, but it is always given after the diagnosis has been determined.

gynec/o	woman, female	gynecology _____
hemat/o **hem/o**	blood	hematology _____

hematoma _____

In this term, -oma means a mass or collection of blood, rather than a growth of cells (tumor). A hematoma occurs when blood escapes from blood vessels and collects as a clot in a cavity, organ, or under the skin.

hemoglobin _____

The suffix -globin means protein. Hemoglobin helps carry oxygen in red blood cells.

hepat/o	liver	hepatitis _____
iatr/o	treatment	iatrogenic _____

The suffix-genic means pertaining to producing, produced by, or produced in. Iatrogenic conditions are adverse side effects that result from treatment or intervention by a physician.

leuk/o	white	leukocyte _____

This blood cell helps the body fight disease.

nephr/o	kidney	nephritis _____
		nephrology _____
neur/o	nerve	neurology _____
onc/o	tumor	oncology _____
		oncologist _____

The suffix -ist means one who specializes in a field of medicine.

ophthalm/o	eye	ophthalmoscope _____

(ŏf-THĂL-mō-skōp) The suffix-scope means an instrument for visual examination.

oste/o	bone	osteitis _____
		osteoarthritis _____

This condition is actually a degeneration of bones and joints that occurs with aging. It is often accompanied by inflammation.

path/o	disease	pathology _____
		pathologist _____

A pathologist examines biopsy samples microscopically and examines a dead body to determine the cause of death.

ped/o	child	pediatric _____

Originally, orthopedists were doctors who straightened (orth/o means straight) children's bones and corrected deformities. Nowadays, orthopedists specialize in disorders of bones and muscles of people of all ages.

psych/o	mind	psychology _____
		psychiatrist _____
radi/o	x-rays	radiology _____
ren/o	kidney	renal _____

Ren/o (Latin) and nephr/o (Greek) both mean kidney. Ren/o is used with -al (Latin) to describe the kidney, whereas nephr/o is used with other suffixes such as -osis, -itis, and -ectomy (Greek) to describe abnormal conditions and operative procedures.

rhin/o	nose	rhinitis _____
sarc/o	flesh	sarcoma _____

This is a cancerous (malignant) tumor. A sarcoma grows from cells of "fleshy" connective tissue such as muscle, bone, and fat, whereas a carcinoma (another type of cancerous tumor) grows from epithelial cells that line the outside of the body or the inside of organs in the body.

sect/o	to cut	resection _____

The prefix re- means back. A resection is a cutting back in the sense of cutting out or removal (excision). A gastric resection is a gastrectomy, or excision of the stomach.

thromb/o	clot, clotting	thrombocyte _____

*Also known as **platelets**, these cells help clot blood. A **thrombus** is the actual clot that forms, and **thrombosis** (-osis means condition) is the condition of clot formation.*

ur/o	urinary tract, urine	urology _____

A urologist is a surgeon who operates on the organs of the urinary tract and the organs of the male reproductive system.

Suffixes

Suffix	Meaning	Terminology	Meaning
-ac	pertaining to	cardiac _____	
-al	pertaining to	neural _____	
-algia	pain	arthralgia _____	
		neuralgia _____	
-cyte	cell	erythrocyte _____	
-ectomy	excision, removal	nephrectomy _____	
-emia	blood condition	leukemia _____	

Literally, this term means "a blood condition of white (blood cells)." Actually, it is a condition of blood in which cancerous white blood cells proliferate (increase in number).

-genic	pertaining to producing, produced by, or produced in	carcinogenic _____	

Cigarette smoke is carcinogenic.

pathogenic _____

A virus or a bacterium is a pathogenic organism.

iatrogenic _____

In this term, -genic means produced by.

-gram	record	electroencephalogram _____	
-ic, -ical	pertaining to	gastric _____	
		neurological _____	
-ion	process	excision _____	
-ist	specialist	gynecologist _____	
-itis	inflammation	cystitis _____	
-logy	study of	endocrinology _____	
-oma	tumor, mass, swelling	hepatoma _____	

A hepatoma (hepatocellular carcinoma) is a malignant tumor of the liver.

-opsy	process of viewing	biopsy _____	
-osis	condition, usually abnormal (slight increase in numbers when used with blood cells)	nephrosis _____	
		leukocytosis _____	
		This condition, a slight increase in normal white blood cells, occurs as white blood cells multiply to fight an infection.	
-pathy	disease condition	enteropathy _____	
		(ĕn-tĕ-RŎP-ă-thē)	
		adenopathy _____	
		(ă-dĕ-NŎP-ă-thē)	
-scope	instrument to visually examine	endoscope _____	
		Endo- means within. A cystoscope is an endoscope.	
-scopy	process of visually examining	endoscopy _____	
		(ĕn-DŎS-kō-pē)	
-sis	state of	prognosis _____	
-tomy	process of cutting, incision	osteotomy _____	
		(ŏs-tē-ŎT-tō-mē)	
-y	process, condition	gastroenterology _____	

Prefixes			
Prefix	Meaning	Terminology	Meaning
a-, an-	no, not, without	anemia _____	
		Anemia is a decreased number of erythrocytes or an abnormality of the hemoglobin (a chemical) within the red blood cells. This results in decreased delivery of oxygen to cells of the body. Originally, anemic patients looked so pale that they were thought to be "without blood."	
auto-	self	autopsy _____	
		This term literally means "to view by one's self." Hence, an autopsy is the examination of a dead body with one's own eyes to determine the cause of death and nature of disease.	
dia-	through, complete	diagnosis _____	

endo-	within	endocrinologist _____
epi-	above, upon	epigastric _____
		epidermis _____
		This outermost layer of skin lies above the middle layer of skin, known as the dermis.
ex-	out	excision _____
exo-	out	exocrine glands _____
hyper-	excessive, above, more than normal	hyperglycemia _____
		The term glyc/o means sugar.
hypo-	deficient, below, under, less than normal	hypogastric _____
		When hypo- is used with a part of the body, it means below.
		hypoglycemia _____
		In this term, hypo- means deficient.
in-	into, in	incision _____
peri-	surrounding, around	pericardium _____
		The suffix -um means a structure. The pericardium is the membrane that surrounds the heart.
pro-	before, forward	prognosis _____
re-	back, backward, again	resection _____
		This is an operation in which an organ is "cut back" or removed.
retro-	behind	retrocardiac _____
sub-	below, under	subhepatic _____
trans-	across, through	transhepatic _____

IV. Practical Applications

This is an opportunity for you to use your skill in understanding medical terms and to increase your knowledge of new terms. Be sure to check your answers with the Answers to Practical Applications on page 24. You should find helpful explanations there.

Specialists

Match the **abnormal condition** in COLUMN I with the **physician (specialist) who treats** it in COLUMN II.

Column I

1. heart attack　_____

2. ovarian cysts　_____

3. bipolar (manic-depressive) disorder　_____

4. breast adenocarcinoma　_____

5. iron-deficiency anemia　_____

6. retinopathy　_____

7. cerebrovascular accident　_____

8. renal failure　_____

9. inflammatory bowel disease　_____

10. cystitis　_____

Column II

A. gastroenterologist
B. hematologist
C. nephrologist
D. cardiologist
E. oncologist
F. gynecologist
G. urologist
H. ophthalmologist
I. neurologist
J. psychiatrist

V. Exercises

The exercises that follow are designed to help you learn the terms presented in the chapter. Writing terms over and over again is a good way to remember this new language. You will find answers to each exercise in Section VI. This makes it easy to check your work. As you check each answer, you will not only reinforce your understanding of a term, but often gain additional information from the answer. Each exercise is designed not as a test, but rather as an opportunity for you to learn the material.

A. Complete the following sentences.

1. Word beginnings are called _____.

2. Word endings are called _____.

3. The foundation of a word is known as the _____.

4. A letter linking a suffix and a root, or linking two roots, in a term is the

   _____.

5. The combination of a root and a combining vowel is known as the _____.

B. Give the meanings of the following combining forms.

1. cardi/o _____

2. aden/o _____

3. bi/o _____

4. cerebr/o _____

5. cephal/o _____

6. arthr/o _____

7. carcin/o _____

8. cyst/o _____

9. cyt/o _____

10. derm/o or dermat/o _____

11. encephal/o _____

12. electr/o _____

C. Give the meanings of the following suffixes.

1. -oma _____

2. -al _____

3. -itis _____

4. -logy _____

5. -scopy _____

6. -ic _____

7. -gram _____

8. -opsy _____

D. Using slashes, divide the following terms into parts and give the meaning of the entire term.

1. cerebral _____

2. biopsy _____

3. adenitis _____

4. cephalic _____

5. carcinoma _____

6. cystoscopy _____

7. electrocardiogram _____

8. cardiology _____

9. electroencephalogram _____

10. dermatitis _____

11. arthroscopy _____

12. cytology _____

E. Give the meanings of the following combining forms.

1. erythr/o _____ 7. nephr/o _____

2. enter/o _____ 8. leuk/o _____

3. gastr/o _____ 9. iatr/o _____

4. gnos/o _____ 10. hepat/o _____

5. hemat/o _____ 11. neur/o _____

6. cis/o _____ 12. gynec/o _____

F. Complete the medical term based on its meaning, as provided.

1. white blood cell: _____ cyte

2. inflammation of the stomach: gastr _____

3. pertaining to being produced by treatment: _____ genic

4. study of kidneys: _____ logy

5. red blood cell: _____ cyte

6. mass of blood: _____ oma

7. view of living tissue: bi _____

8. pain of nerves: neur _____

9. process of viewing the eye: _____ scopy

10. inflammation of the small intestine: _____ itis

G. Match the English term in column I with its combining form in column II.

Column I
English Term

Column II
Combining Form

1. kidney _____

2. disease _____

3. eye _____

4. to cut _____

5. nose _____

6. flesh _____

7. mind _____

8. urinary tract _____

9. bone _____

10. x-rays _____

11. clotting _____

12. tumor _____

onc/o
ophthalm/o
oste/o
path/o
psych/o
radi/o
ren/o
rhin/o
sarc/o
sect/o
thromb/o
ur/o

H. Underline the suffix in each term and give the meaning of the entire term.

1. ophthalmoscopy _____

2. ophthalmoscope _____

3. oncology _____

4. osteitis _____

5. psychosis _____

6. thrombocyte _____

7. renal _____

8. nephrectomy _____

9. osteotomy _____

10. resection _____

11. carcinogenic _____

12. sarcoma _____

I. Match the suffix in column I with its meaning in column II. Write the meaning in the space provided.

Column I
Suffix

1. -algia _____

2. -ion _____

3. -emia _____

4. -gram _____

5. -scope _____

6. -osis _____

7. -ectomy _____

8. -genic _____

9. -pathy _____

10. -tomy _____

11. -itis _____

12. -cyte _____

Column II
Meaning

abnormal condition
blood condition
cell
disease condition
incision, process of cutting into
inflammation
instrument to visually examine
pain
pertaining to producing, produced by, or produced in
process
record
removal, excision, resection

J. **Select from the following terms to complete the sentences below.**

arthralgia   enteropathy   iatrogenic
carcinogenic   exocrine   leukemia
cystitis   hematoma   leukocytosis
endocrine   hepatoma   neuralgia

1. When Paul smoked cigarettes, he inhaled a _____ substance with each puff.

2. Sally's sore throat, fever, and chills made her doctor order a white blood cell count. Results, indicating infection, showed a slight increase in normal cells, a condition

   called _____.

3. Mr. Smith's liver enlarged, giving him abdominal pain and fullness in his RUQ. His radiological

   tests and biopsy revealed a malignant tumor or _____.

4. Mrs. Rose complained of pain in her hip joints, knees, and shoulders each morning. She was told

   that she had painful joints or _____.

5. Dr. Black was trained to treat disorders of the pancreas, thyroid gland, adrenal glands, and pituitary

   gland. Thus, he was an expert in the _____ glands.

6. Ms. Walsh told her doctor she had pain when urinating. After tests, the doctor's diagnosis was

   inflammation of the urinary bladder, or _____.

7. Elizabeth's overhead tennis shot hit David in the thigh and produced a large _____.
   His skin looked bruised and was tender.

8. Mr. Bell's white blood cell count is 10 times higher than normal. Examination of his blood shows

   cancerous white blood cells. His diagnosis is _____.

9. Mr. Kay was resuscitated (revived from potential or apparent death) in the emergency room after
   experiencing a heart attack. Unfortunately, he suffered a broken rib as a result of the physician's

   chest compressions. This is an example of a (an) _____ fracture.

10. After coming back from a trip during which he had eaten strange foods, Mr. Cameron had disease

    of his intestines called _____.

K. Give the meanings of the following prefixes.

1. dia- _____

2. pro- _____

3. auto- _____

4. a-, an- _____

5. hyper- _____

6. hypo- _____

7. epi- _____

8. endo- _____

9. retro- _____

10. trans- _____

11. peri- _____

12. ex- _____

13. sub- _____

14. re- _____

L. Underline the prefix in the following terms and give the meaning of the entire term.

1. diagnosis _____

2. prognosis _____

3. subhepatic _____

4. pericardium _____

5. hyperglycemia _____

6. hypodermic _____

7. epigastric _____

8. resection _____

9. hypoglycemia _____

10. anemia _____

M. Complete the following terms (describing areas of medicine) based on their meanings as given below.

1. study of urinary tract: _____ logy

2. study of women and women's diseases: _____ logy

3. study of blood: _____ logy

4. study of tumors: _____ logy

5. study of the kidneys: _____ logy

6. study of nerves: _____ logy

7. treatment of children: _____ iatrics

8. study of x-rays: _____ logy

9. study of the eyes: _____ logy

10. study of the stomach and intestines: _____ logy

11. study of glands that secrete hormones: _____ logy

12. treatment of the mind: _____ iatry

13. study of disease: _____ logy

14. study of the heart: _____ logy

N. Give the meaning of the underlined word part and then define the term.

1. <u>cerebro</u>vascular accident _____

2. <u>encephal</u>itis _____

3. <u>cysto</u>scope _____

4. <u>trans</u>hepatic _____

5. <u>iatro</u>genic _____

6. <u>hypo</u>gastric _____

7. <u>endo</u>crine glands _____

8. nephr<u>ectomy</u> _____

9. <u>exo</u>crine glands _____

10. neur<u>algia</u> _____

O. Select from the following terms to complete the sentences below.

anemia   oncogenic   psychiatrist
biopsy   oncologist   psychologist
diagnosis   osteoarthritis   thrombocyte
leukemia   pathogenic   thrombosis
nephrologist   prognosis   urologist
neuropathy

1. Seventy-two-year-old Ms. Crick suffers from a degenerative joint disease that is caused by the wearing away of tissue around her joints. This condition, which literally means "inflammation of

   bones and joints," is _____.

2. The _____ sample was removed during surgery and sent to a pathologist to be examined under a microscope for a proper diagnosis.

3. A (an) _____ performed surgery to remove Mr. Simon's cancerous kidney.

4. Ms. Rose has suffered from hyperglycemia (diabetes) for many years. This condition can lead to

   long-term complications, such as the disease of nerves called diabetic _____.

5. A virus or a bacterium produces disease and is therefore a (an) _____ organism.

6. Jordan has a disease caused by abnormal hemoglobin in his erythrocytes. The erythrocytes change shape, collapsing to form sickle-shaped cells that can become clots and stop the flow of

   blood. His condition is sickle-cell _____.

7. Dr. Shelby is a physician who treats carcinomas and sarcomas. He is a (an) _____.

8. Bill had difficulty stopping the bleeding from a cut on his face while shaving. He knew his

   medication caused him to have decreased platelets or a low _____
   count and that was probably the reason his blood was not clotting very well.

9. Dr. Susan Parker told Paul that his condition would improve with treatment in a few weeks.

   She said his _____ is excellent and he can expect total recovery.

10. After fleeing the World Trade Center on September 11, 2001, Mrs. Jones had many problems with

    her job, her boyfriend, and her family relationships. She called a _____
    who prescribed drugs to treat her depression.

P. Circle the correct term to complete each sentence.

1. Ms. Brody had a cough and fever. Her doctor instructed her to go to the **(pathology, radiology, hematology)** department for a chest x-ray.

2. After delivery of her third child, Ms. Thompson had problems holding her urine (a condition known as urinary incontinence). She made an appointment with a **(gastroenterologist, pathologist, urologist)** to evaluate her condition.

3. Dr. Monroe told a new mother she had lost much blood during delivery of her child. She had **(anemia, leukocytosis, adenitis)** and needed a blood transfusion immediately.

4. Mr. Preston was having chest pain during his morning walks. He made an appointment to discuss his new symptom with a **(nephrologist, neurologist, cardiologist)**.

5. After the skiing accident, Dr. Curtin suggested **(cystoscopy, biopsy, arthroscopy)** to visually examine my swollen, painful knee.

VI. Answers to Exercises

A

1. prefixes
2. suffixes
3. root
4. combining vowel
5. combining form

B

1. heart
2. gland
3. life
4. cerebrum, largest part of the brain
5. head
6. joint
7. cancer, cancerous
8. urinary bladder
9. cell
10. skin
11. brain
12. electricity

C

1. tumor, mass, swelling
2. pertaining to
3. inflammation
4. process of study
5. process of visual examination
6. pertaining to
7. record
8. process of viewing

D

1. cerebr/al—pertaining to the cerebrum or largest part of the brain
2. bi/opsy—process of viewing life (removal of living tissue and viewing it under the microscope)
3. aden/itis—inflammation of a gland
4. cephal/ic—pertaining to the head
5. carcin/oma—tumor that is cancerous (cancerous tumor)
6. cyst/o/scopy—process of visually examining the urinary bladder
7. electr/o/cardi/o/gram—record of the electricity in the heart
8. cardi/o/logy—process of study of the heart
9. electr/o/encephal/o/gram—record of the electricity in the brain
10. dermat/itis—inflammation of the skin
11. arthr/o/scopy—process of visual examination of a joint
12. cyt/o/logy—process of study of cells

E

1. red
2. intestines (usually small intestine)
3. stomach
4. knowledge
5. blood
6. to cut
7. kidney
8. white
9. treatment
10. liver
11. nerve
12. woman, female

F

1. leukocyte
2. gastritis
3. iatrogenic
4. nephrology

5. erythrocyte
6. hematoma
7. biopsy
8. neuralgia

9. ophthalmoscopy
10. enteritis

G

1. ren/o
2. path/o
3. ophthalm/o
4. sect/o

5. rhin/o
6. sarc/o
7. psych/o
8. ur/o

9. oste/o
10. radi/o
11. thromb/o
12. onc/o

H

1. ophthalmoscopy—process of visual examination of the eye
2. ophthalmoscope—instrument to visually examine the eye
3. oncology—study of tumors
4. osteitis—inflammation of bone
5. psychosis—abnormal condition of the mind

6. thrombocyte—clotting cell (platelet)
7. renal—pertaining to the kidney
8. nephrectomy—removal (excision) of the kidney
9. osteotomy—incision of (to cut into) a bone
10. resection—process of cutting back (in the sense of "out" or removal)

11. carcinogenic—pertaining to producing cancer
12. sarcoma—tumor of flesh (cancerous tumor of flesh tissue, such as bone, fat, and muscle)

I

1. pain
2. process
3. blood condition
4. record
5. instrument to visually examine

6. abnormal condition
7. removal, excision, resection
8. pertaining to producing, produced by, or produced in
9. disease condition

10. incision, process of cutting into
11. inflammation
12. cell

J

1. carcinogenic
2. leukocytosis
3. hepatoma
4. arthralgia

5. endocrine
6. cystitis
7. hematoma
8. leukemia

9. iatrogenic
10. enteropathy

K

1. complete, through
2. before
3. self
4. no, not, without
5. excessive, above, more than normal

6. deficient, below, less than normal
7. above, upon
8. within
9. behind
10. across, through

11. surrounding
12. out
13. below, under
14. back

L

1. diagnosis—complete knowledge; a decision about the nature of the patient's condition after the appropriate tests are done
2. prognosis—before knowledge; a prediction about the outcome of treatment, and given after the diagnosis
3. subhepatic—pertaining to below the liver. A combining vowel is not needed between the prefix and the root.

4. pericardium—the membrane surrounding the heart
5. hyperglycemia—condition of excessive sugar in the blood
6. hypodermic—pertaining to under the skin
7. epigastric—pertaining to above the stomach
8. resection—process of cutting back (in the sense of cutting out)

9. hypoglycemia—condition of deficient (low) sugar in the blood
10. anemia—blood condition of low numbers of erythrocytes or deficient hemoglobin in the red blood cells. Notice that the root in this term is *em*, which is shortened from *hem*, meaning blood

M

1. urology
2. gynecology
3. hematology
4. oncology
5. nephrology

6. neurology
7. pediatrics (combining vowel *o* has been dropped between ped and iatr)
8. radiology
9. ophthalmology

10. gastroenterology
11. endocrinology
12. psychiatry
13. pathology
14. cardiology

N

1. <u>cerebrum</u> (largest part of the brain). A cerebrovascular accident is damage to the blood vessels of the cerebrum leading to death of brain cells; also called a stroke.
2. <u>brain.</u> Encephalitis is inflammation of the brain.
3. <u>urinary bladder.</u> A cystoscope is an instrument used to visually examine the urinary bladder. The cystoscope is placed through the urethra into the bladder.
4. <u>across, through.</u> Transhepatic means pertaining to across or through the liver.
5. <u>treatment.</u> Iatrogenic means pertaining to an adverse side effect produced by treatment.
6. <u>under, below, deficient.</u> Hypogastric means pertaining to below the stomach.
7. <u>within.</u> Endocrine glands secrete hormones within the body. Examples of these are the pituitary, thyroid, and adrenal glands.
8. <u>excision.</u> Nephrectomy is the removal of a kidney.
9. <u>outside.</u> Exocrine glands secrete chemicals to the outside of the body (sweat, tear, salivary glands).
10. <u>pain.</u> Neuralgia is nerve pain.

O

1. osteoarthritis
2. biopsy
3. urologist (a nephrologist is a medical doctor who treats kidney disorders but does not operate on patients)
4. neuropathy
5. pathogenic
6. anemia
7. oncologist
8. thrombocyte
9. prognosis
10. psychiatrist (a psychologist can treat mentally ill patients but is not a medical doctor and cannot prescribe medications)

P

1. radiology
2. urologist
3. anemia
4. cardiologist
5. arthroscopy

Answers to Practical Applications

1. **D** A **cardiologist** is an internal medicine specialist who takes additional (fellowship) training in the diagnosis and treatment of heart disease.
2. **F** A **gynecologist** trains in both surgery and internal medicine in order to diagnose and treat disorders of the female reproductive system. Ovarian cysts are sacs of fluid that form on and in the ovaries (female organs that produce eggs and hormones).
3. **J** A **psychiatrist** is a specialist in diagnosing and treating mental illness. In bipolar disorder (manic-depressive illness), the mood switches periodically from excessive mania (excitability) to deep depression (sadness, despair, and discouragement).
4. **E** An **oncologist** is an internal medicine specialist who takes fellowship training in the diagnosis and medical (drug) treatment of cancer.
5. **B** A **hematologist** is an internal medicine specialist who takes fellowship training in the diagnosis and treatment of blood disorders such as anemia and clotting diseases.
6. **H** An **ophthalmologist** trains in both surgery and internal medicine to diagnose and treat disorders of the eye. The retina is a sensitive layer of light-receptor cells in the back of the eye. Retinopathy can occur as a secondary complication of chronic diabetes (hyperglycemia).
7. **I** A **neurologist** is an internal medicine specialist who takes fellowship training in the diagnosis and treatment of disorders of nervous tissue (brain, spinal cord, and nerves). A CVA causes damage to areas of the brain and results in loss of function.
8. **C** A **nephrologist** is an internal medicine specialist who takes fellowship training in the diagnosis and medical treatment of kidney disease. A nephrologist does not perform surgery on the urinary tract, but treats kidney disease with drugs.
9. **A** A **gastroenterologist** is an internal medicine specialist who takes fellowship training in the diagnosis and treatment of disorders of the gastrointestinal tract. Examples of inflammatory bowel disease are ulcerative colitis (inflammation of the large intestine) and Crohn's disease (inflammation of the last part of the small intestine).
10. **G** A **urologist** is a surgical specialist who treats and operates on organs of the urinary tract (such as the urinary bladder) and the male reproductive system.

VII. Pronunciation of Terms

The markings ‾ and ˘ above the vowels (a, e, i, o, and u) indicate the proper sounds of the vowels. When ‾ is above a vowel, its sound is long—that is, exactly like its name. For example:

> ā as in āpe
> ē as in ēven
> ī as in īce
> ō as in ōpen
> ū as in ūnit

The ˘ marking indicates a short vowel sound, as in the following examples:

> ă as in ăpple
> ĕ as in ĕvery
> ĭ as in ĭnterest
> ŏ as in pŏt
> ŭ as in ŭnder

To test your understanding of the terminology in this chapter, write the meaning of each term in the space provided. In addition, you may wish to cover the terms and write them by looking at your definitions. Make sure your spelling is correct. The page number after each term indicates where it is defined or used in the text so you can easily check your responses.

Term	Pronunciation	Meaning
adenitis (6)	ăd-ĕ-NĪ-tĭs	_____
adenoma (6)	ăd-ĕ-NŌ-mă	_____
adenopathy (11)	ăd-ĕ-NŎP-ă-thē	_____
anemia (11)	ă-NĒ-mē-ă	_____
arthralgia (10)	ăr-THRĂL-jă	_____
arthritis (6)	ăr-THRĪ-tĭs	_____
autopsy (11)	ĂW-tŏp-sē	_____
biology (6)	bī-ŎL-ō-jē	_____
biopsy (6)	BĪ-ŏp-sē	_____
carcinogenic (10)	kăr-sĭ-nō-JĔN-ĭk	_____
carcinoma (6)	kăr-sĭ-NŌ-mă	_____
cardiac (10)	KĂR-dē-ăk	_____
cardiology (6)	kăr-dē-ŎL-ō-jē	_____
cephalic (6)	sĕ-FĂL-ĭk	_____

cerebral (6)	sĕ-RĒ-brăl or SĔR-ĕ-brăl	_____
cystitis (10)	sĭs-TĪ-tĭs	_____
cystoscopy (7)	sĭs-TŎS-kō-pē	_____
cytology (7)	sī-TŎL-ō-jē	_____
dermatitis (7)	dĕr-mă-TĪ-tĭs	_____
dermatology (7)	dĕr-mă-TŎL-ō-jē	_____
diagnosis (7)	dī-ăg-NŌ-sĭs	_____
electrocardiogram (7)	ē-lĕk-trō-KĂR-dē-ō-grăm	_____
electroencephalogram (7)	ē-lĕk-trō-ĕn-SĔF-ă-lō-grăm	_____
endocrine glands (7)	ĔN-dō-krĭn glăndz	_____
endocrinologist (12)	ĕn-dō-krĭ-NŎL-ō-jĭst	_____
endocrinology (10)	ĕn-dō-krĭ-NŎL-ō-jē	_____
endoscope (11)	ĔN-dō-skōp	_____
endoscopy (11)	ĕn-DŎS-kō-pē	_____
enteritis (7)	ĕn-tĕ-RĪ-tĭs	_____
enteropathy (11)	ĕn-tĕ-RŎP-ă-thē	_____
epidermis (12)	ĕp-ĭ-DĔR-mĭs	_____
epigastric (12)	ĕp-ĭ-GĂS-trĭk	_____
erythrocyte (7)	ĕ-RĬTH-rō-sīt	_____
excision (7)	ĕk-SĬZH-ŭn	_____
exocrine glands (12)	ĔK-sō-krĭn glăndz	_____
gastrectomy (7)	găs-TRĔK-tō-mē	_____
gastric (10)	GĂS-trĭk	_____
gastroenterology (11)	găs-trō-ĕn-tĕr-ŎL-ō-jē	_____
gastrotomy (7)	găs-TRŎT-ō-mē	_____
gynecologist (10)	gī-nĕ-KŎL-ō-jĭst	_____
gynecology (8)	gī-nĕ-KŎL-ō-jē	_____

hematology (8)	hē-mă-TŎL-ō-jē	
hematoma (8)	hē-mă-TŌ-mă	
hemoglobin (8)	HĒ-mō-glō-bĭn	
hepatitis (8)	hĕp-ă-TĪ-tĭs	
hepatoma (10)	hĕp-ă-TŌ-mă	
hyperglycemia (12)	hī-pĕr-glī-SĒ-mē-ă	
hypodermic (7)	hī-pō-DĔR-mĭk	
hypogastric (12)	hī-pō-GĂS-trĭk	
hypoglycemia (12)	hī-pō-glī-SĒ-mē-ă	
iatrogenic (8)	ī-ăt-rō-JĔN-ĭk	
incision (6)	ĭn-SĬZH-ŭn	
leukemia (10)	lū-KĒ-mē-ă	
leukocyte (8)	LŪ-kō-sīt	
leukocytosis (11)	lū-kō-sī-TŌ-sĭs	
nephrectomy (10)	nĕ-FRĔK-tō-mē	
nephritis (8)	nĕ-FRĪ-tĭs	
nephrology (8)	nĕ-FRŎL-ō-jē	
nephrosis (11)	nĕ-FRŌ-sĭs	
neural (10)	NŪ-răl	
neuralgia (10)	nū-RĂL-jă	
neurological (10)	nū-rō-LŎJ-ĭk-ăl	
neurology (8)	nū-RŎL-ō-jē	
oncologist (8)	ŏn-KŎL-ō-jĭst	
oncology (8)	ŏn-KŎL-ō-jē	
ophthalmologist (24)	ŏf-thăl-MŎL-ō-jĭst	
ophthalmoscope (8)	ŏf-THĂL-mō-skōp	
osteitis (8)	ŏs-tē-Ī-tĭs	

osteoarthritis (9)	ŏs-tē-ō-ăr-THRĪ-tĭs	_____
osteotomy (11)	ŏs-tē-ŎT-ō-mē	_____
pathogenic (10)	păth-ō-JĔN-ĭk	_____
pathologist (9)	pă-THŎL-ŏ-jĭst	_____
pathology (9)	pă-THŎL-ō-jē	_____
pediatric (9)	pē-dē-ĂT-rĭk	_____
pericardium (12)	pĕr-ĭ-KĂR-dē-ŭm	_____
prognosis (8)	prŏg-NŌ-sĭs	_____
psychiatrist (9)	sī-KĪ-ă-trĭst	_____
psychiatry (9)	sī-KĪ-ă-trē	_____
psychology (9)	sī-KŎL-ō-jē	_____
radiology (9)	rā-dē-ŎL-ō-jē	_____
renal (9)	RĒ-năl	_____
resection (9)	rē-SĔK-shŭn	_____
retrocardiac (12)	rĕ-trō-KĂR-dē-ăc	_____
rhinitis (9)	rī-NĪ-tĭs	_____
sarcoma (9)	săr-KŌ-mă	_____
subhepatic (12)	sŭb-hĕ-PĂT-ĭk	_____
thrombocyte (9)	THRŎM-bō-sīt	_____
transhepatic (12)	trănz-hĕ-PĂT-ĭk	_____
urology (9)	ū-RŎL-ō-jē	_____

VIII. Review Sheet

This review sheet and the others that follow each chapter are complete lists of the word elements contained in that chapter. The review sheets are designed to pull together the terminology and to reinforce your learning by giving you the opportunity to write the meanings of each word part in the spaces provided and to test yourself. Check your answers with the information in the chapter or in the Glossary (Medical Terms—English) at the end of the book.

COMBINING FORMS

Combining Form	Meaning	Combining Form	Meaning
aden/o		hem/o, hemat/o	
arthr/o		hepat/o	
bi/o		iatr/o	
carcin/o		leuk/o	
cardi/o		log/o	
cephal/o		nephr/o	
cerebr/o		neur/o	
cis/o		onc/o	
crin/o		ophthalm/o	
cyst/o		oste/o	
cyt/o		path/o	
derm/o, dermat/o		ped/o	
electr/o		psych/o	
encephal/o		radi/o	
enter/o		ren/o	
erythr/o		rhin/o	
gastr/o		sarc/o	
glyc/o		sect/o	
gnos/o		thromb/o	
gynec/o		ur/o	

Continued on following page

SUFFIXES

Suffix	Meaning	Suffix	Meaning
-ac	_____	-itis	_____
-al	_____	-logy	_____
-algia	_____	-oma	_____
-cyte	_____	-opsy	_____
-ectomy	_____	-osis	_____
-emia	_____	-pathy	_____
-genic	_____	-scope	_____
-globin	_____	-scopy	_____
-gram	_____	-sis	_____
-ic, -ical	_____	-tomy	_____
-ion	_____	-y	_____
-ist	_____		

PREFIXES

Prefix	Meaning	Prefix	Meaning
a-, an-	_____	hypo-	_____
auto-	_____	in-	_____
dia-	_____	peri-	_____
endo-	_____	pro-	_____
epi-	_____	re-	_____
ex-	_____	retro-	_____
exo-	_____	sub-	_____
hyper-	_____	trans-	_____

chapter

Terms Pertaining to the Body as a Whole

This chapter is divided into the following sections

In this chapter you will

- Define terms that apply to the structural organization of the body.
- Identify the body cavities and recognize the organs contained within those cavities.
- Locate and identify the anatomical and clinical divisions of the abdomen.
- Locate and name the anatomical divisions of the back.
- Become acquainted with terms that describe positions, directions, and planes of the body.
- Identify the meanings for new word elements and use them to understand new medical terms.

I. Structural Organization of the Body

Cells

The cell is the fundamental unit of all living things (animal or plant). Cells are everywhere in the human body—every tissue, every organ is made up of these individual units.

Similarity in Cells. All cells are similar in that they contain a gelatinous substance composed of water, protein, sugar, acids, fats, and various minerals. Several parts of a cell are described below and pictured in Figure 2–1 as they might look when photographed with an electron microscope. Label the structures on Figure 2–1. Throughout the book, numbers in brackets indicate that the boldfaced term preceding it is to be used in labeling.

The **cell membrane** [1] not only surrounds and protects the cell, but also regulates what passes into and out of the cell.

The **nucleus** [2] controls the operations of the cell. It directs cell division and determines the structure and function of the cell.

Chromosomes [3] are rod-like structures within the nucleus. All human body cells (except for the sex cells, the egg and sperm) contain 23 pairs of chromosomes. Each sperm and egg cell has only 23 unpaired chromosomes. After the egg and sperm cells unite to form the embryo, each cell of the embryo then has 46 chromosomes (23 pairs) (Fig. 2–2).

Chromosomes contain regions called **genes.** There are several thousand genes, in an orderly sequence, on every chromosome. Each gene is composed of a chemical called **DNA** (deoxyribonucleic acid). DNA regulates the activities of the cell by its sequence (arrangement into genes) on each chromosome. The DNA sequence resembles a series of recipes in code. The code, when passed out of the nucleus to the rest of the cell, directs the activities of the cell, such as cell division and synthesis of proteins.

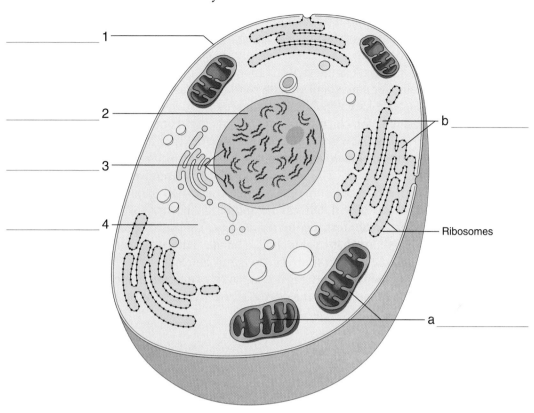

Figure 2-1

Major parts of a cell. Ribosomes (RĪ-bō-sōmz) are small granules that help the cell make proteins.

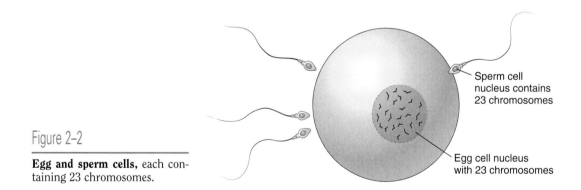

Figure 2-2

Egg and sperm cells, each containing 23 chromosomes.

Chromosomes within the nucleus are analyzed in terms of their size, arrangement, and number by performing a **karyotype.** Karyotyping of chromosomes determines whether the chromosomes are normal in number and structure. For example, obstetricians often recommend an amniocentesis (puncture of the sac around the fetus for removal of fluid and cells) for a pregnant woman so that the karyotype of the baby can be examined. Figure 2–3 shows a karyotype, or chromosome map, of a normal male. The chromosomes have been treated with chemicals so that bands (light and dark areas) can be seen.

If a baby is born with an abnormal number of chromosomes, serious problems can result. In Down syndrome, the karyotype shows 47 chromosomes instead of the normal number of 46. The extra number 21 chromosome results in the development of a child with Down syndrome (also called trisomy-21 syndrome). Its incidence is about 1 in every 750 live births, but as the mother's age increases, the presence of the chromosomal (genetic) abnormality increases. A typical Down syndrome infant is born with physical malformations that may include a small, flattened skull; a short, flat-bridged nose; wide-set, slanted eyes; and short, broad hands and feet with a wide gap between the first and second toes. Reproductive organs are often underdeveloped, congenital heart defects are not uncommon, and some degree of mental retardation is evident (Fig. 2–4).

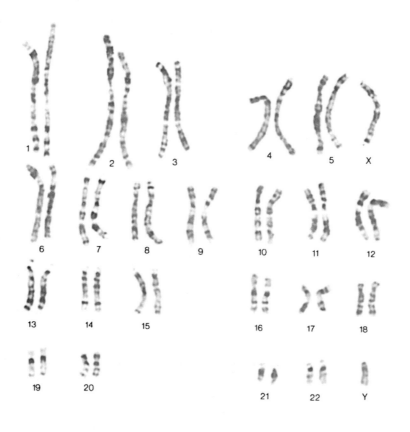

Figure 2-3

Karyotype of a normal male showing 23 pairs of chromosomes. The 23rd pair is the XY pair. In a normal female karyotype, the 23rd pair is XX. (X chromosome is near number 5 pair and Y chromosome is near number 22 pair.) (From Behrman RE, Kliegman RM, Jensen HB: Nelson Textbook of Pediatrics, 16th ed. Philadelphia, WB Saunders, 2000, p 326.)

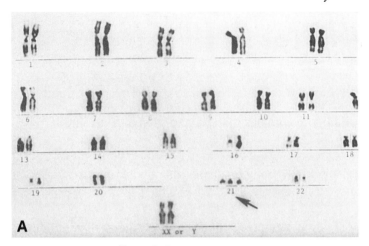
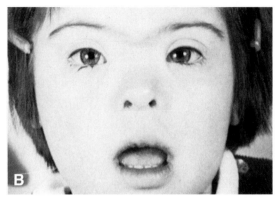

Figure 2-4

(A) Karyotype of a Down syndrome female patient showing trisomy 21. **(B) Photograph of a 3½-year-old girl with the typical facial appearance that occurs in Down syndrome.** This includes a flat nasal bridge, an upward slant of the eyes, and a protruding tongue. Other characteristics of Down syndrome patients are mental deficiency and heart defects. (**A,** From Zitelli BJ, Davis HW [eds]: Atlas of Pediatric Physical Diagnosis, 3rd ed. St. Louis, Mosby-Wolfe, 1997, p 10; **B,** From Jarvis C: Physical Examination and Health Assessment, 3rd ed. Philadelphia, WB Saunders, 2000, p 293.)

Continue labeling Figure 2–1.

Cytoplasm [4] (cyt/o = cell, -plasm = formation) includes all the material outside the nucleus and enclosed by the cell membrane. It carries on the work of the cell (i.e., in a muscle cell, it does the contracting; in a nerve cell, it transmits impulses). The cytoplasm contains:

Mitochondria [a] are small, sausage-shaped bodies that, like miniature power plants, produce energy by burning food in the presence of oxygen. During this chemical process, called **catabolism** (cata = down, bol = to cast, -ism = process), complex foods (sugar and fat) are broken down into simpler substances. The catabolism of sugar and fat releases needed energy to do the work of the cell.

Endoplasmic reticulum [b] is a network (reticulum) of canals within the cell. These canals (containing small structures called ribosomes) are a cellular tunnel system in which proteins are manufactured for use in the cell. This process of building up complex materials, such as proteins, from simpler parts is called **anabolism** (ana = up, bol = to cast, -ism = process). During anabolism, small pieces of protein (called amino acids) are fitted together like links in a chain to make larger proteins.

The two processes, anabolism and catabolism, are known as **metabolism** (meta = change, bol = to cast, -ism = process). Metabolism is the total of the chemical processes occurring in a cell. If a person has a "fast metabolism," then foods, such as sugar and fat, are thought to be used up very quickly, and energy is released. If a person has a "slow metabolism," foods are thought to be burned slowly, and fat accumulates in cells.

Study Section 1

Practice spelling each term, and know its meaning.

anabolism
Process of building up complex materials (proteins) from simple materials.

catabolism
Process of breaking down complex materials (foods) to form simpler substances and release energy.

cell membrane
Structure surrounding and protecting the cell. It determines what enters and leaves the cell.

chromosomes
Rod-shaped structures in the nucleus that contain regions of DNA called genes. There are 46 chromosomes (23 pairs) in every cell except for the egg and sperm cells, which contain only 23 individual, unpaired chromosomes.

cytoplasm
All the material that is outside the nucleus and yet contained within the cell membrane.

DNA
Chemical found within each chromosome. Arranged like a sequence of recipes in code, it directs the activities of the cell.

endoplasmic reticulum
Structure (canals) within the cytoplasm. Site in which large proteins are made from smaller protein pieces. **Ribosomes** are found on the endoplasmic reticulum.

genes
Regions of DNA within each chromosome.

karyotype
Picture of chromosomes in the nucleus of a cell. The chromosomes are arranged in numerical order to determine their number and structure.

metabolism
The total of the chemical processes in a cell. It includes both catabolism and anabolism.

mitochondria
Structures in the cytoplasm in which foods are burned to release energy.

nucleus
Control center of the cell. It contains chromosomes and directs the activities of the cell.

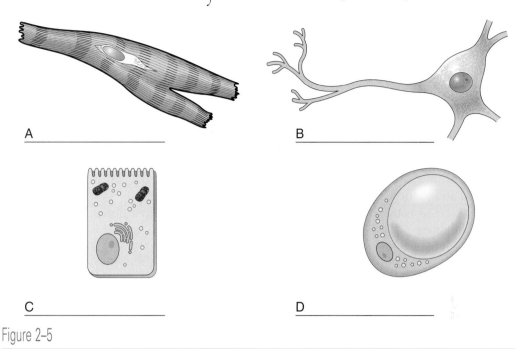

A _____ B _____

C _____ D _____

Figure 2–5

Types of cells. Label **(A)** muscle cell, **(B)** nerve cell, **(C)** epithelial cell, and **(D)** fat cell.

Differences in Cells. Cells are different, or specialized, throughout the body to carry out their individual functions. For example, a **muscle cell** is long and slender and contains fibers that aid in contracting and relaxing; an **epithelial cell** (a lining and skin cell) may be square and flat to provide protection; a **nerve cell** may be long and have various fibrous extensions that aid in its job of carrying impulses; a **fat cell** contains large, empty spaces for fat storage. These are only a few of the many types of cells in the body. Figure 2–5 illustrates the different sizes and shapes of muscle, nerve, fat, and epithelial cells.

Tissues

A tissue is a group of similar cells working together to do a specific job. A **histologist** (hist/o = tissue) is a scientist who specializes in the study of tissues. Different types of tissues include:

Epithelial Tissue. Epithelial tissue, located all over the body, forms the linings of internal organs, and the outer surface of the skin covering the body. It also lines exocrine and endocrine glands. The term **epithelial** originally referred to the tissue above (epi-) the breast nipple (thel/o). Now it describes all tissue that covers the outside of the body and lines the inner surface of internal organs.

Muscle Tissue. Voluntary muscle found in arms and legs and parts of the body where movement is under conscious control. Involuntary muscle, found in the heart and digestive system, as well as other organs, allows movement that is not under conscious control. Cardiac muscle is a specialized type of muscle found only in the heart and can be seen beating in a 6-week-old fetus.

Connective Tissue. Examples are **fat** (adipose tissue), **cartilage** (elastic, fibrous tissue attached to bones), bone, and blood.

Nerve Tissue. Nerve tissue conducts impulses all over the body.

Organs

Organs are structures composed of several kinds of tissue. For example, an organ such as the stomach is composed of muscle tissue, nerve tissue, and glandular epithelial tissue. The medical term for internal organs is **viscera** (singular: **viscus**). Examples of abdominal viscera (organs located in the abdomen) are the liver, stomach, intestines, pancreas, spleen, and gallbladder.

Systems

Systems are groups of organs working together to perform complex functions. For example, the mouth, esophagus, stomach, and small and large intestines are organs that do the work of the digestive system to digest food and absorb it into the bloodstream.

Examine the body systems listed below with their individual organs. Learn to spell and identify the organs in boldface.

System	Organs
Digestive	mouth, **pharynx** (throat), esophagus, stomach, intestines (small and large), liver, gallbladder, pancreas
Urinary or excretory	kidneys, **ureters** (tubes from the kidneys to the urinary bladder), urinary bladder, **urethra** (tube from the bladder to the outside of the body)
Respiratory	nose, pharynx, **larynx** (voice box), **trachea** (windpipe), bronchial tubes, lungs (where the exchange of gases takes place)
Reproductive	female: ovaries, fallopian tubes, **uterus** (womb), vagina, mammary glands; male: testes and associated tubes, urethra, penis, prostate gland
Endocrine	**thyroid gland** (in the neck), **pituitary gland** (at the base of the brain), sex glands (ovaries and testes), adrenal glands, pancreas (islets of Langerhans), parathyroid glands
Nervous	brain, spinal cord, nerves, and collections of nerves
Circulatory	heart, blood vessels (arteries, veins, and capillaries), lymphatic vessels and nodes, spleen, thymus gland
Musculoskeletal	muscles, bones, and joints
Skin and sense organs	skin, hair, nails, sweat glands, and sebaceous (oil) glands; eye, ear, nose, and tongue

Study Section 2

Practice spelling each term, and know its meaning.

adipose tissue   Collection of fat cells.

cartilage   Flexible connective tissue attached to bones at joints. For example, it surrounds the trachea and forms part of the external ear and nose.

epithelial cell   Skin cells that cover the external body surface and line the internal surfaces of organs.

histologist   Specialist in the study of tissues.

larynx (LĂR-ĭnks)   Voice box; located at the upper part of the trachea.

pharynx (FĂR-ĭnks)   Throat. The pharynx is the common passageway for food (from the mouth going to the esophagus) and air (from the nose to the trachea).

pituitary gland   Endocrine gland at the base of the brain.

thyroid gland   Endocrine gland that surrounds the trachea in the neck.

trachea   Windpipe (tube leading from the throat to the bronchial tubes).

ureter   One of two tubes, each leading from a single kidney to the urinary bladder. Spelling clue: Ureter has two e's and there are two of them.

urethra   Tube from the urinary bladder to the outside of the body. Spelling clue: Urethra has one e and there is only one urethra.

uterus   The womb. The organ that holds the embryo and fetus as it develops.

viscera   Internal organs.

II. Body Cavities

A body cavity is a space within the body that contains internal organs (viscera). Label Figure 2–6 as you learn the names of the body cavities. Some of the important viscera contained within those cavities are listed as well.

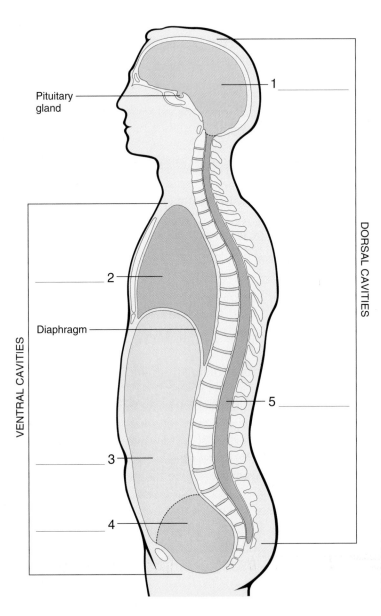

Figure 2–6

Body cavities. Ventral (anterior) cavities are in the front of the body. Dorsal (posterior) cavities are in the back.

Cavity	Organs
Cranial [1]	Brain, pituitary gland.
Thoracic [2]	Lungs, heart, esophagus, trachea, bronchial tubes, thymus gland, aorta (large artery).

The thoracic cavity is divided into two smaller cavities (Fig. 2–7):

    a. **Pleural cavity**—space surrounding each lung. A double-folded membrane, or **pleura**, lines the pleural cavity. If the pleura becomes inflamed (as in pleuritis or pleurisy), the pleural cavity can fill with fluid.

    b. **Mediastinum**—centrally located area outside of and between the lungs. It contains the heart, aorta, trachea, esophagus, thymus gland, bronchial tubes, and many lymph nodes.

Abdominal [3]	Stomach, small and large intestines, spleen, pancreas, liver, and gallbladder.

The **peritoneum** is the double-folded membrane surrounding the abdominal cavity (Fig. 2–8). The kidneys are two bean-shaped organs situated behind (retroperitoneal area) the abdominal cavity on either side of the backbone (see Fig. 2–10).

Pelvic [4]	Portions of the small and large intestines, rectum, urinary bladder, urethra, and ureters; uterus and vagina in the female.
Spinal [5]	Nerves of the spinal cord.

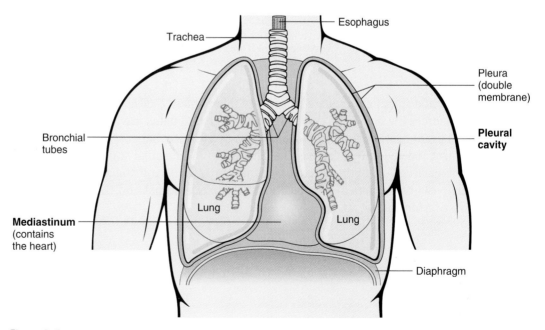

Figure 2–7

Divisions of the thoracic cavity.

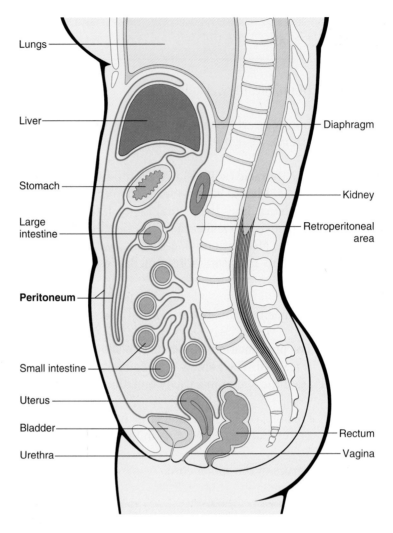

Figure 2–8

Abdominal cavity (side view). Notice the **peritoneum,** which is a membrane surrounding the organs in the abdominal cavity. The retroperitoneal area is behind the peritoneum and contains the kidneys.

The cranial and spinal cavities are considered **dorsal** body cavities because of their location on the back (posterior) portion of the body. The thoracic, abdominal, and pelvic cavities are **ventral** body cavities because they are on the front (anterior) portion of the body. See Figure 2–6.

The thoracic and abdominal cavities are separated by a muscular wall called the **diaphragm.** The abdominal and pelvic cavities are not separated by a muscular wall, and together they are frequently called the **abdominopelvic cavity.** Figures 2–9 and 2–10 show the abdominal and thoracic viscera from anterior (ventral) and posterior (dorsal) views.

Study Section 3

Practice spelling each term, and know its meaning.

abdominal cavity	Space below the chest containing organs such as the liver, stomach, gallbladder, and intestines; also called the **abdomen.**
cranial cavity	Space in the head containing the brain and surrounded by the skull. **Cranial** means **pertaining to the skull.**
diaphragm	Muscle separating the abdominal and thoracic cavities.
dorsal (posterior)	Pertaining to the back.
mediastinum	Centrally located space between the lungs.
pelvic cavity	Space below the abdomen containing portions of the intestines, rectum, urinary bladder, and reproductive organs. **Pelvic** means **pertaining to the hip bone,** which surrounds the pelvic cavity.
peritoneum	Membrane surrounding the organs in the abdomen.
pleura	A double-layered membrane surrounding each lung.
pleural cavity	Space between the pleural membranes and surrounding each lung.
spinal cavity	Space within the spinal column (backbones) and containing the spinal cord. Also called the **spinal canal.**
thoracic cavity	Space in the chest containing the heart, lungs, bronchial tubes, trachea, esophagus, and other organs.
ventral (anterior)	Pertaining to the front.

RIGHT SIDE   LEFT SIDE

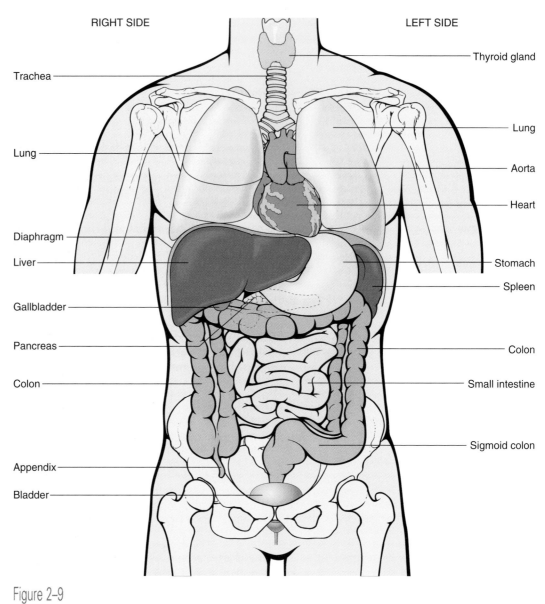

Trachea

Lung

Diaphragm

Liver

Gallbladder

Pancreas

Colon

Appendix

Bladder

Thyroid gland

Lung

Aorta

Heart

Stomach

Spleen

Colon

Small intestine

Sigmoid colon

Figure 2–9

Organs of the abdominopelvic and thoracic cavities, anterior view.

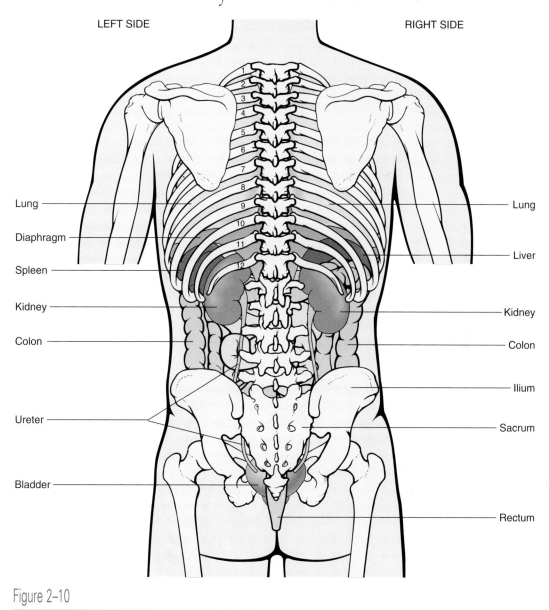

LEFT SIDE   RIGHT SIDE

Lung —   — Lung

Diaphragm —   — Liver

Spleen —

Kidney —   — Kidney

Colon —   — Colon

              — Ilium

Ureter —   — Sacrum

Bladder —

              — Rectum

Figure 2–10

Organs of the abdominopelvic and thoracic cavities, posterior view.

III. Abdominopelvic Regions and Quadrants

Regions

Doctors divide the abdominopelvic area into nine regions. Study the names of these regions, which are found in Figure 2–11.

Hypochondriac regions: two upper right and left regions below the cartilage (chondr/o) of the ribs that extend over the abdomen.

Epigastric region: region above the stomach.

Lumbar regions: two middle right and left regions near the waist.

Umbilical region: region of the navel or umbilicus.

Inguinal regions: two lower right and left regions near the groin (inguin/o = groin), which is the area where the legs join the trunk of the body. These regions are also known as **iliac** regions because they are near the ilium, which is the upper portion of the hip bone on each side of the body.

Hypogastric region: lower middle region below the umbilical region.

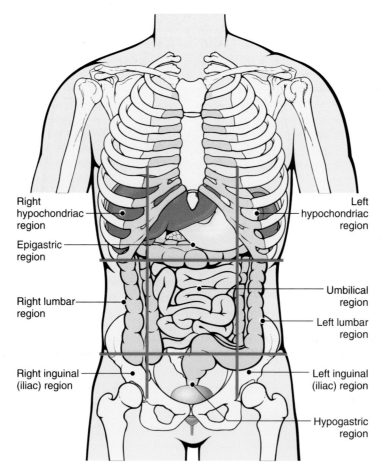

Right
hypochondriac
region

Epigastric
region

Right lumbar
region

Right inguinal
(iliac) region

Left
hypochondriac
region

Umbilical
region

Left lumbar
region

Left inguinal
(iliac) region

Hypogastric
region

Figure 2–11

Abdominopelvic regions. These regions can be used clinically to locate internal organs.

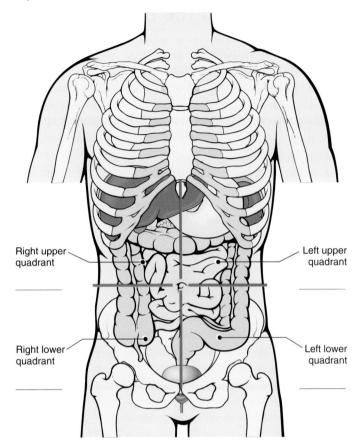

Right upper
quadrant

Left upper
quadrant

Right lower
quadrant

Left lower
quadrant

Figure 2–12

Abdominopelvic quadrants. Give the abbreviation for each quadrant on the line provided.

Quadrants

The abdominopelvic area is divided into four quadrants by drawing two imaginary lines—one horizontally and one vertically through the body. Figure 2–12 shows these quadrants. You add the proper abbreviation on the line under each label on the diagram.

Right upper quadrant (RUQ) contains the liver (right lobe), gallbladder, part of the pancreas, parts of the small and large intestines.

Left upper quadrant (LUQ) contains the liver (left lobe), stomach, spleen, part of the pancreas, parts of the small and large intestines.

Right lower quadrant (RLQ) contains parts of the small and large intestines, right ovary, right fallopian tube, appendix, right ureter.

Left lower quadrant (LLQ) contains parts of the small and large intestines, left ovary, left fallopian tube, left ureter.

IV. Divisions of the Back (Spinal Column)

The spinal column is composed of a series of bones that extend from the neck to the tailbone. Each bone is a **vertebra** (plural: **vertebrae**).

Label the divisions of the back on Figure 2–13 as you study the following:

Division of the Back	Abbreviation	Location
Cervical [1]	C	Neck region. There are seven cervical vertebrae (C1–C7).
Thoracic [2]	T	Chest region. There are twelve thoracic vertebrae (T1–T12). Each bone is joined to a rib.
Lumbar [3]	L	Loin (waist) or flank region (between the ribs and the hipbone). There are five lumbar vertebrae (L1–L5).
Sacral [4]	S	Five bones (S1–S5) are fused to form one bone, the **sacrum**.
Coccygeal [5]		The **coccyx** (tailbone) is a small bone composed of four fused pieces.

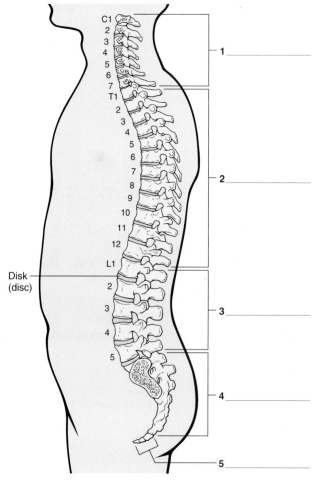

Figure 2-13

Anatomical divisions of the back (spinal column). A disk (disc) is a small pad of cartilage between each backbone (vertebra).

Do not confuse the **spinal column** (back bones or vertebrae) and the **spinal cord** (nerves surrounded by the column). The column is bone tissue, whereas the cord is nervous tissue.

The spaces between the vertebrae (intervertebral spaces) are identified according to the two vertebrae between which they lie; for example, L5–S1 lies between the fifth lumbar and the first sacral vertebrae. Within the space and between vertebrae is a small pad called a **disk** or **disc**. The disk, composed of water and cartilage, is a shock absorber. Occasionally, it moves out of place (ruptures) and puts pressure on a nerve. This is a **slipped disk**, which causes back pain.

▬ Study Section 4

Practice spelling each term, and know its meaning.

ABDOMINOPELVIC REGIONS

hypochondriac	Upper right and left regions beneath the ribs.
epigastric	Upper middle region above the stomach.
lumbar	Middle right and left regions near the waist.
umbilical	Central region near the navel.
inguinal	Lower right and left regions near the groin. Also called **iliac regions.**
hypogastric	Lower middle region below the umbilical region.

ABDOMINOPELVIC QUADRANTS

RUQ	Right upper quadrant
LUQ	Left upper quadrant
RLQ	Right lower quadrant
LLQ	Left lower quadrant

DIVISIONS OF THE BACK

cervical	Neck region (C1–C7)
thoracic	Chest region (T1–T12)
lumbar	Loin (waist) region (L1–L5)
sacral	Region of the sacrum (S1–S5)
coccygeal	Region of the coccyx (tailbone)

Continued on following page

RELATED TERMS

vertebra	A single backbone.
vertebrae	Backbones.
spinal column	Bone tissue surrounding the spinal cavity.
spinal cord	Nervous tissue within the spinal cavity.
disk (disc)	A pad of cartilage between vertebrae.

V. Positional and Directional Terms

The following terms (illustrated in Figure 2–14) describe the locations of organs in relationship to one another throughout the body.

Location	Relationship
Anterior (ventral)	Front side of the body. *Example:* The forehead is on the **anterior** side of the body.
Posterior (dorsal)	The back side of the body. *Example:* The back of the head is **posterior** (**dorsal**) to the face.
Deep	Away from the surface. *Example:* The stab wound penetrated **deep** into the abdomen.
Superficial	On the surface. *Example:* **Superficial** veins can be viewed through the skin.
Proximal	Near the point of attachment to the trunk or near the beginning of a structure. *Example:* The **proximal** end of the upper armbone (humerus) joins with the shoulder bone.
Distal	Far from the point of attachment to the trunk or far from the beginning of a structure. *Example:* At its **distal** end, the humerus joins with the lower armbones at the elbow.
Inferior	Below another structure. *Example:* The feet are at the **inferior** part of the body. They are **inferior** to the knees. The term **caudal** (pertaining to the tail) means inferior.
Superior	Above another structure. *Example:* The head is **superior** to the neck of the body. The term **cephalic** (pertaining to the head) is also used to mean superior.

Medial	Pertaining to the middle or nearer the medial plane of the body. *Example:* In the anatomical position (see Fig. 2–14), the palms of the hands face outward, and the fifth finger is **medial** to the other fingers.
Lateral	Pertaining to the side. *Example:* In the anatomical position, the thumb is **lateral** to the other fingers.
Supine	Lying on the back. *Example:* The patient lies **supine** during an examination of the abdomen. The face is **up** in the s**up**ine position.
Prone	Lying on the belly. *Example:* The backbones are examined with the patient in a **prone** position. The patient is lying **on** his or her face in the pr**on**e position.

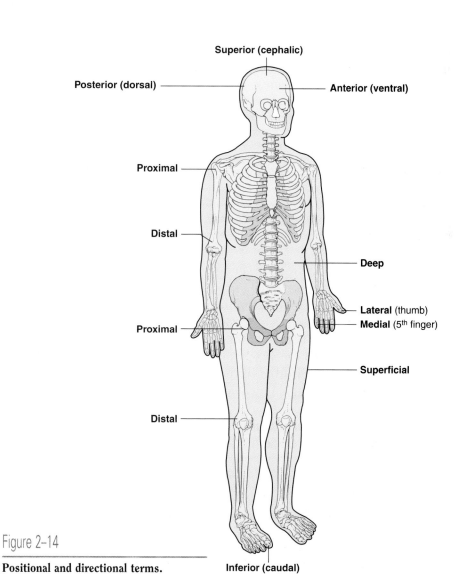

Figure 2–14

Positional and directional terms.

VI. Planes of the Body

A plane is an imaginary flat surface. Label Figure 2–15 as you study the terms for the planes of the body:

Plane	Location
Frontal (coronal) [1]	Vertical plane dividing the body or structure into anterior and posterior portions. A common chest x-ray is a PA (posterior-anterior) view, which is in the **frontal (coronal)** plane.
Sagittal (lateral) [2]	Lengthwise vertical plane dividing the body or structure into right and left sides. The **midsagittal** plane divides the body into right and left halves. A **lateral** (side to side) chest x-ray film is taken in the **sagittal** plane.
Transverse [3] (cross-sectional or axial)	Plane running across the body parallel to the ground (horizontal). This **cross-sectional** plane divides the body or structure into upper and lower portions. A CT (computed tomography) scan is one of a series of x-ray pictures taken in the transverse plane.

— Study Section 5 —

Practice spelling each term, and know its meaning.

anterior (ventral)	Front side of the body.
deep	Away from the surface.
distal	Far from the point of attachment to the trunk or far from the beginning of a structure.
frontal (coronal) plane	Vertical plane dividing the body or structure into anterior and posterior portions.
inferior (caudal)	Below another structure.
lateral	Pertaining to the side.
medial	Pertaining to the middle or near the medial plane of the body.

Continued on page 54

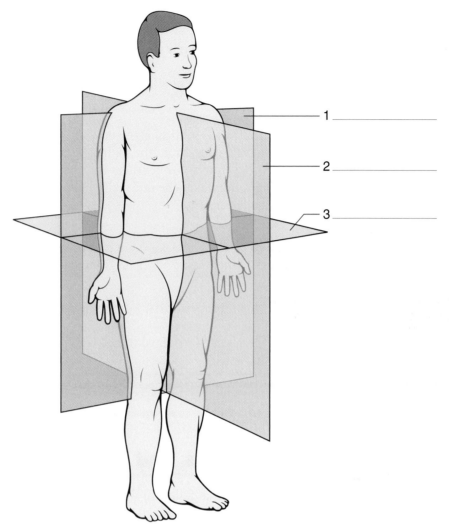

Figure 2–15

Planes of the body. The figure is standing in the anatomical position with the palms of the hands facing outward and the fifth finger lying medial to the other fingers.

posterior (dorsal)	Back side of the body.
prone	Lying on the belly (face down, palm down).
proximal	Near the point of attachment to the trunk or near the beginning of a structure.
sagittal (lateral) plane	Lengthwise, vertical plane dividing the body or structure into right and left sides. From the Latin *sagitta,* meaning arrow. As an arrow is shot from a bow it enters the body in the sagittal plane, dividing right from left. The **midsagittal plane** divides the body into right and left halves.
superficial	On the surface.
superior (cephalic)	Above another structure.
supine	Lying on the back (face up, palm up).
transverse (cross-sectional or axial) plane	Horizontal plane dividing the body into upper and lower portions.

VII. Combining Forms, Prefixes, and Suffixes

Write the meaning of the medical terms that follow in the spaces provided.

Combining Forms

Combining Form	Meaning	Terminology	Meaning
abdomin/o	abdomen	abdominal	_____
		The abdomen is the region below the chest containing internal organs (liver, intestines, stomach, gallbladder, etc.).	
adip/o	fat	adipose	_____
		The suffix -ose means pertaining to or full of.	
anter/o	front	anterior	_____
		The suffix -ior means pertaining to.	

bol/o	to cast (throw)	ana<u>bol</u>ism _____

The prefix ana- means up. The suffix -ism means process. In this cellular process, proteins are built up (protein synthesis).

cervic/o	neck (of the body or of the uterus)	<u>cervic</u>al _____

The cervix is the neck of the uterus. The term cervical can mean pertaining to the neck of the body or the neck (lower part) of the uterus.

chondr/o	cartilage (type of connective tissue)	<u>chondr</u>oma _____

This is a benign tumor.

<u>chondr</u>osarcoma _____

This is a malignant tumor. The term sarc indicates that the malignant tumor is a type of flesh or connective tissue.

chrom/o	color	<u>chrom</u>osomes _____

These nuclear structures absorb the color of dyes used to stain the cell. The suffix -somes means bodies. Literally, this term means "bodies of color," which is how they first appeared to doctors who saw them under the microscope.

coccyg/o	coccyx (tailbone)	<u>coccyg</u>eal _____
crani/o	skull	<u>crani</u>otomy _____
cyt/o	cell	<u>cyt</u>oplasm _____

The suffix -plasm means formation.

dist/o	far, distant	<u>dist</u>al _____
dors/o	back portion of the body	<u>dors</u>al _____

The dorsal fin of a fish is on its back side.

hist/o	tissue	<u>hist</u>ology _____
ili/o	ilium (part of the pelvic bone)	<u>ili</u>ac _____

See Figure 2–10 for a picture of the ilium.

inguin/o	groin	<u>inguin</u>al _____
kary/o	nucleus	<u>kary</u>otype _____

The suffix -type means classification or picture.

later/o	side	lateral _____
lumb/o	lower back (side and back between the ribs and the pelvis)	lumbosacral _____
medi/o	middle	medial _____
nucle/o	nucleus	nucleic _____
pelv/o	hip, pelvic cavity	pelvic _____
poster/o	back, behind	posterior _____
proxim/o	nearest	proximal _____
sacr/o	sacrum	sacral _____
sarc/o	flesh	sarcoma _____
spin/o	spine, backbone	spinal _____
thel/o	nipple	epithelial cell _____

This cell, originally identified as covering nipples, lies upon body surfaces, externally (outside the body) and internally (lining cavities and organs).

thorac/o	chest	thoracic _____
		thoracotomy _____
trache/o	trachea, windpipe	tracheal _____
umbilic/o	navel, umbilicus	umbilical _____
ventr/o	belly side of the body	ventral _____

The ventral fin of a fish is on its belly side.

| **vertebr/o** | vertebrae, backbones | vertebral _____ |
| **viscer/o** | internal organs | visceral _____ |

Prefixes

Prefix	Meaning	Terminology	Meaning
ana-	up	anabolic	_____
cata-	down	catabolism	_____

The cellular process of breaking down foods to release energy.

epi-	above	epigastric	_____
hypo-	below	hypochondriac regions	_____

The Greeks thought organs (liver and spleen) in the hypochondriac region of the abdomen were the origin of imaginary illnesses. Hence the term hypochondriac, a person with unusual anxiety about his or her health and with symptoms not attributable to any disease process.

inter-	between	intervertebral	_____

A disk (disc) is an intervertebral structure.

meta-	change	metabolism	_____

Literally, to cast (bol/o) a change (meta-), meaning the chemical changes (processes) that occur in a cell.

Suffixes

The following are some new suffixes introduced in this chapter.

Suffix	Meaning	Suffix	Meaning
-eal	pertaining to	**-ose**	pertaining to, full of
-iac	pertaining to	**-plasm**	formation
-ior	pertaining to	**-somes**	bodies
-ism	process	**-type**	picture, classification

VIII. Practical Applications

Be sure to check your answers with the Answers to Practical Applications on page 66.

Surgical Procedures

Match the **surgical procedure** in COLUMN I with a **reason for performing** it in COLUMN II:

Column I

1. Craniotomy _____
2. Thoracotomy _____
3. Diskectomy _____
4. Mediastinoscopy _____
5. Tracheotomy _____
6. Laryngectomy _____
7. Arthroscopy _____
8. Peritoneoscopy _____

Column II

A. Emergency effort to remove foreign material from the windpipe

B. Inspection and repair of torn cartilage in the knee

C. Removal of a diseased or injured portion of the brain

D. Inspection of lymph nodes* in the region between the lungs

E. Removal of a squamous cell† carcinoma in the voicebox

F. Open-heart surgery; or removal of lung tissue

G. Inspection of abdominal organs and removal of diseased tissue

H. Relieving of symptoms of a bulging intervertebral pad of cartilage

*Lymph nodes are collections of tissue containing white blood cells called lymphocytes.
†A squamous cell is a type of epithelial cell.

IX. Exercises

Remember to check your answers carefully with those given in Section X, Answers to Exercises.

A. *The following terms are parts of a cell. Match each term with its meaning below.*

cell membrane   DNA   mitochondria
chromosomes   endoplasmic reticulum   nucleus
cytoplasm   genes

1. material of the cell located outside the nucleus and yet enclosed by the cell membrane

   _____

2. regions of DNA within each chromosome _____

3. small, sausage-shaped structures; the place where food is burned to release energy

   _____

4. canal-like structure in the cytoplasm; the site of protein synthesis _____

5. structure that surrounds and protects the cell _____

6. control center of the cell, containing chromosomes _____

7. chemical found within each chromosome _____

8. rod-shaped structures in the nucleus that contain regions called genes _____

B. *Use medical terms or numbers to complete the following sentences.*

1. A picture of chromosomes in the nucleus of a cell is a (an) _____

2. The number of chromosomes in a normal male's muscle cell is _____

3. The number of chromosomes in a female's egg cell is _____

4. The process of building up proteins in a cell is _____

5. The process of chemically burning or breaking down foods to release energy in cells is

   _____

6. The total of the chemical processes in a cell is _____

7. A scientist who studies tissues is a (an) _____

8. The medical term for internal organs is _____

C. Match the following body parts or tissues with their descriptions.

adipose tissue   pharynx   trachea
cartilage   pituitary gland   ureter
epithelial tissue   pleura   urethra
larynx   thyroid gland   uterus

1. voice box _____

2. membrane surrounding the lungs _____

3. throat _____

4. tube from the kidney to the urinary bladder _____

5. collection of fat cells _____

6. endocrine organ located at the base of the brain _____

7. windpipe _____

8. flexible connective tissue attached to bones at joints _____

9. surface cells covering the outside of the body and lining internal organs _____

10. endocrine gland surrounding the windpipe in the neck _____

11. womb _____

12. tube leading from the urinary bladder to the outside of the body _____

D. Name the five cavities of the body.

1. cavity surrounded by the skull _____

2. cavity in the chest surrounded by the ribs _____

3. cavity below the chest containing the stomach, liver, and gallbladder _____

4. cavity surrounded by the hip bone _____

5. cavity surrounded by the bones of the back _____

E. Select from the following definitions to complete the sentences below (1–11).

space surrounding each lung
space between the lungs
muscle separating the abdominal and thoracic cavities
membrane surrounding the abdominal organs
area below the umbilicus (as well as below the stomach)
area above the stomach
area of the navel
areas near the groin
nervous tissue within the spinal cavity
bone tissue surrounding the spinal cavity
pad of cartilage between each vertebra

1. The hypogastric region is the _____

2. The mediastinum is the _____

3. The spinal cord is _____

4. The diaphragm is a (an) _____

5. An intervertebral disk is _____

6. The pleural cavity is _____

7. The spinal column is _____

8. Inguinal areas are the _____

9. The peritoneum is the _____

10. The umbilical region is the _____

11. The epigastric region is the _____

F. Name the five divisions of the back.

1. region of the neck _____

2. region of the chest _____

3. region of the waist _____

4. region of the sacrum _____

5. region of the tailbone _____

G. Give the meanings of the following abbreviations.

1. LLQ _____

2. L5–S1 _____

3. RUQ _____

4. C3–C4 _____

5. RLQ _____

H. Give the opposites of the following terms.

1. deep _____   4. medial _____

2. proximal _____   5. dorsal _____

3. supine _____   6. superior _____

I. Select from the following medical terms to complete the sentences below.

distal	midsagittal	transverse (cross-sectional)
frontal (coronal)	proximal	vertebra
inferior (caudal)	superior (cephalic)	vertebrae
lateral		

1. The kidney lies _____ to the spinal cord.

2. The _____ end of the thigh bone (femur) joins with the knee cap (patella).

3. The _____ plane divides the body into an anterior and a posterior portion.

4. Each backbone is a (an) _____.

5. Several backbones are _____.

6. The diaphragm lies _____ to the organs in the thoracic cavity.

7. The _____ plane divides the body into right and left halves.

8. The _____ end of the upper armbone (humerus) is at the shoulder.

9. The _____ plane divides the body into upper and lower portions.

10. The pharynx is located _____ to the esophagus.

J. Give the meanings of the following medical terms.

1. craniotomy _____

2. cervical _____

3. chondroma _____

4. chondrosarcoma _____

5. nucleic _____

K. Give the medical term for the following definitions. Pay attention to spelling!

1. space below the chest containing the liver, stomach, gallbladder, and intestines:

   _____   _____

2. flexible connective tissue attached to bones at joints: _____

3. rod-shaped structures in the cell nucleus, containing regions of DNA: _____

4. muscle separating the abdominal and thoracic cavities: _____

5. voice box: _____

6. vertical plane dividing the body into right and left sides: _____

7. pertaining to the neck: _____

8. tumor (benign) of cartilage: _____

9. control center of the cell; directs the activities of the cell: _____

10. pertaining to the windpipe: _____

L. Complete each term based on the meaning provided.

1. pertaining to internal organs: _____ al

2. tumor of flesh tissue (malignant): _____ oma

3. pertaining to the chest: _____ ic

4. picture of the chromosomes in the cell nucleus: _____ type

5. sausage-shaped cellular structures in which catabolism takes place: mito _____

6. space between the lungs: media _____

7. endocrine gland at the base of the brain: _____ ary gland

8. pertaining to skin (surface) cells: epi _____

M. Circle the correct term to complete each sentence.

1. Dr. Curnen said the **(inguinal, superior, superficial)** wound barely scratched the surface.

2. Because the liver and spleen are on opposite sides of the body. The liver is in the **(RUQ, LUQ, LLQ)** of the abdominopelvic cavity and the spleen is in the **(RUQ, LUQ, RLQ)**.

3. When a gynecologist examines a patient's pelvis, the patient lies on her back in the **(ventral, dorsal, medial)** lithotomy position. (Lithotomy = incision of an organ to remove a stone—the position also used for removal of ureteral or kidney stones.)

4. Sally complained of pain surrounding her navel. The doctor described the pain as **(periumbilical, epigastric, hypogastric)**.

5. After sampling the fluid surrounding her 16-week-old fetus and reviewing the chromosomal picture, the doctor explained to Mrs. Jones that the fetus had trisomy-21 syndrome. The diagnosis was made by analysis of an abnormal **(urine sample, x-ray, karyotype)**.

6. The **(spinal, sagittal, abdominal)** cavity contains digestive organs.

7. The emergency department physician suspected appendicitis when Brandon was admitted with sharp **(LLQ, RLQ, RUQ)** pain.

8. Susan had hiccups after rapidly eating spicy Indian food. Her physician explained that the hiccups were involuntary contractions or spasms of the **(umbilicus, diaphragm, mediastinum)** resulting in uncontrolled breathing in of air.

9. Everyone in the society pages looked slimmer this year. Could the popularity of liposuction surgery to remove unwanted **(cartilage, epithelial tissue, adipose tissue)** have something to do with this phenomenon?

10. Maria's coughing and sneezing was a result of an allergy to animal dander that affected her **(respiratory, cardiovascular, urinary)** system.

11. While ice skating, Natalie fell and landed on her buttocks. She had persistent **(cervical, thoracic, coccygeal)** pain for a few weeks but no broken bones on x-ray examination.

X. Answers to Exercises

A

1. cytoplasm
2. genes
3. mitochondria
4. endoplasmic reticulum
5. cell membrane
6. nucleus
7. DNA
8. chromosomes

B

1. karyotype
2. 46 (23 pairs)
3. 23
4. anabolism
5. catabolism
6. metabolism
7. histologist
8. viscera

C

1. larynx
2. pleura
3. pharynx
4. ureter
5. adipose tissue
6. pituitary gland
7. trachea
8. cartilage
9. epithelial tissue
10. thyroid gland
11. uterus
12. urethra

D

1. cranial
2. thoracic
3. abdominal
4. pelvic
5. spinal

E

1. area below the umbilicus
2. space between the lungs
3. nervous tissue within the spinal cavity
4. muscle separating the abdominal and thoracic cavities
5. a pad of cartilage between each vertebra
6. space surrounding each lung
7. bone tissue surrounding the spinal cavity
8. areas near the groin
9. membrane surrounding the abdominal organs
10. area of the navel
11. area above the stomach

F

1. cervical
2. thoracic
3. lumbar
4. sacral
5. coccygeal

G

1. left lower quadrant (of the abdominopelvic cavity)
2. between the fifth lumbar vertebra and the first sacral vertebra (a common place for a slipped disk)
3. right upper quadrant (of the abdominopelvic cavity)
4. between the third cervical vertebra and the fourth cervical vertebra
5. right lower quadrant (of the abdominopelvic cavity)

H

1. superficial
2. distal
3. prone
4. lateral
5. ventral (anterior)
6. inferior (caudal)

I

1. lateral
2. distal
3. frontal (coronal)
4. vertebra
5. vertebrae
6. inferior (caudal)
7. midsagittal
8. proximal
9. transverse
10. superior (cephalic)

J

1. incision of the skull
2. pertaining to the neck (of the body or the cervix of the uterus)
3. tumor of cartilage (benign or noncancerous tumor)
4. flesh tumor of cartilage (cancerous, malignant tumor)
5. pertaining to the nucleus

K

1. abdomen or abdominal cavity
2. cartilage
3. chromosomes
4. diaphragm
5. larynx
6. sagittal—note spelling with two t's
7. cervical
8. chondroma
9. nucleus
10. tracheal

L

1. visceral
2. sarcoma
3. thoracic
4. karyotype
5. mitochondria—memory tip: catabolism and mitochondria and cat and mouse!
6. mediastinum
7. pituitary gland
8. epithelial

M

1. superficial
2. RUQ; LUQ
3. dorsal; often called the dorsolithotomy position
4. periumbilical
5. karyotype
6. abdominal
7. RLQ
8. diaphragm
9. adipose tissue
10. respiratory
11. coccygeal

Answers to Practical Applications

1. **C** A trephine is a type of circular saw used for craniotomy.
2. **F**
3. **H** Endoscopic diskectomy is performed through a small incision on the back, lateral to the spine. All or a portion of the disk is removed.
4. **D** A small incision is made above the breastbone and an endoscope is inserted to inspect the lymph nodes around the trachea.
5. **A**
6. **E**
7. **B**
8. **G** A small incision is made near the navel, and a laparoscope is inserted. The procedure, also called laparoscopy (lapar/o means abdomen) or minimally invasive surgery, is used to examine organs and perform surgical operations, such as the removal of the gallbladder or appendix or the tying off of the fallopian tubes.

XI. Pronunciation of Terms

Pronunciation Guide

ā as in āpe   ă as in ăpple
ē as in ēven   ĕ as in ĕvery
ī as in īce   ĭ as in ĭnterest
ō as in ōpen   ŏ as in pŏt
ū as in ūnit   ŭ as in ŭnder

To test your understanding of the terminology in this chapter, write the meaning of each term in the space provided. In addition, you may wish to cover the terms and write them by looking at your definitions. Make sure your spelling is correct. The page number after each term indicates where it is defined or used in the text so you can easily check your responses.

Term	Pronunciation	Meaning
abdomen (43)	ĂB-dō-mĕn or ăb-DŌ-mĕn	
abdominal cavity (43)	ăb-DŎM-ĭ-năl KĂ-vĭ-tē	
adipose (54)	ĂD-ĭ-pōs	
anabolism (36)	ă-NĂB-ō-lĭzm	
anterior (43)	an-TĒ-rē-ŏr	
cartilage (39)	KĂR-tĭ-lĭj	
catabolism (36)	kă-TĂB-ō-lĭsm	
caudal (52)	KAWD-ăl	
cell membrane (36)	sĕl MĔM-brān	
cephalic (54)	sĕ-FĂL-ĭk	
cervical (55)	SĔR-vĭ-kăl	
chondroma (55)	kŏn-DRŌ-mă	
chondrosarcoma (55)	kŏn-drō-săr-KŌ-mă	
chromosomes (36)	KRŌ-mō-sōm	
coccygeal (49)	kŏk-sĭ-JĒ-ăl	
coccyx (48)	KŎK-sĭks	
cranial cavity (43)	KRĀ-nē-ăl KĂ-vĭ-tē	
craniotomy (55)	krā-nē-ŎT-ō-mē	
cytoplasm (36)	SĪ-tō-plăzm	
diaphragm (43)	DĪ-ă-frăm	
disk (disc) (50)	dĭsk	
distal (52)	DĬS-tăl	
dorsal (43)	DŎR-săl	
endoplasmic reticulum (36)	ĕn-dō-PLĂZ-mĭk rē-TĬK-ū-lŭm	
epigastric region (49)	ĕp-ĭ-GĂS-trĭk RĒ-jŭn	

epithelial cell (39)	ĕp-ĭ-THĒ-lē-ăl sĕl	_____
frontal plane (52)	FRŬN-tăl plān	_____
genes (36)	jēnz	_____
histology (55)	hĭs-TŎL-ō-jē	_____
hypochondriac region (49)	hī-pō-KŎN-drē-ăk RĒ-jŭn	_____
hypogastric region (49)	hĭ-pō-GĂS-trĭk RĒ-jŭn	_____
iliac (55)	ĬL-ē-ăk	_____
inguinal region (49)	ĬNG-gwĭ-năl RĒ-jŭn	_____
intervertebral (57)	ĭn-tĕr-VĔR-tĕ-brăl or ĭn-tĕr-vĕr-TĒ-brăl	_____
karyotype (36)	KĂR-ē-ō-tīp	_____
larynx (39)	LĂR-ĭnks	_____
lateral (52)	LĂT-ĕr-al	_____
lumbar region (49)	LŬM-băr RĒ-jŭn	_____
lumbosacral (56)	lŭm-bō-SĀ-krăl	_____
medial (52)	MĒ-dē-ăl	_____
mediastinum (43)	mē-dē-ă-STĪ-nŭm	_____
metabolism (36)	mĕ-TĂB-ō-lĭzm	_____
mitochondria (36)	mī-tō-KŎN-drē-ă	_____
nucleic (56)	nū-KLĒ-ĭk	_____
nucleus (36)	NŪ-klē-ŭs	_____
pelvic cavity (43)	PĔL-vĭk KĂ-vĭ-tē	_____
peritoneum (43)	pĕ-rĭ-tō-NĒ-um	_____
pharynx (39)	FĂR-ĭnks	_____
pituitary gland (39)	pĭ-TŪ-ĭ-tăr-ē glănd	_____
pleura (43)	PLOO-ră	_____
pleural cavity (43)	PLOOR-ăl KĂ-vĭ-tē	_____
posterior (43)	pōs-TĒR-ē-ŏr	_____

prone (54)	prōn	
proximal (54)	PRŎK-sĭ-măl	
sacral (49)	SĀ-krăl	
sacrum (48)	SĀ-krŭm	
sagittal plane (54)	SĂJ-ĭ-tăl plān	
sarcoma (56)	săr-KŌ-mă	
spinal cavity (43)	SPĪ-năl KĂ-vĭ-tē	
spinal column (50)	SPĪ-năl KŎL-ŭm	
spinal cord (50)	SPĪ-năl kŏrd	
superficial (54)	sū-pĕr-FĬSH-ăl	
supine (54)	SŪ-pīn	
thoracic cavity (43)	thō-RĂS-ĭk KĂ-vĭ-tē	
thoracotomy (56)	thō-ră-KŎT-ō-mē	
thyroid gland (39)	THĪ-royd glănd	
trachea (39)	TRĀ-kē-ă	
tracheal (56)	TRĀ-kē-ăl	
transverse plane (54)	trănz-VĔRS plān	
umbilical region (49)	ŭm-BĬL-ĭ-kăl RĒ-jŭn	
ureter (39)	Ū-rĕ-tĕr or ū-RĒ-tĕr	
urethra (39)	ū-RĒ-thră	
uterus (39)	Ū-tĕ-rŭs	
ventral (43)	VĔN-trăl	
vertebra (50)	VĔR-tĕ-bră	
vertebrae (50)	VĔR-tĕ-brā	
vertebral (56)	VĔR-tĕ-brăl or vĕr-TĒ-brăl	
viscera (39)	VĬS-ĕr-ă	
visceral (56)	VĬS-ĕr-ăl	

XII. Review Sheet

Write the meaning of each combining form in the space provided and test yourself. Check your answers with the information in the chapter or in the Glossary (Medical Terms—English) at the end of the book.

COMBINING FORMS

Combining Form	Meaning	Combining Form	Meaning
abdomin/o		lumb/o	
adip/o		medi/o	
anter/o		nucle/o	
bol/o		pelv/o	
cervic/o		poster/o	
chondr/o		proxim/o	
chrom/o		sacr/o	
coccyg/o		sarc/o	
crani/o		spin/o	
cyt/o		thel/o	
dist/o		thorac/o	
dors/o		trache/o	
hist/o		umbilic/o	
ili/o		ventr/o	
inguin/o		vertebr/o	
kary/o		viscer/o	
later/o			

PREFIXES

Prefix	Meaning	Prefix	Meaning
ana-	_____	hypo-	_____
cata-	_____	inter-	_____
epi-	_____	meta-	_____

SUFFIXES

Suffix	Meaning	Suffix	Meaning
-eal	_____	-ose	_____
-ectomy	_____	-plasm	_____
-iac	_____	-somes	_____
-ior	_____	-tomy	_____
-ism	_____	-type	_____
-oma	_____		

Label the regions and quadrants of the abdominopelvic cavity.

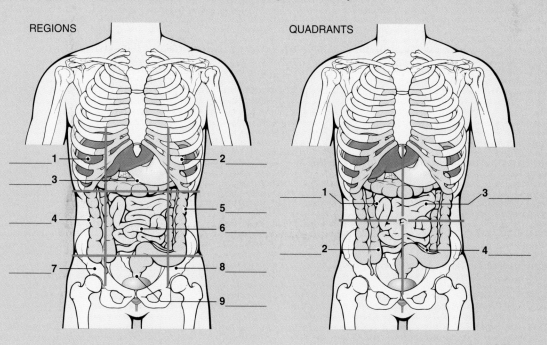

REGIONS

QUADRANTS

Continued on following page

Name the divisions of the spinal column.

neck region (C1–C7) _____

chest region (T1–T12) _____

lower back (loin) region (L1–L5) _____

region of the sacrum (S1–S5) _____

tailbone region _____

Name the planes of the head as pictured below:

Brain

vertical plane that divides the body into anterior and posterior portions

_____

Brain

horizontal plane that divides the body into upper and lower portions

_____

Brain

vertical plane that divides the body into right and left portions

_____

Name the positional and directional terms.

front of the body _____

back of the body _____

away from the surface of the body _____

on the surface of the body _____

far from the point of attachment to the trunk or far from the beginning of a structure

_____

near the point of attachment to the trunk or near the beginning of a structure

_____

below another structure _____

above another structure _____

pertaining to the side _____

pertaining to the middle _____

lying on the belly _____

lying on the back _____

Give the meanings of the following terms that pertain to the cell.

chromosomes _____

mitochondria _____

nucleus _____

DNA _____

endoplasmic reticulum _____

cell membrane _____

catabolism _____

anabolism _____

metabolism _____

Continued on following page

Give the term that suits the meaning provided.

membrane surrounding the lungs _____

membrane surrounding the abdominal viscera _____

muscular wall separating the thoracic and abdominal cavities _____

space between the lungs, containing the heart, windpipe, aorta _____

a backbone _____

a pad of cartilage between each backbone and the next _____

chapter

Suffixes

This chapter is divided into the following sections

In this chapter you will

- Define new suffixes and review those presented in previous chapters.
- Gain practice in word analysis by using these suffixes with combining forms to build and understand terms.
- Name and know the functions of the different types of blood cells in the body.

I. Introduction

This chapter has three purposes. The first purpose is to teach many of the most common suffixes in the medical language. As you work through the entire book, the suffixes mastered in this chapter will appear often. An additional group of suffixes is presented in Chapter 6.

The second purpose is to introduce new combining forms and use them to make words with suffixes. Your analysis of the terminology in Section III of this chapter will increase your medical language vocabulary.

The third purpose is to expand your understanding of terminology beyond basic word analysis. The appendices in Section IV present illustrations and additional explanations of new terms. You should refer to these appendices as you complete the meanings of terms in Section III.

II. Combining Forms

Read this list and underline those combining forms that are unfamiliar.

Combining Forms		Combining	
Combining Form	Meaning	Combining Form	Meaning
abdomin/o	abdomen	**encephal/o**	brain
acr/o	extremities, top, extreme point	**hydr/o**	water, fluid
acu/o	sharp, severe, sudden	**inguin/o**	groin
aden/o	gland	**isch/o**	to hold back
agor/a	marketplace	**lapar/o**	abdomen, abdominal wall
amni/o	amnion (sac surrounding the embryo in the uterus)	**laryng/o**	larynx (voice box)
angi/o	vessel	**lymph/o**	lymph
arteri/o	artery		*Lymph, a clear fluid that bathes tissue spaces, is contained in special lymph vessels and nodes throughout the body.*
arthr/o	joint		
axill/o	armpit	**mamm/o**	breast
blephar/o	eyelid	**mast/o**	breast
bronch/o	bronchial tubes (two tubes, one right and one left, that branch from the trachea to enter the lungs)	**morph/o**	shape, form
		muc/o	mucus
		my/o	muscle
carcin/o	cancer	**myel/o**	spinal cord, bone marrow
chem/o	drug, chemical		*Context of usage indicates the meaning intended.*
chondr/o	cartilage		
chron/o	time	**necr/o**	death (of cells or whole body)
col/o	colon (large intestine)	**nephr/o**	kidney
cyst/o	urinary bladder	**neur/o**	nerve

neutr/o	neutrophil (a white blood cell)	**pulmon/o**	lungs
ophthalm/o	eye	**rect/o**	rectum
oste/o	bone	**ren/o**	kidney
ot/o	ear	**sarc/o**	flesh
path/o	disease	**splen/o**	spleen
peritone/o	peritoneum	**staphyl/o**	clusters
phag/o	to eat, swallow	**strept/o**	twisted chains
phleb/o	vein	**thorac/o**	chest
plas/o	formation, development	**thromb/o**	clot
pleur/o	pleura (membranes surrounding lungs and adjacent to chest wall muscles)	**tonsill/o**	tonsils
		trache/o	trachea (windpipe)
pneumon/o	lungs	**ven/o**	vein

III. Suffixes and Terminology

Noun Suffixes

The following list includes common noun suffixes. After the meaning of each suffix, terminology illustrates the use of the suffix in various words. Remember the basic rule for building a medical term: Use a combining vowel, such as **o,** to connect the root to the suffix. However, drop the combining vowel if the suffix begins with a vowel. For example: **gastr/itis**, *not* **gastr/o/itis**.

Numbers after certain terms direct you to the Appendices that follow this list. These Appendices contain additional information to help you understand the terminology.

Suffix	Meaning	Terminology	Meaning
-algia	pain	arthr<u>algia</u>	_____
		ot<u>algia</u>	_____
		neur<u>algia</u>	_____
		my<u>algia</u>	_____

-cele	hernia[1]	rectocele _____
		cystocele _____
-centesis	surgical puncture to remove fluid	thoracentesis _____

Notice that this term is shortened from thoracocentesis.

amniocentesis[2] _____

abdominocentesis _____

*This procedure is more commonly known as a **paracentesis** (para-means beside). A tube is placed through an incision of the abdomen and fluid is removed from the peritoneal cavity (**beside** the abdominal organs).*

-coccus (plural: **-cocci**)[3]	berry-shaped bacterium (plural: bacteria)	streptococcus[4] _____
		staphylococci _____
-cyte	cell	erythrocyte[5] _____
		leukocyte _____
		thrombocyte _____
-dynia	pain	pleurodynia _____

Pain in the chest wall muscles that is aggravated by breathing.

-ectomy	excision, removal, resection	laryngectomy[6] _____
		mastectomy _____
-emia	blood condition	anemia[7] _____
		ischemia[8] _____
-genesis	condition of producing, forming	carcinogenesis _____
		pathogenesis _____
		angiogenesis _____

---

[1]See Appendix A.
[2]See Appendix B.
[3]See Appendix C.
[4]See Appendix D.
[5]See Appendix E.
[6]See Appendix F.
[7]See Appendix G.
[8]See Appendix H.

| **-genic** | pertaining to producing, produced by, or in | carcino<u>genic</u> _____ |
| | | osteo<u>genic</u> _____ |

An osteogenic sarcoma is a tumor produced in bone tissue.

| **-gram** | record | electroencephalo<u>gram</u> _____ |
| | | myelo<u>gram</u> _____ |

Myel/o means spinal cord in this term. This is an x-ray record taken after contrast material is injected into membranes around the spinal cord.

mammo<u>gram</u> _____

| **-graph** | instrument for recording | electroencephalo<u>graph</u> _____ |

| **-graphy** | process of recording | electroencephalo<u>graphy</u> _____ |
| | | angio<u>graphy</u> _____ |

-itis	inflammation	bronch<u>itis</u> _____
		tonsill<u>itis</u>[9] _____
		thrombophleb<u>itis</u> _____

Also called phlebitis.

| **-logy** | study of | ophthalmo<u>logy</u> _____ |
| | | morpho<u>logy</u> _____ |

| **-lysis** | breakdown, destruction, separation | hemo<u>lysis</u> _____ |

Breakdown of red blood cells with release of hemoglobin.

| **-malacia** | softening | osteo<u>malacia</u> _____ |
| | | chondro<u>malacia</u> _____ |

| **-megaly** | enlargement | acro<u>megaly</u>[10] _____ |
| | | spleno<u>megaly</u>[11] _____ |

[9]See Appendix I.
[10]See Appendix J.
[11]See Appendix K.

-oma   tumor, mass,   myoma _____
                collection of fluid *A benign tumor.*

                                    myosarcoma _____
                                    A malignant tumor. Muscle is a type of flesh (sarc/o) tissue.

                                    multiple myeloma _____
                                    Myel/o means bone marrow in this term. This malignant tumor occurs
                                    in bone marrow tissue throughout the body.

                                    hematoma _____

-opsy   to view   biopsy _____

                                    necropsy _____
                                    This is an autopsy or postmortem examination.

-osis   condition, usually necrosis _____
                abnormal
                                    hydronephrosis _____

                                    leukocytosis[12] _____

-pathy   disease condition   cardiomyopathy _____
                                    Primary disease of the heart muscle in the absence of a known
                                    underlying etiology (cause).

-penia   deficiency   erythropenia _____

                                    neutropenia _____
                                    In this term, neutr/o means neutrophil (a type of white blood cell).

                                    thrombocytopenia _____

-phobia   fear   acrophobia _____
                                    Fear of heights.

                                    agoraphobia _____
                                    An anxiety disorder marked by fear of venturing out into a crowded
                                    place.

---

[12]See Appendix L.

-plasia	development, formation, growth	achondroplasia[13] _____
-plasty	surgical repair	angioplasty _____

A cardiologist opens a narrowed blood vessel (artery) using a balloon that is inflated after insertion into the vessel. Stents, or slotted tubes, are then put in place to keep the artery open.

-ptosis[14]	drooping, sagging, prolapse	blepharoptosis _____

*Physicians use **ptosis** (TŌ-sĭs) alone, to indicate prolapse of the upper eyelid.*

nephroptosis _____

-sclerosis	hardening	arteriosclerosis _____

In atherosclerosis (a form of arteriosclerosis) deposits of fat (ather/o means fatty material) collect in an artery.

-scope	instrument for visual examination	laparoscope _____
-scopy	process of visual examination	laparoscopy[15] _____
-stasis	stopping, controlling	metastasis _____

Meta- means beyond. A metastasis is the spread of a malignant tumor beyond its original site to a secondary organ or location.

hemostasis _____

Blood flow is stopped naturally by clotting or artificially by compression or suturing of a wound.

-stomy	opening to form a mouth (stoma)	colostomy _____
		tracheostomy _____
-therapy	treatment	hydrotherapy _____
		chemotherapy _____
		radiotherapy _____

---

[13]See Appendix M.
[14]See Appendix N.
[15]See Appendix O.

IV. Appendices

Appendix A: Hernia

A **hernia** is protrusion of an organ or the muscular wall of an organ through the cavity that normally contains it. A **hiatal hernia** occurs when the stomach protrudes upward into the mediastinum through the esophageal opening in the diaphragm (see Fig. 5–21, page 165), and an **inguinal hernia** occurs when part of the intestine protrudes downward into the groin region and commonly into the scrotal sac in the male (see Fig. 5–21, page 165). A **rectocele** is the protrusion of a portion of the rectum toward the vagina through a weak part of the vaginal wall muscles. An **omphalocele** (omphal/o = umbilicus, navel) is a herniation of the intestines through the navel occurring in infants at birth. A **cystocele** occurs when part of the urinary bladder herniates through the vaginal wall due to weakened pelvic muscles (Fig. 3–1).

Appendix B: Amniocentesis

The amnion is the sac (membrane) that surrounds the embryo (called the fetus after the 8th week) in the uterus. Fluid accumulates within the sac and can be withdrawn **(amniocentesis)** for analysis between the 12th and 18th weeks of pregnancy. The fetus sheds cells into the fluid, and these cells are grown (cultured) for microscopic analysis. A karyotype is made to analyze chromosomes, and the fluid can be examined for high levels of chemicals that indicate defects in the developing spinal cord and spinal column of the fetus (Fig. 3–2).

Appendix C: Plurals

Words ending in **-us** commonly form their plural by dropping the **-us** and adding **-i.** Thus, nucleus becomes nuclei and coccus becomes cocci (KŎK-sī). For additional information on formation of plurals, please refer to Appendix I, page 949, at the end of the book.

Appendix D: Streptococcus and Staphylococcus

Streptococcus, a berry-shaped bacterium, grows in twisted chains. One group of streptococci causes such conditions as "strep" throat, tonsillitis, rheumatic fever, and certain kidney ailments, whereas another group causes infections in teeth, in the sinuses (cavities) of the nose and face, and in the valves of the heart.

Staphylococci, other berry-shaped bacteria, grow in small clusters, like grapes. Staphylococcal lesions may be external (skin abscesses, boils, styes) or internal (abscesses in bone and kidney). An **abscess** is a collection of pus, white blood cells, and protein that is present at the site of infection.

Examples of **diplococci** (berry-shaped bacteria organized in pairs) are **pneumococci** (pneum/o = lungs) and **gonococci** (gon/o = seed). Pneumococci cause bacterial pneumonia, and gonococci invade the reproductive organs causing gonorrhea. Figure 3–3 illustrates the different growth patterns of streptococci, staphylococci, and diplococci.

CYSTOCELE

RECTOCELE

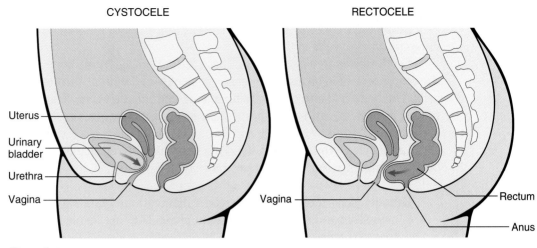

Figure 3–1

Cystocele and **rectocele.**

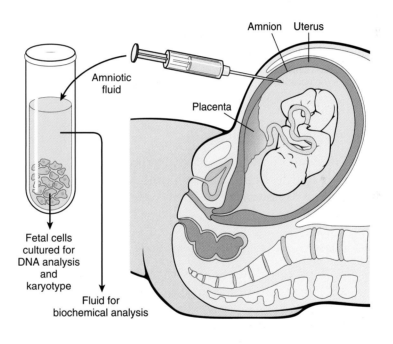

Figure 3–2

Amniocentesis. Under ultrasound (sound wave images) guidance, a physician inserts a needle through the uterine wall and amnion (membrane surrounding the fetus) into the amniotic cavity. Amniotic fluid, containing fetal cells, is withdrawn for analysis. The physician uses continuous ultrasound pictures to locate the fetus and other structures within the uterus, and to ensure the proper placement of the needle.

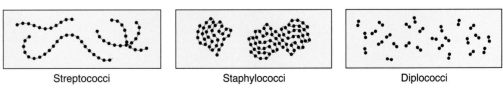

Streptococci

Staphylococci

Diplococci

Figure 3–3

Types of coccal bacteria.

Appendix E: Blood Cells

Study Figure 3–4 as you read the following to note the differences among the three different types of cells in the blood.

Erythrocytes (red blood cells). These cells are made in the bone marrow (soft tissue in the center of certain bones). They carry oxygen from the lungs through the blood to all body cells. The body cells use oxygen to burn food and release energy (catabolism). **Hemoglobin** (globin = protein), an important protein in erythrocytes, carries the oxygen through the bloodstream.

Leukocytes (white blood cells). There are five different leukocytes (three granulocytes or polymorphonuclear cells and two mononuclear cells):

Granulocytes (polymorphonuclear cells) contain dark-staining granules in their cytoplasm and have a multilobed nucleus. They are formed in the bone marrow and there are three types:

1. **Eosinophils** (granules stain red [eosin/o = rosy] with acidic stain) are active and elevated in allergic conditions such as asthma. About 3 percent of leukocytes are eosinophils.
2. **Basophils** (granules stain blue with basic [bas/o = basic] stain). The function of basophils is not clear, but they play a role in inflammation. Less than 1 percent of leukocytes are basophils.

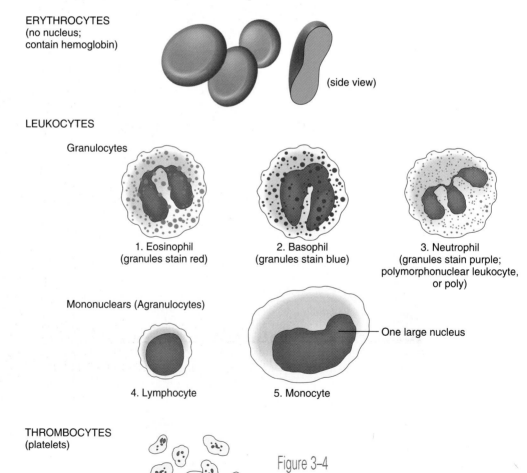

ERYTHROCYTES
(no nucleus;
contain hemoglobin)

(side view)

LEUKOCYTES

Granulocytes

1. Eosinophil
(granules stain red)

2. Basophil
(granules stain blue)

3. Neutrophil
(granules stain purple;
polymorphonuclear leukocyte,
or poly)

Mononuclears (Agranulocytes)

One large nucleus

4. Lymphocyte

5. Monocyte

THROMBOCYTES
(platelets)

Figure 3–4

Types of blood cells. An easy way to remember the names of the five leukocytes is: **N**ever (neutrophil) **L**et (lymphocyte) **M**onkeys (monocyte) **E**at (eosinophil) **B**ananas (basophil).

3. **Neutrophils** (granules stain blue and red [purple] with neutral stain) are important disease-fighting cells. They are **phagocytes** (phag/o = eating, swallowing) because they engulf and digest bacteria. They are the most numerous disease-fighting "soldiers" (50 to 60 percent of leukocytes are neutrophils), and are referred to as "polys" or **polymorphonuclear leukocytes** (poly = many, morph/o = shape) because of their multilobed nucleus.

Mononuclear leukocytes have one large nucleus and only a few granules in their cytoplasm. They are produced in lymph nodes and the spleen. There are two types of mononuclear leukocytes (see Fig. 3-4):

4. **Lymphocytes** (lymph cells) fight disease by producing antibodies and thus destroying foreign cells. They may also attach directly to foreign cells and destroy them. Two types of lymphocytes are T cells and B cells. About 32 percent of leukocytes are lymphocytes.

5. **Monocytes** (cells with one [mon/o = one] very large nucleus) engulf and destroy cellular debris after neutrophils have attacked foreign cells. Monocytes leave the bloodstream and enter tissues (such as lung and liver) to become **macrophages,** which are large phagocytes. Monocytes make up about 4 percent of all leukocytes.

Thrombocytes or **platelets** (clotting cells). These tiny fragments of blood cells are formed in the bone marrow and are necessary for blood clotting.

Appendix F: Pronunciation Clue

Pronunciation clue: The letters **g** and **c** are soft (as in ginger and cent) when followed by an **i** or **e,** and are hard (as in good and can) when followed by an **o** or **a.**

For example: laryngitis (lăr-ĭn-JĪ-tĭs)
laryngotomy (lă-rĭn-GŎT-ō-mē)

Appendix G: Anemia

Anemia literally means no blood. However, in medical language and usage, anemia is a condition of *reduction* in the number of erythrocytes or amount of hemoglobin in the circulating blood. Anemias are classified according to the different problems that arise with red blood cells. **Aplastic** (a- = no, plas/o = formation) **anemia,** a severe type, occurs when bone marrow fails to produce not only erythrocytes but leukocytes and thrombocytes as well.

Appendix H: Ischemia

Ischemia literally means to hold back (isch/o) blood (-emia) from a part of the body. Tissue that becomes **ischemic** loses its normal flow of blood and becomes deprived of oxygen. The ischemia can be caused by mechanical injury to a blood vessel, by blood clots lodging in a vessel, or by the progressive and gradual closing off (occlusion) of a vessel caused by collection of fatty material.

Appendix I: Tonsillitis

The tonsils (notice the spelling with one letter l, whereas the combining form has a double letter l) are lymphatic tissue in back of the throat. They contain white blood cells (lymphocytes), which filter and fight bacteria. However, tonsils can also become infected and inflamed. Streptococcal infection of the throat causes **tonsillitis,** which may require **tonsillectomy.**

Appendix J: Acromegaly

Acromegaly is an endocrine disorder. It occurs when the **pituitary gland,** attached to the base of the brain, produces an excessive amount of growth hormone *after* the completion of puberty. The excess growth hormone most often results from a benign tumor of the pituitary gland. A person with acromegaly is of normal height because the long bones have stopped growth after puberty, but bones and soft tissue in the hands, feet, and face grow abnormally. High levels of growth hormone *before* completion of puberty produce excessive growth of long bones (gigantism) as well as acromegaly.

Appendix K: Splenomegaly

The spleen is an organ in the left upper quadrant (LUQ) of the abdomen (below the diaphragm and to the side of the stomach). Composed of lymph tissue and blood vessels, it disposes of dying red blood cells and manufactures white blood cells (lymphocytes) to fight disease. If the spleen is removed (splenectomy), other organs carry out these functions.

Appendix L: Leukocytosis

When **-osis** is a suffix with blood cells, it is an abnormal condition of increase in normal circulating blood cells. Thus, in leukocytosis an elevation in numbers of *normal* white blood cells occurs in response to the presence of infection (bacterial). When **-emia** is a suffix with blood cells (**-cyte** is usually dropped, as in leukemia), the condition is an *abnormally* high, excessive increase in number of cancerous blood cells.

Appendix M: Achondroplasia

Achondroplasia is an inherited disorder in which the bones of the arms and legs fail to grow to normal size because of a defect in both cartilage and bone. It results in a type of dwarfism characterized by short limbs, a normal-sized head and body, and normal intelligence (Fig. 3–5).

Appendix N: -ptosis

The suffix **-ptosis** is pronounced TŌ-sĭs. When two consonants begin a word, the first is silent. If the two consonants are found in the middle of a word, both are pronounced—for example, blepharoptosis (blĕ-făr-ŏp-TŌ-sĭs). This condition occurs when eyelid muscles weaken, and a person has difficulty lifting the eyelid to keep it open (Fig. 3–6).

Appendix O: Laparoscopy

Laparoscopy (**peritoneoscopy** or **MIS, minimally invasive surgery**) is visual examination of the abdominal (peritoneal) cavity using a laparoscope. The laparoscope, a lighted telescopic instrument, is inserted through an incision in the abdomen near the navel, and gas (carbon dioxide) is infused into the peritoneal cavity to prevent injury to abdominal structures during surgery. Surgeons use laparoscopy to examine abdominal viscera for evidence of disease (performing biopsies) or for procedures such as removal of the appendix, gallbladder, adrenal gland, spleen, or colon, and repair of hernias. It is also used to clip and collapse the fallopian tubes (tubal ligation), which prevents sperm cells from reaching eggs that leave the ovary (Fig. 3–7).

Figure 3–5

A boy with achondroplasia showing short stature, short limbs and fingers, normal length of the trunk, bowed legs, a relatively large head, a prominent forehead, and a depressed nasal bridge. (Courtesy of Dr. A.E. Chudley, Professor of Pediatrics and Child Health, Children's Hospital and University of Manitoba, Winnipeg, Manitoba, Canada.)

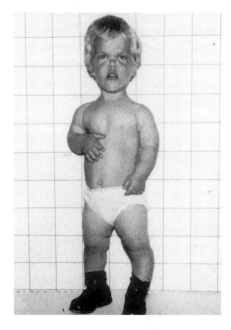

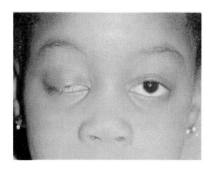

Figure 3–6

Ptosis of the upper eyelid (blepharoptosis) can occur with aging or may be associated with cerebrovascular accidents, cranial nerve damage, and other neurological disorders. (From Seidel HM, et al: Mosby's Guide to Physical Examination, 5th ed. St. Louis, Mosby, 2003, p. 286.)

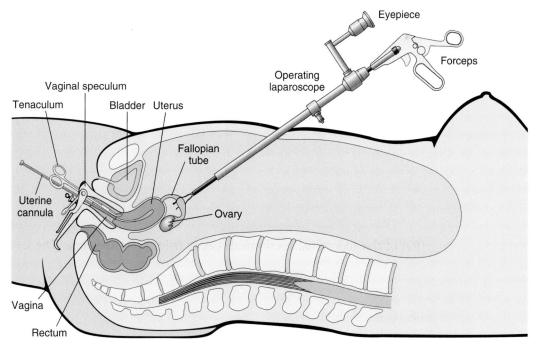

Figure 3–7

Laparoscopy for tubal ligation (interruption of the continuity of the fallopian tubes) as a means of preventing future pregnancy. The **tenaculum** grasps the cervix. The **vaginal speculum** keeps the vaginal cavity open. The **uterine cannula** is a tube placed into the uterus to manipulate the uterus during the procedure. **Forceps,** placed through the laparoscope, grasp or move tissue.

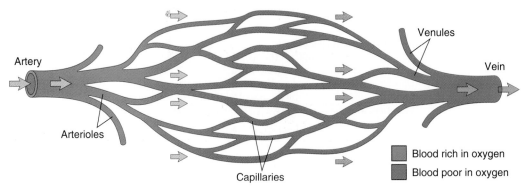

Figure 3–8

Relationship of blood vessels. An artery carries blood rich in oxygen from the heart to the organs of the body. In the organs, the artery narrows to form **arterioles** (small arteries), which branch into **capillaries** (the smallest blood vessels). Through the thin walls of capillaries, oxygen leaves the blood and enters cells. Thus, the capillaries branching into **venules** (small veins) carry blood poor in oxygen. Venules lead to a **vein** that brings oxygen-poor blood back to the heart.

Appendix P: Arteriole

Notice the relationship among an artery, **arterioles,** capillaries (the tiniest of blood vessels), **venules** (small veins), and a vein as illustrated in Figure 3–8.

Appendix Q: Adenoids

The **adenoids** are lymphatic tissue in the part of the pharynx (throat) near the nose and nasal passages. The literal meaning "resembling glands" is appropriate because they are neither endocrine nor exocrine glands. Enlargement of adenoids may cause blockage of the airway from the nose to the pharynx, and adenoidectomy may be advised. The tonsils are also lymphatic tissue, and their location as well as that of the adenoids is indicated in Figure 3–9.

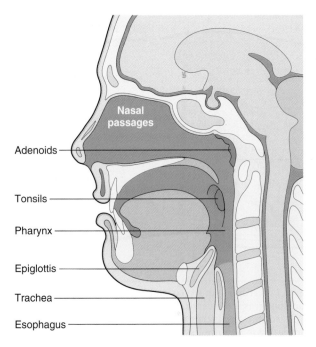

Figure 3–9

Adenoids and tonsils.

V. Practical Applications

Check your answers with the Answers to Practical Applications on page 100.

Procedures

Match the diagnostic or treatment procedures with their descriptions:

amniocentesis	colostomy	mastectomy	tonsillectomy
angiography	laparoscopy	paracentesis	tracheotomy
angioplasty	laparotomy	thoracentesis	

1. Removal of abdominal fluid from the peritoneal space.

   _____

2. Large abdominal incision to remove an ovarian adenocarcinoma.

   _____

3. Removal of an adenocarcinoma of the breast.

   _____

4. A method used to determine the karyotype of a fetus.

   _____

5. Establishment of an emergency airway path.

   _____

6. Surgical procedure to remove pharyngeal lymphatic tissue.

   _____

7. Surgical procedure to open clogged coronary arteries.

   _____

8. Method of removing fluid from the chest (pleural effusion).

   _____

9. Procedure to drain feces from the body after bowel resection.

   _____

10. X-ray procedure used to examine blood vessels before surgery.

    _____

11. Minimally invasive surgery within the abdomen.

    _____

VI. Exercises

Remember to check your answers carefully with those given in Section VII, Answers to Exercises.

A. *Give the meanings for the following suffixes.*

1. -cele _____
2. -emia _____
3. -coccus _____
4. -gram _____
5. -cyte _____
6. -algia _____

7. -ectomy _____
8. -centesis _____
9. -genesis _____
10. -graph _____
11. -itis _____
12. -graphy _____

B. *Using the following combining forms and your knowledge of suffixes, build the following medical terms.*

amni/o	isch/o	ot/o
angi/o	laryng/o	rect/o
arthr/o	mast/o	staphyl/o
bronch/o	my/o	strept/o
carcino/o	myel/o	thorac/o
cyst/o		

1. hernia of the urinary bladder _____

2. pain of muscle _____

3. process of producing cancer _____

4. record (x-ray) of the spinal cord _____

5. berry-shaped bacteria in twisted chains _____

6. surgical puncture to remove fluid from the chest _____

7. removal of the breast _____

8. inflammation of the tubes leading from the windpipe to the lungs _____

9. to hold back blood from cells _____

10. process of recording (x-ray) blood vessels _____

11. visual examination of joints _____

12. berry-shaped bacteria in clusters _____

13. resection of the voice box _____

14. surgical procedure to remove fluid from the sac around the fetus _____

C. Match the following terms, which describe blood cells, with their meanings below.

basophil   lymphocyte   neutrophil
eosinophil   monocyte   thrombocyte
erythrocyte

1. granulocytic white blood cell (granules stain purple) that destroys foreign cells by engulfing and

   digesting them; also called a polymorphonuclear leukocyte _____

2. mononuclear white blood cell that destroys foreign cells by making antibodies

   _____

3. clotting cell; also called a platelet _____

4. leukocyte with reddish-staining granules and numbers elevated in allergic reactions

   _____

5. red blood cell _____

6. mononuclear white blood cell that engulfs and digests cellular debris; contains one large nucleus

   _____

7. granulocytic (granules stain blue) white blood cell prominent in inflammatory reactions

   _____

D. Give the meanings of the following suffixes.

1. -logy _____   8. -megaly _____

2. -lysis _____   9. -oma _____

3. -pathy _____   10. -opsy _____

4. -penia _____   11. -plasia _____

5. -malacia _____   12. -plasty _____

6. -osis _____   13. -sclerosis _____

7. -phobia _____   14. -stasis _____

E. Using the following combining forms and your knowledge of suffixes, build the following medical terms.

acr/o	chondr/o	nephr/o
agor/a	hem/o	phleb/o
arteri/o	hydr/o	rhin/o
bi/o	morph/o	sarc/o
blephar/o	my/o	splen/o
cardi/o	myel/o	

1. fear of the marketplace (crowds) _____

2. enlargement of the spleen _____

3. study of the shape (of cells) _____

4. softening of cartilage _____

5. abnormal condition of water (fluid) in the kidney _____

6. disease condition of heart muscle _____

7. hardening of arteries _____

8. tumor (benign) of muscle _____

9. flesh tumor (malignant) of muscle _____

10. surgical repair of the nose _____

11. tumor of bone marrow _____

12. fear of heights _____

13. view of living tissue under the microscope _____

14. stoppage of the flow of blood (by mechanical or natural means) _____

15. inflammation of the eyelid _____

16. incision of a vein _____

F. Match the following terms with their meanings below.

achondroplasia   colostomy   laparoscopy
acromegaly   hydrotherapy   metastasis
atrophy   hypertrophy   necrosis
chemotherapy   laparoscope   osteomalacia

1. treatment using drugs _____

2. condition of death (of cells) _____

3. softening of bone _____

4. opening of the large intestine to the outside of the body _____

5. no development; shrinkage of cells _____

6. beyond control; spread of a cancerous tumor to another organ _____

7. instrument to visually examine the abdomen _____

8. enlargement of extremities; an endocrine disorder that causes excess growth hormone to be

   produced by the pituitary gland after puberty _____

9. condition of improper formation of cartilage in the embryo that leads to short bones and dwarf-

   like deformities _____

10. process of viewing the peritoneal (abdominal) cavity _____

11. treatment using water _____

12. excessive development of cells (increase in size of individual cells) _____

G. Give the meanings of the following suffixes.

1. -ia _____   7. -um _____

2. -trophy _____   8. -ule _____

3. -stasis _____   9. -y _____

4. -stomy _____   10. -oid _____

5. -tomy _____   11. -genic _____

6. -ole _____   12. -ptosis _____

H. Using the following combining forms and suffixes, build the following medical terms.

Combining Forms   *Suffixes*

arteri/o   pleur/o   -dynia   -ole   -therapy
lapar/o   pneumon/o   -ectomy   -pathy   -tomy
mamm/o   radi/o   -gram   -plasty   -ule
nephr/o   ven/o   -ia   -scopy

1. incision of the abdomen _____

2. process of visual examination of the abdomen _____

3. a small artery _____

4. condition of the lungs _____

5. treatment using x-rays _____

6. record (x-ray) of the breast _____

7. pain of the chest wall and the membranes surrounding the lungs _____

8. a small vein _____

9. disease condition of the kidney _____

10. surgical repair of the breast _____

I. Underline the suffix in the following terms and give the meaning of the entire term.

1. laryngeal _____

2. inguinal _____

3. chronic _____

4. pulmonary _____

5. adipose _____

6. peritoneal _____

7. axillary _____

8. necrotic _____

9. mucoid _____

10. mucous _____

J. Select from the following terms relating to blood and blood vessels to complete the sentences below.

anemia	hemolysis	leukocytosis
angioplasty	hemostasis	multiple myeloma
arterioles	ischemia	thrombocytopenia
hematoma	leukemia	venules

1. Billy was diagnosed with excessively high numbers of cancerous white blood cells,

   or _____. His doctor prescribed chemotherapy and expected an
   excellent prognosis.

2. Mr. Clark's angiogram showed that he had serious atherosclerosis of one of the arteries supplying

   blood to his heart. His doctor recommended that _____ would be
   helpful to open up his clogged artery by threading a catheter (tube) through his artery and
   opening a balloon at the end of the catheter to widen the artery.

3. Mrs. Jackson's blood count showed a reduced number of red blood cells, indicating

   _____. Her erythrocytes were being destroyed by _____.

4. Doctors refused to operate on Joe Hite because of his low platelet count, a condition called

   _____.

5. Blockage of an artery leading to Mr. Stein's brain led to the holding back of blood flow to nerve

   tissue in his brain. This condition, called _____, could lead to necrosis of
   tissue and a cerebrovascular accident.

6. Small arteries, or _____, were broken under Ms. Bein's scalp
   when she was struck on the head with a rock. She soon developed a mass of blood, a (an)

   _____, under the skin in that region of her head.

7. Sarah Jones had a staphylococcal infection causing elevation of her white blood cell count.

   She was treated with antibiotics and the _____ returned to normal.

8. Within the body, the bone marrow (soft tissue within bones) is the "factory" for making

   blood cells. Mr. Scott developed _____, a malignant condition of the bone
   marrow cells in his hip, upper arm, and thigh bones.

9. During operations, surgeons use clamps to close off blood vessels and prevent blood loss.

   Thus, they maintain _____ and avoid blood transfusions.

10. Small vessels that carry blood toward the heart from capillaries and tissues are

    _____.

K. Complete the medical term for the following definitions.

Definition   *Medical Term*

1. The membrane surrounding the heart   peri _____

2. Hardening of arteries   arterio _____

3. Enlargement of the liver   hepato _____

4. New opening of the windpipe to the outside of the body   tracheo _____

5. Inflammation of the tonsils   _____itis

6. Surgical puncture to remove fluid from the abdomen   abdomino _____

7. Muscle pain   my _____

8. Pertaining to the membranes surrounding the lungs   _____ al

9. Study of the eye   _____ logy

10. Berry-shaped bacteria in clusters   _____ cocci

11. Beyond control (spread of a cancerous tumor)   meta _____

12. Pertaining to the voice box   _____ eal

L. Circle the correct term to complete the following sentences.

1. Ms. Daley has nine children and presents to her doctor complaining of problems urinating. After
   examining her, the doctor finds her bladder protruding into her vagina and tells her she has a
   (rectocele, cystocele, hiatal hernia).

2. Suzy coughed constantly for a week. Her doctor told her that her chest x-ray showed pneumonia.
   Her sputum (material coughed up from her chest) demonstrated **(ischemic, pleuritic,
   pneumococcal)** bacteria.

3. Mr. Manion went to the doctor complaining that he couldn't keep his left upper eyelid from
   sagging. His doctor told him that he had a neurological problem called Horner syndrome,
   characterized by **(necrosis, hydronephrosis, ptosis)** of his eyelid.

4. After six weeks in a cast to set her broken arm, Jill's arm muscles were smaller and weaker. They
   had **(atrophied, hypertrophied, metastasized)**. Her physician recommended physical therapy to
   strengthen her arm.

5. Ms. Brody was diagnosed with breast cancer. The first phase of her treatment included a
   (nephrectomy, mastectomy, pulmonary resection) to remove her breast and the tumor. Following
   the surgery her doctors recommended **(chemotherapy, radiotherapy, hydrotherapy)** using drugs
   such as adriamycin and taxol.

6. At age 29, Kevin's facial features became coarser and his hands and tongue enlarged. After a head CT scan, doctors diagnosed him with **(hyperglycemia, hyperthyroidism, acromegaly)**, a slowly progressive endocrine condition involving the pituitary gland.

7. Each winter, when cold and flu season occurred, Daisy developed **(chondromalacia, bronchitis, cardiomyopathy)**. Her doctor prescribed antibiotics and respiratory therapy to help her recover.

8. After **(arthroscopy, laparotomy, radiotherapy)** on her knee, Ellen had swelling and inflammation near the small incisions. Dr. Nicholas assured her that this was a common side effect of the surgery that would resolve spontaneously.

9. Under the microscope, Dr. Vance could see grape-like clusters of bacteria called **(eosinophils, streptococci, staphylococci)**. He made the diagnosis of **(staphylococcemia, eosinophilia, streptococcemia)** and antibiotics were started.

10. David enjoyed lifting weights, but recently noticed a bulging in his right groin region. He visited his doctor, who made the diagnosis of **(hiatal hernia, rectocele, inguinal hernia)** and recommended surgical repair.

VII. Answers to Exercises

A

1. hernia
2. blood condition
3. berry-shaped bacterium
4. record
5. cell
6. pain
7. removal, excision, resection
8. surgical puncture to remove fluid
9. process of producing, forming
10. instrument to record
11. inflammation
12. process of recording

B

1. cystocele
2. myalgia (myodynia is not used)
3. carcinogenesis
4. myelogram
5. streptococci (bacteria is a plural term)
6. thoracocentesis or thoracentesis
7. mastectomy
8. bronchitis
9. ischemia
10. angiography
11. arthroscopy
12. staphylococci
13. laryngectomy
14. amniocentesis

C

1. neutrophil
2. lymphocyte
3. thrombocyte
4. eosinophil
5. erythrocyte
6. monocyte
7. basophil

D

1. process of study
2. breakdown, separation, destruction
3. process of disease
4. deficiency, less than normal
5. softening
6. condition, abnormal condition
7. fear of
8. enlargement
9. tumor, mass
10. process of viewing
11. condition of formation, growth
12. surgical repair
13. hardening, to harden
14. to stop, control

E

1. agoraphobia
2. splenomegaly
3. morphology
4. chondromalacia
5. hydronephrosis
6. cardiomyopathy
7. arteriosclerosis
8. myoma
9. myosarcoma
10. rhinoplasty
11. myeloma (called multiple myeloma)
12. acrophobia
13. biopsy
14. hemostasis
15. blepharitis
16. phlebotomy

Continued on following page

F

1. chemotherapy
2. necrosis
3. osteomalacia
4. colostomy
5. atrophy
6. metastasis
7. laparoscope
8. acromegaly
9. achondroplasia
10. laparoscopy
11. hydrotherapy
12. hypertrophy

G

1. condition
2. development, nourishment
3. to stop, control
4. new opening
5. incision, cut into
6. small, little
7. structure
8. small, little
9. condition, process
10. resembling
11. pertaining to producing, produced by or in
12. prolapse, drooping, sagging

H

1. laparotomy
2. laparoscopy
3. arteriole
4. pneumonia (this condition is actually pneumonitis)
5. radiotherapy
6. mammogram
7. pleurodynia
8. venule
9. nephropathy
10. mammoplasty

I

1. laryngeal—pertaining to the voice box
2. inguinal—pertaining to the groin
3. chronic—pertaining to time (over a long period of time)
4. pulmonary—pertaining to the lung
5. adipose—pertaining to (or full of) fat
6. peritoneal—pertaining to the peritoneum (membrane around the abdominal organs)
7. axillary—pertaining to the armpit, under arm
8. necrotic—pertaining to death
9. mucoid—resembling mucus
10. mucous—pertaining to mucus

J

1. leukemia
2. angioplasty
3. anemia; hemolysis
4. thrombocytopenia
5. ischemia
6. arterioles; hematoma
7. leukocytosis
8. multiple myeloma
9. hemostasis
10. venules

K

1. pericardium
2. arteriosclerosis
3. hepatomegaly
4. tracheostomy
5. tonsillitis
6. abdominocentesis (this procedure is also known as a paracentesis)
7. myalgia
8. pleural
9. ophthalmology
10. staphylococci
11. metastasis
12. laryngeal

L

1. cystocele
2. pneumococcal
3. ptosis
4. atrophied
5. mastectomy; chemotherapy
6. acromegaly
7. bronchitis
8. arthroscopy
9. staphylococci; staphylococcemia
10. arterioles

Answers to Practical Applications

1. paracentesis
2. laparotomy
3. mastectomy
4. amniocentesis
5. tracheotomy
6. tonsillectomy
7. angioplasty
8. thoracentesis
9. colostomy
10. angiography
11. laparoscopy

VIII. Pronunciation of Terms

Pronunciation Guide

ā as in āpe   ă as in ăpple
ē as in ēven   ĕ as in ĕvery
ī as in īce   ĭ as in ĭnterest
ō as in ōpen   ŏ as in pŏt
ū as in ūnit   ŭ as in ŭnder

To test your understanding of the terminology in this chapter, write the meaning of each term in the space provided. In addition, you may wish to cover the terms and write them by looking at your definitions. Check your spelling! The page number after each term indicates where it is defined or used in the text so you can check your responses.

Term	Pronunciation	Meaning
abdominocentesis (78)	ăb-dŏm-ĭ-nō-sĕn-TĒ-sĭs	
achondroplasia (81)	ā-kŏn-drō-PLĀ-zē-ă	
acromegaly (79)	ăk-rō-MĔG-ă-lē	
acrophobia (80)	ăk-rō-FŌ-bē-ă	
acute (83)	ă-KŪT	
adenoids (83)	ĂD-ĕ-noydz	
adipose (83)	Ă-dĭ-pōs	
agoraphobia (80)	ă-gŏr-ă-FŌ-bē-ă	
amniocentesis (78)	ăm-nē-ō-sĕn-TĒ-sĭs	
anemia (78)	ă-NĒ-mē-ă	
angiogenesis (78)	ăn-jē-ō-JĔN-ĕ-sĭs	
angiography (79)	ăn-jē-ŎG-ră-fē	
angioplasty (81)	ăn-jē-ō-PLĂS-tē	
arteriole (82)	ăr-TĒR-ē-ōl	
arteriosclerosis (81)	ăr-tē-rē-ō-sklĕ-RŌ-sĭs	
arthralgia (77)	ăr-THRĂL-jă	
atrophy (82)	ĂT-rō-fē	
axillary (83)	ĂK-sĭ-lār-ē	
basophil (86)	BĀ-sō-fĭl	
biopsy (80)	BĪ-ŏp-sē	
blepharoptosis (81)	blĕ-fă-rŏp-TŌ-sĭs	

bronchitis (79)	brŏng-KĪ-tĭs	_____
carcinogenesis (78)	kăr-sĭ-nō-JĔN-ĕ-sĭs	_____
cardiomyopathy (80)	kăr-dē-ō-mī-ŎP-ă-thē	_____
chemotherapy (81)	kē-mō-THĔR-ĕ-pē	_____
chondromalacia (79)	kŏn-drō-mă-LĀ-shă	_____
chronic (83)	KRŎN-ĭk	_____
colostomy (81)	kō-LŎS-tō-mē	_____
cystocele (78)	SĬS-tō-sēl	_____
electroencephalogram (79)	ē-lĕk-trō-ĕn-SĔF-ă-lō-grăm	_____
electroencephalograph (79)	ē-lĕk-trō-ĕn-SĔF-ă-lō-grăf	_____
electroencephalography (79)	ē-lĕk-trō-ĕn-sĕf-ă-LŎG-ră-fē	_____
eosinophil (86)	ē-ō-SĬN-ō-fĭl	_____
erythrocyte (78)	ĕ-RĬTH-rō-sīt	_____
erythropenia (80)	ĕ-rĭth-rō-PĒ-nē-ă	_____
hematoma (80)	hē-mă-TŌ-mă	_____
hemolysis (79)	hē-MŎL-ĭ-sĭs	_____
hemostasis (81)	hē-mō-STĀ-sĭs	_____
hydronephrosis (80)	hī-drō-nĕ-FRŌ-sīs	_____
hydrotherapy (81)	hī-drō-THĔR-ă-pē	_____
hypertrophy (82)	hī-PĔR-trō-fē	_____
inguinal (83)	ĬNG-wă-năl	_____
ischemia (78)	ĭs-KĒ-mē-ă	_____
laparoscope (81)	LĂP-ă-rō-skōp	_____
laparoscopy (81)	lă-pă-RŎS-kō-pē	_____
laparotomy (82)	lăp-ă-RŎT-ō-mē	_____
laryngeal (83)	lă-RĬN-jē-ăl or lăr-ĭn-JĒ-ăl	_____
laryngectomy (78)	lăr-ĭn-JĔK-tō-mē	_____
leukemia (82)	lū-KĒ-mē-ă	_____

leukocytosis (80)	lū-kō-sī-TŌ-sĭs	
lymphocyte (87)	LĬM-fō-sīt	
mammogram (79)	MĂM-mō-grăm	
mastectomy (78)	măs-TĔK-tō-mē	
metastasis (81)	mĕ-TĂS-tă-sĭs	
monocyte (87)	MŎN-ō-sīt	
morphology (79)	mŏr-FŎL-ō-jē	
mucous (83)	MŪ-kŭs	
myalgia (77)	mī-ĂL-jă	
myelogram (79)	MĪ-ĕ-lō-grăm	
myeloma (80)	mī-ĕ-LŌ-mă	
myoma (80)	mī-Ō-mă	
myosarcoma (80)	mī-ō-săr-KŌ-mă	
necropsy (80)	NĔ-krŏp-sē	
necrosis (80)	nĕ-KRŌ-sĭs	
necrotic (83)	nĕ-KRŎT-ĭk	
nephrologist (82)	nĕ-FRŎL-ō-jĭst	
nephropathy (82)	nĕ-FRŎP-ă-thē	
nephroptosis (81)	nĕ-Frŏp-TŌ-sĭs	
neuralgia (77)	nū-RĂL-jă	
neutropenia (80)	nū-trō-PĒ-nē-ă	
neutrophil (87)	NŪ-trō-fĭl	
ophthalmology (79)	ŏf-thăl-MŎL-ō-jē	
osteogenic (79)	ŏs-tē-ō-JĔN-ĭk	
osteomalacia (79)	ŏs-tē-ō-mă-LĀ-shă	
otalgia (77)	ō-TĂL-jă	
paracentesis (78)	pă-ră-cĕn-TĒ-sĭs	
pathogenesis (78)	păth-ŏ-JĔN-ĕ-sĭs	

pathological (83)	păth-ō-LŎJ-ĭk-ăl
pericardium (82)	pĕr-ē-KĂR-dē-ŭm
peritoneal (83)	pĕr-ĭ-tō-NĒ-ăl
peritoneoscopy (88)	pĕr-ĭ-tō-nē-ŎS-kō-pē
phlebotomy (82)	flĕ-BŎT-ō-mē
platelet (87)	PLĀT-lĕt
pleurodynia (78)	plŭr-ō-DĬN-ē-ă
pneumonia (82)	nū-MŌN-yă
polymorphonuclear leukocyte (87)	pŏl-ē-mŏr-fō-NŪ-klē-ăr LŪ-kō-sīt
ptosis (81)	Tō-sĭs
pulmonary (83)	PŬL-mō-nă-rē
radiographer (82)	rā-dē-ŎG-ră-fĕr
radiotherapy (81)	rā-dē-ō-THĔ-ră-pē
rectocele (78)	RĔK-tō-sēl
splenomegaly (79)	splē-nō-MĔG-ă-lē
staphylococci (78)	stăf-ĭ-lō-KŎK-sī
streptococcus (78)	strĕp-tō-KŎK-ŭs
thoracentesis (78)	thō-ră-sĕn-TĒ-sĭs
thrombocytopenia (80)	thrŏm-bō-sī-tō-PĒ-nē-ă
thrombophlebitis (79)	thrŏm-bō-flĕ-BĪ-tĭs
tonsillitis (79)	tŏn-sĭ-LĪ-tĭs
tracheostomy (81)	trā-kē-ŎS-tō-mē
venule (82)	VĔN-ūl

IX. Review Sheet

Write the meanings of each word part in the space provided and test yourself. Check your answers with the information in the chapter or in the glossary (Medical Terms—English) at the end of the book.

NOUN SUFFIXES

Suffix	Meaning	Suffix	Meaning
-algia		-ole	
-cele		-oma	
-centesis		-opsy	
-coccus		-osis	
-cyte		-pathy	
-dynia		-penia	
-ectomy		-phobia	
-emia		-plasia	
-er		-plasty	
-genesis		-ptosis	
-genic		-sclerosis	
-gram		-scope	
-graph		-scopy	
-graphy		-stasis	
-ia		-stomy	
-ist		-therapy	
-itis		-tomy	
-logy		-trophy	
-lysis		-ule	
-malacia		-um, -ium	
-megaly		-y	

Continued on following page

chapter

Prefixes

This chapter is divided into the following sections

In this chapter you will
- Define basic prefixes used in the medical language.
- Analyze medical terms that combine prefixes and other word elements.
- Learn about the Rh condition as an example of an antigen-antibody reaction.

I. Introduction

This chapter on prefixes, like the preceding chapter on suffixes, gives you practice in word analysis and provides a foundation for the study of the terminology of body systems that follows.

The list of combining forms, suffixes, and meanings in Section II helps you analyze terminology in the rest of the chapter. The appendices (Section IV) are included to provide more complete understanding of the terms and to explain the words with reference to the anatomy, physiology, and pathology of the body.

II. Combining Forms and Suffixes

Combining Forms

Combining Form	Meaning	Combining Form	Meaning
carp/o	wrist bones	**nect/o**	to bind, tie, connect
cib/o	meals	**norm/o**	rule, order
cis/o	to cut	**ox/o**	oxygen
cost/o	rib	**pub/o**	pubis (pubic bone); anterior portion of the pelvic or hipbone
cutane/o	skin		
dactyl/o	fingers, toes	**seps/o**	infection
duct/o	to lead, carry	**somn/o**	sleep
flex/o	to bend	**son/o**	sound
furc/o	forking, branching	**the/o**	to put, place
gloss/o	tongue	**thel/o**	nipple
glyc/o	sugar	**thyr/o**	shield; the shape of the thyroid gland resembled (-oid) a shield to those who named it
immun/o	protection		
morph/o	shape, form	**top/o**	place, position, location
mort/o	death	**tox/o**	poison
nat/i	birth	**trache/o**	windpipe, trachea
		urethr/o	urethra

Suffixes

Suffix	Meaning	Suffix	Meaning
-blast	embryonic, immature	**-gen**	producing, forming
-cyesis	pregnancy	**-lapse**	to slide, fall, sag
-drome	to run	**-lysis**	breakdown, separation, loosening
-fusion	coming together; to pour	**-meter**	to measure

-mission	to send	**-plasm**	development, formation
-or	one who	**-pnea**	breathing
-partum	birth, labor	**-ptosis**	droop, sag, prolapse
-phoria	to bear, carry; feeling (mental state)	**-rrhea**	flow, discharge
		-stasis	stop, control; place
-physis	to grow	**-trophy**	nourishment, development
-plasia	development, formation		

III. Prefixes and Terminology

Write the meaning of the medical term in the space provided.

Prefix	Meaning	Terminology	Meaning
a-, an-	no, not, without	apnea _____	
		anoxia _____	
ab-	away from (notice that the "b" faces away from the "a.")	abnormal _____	
		abductor _____	
		A muscle that draws a limb away from the body.	
ad-	toward (notice that the "d" faces toward the "a.")	adductor _____	
		adrenal glands[1] _____	
ana-	up, apart	anabolism _____	
		analysis _____	
		Urinalysis (urin/o + [an]alysis) is a laboratory examination of urine that aids in the diagnosis of many medical conditions.	
ante-	before, forward	ante cibum _____	
		a. c. is a notation on prescription orders. It means before meals.	
		anteflexion _____	
		antepartum _____	

[1]See Appendix A.

anti-	against	antisepsis _____

An antiseptic (-sis changes to -tic to form an adjective) substance fights infection. Anti- is pronounced ăn-tŭh.

antibiotic[2] _____

antigen[3] _____

In this word, anti- stands for antibody.

antibody _____

antitoxin _____

This is an antibody, often from an animal (such as a horse), which acts against a toxin.

auto-	self, own	autoimmune[4] _____
bi-	two	bifurcation _____

Normal splitting into two branches, such as the trachea bifurcating to form bronchi.

bilateral _____

brady-	slow	bradycardia _____

Usually a pulse of less than 60 beats per minute.

cata-	down	catabolism _____
con-	with, together	congenital anomaly[5] _____

connective _____

Connective tissue supports and binds other body tissue and parts. Bone, cartilage, and fibrous tissue are connective tissues.

contra-	against, opposite	contraindication _____

Contra- means against in this term.

contralateral[6] _____

Contra- means opposite in this term.

de-	down, lack of	dehydration _____

---

[2]See Appendix B.
[3]See Appendix C.
[4]See Appendix D.
[5]See Appendix E.
[6]See Appendix F.

dia-	through, complete	diameter _____
		diarrhea _____
		dialysis[7] _____
dys-	bad, painful, difficult, abnormal	dyspnea _____

Often caused by respiratory or cardiac conditions, strenuous exercise, or anxiety.

dysplasia _____

ec-, ecto-	out, outside	ectopic pregnancy[8] _____
en-, endo-	in, within	endocardium _____
		endoscope _____
		endotracheal _____

An endotracheal tube, placed through the mouth into the trachea, is used for giving oxygen and in general anesthesia procedures.

| epi- | upon, on, above | epithelium _____ |
| eu- | good, normal | euphoria _____ |

Exaggerated feeling of well-being.

euthyroid _____

Normal thyroid function.

| ex- | out, away from | exophthalmos _____ |

Protrusion of the eyeball associated with enlargement and overactivity of the thyroid gland; also called proptosis (pro = forward, -ptosis = prolapse).

hemi-	half	hemiglossectomy _____
hyper-	excessive, above	hyperglycemia _____
		hyperplasia _____

Increase in cell numbers. Hyperplasia is a characteristic of tumor growth.

hypertrophy _____

Increase in size of individual cells. Muscle, cardiac, and renal cells exhibit hypertrophy when workload is increased.

[7]See Appendix G.
[8]See Appendix H.

hypo-	deficient, under	hypodermic _____
		hypoglycemia _____
in-	not	insomniac _____
in-	into, within	incision _____
infra-	beneath	infracostal _____
inter-	between	intercostal _____

Intercostal muscles lie between adjacent ribs.

intra-	into, within	intravenous _____
macro-	large	macrocephaly _____

This is a congenital anomaly.

mal-	bad	malignant _____

*From the Latin "ignis," meaning "fire." **Benign** (ben- = good) tumors are noncancerous, whereas malignant tumors are cancerous.*

malaise _____

From the French "malaise," meaning "a vague feeling of bodily discomfort."

meta-	beyond, change	metacarpal bones _____

The five hand bones lie beyond the wrist bones but before the finger bones (phalanges).

metamorphosis _____

Meta- means change in this term. The change in development from the larval (caterpillar) stage to the adult (butterfly) is metamorphosis.

metastasis _____

Meta = beyond and -stasis = control, or meta = change and -stasis = place. A metastasis is a cancerous tumor that has spread to a secondary location.

micro-	small	microscope _____
neo-	new	neonatal _____

The neonatal period is the interval from birth to 28 days.

neoplasm _____

A neoplasm may be benign or malignant.

pan-   all   pan<u>cyto</u>penia _____

Deficiency of erythrocytes, leukocytes, and thrombocytes.

para-   abnormal, beside,   para<u>lysis</u> _____
              near

Abnormal disruption of the connection between nerve and muscle. Originally from the Greek "paralusis," meaning "to separate, loosen on one side," describing the loss of movement on one side of the body (occurring in stroke patients).

para<u>thyroid</u> glands[9] _____

per-   through   per<u>cutaneous</u> _____

peri-   surrounding   peri<u>cardium</u> _____

peri<u>osteum</u> _____

poly-   many, much   poly<u>morphonuclear</u> _____

poly<u>neuritis</u> _____

post-   after, behind post<u>mortem</u> _____

post<u>partum</u> _____

pre-   before, in front of   pre<u>cancerous</u> _____

pre<u>natal</u> _____

pro-   before, forward   pro<u>drome</u> _____

Prodromal symptoms (rash, fever) appear before the actual illness and signal its onset.

pro<u>lapse</u>[10] _____

pseudo-   false   pseudo<u>cyesis</u> _____

Development of signs of pregnancy but without the presence of an embryo. The origin of this condition may be psychogenic, or caused by tumor and endocrine dysfunction.

re-   back, again   re<u>lapse</u> _____

A disease or its symptoms return after an apparent recovery.

re<u>mission</u> _____

Symptoms lessen and the patient feels better. Remission may be spontaneous or the result of treatment. In some cases the remission is permanent and the disease is cured.

---

[9]See Appendix I.
[10]See Appendix J.

recombinant DNA[11] _____

Genetic engineering uses recombinant DNA techniques.

retro-	behind, backward	retroperitoneal _____

retroflexion _____

An abnormal position of an organ, such as the uterus, bent or tilted backward.

sub-	under	subcutaneous _____
supra-	above, upper	suprapubic _____

The pubis is one of a pair of pubic bones that forms the anterior part of the pelvic (hip) bone.

syn-, sym-	together, with	syndactyly _____

Webbed fingers or toes.

synthesis _____

In protein synthesis, complex proteins are built up from simpler amino acids.

syndrome[12] _____

Before the letters b, m, and p, syn becomes sym.

symbiosis[13] _____

symmetry _____

Equality of parts on opposite sides of the body. What is asymmetry?

symphysis[14] _____

tachy-	fast	tachypnea _____
		(tă-KĬP-nē-ă)
trans-	across, through	transfusion _____

Transfer of blood or blood parts from one person to another.

transurethral[15] _____

ultra-	beyond, excess	ultrasonography[16] _____
uni-	one	unilateral _____

---

[11]See Appendix K.
[12]See Appendix L.
[13]See Appendix M.
[14]See Appendix N.
[15]See Appendix O.
[16]See Appendix P.

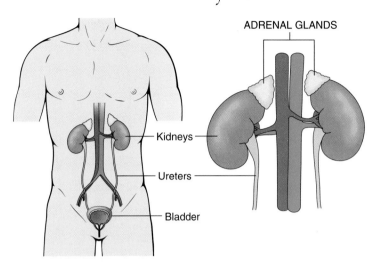

ADRENAL GLANDS

— Kidneys

— Ureters

— Bladder

Figure 4–1

Adrenal glands.

IV. Appendices

Appendix A: Adrenal Glands

The **adrenal glands** are endocrine glands located above each kidney. They secrete chemicals (hormones) that affect the body's functioning. One of these hormones is adrenaline (epinephrine). It causes the bronchial tubes to widen, the heart to beat more rapidly, and blood pressure to rise (Fig. 4–1).

Appendix B: Antibiotic

An **antibiotic** destroys or inhibits the growth of microorganisms (small living things) such as bacteria. Penicillin, the first antibiotic, was cultured from immature plants (molds) and found to inhibit bacterial growth.

Appendix C: Antigens and Antibodies; the Rʜ Condition

An **antigen** is a substance, usually foreign to the body (such as a poison, virus, or bacterium), that stimulates the production of **antibodies**. Antibodies are protein substances made by white blood cells in response to the presence of foreign antigens. For example, the flu virus (antigen) enters the body, causing the production of antibodies in the bloodstream. These antibodies then attach to and destroy the antigens (viruses) that produced them. The reaction between an antigen and an antibody is called an immune reaction (immun/o means protection).

Another example of an antigen-antibody is the **Rh condition.** A person who is Rh$^+$ has a protein coating (antigen) on his or her red blood cells (RBCs). This specific antigen factor is something that the person is born with and is normal. People who are Rh$^-$ have normal RBCs as well, but their red cells lack the Rh factor antigen.

If an Rh$^-$ woman and an Rh$^+$ man conceive an embryo, the embryo may be Rh$^-$ or Rh$^+$. A dangerous condition arises only when the embryo is Rh$^+$ (because this is different from the Rh$^-$ mother). During delivery of the first Rh$^+$ baby, some of the baby's blood cells containing Rh$^+$ antigens can escape into the mother's bloodstream. This sensitizes the mother so that she produces a low level of antibodies to the Rh$^+$ antigen. Because this occurs at delivery, the first baby is generally not affected and is normal at birth. Sensitization can also occur after a miscarriage or an abortion.

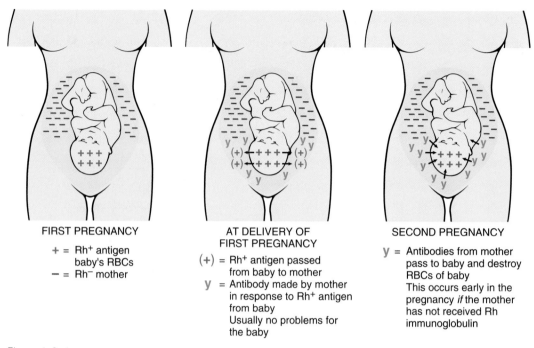

FIRST PREGNANCY

+ = Rh⁺ antigen
  baby's RBCs
− = Rh⁻ mother

AT DELIVERY OF
FIRST PREGNANCY

(+) = Rh⁺ antigen passed
  from baby to mother
y = Antibody made by mother
  in response to Rh⁺ antigen
  from baby
  Usually no problems for
  the baby

SECOND PREGNANCY

y = Antibodies from mother
  pass to baby and destroy
  RBCs of baby
  This occurs early in the
  pregnancy *if* the mother
  has not received Rh
  immunoglobulin

Figure 4-2

Rh condition as an example of an antigen-antibody reaction.

Difficulties arise with the second Rh⁺ pregnancy. If the embryo is Rh⁺ again, during pregnancy the mother's acquired antibodies (from the first pregnancy) enter the embryo's bloodstream. These antibodies attack and destroy the embryo's Rh⁺ RBCs. The embryo attempts to compensate for this loss by making many new, but immature RBCs (erythroblasts). The infant is born with **hemolytic disease of the newborn (HDN)** or **erythroblastosis fetalis.**

One of the clinical symptoms of HDN is **jaundice** (yellow skin pigmentation). Jaundice results from excessive destruction of RBCs. When RBCs break down (hemolysis), the hemoglobin within the cells produces **bilirubin** (a chemical pigment). High levels of bilirubin in the bloodstream (hyperbilirubinemia) cause jaundice. To prevent bilirubin from affecting the brain cells of the infant, newborns are treated with exposure to bright lights (phototherapy). The light decomposes the bilirubin, which is excreted from the infant's body.

Physicians administer Rh immune globulin to an Rh⁻ woman within 72 hours after each Rh⁺ delivery, abortion, or miscarriage. The globulin binds to Rh⁺ cells that escape into the mother's circulation and prevents formation of Rh⁺ antibodies. This protects future babies from developing HDN. Figure 4–2 reviews the Rh antigen-antibody reaction.

Appendix D: Autoimmune

Part of the normal immune reaction (protecting the body against foreign invaders) involves making antibodies to fight against viruses and bacteria. However, in an **autoimmune** disease, the body makes antibodies against its own good cells and tissues, causing inflammation and injury. Examples of autoimmune disorders are rheumatoid arthritis, affecting joints; systemic lupus erythematosus, affecting connective tissues, skin, and internal organs; and Graves disease, causing hyperthyroidism.

Appendix E: Congenital Anomaly

An anomaly is an irregularity in a structure or organ. Examples of **congenital anomalies** (those that an infant is born with) include webbed fingers or toes (syndactyly) and heart defects. Some congenital anomalies are hereditary (passed to the infant through chromosomes from the father or mother, or both), whereas others are produced by factors present during pregnancy. For example, cocaine addiction in the pregnant mother produces addiction and brain damage in the infant at birth.

Appendix F: Contralateral

After a stroke involving the motor (movement) area of the brain, the **contralateral** side of the body often demonstrates a deficit. This means that if brain damage is on the right side of the brain, the patient will have paralysis on the left side of the body. Muscles on one side of the body are controlled by nerves on the opposite (contralateral) side of the brain. **Ipsilateral** (**ipsi-** means same) means the same side.

Appendix G: Dialysis

Dialysis literally means complete separation. A dialysis machine (artificial kidney) can completely separate out from the blood the harmful waste products of the body that are normally removed by the urine.

Appendix H: Ectopic Pregnancy

In a normal pregnancy, the embryo develops within the uterus. In an **ectopic pregnancy,** the embryo implants outside the uterus—most often in the fallopian tubes and sometimes on the ovary or within abdominal cavity (Fig. 4–3).

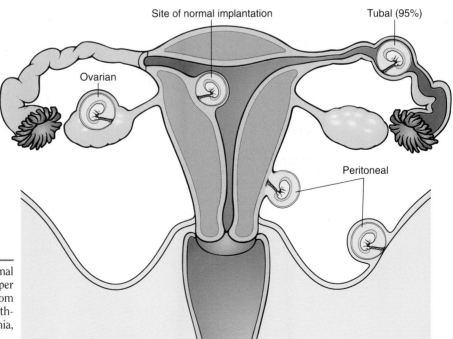

Figure 4–3

Sites of ectopic pregnancies. Normal pregnancy implantation is in the upper portion of the uterus. (Modified from Damjanov I: Pathology for the Health-Related Professions, 2nd ed. Philadelphia, WB Saunders, 2000, p. 383.)

Appendix I: Parathyroid Glands

There are four **parathyroid glands** located on the dorsal side of the thyroid gland. They are endocrine glands that produce a hormone and function entirely separately from the thyroid gland. **Parathyroid hormone** increases blood calcium and maintains it at a normal level.

Appendix J: Prolapse

The suffix **-lapse** means "to slide, sag, or fall." If an organ or tissue **prolapses,** it slides forward or downward. For example, if the muscles that hold the uterus in place become weak, the uterus may slide downward, or prolapse toward the vagina (Fig. 4–4).

Appendix K: Recombinant DNA

This is the process of taking a gene (a region of DNA) from one organism and inserting it (recombining it) into the DNA of another organism. An example is the **recombinant DNA** technique used to manufacture insulin outside the body. The gene that codes for insulin (i.e., contains the recipe for making insulin) is cut out of a human chromosome (using special enzymes) and transferred into a bacterium, such as *Escherichia coli.* The bacterium then contains the gene for making human insulin and, because it divides very rapidly, can produce insulin in large quantities. Diabetic patients, unable to make their own insulin, can use this synthetic product. Scientists have also developed the technique of *polymerase chain reaction* (*PCR*), a method of producing multiple copies of a single gene, which is an important tool in recombinant DNA technology.

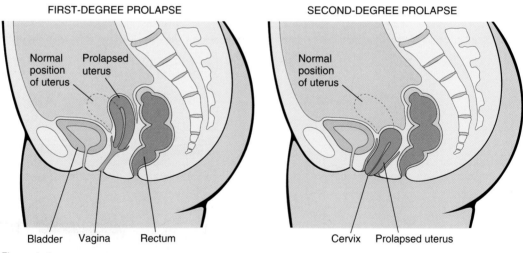

Figure 4–4

First- and second-degree prolapse of the uterus. In **first-degree** prolapse, the uterus descends into the vaginal canal. In **second-degree** prolapse, the body of the uterus is still within the vagina, but the cervix protrudes from the vaginal orifice (opening). In **third-degree** prolapse (not pictured), the entire uterus projects permanently outside the orifice. As treatment, the uterus may be held in position by a plastic pessary (oval supporting object) that is inserted into the vagina. Some patients may require hysterectomy (removal of the uterus).

Appendix L: Syndrome

A **syndrome** is a group of signs or symptoms that commonly occur together and indicate a particular disease or abnormal condition. For example, Reye syndrome is characterized by vomiting, swelling of the brain, increased intracranial pressure, hypoglycemia, and dysfunction of the liver. It may occur in children following a viral infection that has been treated with aspirin.

Fetal alcohol syndrome, a group of symptoms (pre- and postnatal growth deficiency and craniofacial anomalies such as microcephaly and limb and heart defects) in an infant, results from a mother's intake of alcohol during pregnancy.

Appendix M: Symbiosis

Symbiosis refers to two organisms living together in close association, either for mutual benefit or not. The bacteria that normally live in the digestive tract of humans live in symbiosis with the cells lining the intestine. **Parasitism,** another example of symbiosis, occurs when one organism benefits and the other does not.

In psychiatry, symbiosis is a relationship between two persons who are emotionally dependent on each other.

Appendix N: Symphysis

A **symphysis** is a joint in which the bony surfaces are firmly united by a layer of fibrocartilage. The pubic symphysis is where the pubic bones of the pelvis have grown together. The two halves of the lower jaw bone (mandible) unite before birth and form a symphysis. Notice the placement of a suprapubic catheter above the pubic symphysis in Figure 4–5.

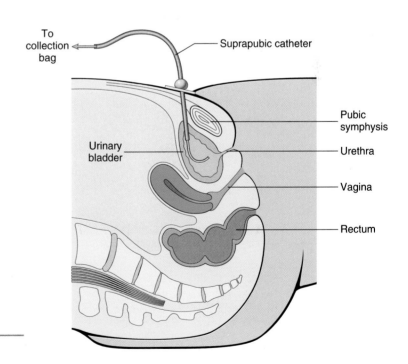

Figure 4–5

Suprapubic catheter.

Appendix O: Transurethral

A **transurethral** resection of the prostate gland (TURP) is removal of a portion of the prostate gland with an instrument passed through **(trans-)** the urethra. The procedure is indicated when prostatic tissue enlarges (hypertrophies) and interferes with urination. Figure 4–6 shows the location of the prostate gland at the base of the urinary bladder.

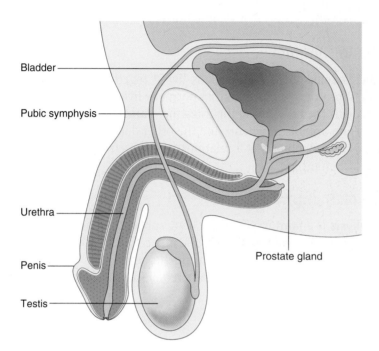

Bladder

Pubic symphysis

Urethra

Penis

Testis

Prostate gland

Figure 4–6

Location of the prostate gland.

Appendix P: Ultrasonography

Ultrasonography is a diagnostic technique using ultrasound waves (inaudible sound waves) to produce an image or photograph of an organ or tissue. A machine records ultrasonic echoes as they pass through different types of tissue. **Echocardiograms** are ultrasound images of the heart. Figure 4–7 shows a fetal ultrasound image **(sonogram)**.

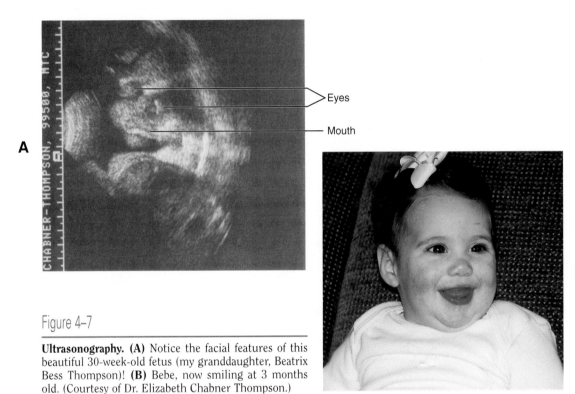

Figure 4–7

Ultrasonography. (A) Notice the facial features of this beautiful 30-week-old fetus (my granddaughter, Beatrix Bess Thompson)! **(B)** Bebe, now smiling at 3 months old. (Courtesy of Dr. Elizabeth Chabner Thompson.)

V. Practical Applications

Check your answers with the Answers to Practical Applications on page 131.

Procedures

Match the **procedure** or **treatment** in COLUMN I with the best **reason for using it** in COLUMN II:

Column I

1. Ultrasonography   _____

2. Hemiglossectomy   _____

3. Percutaneous liver biopsy _____

4. Transfusion of blood cells _____

5. Gastric endoscopy   _____

6. Autopsy   _____

7. Endotracheal intubation _____

8. Dialysis   _____

9. Antibiotics   _____

10. Transurethral resection _____
    of a gland below the
    bladder in a male

Column II

A. Diagnose hepatopathy

B. Treat renal failure

C. Obtain prenatal images

D. Determine the postmortem
   status of organs

E. Treat carcinoma of the tongue

F. Treat benign prostatic
   hypertrophy

G. Diagnose disease in the stomach

H. Establish an airway during
   surgery

I. Treat pancytopenia

J. Treat staphylococcemia

VI. Exercises

Remember to check your answers carefully with those given in Section VII, Answers to Exercises.

A. *Give the meanings of the following prefixes.*

1. ante- _____

2. ab- _____

3. ana- _____

4. anti- _____

5. a-, an- _____

6. ad- _____

7. auto- _____

8. cata- _____

9. brady- _____

10. contra- _____

11. bi- _____

12. con- _____

B. *Match the following terms with their meanings below.*

adductor	anteflexion	bilateral
adrenal	antepartum	bradycardia
analysis	antisepsis	congenital anomaly
anoxia	apnea	contralateral

1. bending forward _____

2. muscle that carries the limb toward the body _____

3. before birth _____

4. slow heartbeat _____

5. gland located near (above) each kidney _____

6. not breathing _____

7. pertaining to the opposite side _____

8. against infection _____

9. to separate apart _____

10. pertaining to two (both) sides _____

11. condition of no oxygen in tissues _____

12. irregularity present at birth _____

C. Select from the following terms to match the descriptions below.

anabolism   antigen   catabolism
antibiotic   antitoxin   contraindication
antibody   autoimmune

1. Chemical substance, such as erythromycin (-mycin = mold), made from molds and used against

   bacterial life _____.

2. Process of burning food (breaking it down) and releasing the energy stored in the food

   _____.

3. Reason that a doctor would advise against taking a specific medication _____.

4. Disorder in which the body's own leukocytes make antibodies that damage its own good tissue

   _____.

5. A foreign agent (virus or bacterium) that causes production of antibodies _____.

6. An antibody that acts against poisons that enter the body _____.

7. Process of building up proteins in cells by putting together small pieces of proteins, called amino

   acids _____.

8. Protein made by lymphocytes in response to the presence in the blood of a specific antigen is a (an)

   _____.

D. Give the meanings of the following prefixes.

1. ec- _____   9. en- _____

2. dys- _____   10. eu- _____

3. de- _____   11. in- _____

4. dia- _____   12. inter- _____

5. hemi- _____   13. intra- _____

6. hypo- _____   14. infra- _____

7. epi- _____   15. macro- _____

8. hyper- _____

E. Complete the following terms based on their meanings as given below.

1. normal thyroid function: _____ thyroid

2. painful breathing: _____ pnea

3. pregnancy that is out of place (outside the uterus): _____ topic

4. instrument to visually examine within the body: endo _____

5. removal of half of the tongue: _____ glossectomy

6. good (exaggerated) feeling (of well-being): _____ phoria

7. pertaining to within the windpipe: endo _____

8. blood condition of less than normal sugar: _____ glycemia

9. condition (congenital anomaly) of large head: _____ cephaly

10. pertaining to between the ribs: _____ costal

11. pertaining to within a vein: intra _____

12. condition of bad (abnormal) formation (of cells): dys _____

13. condition of excessive formation (numbers of cells): _____ plasia

14. structure (membrane) that forms the inner lining of the heart: endo _____

15. pertaining to below the ribs: infra _____

16. blood condition of excessive amount of sugar: hyper _____

F. Match the following terms with their meanings below.

dehydration	incision	metamorphosis
dialysis	insomnia	metastasis
diarrhea	malaise	microscope
exophthalmos	malignant	pancytopenia

1. vague feeling of bodily discomfort _____

2. not able to sleep _____

3. lack of water _____

4. spread of a cancerous tumor to a secondary organ or tissue _____

5. instrument used to see small objects _____

6. to cut into an organ or tissue _____

7. eyeballs that bulge outward (proptosis) _____

8. condition of change in shape or form _____

9. watery discharge (of wastes from the colon) _____

10. deficiency of all (blood) cells _____

11. separation of wastes from the blood by using a machine that does the job of the kidney

_____

12. harmful, cancerous _____

G. Give the meanings of the following prefixes.

1. mal- _____ 11. sub- _____

2. pan- _____ 12. supra- _____

3. per- _____ 13. re- _____

4. meta- _____ 14. retro- _____

5. para- _____ 15. tachy- _____

6. peri- _____ 16. syn- _____

7. poly- _____ 17. uni- _____

8. post- _____ 18. trans- _____

9. pro- _____ 19. neo- _____

10. pre- _____ 20. epi- _____

H. Underline the prefix in the following terms and give the meaning of the entire term.

1. periosteum _____

2. percutaneous _____

3. retroperitoneal _____

4. suprapubic _____

5. polyneuritis _____

6. retroflexion _____

7. transurethral _____

8. subcutaneous _____

9. tachypnea _____

10. unilateral _____

11. pseudocyesis _____

I. Match the following terms with their meanings below.

adrenal	parathyroid	recombinant DNA	syndactyly
neoplasm	prodrome	relapse	syndrome
paralysis	prolapse	remission	ultrasonography

1. return of a disease or its symptoms _____

2. loss of movement in muscles _____

3. congenital anomaly in which fingers or toes are webbed (formed together) _____

4. four endocrine glands that are located near (behind) another endocrine gland in the neck

_____

5. glands that are located above the kidneys _____

6. symptoms that come before the actual illness _____

7. technique of transferring genetic material from one organism into another _____

8. sliding, sagging downward or forward _____

9. new growth or tumor _____

10. process of using sound waves to create an image of organs and structures in the body

_____

11. group of symptoms that occur together and indicate a particular disorder _____

12. symptoms lessen and a patient feels better _____

J. Complete the following terms based on their meanings as given below.

1. pertaining to new birth: neo _____

2. after death: post _____

3. spread of a cancerous tumor: meta _____

4. branching into two: bi _____

5. increase in development (size of cells): hyper _____

6. pertaining to a chemical that works against bacterial life: _____ biotic

7. hand bones (beyond the wrist): _____ carpals

8. protein produced by leukocytes to fight foreign organisms: anti _____

9. group of symptoms that occur together: _____ drome

10. surface or skin tissue of the body: _____ thelium

K. Circle the correct term to complete each sentence.

1. Dr. Tate felt that Mrs. Snow's condition of thrombocytopenia was a clear **(analysis, contraindication, synthesis)** to performing elective surgery.

2. Medical science was revolutionized by the introduction of **(antigens, antibiotics, antibodies)** in the 1940s. Now we occasionally treat an infection with only one dose.

3. The elderly gentleman complained of **(malaise, dialysis, insomnia)** despite taking the sleeping medication that his doctor prescribed.

4. During her pregnancy, Ms. Payne described pressure on her **(pituitary gland, parathyroid gland, pubic symphysis)**, making it difficult for her to find a comfortable position, even when seated.

5. Many times, people with diabetes accidentally take too much insulin. This results in lowering their blood sugar so much that they may be admitted to the emergency department with **(hyperplasia, hypoglycemia, hyperglycemia)**.

6. Before his migraine headaches would begin, John noticed changes in his eyesight, such as bright spots, zigzag lines, and double vision. His physician told him that these were **(symbiotic, exophthalmal, prodromal)** symptoms.

7. After hiking in the Grand Canyon and not carrying water, Julie experienced **(hyperglycemia, dehydration, hypothyroidism)**.

8. Sixty-five-year-old Paul Smith often felt fullness in his urinary bladder but had difficulty urinating. He visited his **(cardiologist, nephrologist, urologist)**, who examined his prostate gland and diagnosed **(hypertrophy, atrophy, ischemia)**. The doctor advised **(intracostal, transurethral, peritoneal)** resection of Paul's prostate.

9. After running the Boston Marathon, Elizabeth felt nauseated and dizzy. She realized that she was experiencing (**malaise, euphoria, hypoglycemia**) and drank a sports drink containing sugar, which made her feel better.

10. While she was taking an antibiotic that reacted with sunlight, Ruth's physician advised her that sunbathing was (**unilateral, contraindicated, contralateral**) and might cause a serious sunburn.

VII. Answers to Exercises

A

1. before, forward	5. no, not, without	9. slow
2. away from	6. toward	10. against, opposite
3. up, apart	7. self, own	11. two
4. against	8. down	12. together, with

B

1. anteflexion	5. adrenal	9. analysis
2. adductor	6. apnea	10. bilateral
3. antepartum	7. contralateral	11. anoxia
4. bradycardia	8. antisepsis	12. congenital anomaly

C

1. antibiotic	4. autoimmune	7. anabolism
2. catabolism	5. antigen	8. antibody
3. contraindication	6. antitoxin	

D

1. out, outside	6. deficient, under	11. in, not
2. bad, painful, difficult	7. upon, on, above	12. between
3. down, lack of	8. excessive, above, beyond	13. within
4. through, complete	9. in, within	14. below, inferior
5. half	10. good, well	15. large

E

1. euthyroid	7. endotracheal	12. dysplasia
2. dyspnea	8. hypoglycemia	13. hyperplasia
3. ectopic	9. macrocephaly	14. endocardium
4. endoscope	10. intercostal	15. infracostal
5. hemiglossectomy	11. intravenous	16. hyperglycemia
6. euphoria		

F

1. malaise	5. microscope	9. diarrhea
2. insomnia	6. incision	10. pancytopenia
3. dehydration	7. exophthalmos (proptosis)	11. dialysis
4. metastasis	8. metamorphosis	12. malignant

G

1. bad	8. after, behind	15. fast
2. all	9. before, forward	16. together, with
3. through	10. before, in front of	17. one
4. change, beyond	11. under	18. across, through
5. near, beside, abnormal	12. above	19. new
6. surrounding	13. back, again	20. above, upon, on
7. many, much	14. behind, backward	

H

1. <u>peri</u>osteum—membrane (structure) surrounding bone
2. <u>per</u>cutaneous—pertaining to through the skin
3. <u>retro</u>peritoneal—pertaining to behind the peritoneum
4. <u>supra</u>pubic—above the pubic bone
5. <u>poly</u>neuritis—inflammation of many nerves
6. <u>retro</u>flexion—bending backward
7. <u>trans</u>urethral—pertaining to through the urethra
8. <u>sub</u>cutaneous—pertaining to below the skin
9. <u>tachy</u>pnea—rapid, fast breathing
10. <u>uni</u>lateral—pertaining to one side
11. <u>pseudo</u>cyesis—false pregnancy (no pregnancy actually occurs)

I

1. relapse
2. paralysis
3. syndactyly
4. parathyroid
5. adrenal
6. prodrome
7. recombinant DNA
8. prolapse
9. neoplasm
10. ultrasonography
11. syndrome
12. remission

J

1. neonatal
2. postmortem
3. metastasis
4. bifurcation
5. hypertrophy
6. antibiotic
7. metacarpals
8. antibody
9. syndrome
10. epithelium

K

1. contraindication
2. antibiotics
3. insomnia
4. pubic symphysis
5. hypoglycemia
6. prodromal
7. dehydration
8. urologist; hypertrophy; transurethral
9. hypoglycemia
10. contraindicated

Answers to Practical Applications

1. **C** Ultrasonography is especially useful to detect fetal structures because no x-rays are used.
2. **E** Malignancies of the oral (mouth) cavity are often treated with surgery to remove the cancerous growth.
3. **A** Diseases such as hepatitis or hepatoma are diagnosed by performing a liver biopsy.
4. **I** Transfusion of leukocytes, erythrocytes, and platelets will increase numbers of these cells in the bloodstream.
5. **G** Placement of an endoscope through the mouth and esophagus and into the stomach is used to diagnose gastric (stomach) disease.
6. **D** A veterinarian performs a postmortem examination of an animal, which is called a necropsy.
7. **H** Endotracheal intubation is necessary during surgery in which general anesthesia is used.
8. **B** Patients experiencing loss of kidney function need dialysis to remove waste materials from the blood.
9. **J** Examples of antibiotics are penicillin, erythromycin, and amoxicillin.
10. **F** A TURP is a transurethral resection of the prostate gland.

VIII. Pronunciation of Terms

Pronunciation Guide

ā as in āpe
ē as in ēven
ī as in īce
ō as in ōpen
ū as in ūnit

ă as in ăpple
ĕ as in ĕvery
ĭ as in ĭnterest
ŏ as in pŏt
ŭ as in ŭnder

To test your understanding of the terminology in this chapter, write the meaning of each term in the space provided. In addition, you may wish to cover the terms and write them by looking at your definitions. Make sure your spelling is correct. The page number after each term indicates where it is defined or used in the text so you can easily check your responses.

Term	Pronunciation	Meaning
abductor (111)	ăb-DŬK-tŏr	_____
adductor (111)	ă-DŬK-tŏr	_____
adrenal glands (111)	ă-DRĒ-năl glăndz	_____
anabolism (111)	ă-NĂ-bō-lĭzm	_____
analysis (111)	ă-NĂL-ĭ-sĭs	_____
anoxia (111)	ă-NŎK-sē-ă	_____
ante cibum (111)	ĂN-tē SĒ-bŭm	_____
anteflexion (111)	ĂN-tē-FLĔK-shŭn	_____
antepartum (111)	ĂN-tē-PĂR-tŭm	_____
antibiotic (112)	ăn-tĭ-bī-ŎT-ĭk	_____
antibody (112)	ĂN-tĭ-bŏd-ē	_____
antigen (112)	ĂN-tĭ-jĕn	_____
antisepsis (112)	ăn-tĭ-SĔP-sĭs	_____
antitoxin (112)	ăn-tĭ-TŎK-sĭn	_____
apnea (111)	ĂP-nē-ă or ăp-NĒ-ă	_____
autoimmune (112)	ăw-tō-ĭ-MŪN	_____
benign (114)	bē-NĪN	_____
bifurcation (112)	bī-fŭr-KĀ-shŭn	_____
bilateral (112)	bī-LĂT-ĕr-ăl	_____
bradycardia (112)	brăd-ē-KĂR-dē-ă	_____
congenital anomaly (112)	kŏn-JĔN-ĭ-tăl ă-NŎM-ă-lē	_____
connective tissue (112)	kŏn-NĔK-tĭv TĬ-shū	_____
contraindication (112)	kŏn-tră-ĭn-dĭ-KĀ-shŭn	_____
contralateral (112)	kŏn-tră-LĂT-ĕr-ăl	_____
dehydration (112)	dē-hī-DRĀ-shŭn	_____
dialysis (113)	dī-ĂL-ĭ-sĭs	_____
diameter (113)	dī-ĂM-ĭ-tĕr	_____
diarrhea (113)	dī-ă-RĒ-ă	_____
dysplasia (113)	dĭs-PLĀ-zē-ă	_____

dyspnea (113)	DĬSP-nē-ă or dĭsp-NĒ-ă	_____
ectopic pregnancy (113)	ĕk-TŎP-ĭk PRĔG-năn-sē	_____
endocardium (113)	ĕn-dō-KĂR-dē-ŭm	_____
endoscope (113)	ĔN-dō-skōp	_____
endotracheal (113)	ĕn-dō-TRĀ-kē-ăl	_____
epithelium (113)	ĕp-ĭ-THĒ-lē-ŭm	_____
euphoria (113)	ū-FŎR-ē-ă	_____
euthyroid (113)	ū-THĪ-royd	_____
exophthalmos (113)	ĕk-sŏf-THĂL-mŏs	_____
hemiglossectomy (113)	hĕm-ē-glŏs-SĔK-tō-mē	_____
hyperglycemia (113)	hī-pĕr-glī-SĒ-mē-ă	_____
hyperplasia (113)	hī-pĕr-PLĀ-zē-ă	_____
hypertrophy (113)	hī-PĔR-trō-fē	_____
hypodermic injection (114)	hī-pō-DĔR-mĭk ĭn-JĔK-shŭn	_____
hypoglycemia (114)	hī-pō-glī-SĒ-mē-ă	_____
infracostal (114)	ĭn-fră-KŎS-tăl	_____
insomniac (114)	ĭn-SŎM-nē-ăk	_____
intercostal (114)	ĭn-tĕr-KŎS-tăl	_____
intravenous (114)	ĭn-tră-VĒ-nŭs	_____
macrocephaly (114)	măk-rō-SĔF-ă-lē	_____
malaise (114)	măl-ĀZ	_____
malignant (114)	mă-LĬG-nănt	_____
metacarpal bones (114)	mĕ-tă-KĂR-păl bōnz	_____
metamorphosis (114)	mĕt-ă-MŎR-fŏ-sĭs	_____
metastasis (114)	mĕ-TĂS-tă-sĭs	_____
microscope (114)	MĪ-krō-skōp	_____
neonatal (114)	nē-ō-NĀ-tăl	_____
neoplasm (114)	NĒ-ō-plăzm	_____
pancytopenia (115)	păn-sī-tō-PĒ-nē-ă	_____
paralysis (115)	pă-RĂL-ĭ-sĭs	_____

parathyroid glands (115)	păr-ă-THĪ-royd glănz	_____
percutaneous (115)	pĕr-kū-TĀ-nē-ŭs	_____
periosteum (115)	pĕr-ē-ŎS-tē-ŭm	_____
polymorphonuclear (115)	pŏl-ĕ-mŏr-fō-NŪ-klē-ăr	_____
polyneuritis (115)	pŏl-ē-nū-RĪ-tĭs	_____
postmortem (115)	pōst-MŎR-tĕm	_____
postpartum (115)	pōst-PĂR-tŭm	_____
precancerous (115)	prē-KĂN-sĕr-ŭs	_____
prenatal (115)	prē-NĀ-tăl	_____
prodrome (115)	PRŌ-drōm	_____
prolapse (115)	PRŌ-lăps	_____
pseudocyesis (115)	sū-dō-sī-Ē-sĭs	_____
recombinant DNA (116)	rē-KŎM-bĭ-nănt DNA	_____
relapse (115)	RĒ-lăps	_____
remission (115)	rē-MĬ-shŭn	_____
retroflexion (116)	rĕt-rō-FLĔK-shŭn	_____
retroperitoneal (116)	rĕt-rō-pĕr-ĭ-tō-NĒ-ăl	_____
subcutaneous (116)	sŭb-kū-TĀ-nē-ŭs	_____
suprapubic (116)	sū-pră-PŪ-bĭk	_____
symbiosis (116)	sĭm-bē-Ō-sĭs	_____
symmetry (116)	SĬM-mĕ-trē	_____
symphysis (116)	SĬM-fĭ-sĭs	_____
syndactyly (116)	sĭn-DĂK-tĭ-lē	_____
syndrome (116)	SĬN-drōm	_____
synthesis (116)	SĬN-thĕ-sĭs	_____
tachypnea (116)	tă-KĬP-nē-ă or tăk-ĭp-NĒ-ă	_____
transfusion (116)	trăns-FŪ-zhŭn	_____
transurethral (116)	trăns-ū-RĒ-thrăl	_____
ultrasonography (116)	ŭl-tră-sŏ-NŎG-ră-fē	_____
unilateral (116)	ū-nē-LĂT-ĕr-ăl	_____

IV. Combining Forms, Suffixes, and Terminology

Check Section VIII of this chapter for help with pronunciation of terms. Write the meaning of the medical term in the space provided.

Parts of the Body Combining Form	Meaning	Terminology	Meaning
an/o	anus	perianal _____	
append/o	appendix	appendectomy _____	
appendic/o	appendix	appendicitis _____	
		See Figure 5–13.	
bucc/o	cheek	buccal mucosa _____	
		A mucosa is composed of epithelial cells.	
cec/o	cecum	cecal _____	
celi/o	belly, abdomen	celiac _____	

Abdomin/o and lapar/o also mean abdomen. When more than one combining form has the same meaning, no rule exists for the proper usage of one or the other. You will learn to recognize each in its proper context.

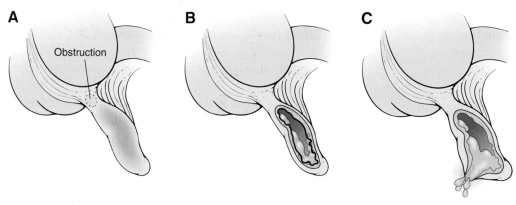

Figure 5–13

Stages of appendicitis. (A) Obstruction and bacterial infection cause red, swollen, and inflamed appendix. **(B)** Pus and bacteria invade the wall of the appendix. **(C)** Pus perforates (ruptures through) the wall of the appendix into the abdomen, leading to peritonitis (inflammation of the peritoneum). (Modified from Damjanov I: Pathology for the Health-Related Professions, 2nd ed. Philadelphia, WB Saunders, 2000, p. 263.)

cheil/o	lip	<u>cheil</u>osis _____
		Labi/o also means lip.
cholecyst/o	gallbladder	<u>cholecyst</u>ectomy _____
choledoch/o	common bile duct	<u>choledoch</u>otomy _____
col/o	colon, large intestine	<u>col</u>ostomy _____
		*-stomy, when used with a combining form for an organ, means an opening to the outside of the body. A **stoma** is an opening between an organ and the surface of the body (Fig. 5–14).*
colon/o	colon	<u>colon</u>ic _____
		<u>colon</u>oscopy _____
dent/i	tooth	<u>dent</u>ibuccal _____
		Odont/o also means tooth.
duoden/o	duodenum	<u>duoden</u>al _____
enter/o	intestines, usually small intestine	<u>enter</u>ocolitis _____
		When two combining forms for gastrointestinal organs are in a term, the one closest to the mouth appears first.

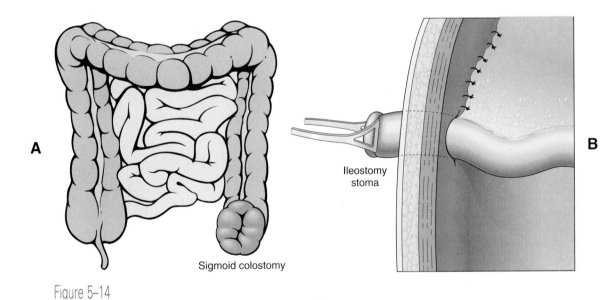

A

B

Ileostomy stoma

Sigmoid colostomy

Figure 5–14

(A) Sigmoid colostomy after resection of the rectum and part of the sigmoid colon. **(B)** Ileostomy after resection of the entire colon. The ileum is drawn through the abdominal wall to form an ileostomy stoma.

enterocolostomy _____

*-stomy, when used with two or more combining forms for organs, means the surgical creation of an opening between those organs inside the body. This is an **anastomosis**, which is any surgical connection between two parts, such as vessels, ducts, or bowel segments (ana = up, stom = opening, -sis = state of) (Fig. 5–15A).*

mesentery _____

Part of the double fold of peritoneum that stretches around the organs in the abdomen, the mesentery holds the organs in place. Literally, it lies in the middle (mes-) of the intestines, a membrane attaching the intestines to the muscle wall at the back of the abdomen (Fig. 5–15B)

parenteral _____

Par (from para-) means apart from in this term. An intravenous line brings parenteral nutrition directly into the bloodstream, bypassing the intestinal tract. Parenteral injections can be subcutaneous and intramuscular, as well.

esophag/o   esophagus   **esophageal** _____

Note: Changing the suffix from –al to –eal softens the final "g" (ĕ-sŏf-ă-JĒ-ăl).

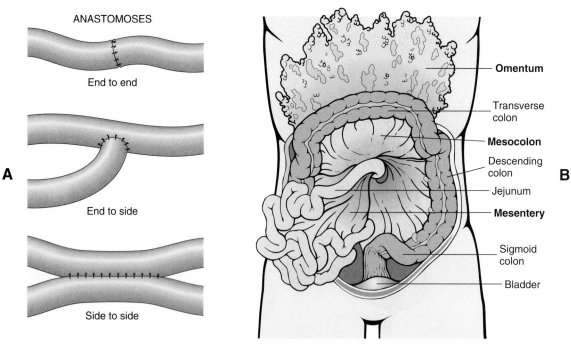

Figure 5–15

(A) Three types of anastomoses. (B) Mesentery. The **omentum** and **mesocolon** are parts of the mesentery. The omentum (raised in this figure) actually hangs down like an apron over the intestines.

faci/o	face	facial _____
gastr/o	stomach	gastrostomy _____
gingiv/o	gums	gingivitis _____
gloss/o	tongue	hypoglossal _____

Lingu/o also means tongue.

hepat/o	liver	hepatoma _____

Also called hepatocellular carcinoma.

hepatomegaly _____

ile/o	ileum	ileocecal sphincter _____

Also called the ileocecal valve.

ileitis _____

ileostomy _____

See Figure 5–14B.

jejun/o	jejunum	choledochojejunostomy _____

An anastomosis.

gastrojejunostomy _____

labi/o	lip	labial _____
lapar/o	abdomen	laparoscopy _____

Minimally invasive surgery (MIS). Examples are laparoscopic cholecystectomy and laparoscopic appendectomy.

lingu/o	tongue	sublingual _____
mandibul/o	lower jaw, mandible	submandibular _____
odont/o	tooth	orthodontist _____

Orth/o means straight.

periodontist _____

endodontist _____

Performs root canal therapy.

or/o	mouth	oral _____

Stomat/o also means mouth.

palat/o	palate	palatoplasty _____
pancreat/o	pancreas	pancreatitis _____
peritone/o	peritoneum	peritonitis _____

The e of the root has been dropped in this term.

pharyng/o	throat	pharyngeal _____
proct/o	anus and rectum	proctologist _____
pylor/o	pyloric sphincter	pyloroplasty _____
rect/o	rectum	rectocele _____
sialaden/o	salivary gland	sialadenitis _____
sigmoid/o	sigmoid colon	sigmoidoscopy _____
stomat/o	mouth	stomatitis _____

Substances

Combining Form	Meaning	Terminology	Meaning
amyl/o	starch	amylase _____	

-ase means enzyme.

bil/i	gall, bile	biliary _____	

The biliary tract includes the organs (liver and gallbladder) and ducts (hepatic, cystic, and common bile ducts) that secrete, store, and empty bile into the duodenum.

bilirubin/o	bilirubin (bile pigment)	hyperbilirubinemia _____	
chol/e	gall, bile	cholelithiasis _____	

Lith/o means stone or calculus; -iasis means abnormal condition.

chlorhydr/o	hydrochloric acid	a<u>chlorhydr</u>ia _____	

Absence of gastric juice is associated with gastric carcinoma.

gluc/o	sugar	<u>gluc</u>oneogenesis _____

Liver cells make new sugar from fats and proteins.

glyc/o	sugar	hyper<u>glyc</u>emia _____
glycogen/o	glycogen, animal starch	<u>glycogen</u>olysis _____

Liver cells change glycogen back to glucose when blood sugar levels drop.

lip/o	fat, lipid	<u>lip</u>oma _____
lith/o	stone	cholecysto<u>lith</u>iasis _____
prote/o	protein	<u>prote</u>ase _____
sial/o	saliva, salivary	<u>sial</u>olith _____
steat/o	fat	<u>steat</u>orrhea _____

Improperly digested (malabsorbed) fats and appear in the feces.

Suffixes

Suffix	Meaning	Terminology	Meaning
-ase	enzyme	lip<u>ase</u> _____	
-chezia	defecation, elimination of wastes	hemato<u>chezia</u> _____	

(hē-mă-tō-KĒ-zē-ă). Bright red blood is found in the feces.

-iasis	abnormal condition	choledocholith<u>iasis</u> _____	
-prandial	meal	post<u>prandial</u> _____	

Post cibum (p.c.) also means after meals.

V. Pathology of the Digestive System

Here are medical terms that describe symptoms (signs of illness) and pathological conditions. Sentences following each definition describe the **etiology** (eti/o = cause) of the illness and its treatment. When the etiology is not understood, it is **idiopathic** (idi/o = unknown). You can find a list of drugs prescribed to treat gastrointestinal symptoms and conditions on page 861 of Chapter 21, Pharmacology.

Symptoms

anorexia

Lack of appetite (-orexia = appetite).

Anorexia is often a sign of malignancy or liver disease. Anorexia nervosa is loss of appetite caused by emotional problems such as anger, anxiety, and fear. It is an eating disorder and is discussed, along with a similar disorder, bulimia nervosa, in Chapter 22.

ascites

Abnormal accumulation of fluid in the abdomen.

This condition, occurs when fluid passes from the bloodstream and collects in the peritoneal cavity. It can be a symptom of neoplasm or inflammatory disorders in the abdomen, venous hypertension (high blood pressure) caused by liver disease (cirrhosis), and heart failure (Fig. 5–16). Patients are treated with drugs (diuretics) and paracentesis to remove abdominal fluid.

borborygmus

Rumbling or gurgling noise produced by the movement of gas, fluid, or both in the gastrointestinal tract.

A sign of hyperactive intestinal peristalsis, borborygmi are often present in cases of gastroenteritis and diarrhea.

constipation

Difficulty in passing stools (feces).

When peristalsis is slow, stools are dry and hard. A diet of fruit, vegetables, and water is helpful. **Laxatives** and **cathartics** are medications to promote movement of stools.

diarrhea

Frequent passage of loose, watery stools.

Abrupt onset of diarrhea immediately after eating suggests acute infection or toxin in the gastrointestinal tract. Untreated, severe diarrhea may lead to dehydration. Antidiarrheal drugs are helpful.

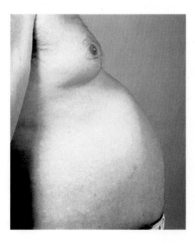

Figure 5–16

Ascites in a male patient. The photograph was taken after a paracentesis (puncture to remove fluid from the abdomen) was performed. Notice the gynecomastia (condition of female breasts) in this patient due to an excess of estrogen that can accompany cirrhosis, especially in alcoholics. (From Lewis SM, Heitkemper MM, Dirksen SR: Medical-Surgical Nursing, 5th ed., St. Louis, Mosby, 2000, p. 1206.)

dysphagia

Difficulty in swallowing.

This sensation occurs when a swallowed bolus fails to progress, either because of a physical obstruction (obstructive dysphagia) or because of a motor disorder in which esophageal peristalsis is not properly coordinated (motor dysphagia). **Odynophagia** means painful swallowing.

eructation

Gas expelled from the stomach through the mouth.

Eructation produces a characteristic sound and is also called **belching.**

flatus

Gas expelled through the anus.

Flatulence is the presence of excessive gas in both the stomach and the intestines.

hematochezia

Passage of bright, fresh, red blood from the rectum.

The cause of hematochezia is usually bleeding from colitis, ulcers, or polyps in the colon or rectum.

jaundice

Yellow-orange coloration of the skin and other tissues caused by high levels of bilirubin in the blood (hyperbilirubinemia).

Jaundice **(icterus)** can occur in three major ways: (1) excessive destruction of erythrocytes, as in **hemolysis,** causes excess bilirubin in the blood; (2) malfunction of liver cells (hepatocytes) because of **liver disease** prevents the liver from excreting bilirubin with bile; (3) **obstruction of bile flow,** such as from choledocholithiasis or tumor, prevents bilirubin in bile from being excreted into the duodenum.

melena

Black, tarry stools; feces containing digested blood.

This symptom usually reflects a condition in which blood has had time to be digested (acted on by intestinal juices) and results from bleeding in the upper gastrointestinal tract (duodenal ulcer). A positive stool guaiac test (see page 191) indicates blood in the stool.

nausea

Unpleasant sensation in the stomach and a tendency to vomit.

Common causes are sea and motion sickness and early pregnancy. Nausea and vomiting may be symptomatic of a perforation (hole in the wall) of an abdominal organ; obstruction of a bile duct, stomach, or intestine; or toxins (poisons).

steatorrhea

Fat in the feces; frothy, foul-smelling, fecal matter.

Improper digestion or absorption of fat can cause fat to remain in the intestine. This may occur with disease of the pancreas (pancreatitis) when pancreatic enzymes are not excreted. It is also a symptom of intestinal disease that involves malabsorption of fat.

Pathological Conditions

Oral Cavity and Teeth

aphthous stomatitis

Inflammation of the mouth with small, painful ulcers.

Commonly called **canker** (KĂNK-ĕr) **sores,** its cause is unknown.

dental caries

Tooth decay (caries means decay).

Dental plaque results from the accumulation of foods, proteins from saliva, and necrotic debris on the tooth enamel. Bacteria grow in the plaque and cause production of acid that dissolves the tooth enamel, resulting in a cavity (area of decay). If the bacterial infection reaches the pulp of the tooth (causing pulpitis), root canal therapy may be necessary.

herpetic stomatitis

Inflammation of the mouth (gingiva, lips, palate, and tongue) **by infection with the herpesvirus.**

Marked by painful fluid-filled blisters on skin and mucous membranes, this is commonly called **fever blisters** or **cold sores.** It is caused by herpes simplex virus (HSV1). Treatment is medication to relieve symptoms. Herpes genitalis (HSV2) occurs on the reproductive organs. Both conditions are highly contagious.

oral leukoplakia

White plaques or patches (-plakia means plaque) **on the mucosa of the mouth.**

This precancerous lesion can result from chronic tobacco (pipe smoking or chewing tobacco) use. Malignant potential is assessed by microscopic study of biopsied tissue.

periodontal disease

Inflammation and degeneration of gums, teeth, and surrounding bone; also called **pyorrhea** (py/o means pus).

Chronic inflammation of gums (gingivitis) occurs as a result of accumulation of **dental plaque** (noncalcified collection of oral microorganisms and their products) and **dental calculus** or **tartar** (a white, brown, or yellow-brown calcified deposit at or below the gingival margin of teeth). In gingivectomy, a periodontist uses a metal instrument to scrape away plaque and tartar from teeth) and remove pockets of pus to allow new tissue to form. Infected areas are treated with antibiotics.

Upper Gastrointestinal Tract

achalasia

Failure of the lower esophagus sphincter (LES) muscle to relax.

Achalasia (-chalasia means relaxation) results from the loss of peristalsis so that food cannot pass easily through the esophagus. Both failure of the LES to relax and the loss of peristalsis cause dilation (widening) of the esophagus (Fig. 5–17A). Physicians recommend a bland diet low in bulk and dilation of the LES to relieve symptoms (Fig. 5–17B).

esophageal varices

Swollen, varicose veins in the distal portion of the esophagus or upper part of the stomach.

Liver disease (such as cirrhosis) can cause increased pressure in veins near and around the liver **(portal hypertension).** This leads to enlarged, tortuous esophageal veins with danger of hemorrhage (bleeding). Treatment includes drug therapy to lower portal hypertension or the use of sclerosing (hardening) agents to close off veins (Fig. 5–18A).

gastric carcinoma

Malignant tumor of the stomach.

Chronic gastritis associated with *H. pylori* (bacterial) infection is a major risk factor for gastric carcinoma. Gastric endoscopy and biopsy diagnose the condition. Cure depends on early detection and surgical removal (Fig. 5–18B).

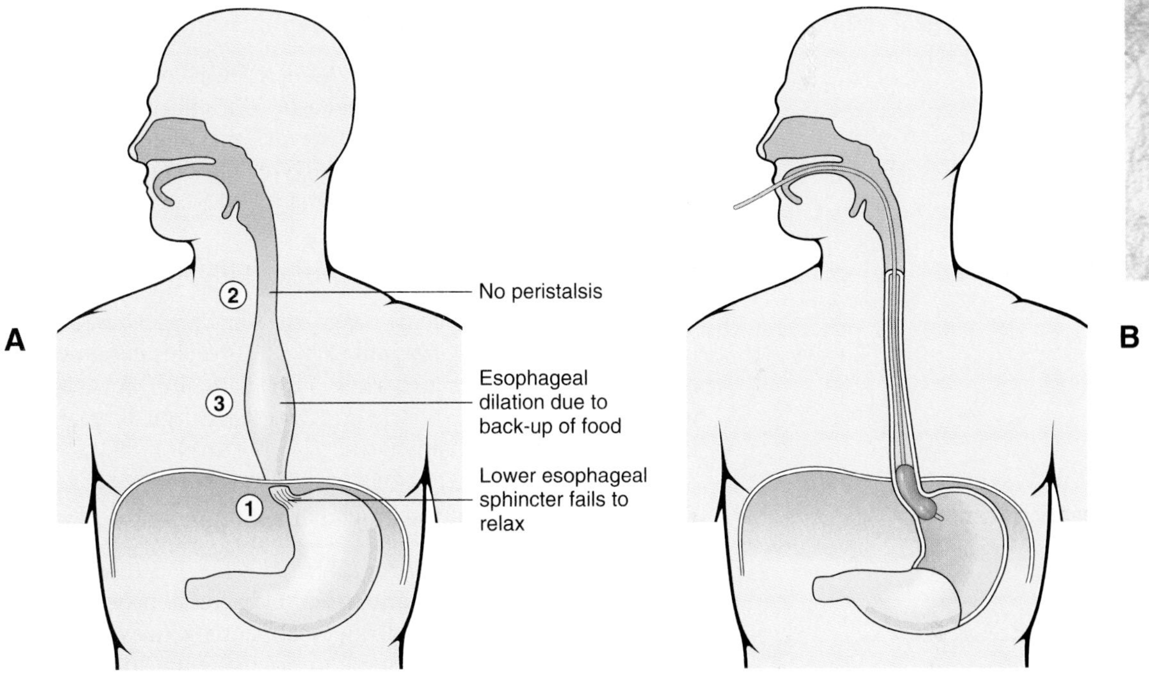

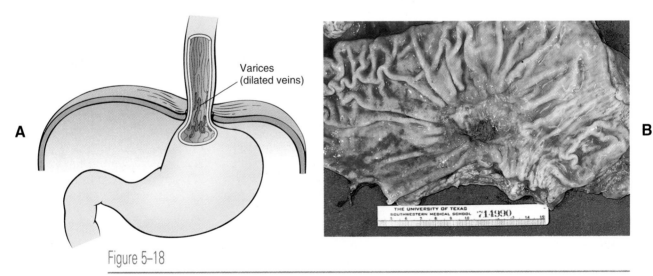

Figure 5–17

(A) Achalasia. Numbers refer to the sequence of events that occur in achalasia. **(B) Balloon dilation (dilatation)** of the lower esophageal sphincter (LES) as treatment for achalasia.

Figure 5–18

(A) Esophageal varices. (B) Advanced gastric carcinoma with a large, irregular ulcer. (A from Damjanov I: Pathology for the Health-Related Professions, 2nd ed, Philadelphia, WB Saunders, 2000, p. 249. B from Kumar V, Cotran RS, Robbins SL: Basic Pathology, 7th ed, Philadelphia, WB Saunders, 2003, p. 562.)

gastroesophageal reflux disease (GERD)

Solids and fluids return to the mouth from the stomach.

Heartburn is the burning sensation caused by regurgitation of hydrochloric acid from the stomach to the esophagus. Chronic exposure of esophageal mucosa to gastric acid and pepsin (an enzyme that digests protein) leads to **reflux esophagitis.** Drug treatment for GERD includes antacid (acid-suppressive) agents and medication to increase the tone of the LES.

hernia

Protrusion of an organ or part through the muscle normally containing it.

A **hiatal hernia** occurs when the upper part of the stomach protrudes upward through the diaphragm (Fig. 5–19A). This condition can lead to GERD. An **inguinal hernia** occurs when a small loop of bowel protrudes through a weak lower abdominal muscle (Fig. 5–19B). Surgical repair of inguinal hernias is known as herniorrhaphy (-rrhaphy = suture).

peptic ulcer

Open sore or lesion of the mucous membrane of the stomach or duodenum.

A bacterium, *Helicobacter pylori* (*H. pylori*), is thought to be responsible for peptic ulcer disease. The combination of bacteria, hyperacidity, and gastric juice damages epithelial linings. Drug treatment includes antibiotics, antacids, and agents to protect the lining of the stomach and intestine.

Lower Gastrointestinal Tract (Small and Large Intestine)

anal fistula

Abnormal tube-like passageway near the anus.

The fistula often results from an abscess (infection) and may or may not open into the rectum (Fig. 5–20A). An **anal fissure** is a painful narrow slit in the mucous membrane of the anus.

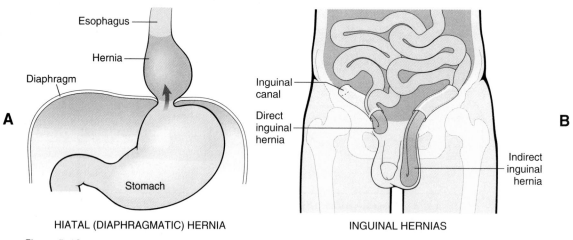

A HIATAL (DIAPHRAGMATIC) HERNIA

B INGUINAL HERNIAS

Figure 5–19

Hernias. (A) Hiatal hernia. (B) Inguinal hernias. A **direct inguinal hernia** passes through the abdominal wall in an area of muscular weakness. An **indirect inguinal hernia** occurs through the inguinal canal (passageway in the lower abdomen) and descends into the scrotal sac.

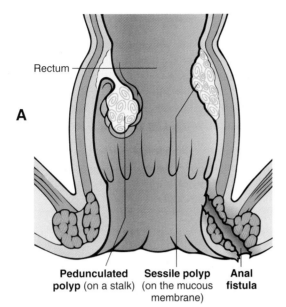

Rectum

A

Pedunculated | Sessile polyp | Anal
polyp (on a stalk) | (on the mucous | fistula
                membrane)

Figure 5–20

(A) Anal fistula and two types of polyps. (B) Multiple polyps of the colon. (Part (B) from Damjanov I: Pathology for the Health-Related Professions, 2nd ed, Philadelphia, WB Saunders, 2000, p. 270.)

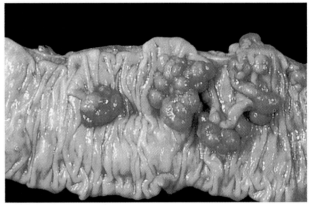

B

colonic polyposis

Polyps (benign growths) protrude from the mucous membrane of the colon.

Figure 5–20A illustrates two types of polyps: **pedunculated** (attached to the membrane by a stalk) and **sessile** (sitting directly on the mucous membrane). Figure 5–20B shows multiple polyps of the colon. Polyps are often removed (polypectomy) for biopsy and to prevent growth leading to malignancy.

colorectal cancer

Adenocarcinoma of the colon or rectum, or both.

Colorectal cancer (Fig. 5–21) can arise from polyps in the colon or rectal region. Diagnosis is determined by detecting melena (blood in stool) and by colonoscopy. Prognosis depends on the stage (extent of spread) of the tumor, including size, depth of invasion, and involvement of lymph nodes. Surgical treatment may require wide resection with colostomy. Chemotherapy and radiotherapy are administered as needed.

Figure 5–21

Adenocarcinoma of the colon. This tumor has heaped up edges and an ulcerated central portion. (From Damjanov I: Pathology for the Health-Related Professions, 2nd ed, Philadelphia, WB Saunders, 2000, p. 272.)

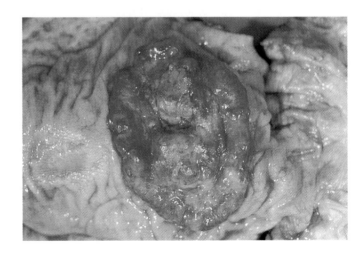

Crohn disease

Chronic inflammation of the intestinal tract (terminal ileum and colon).

Symptoms include diarrhea, severe abdominal pain, fever, anorexia, weakness, and weight loss. Similar to ulcerative colitis, both are forms of **inflammatory bowel disease (IBD).** Treatment is drugs to control symptoms or surgical removal of diseased portions of the intestine, with anastomosis of remaining parts.

diverticulosis

Abnormal side pockets (outpouchings) in the intestinal wall.

Diverticula (Fig. 5–22A) are the pouch-like herniations through the muscular wall of the colon. Rectal bleeding is the primary symptom. When fecal matter becomes trapped in diverticula, **diverticulitis** can occur. Figure 5–22B shows diverticulosis in a section through the sigmoid colon.

dysentery

Painful, inflamed intestines.

Commonly occurring in the colon, dysentery usually results from the ingestion of food or water containing bacteria (salmonellae or shigellae), amebae (one-celled organisms), or viruses. Symptoms are bloody stools and abdominal pain.

hemorrhoids

Swollen, twisted, varicose veins in the rectal region.

Varicose veins can be internal (within the rectum) or external (outside the anal sphincter). Pregnancy and chronic constipation, which put pressure on anal veins, often cause hemorrhoids.

ileus

Failure of peristalsis with obstruction of the intestines.

Mechanical obstruction of the bowel (adhesions, tumor, or stones) is a cause. Surgery, trauma, or bacterial injury to the peritoneum can lead to a **paralytic ileus** (acute, transient loss of peristalsis).

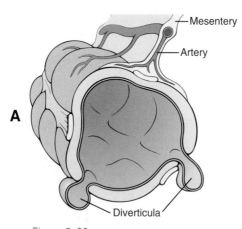

A

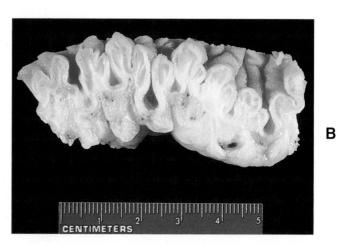

B

Figure 5-22

(A) Diverticula. The mucous membrane lining of the colon bulges through the muscular wall to form diverticula (sing. diverticulum). **(B) Diverticulosis.** Avoidance of foods with seeds and nuts decreases the risk of fecal material lodging in diverticula. (Part B from Kumar V, Cotran RS, Robbins SL: Basic Pathology, 7th ed, Philadelphia, WB Saunders, 2003, p. 577.)

intussusception   **Telescoping of the intestines.**

In this condition, one segment of the bowel collapses into the opening of another segment (Fig. 5–23). It often occurs in children and at the ileocecal region. Intestinal obstruction with pain and vomiting can occur. Surgical removal of the intussusception and anastomosis are frequently necessary to correct the obstruction.

irritable bowel syndrome (IBS)   **Group of gastrointestinal (GI) symptoms associated with stress and tension.**

Gastrointestinal symptoms are diarrhea, constipation, bloating, and lower abdominal pain. Upon extensive examination, the intestines appear normal, yet symptoms persist. Treatment is symptomatic with a diet high in bran and fiber to soften stools and establish regular bowel habits.

ulcerative colitis   **Chronic inflammation of the colon with presence of ulcers.**

This idiopathic, chronic, recurrent diarrheal disease (an **inflammatory bowel disease**) presents with rectal bleeding and pain. Often beginning in the colon, the inflammation spreads proximally, involving the entire colon. Drug treatment and careful attention to diet are recommended. Resection of diseased bowel with ileostomy may be necessary. Patients with ulcerative colitis have a higher risk of colon cancer.

volvulus   **Twisting of the intestine upon itself.**

Volvulus causes intestinal obstruction. Severe pain, nausea and vomiting, and absence of bowel sounds are symptoms. Surgical correction is necessary to prevent necrosis of the affected segment of the bowel (Fig. 5–23).

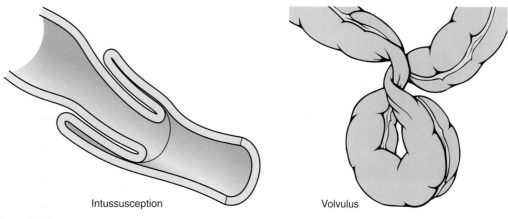

Intussusception   Volvulus

Figure 5–23

Intussusception and volvulus. (From Damjanov I: Pathology for the Health-Related Profession, 2nd ed. Philadelphia, WB Saunders, 2000, p. 264.)

Liver, Gallbladder, and Pancreas

cholelithiasis

Gallstones in the gallbladder (Fig. 5–24A).

> **Calculi** (stones) prevent bile from leaving the gallbladder and bile ducts (Fig. 5–25). Many patients remain asymptomatic and do not require treatment; however, if a patient experiences episodes of **biliary colic** (pain from blocked cystic or common bile duct), treatment may be required. Currently, laparoscopic or minimally invasive surgery **(laparoscopic cholecystectomy)** is performed to remove the gallbladder and stones (Fig. 5–26).

cirrhosis

Chronic degenerative disease of the liver.

> Cirrhosis is commonly the result of chronic alcoholism and often malnutrition, hepatitis, or other causes. Lobes of the liver become covered with fibrous tissue, hepatic cells degenerate, and the liver is infiltrated with fat. Cirrh/o means yellow-orange, which describes the liver's color caused by fat accumulation (Fig. 5–24B). Treatment is dependent on the cause.

pancreatitis

Inflammation of the pancreas.

> Digestive enzymes attack pancreatic tissue and damage the gland. Treatment includes medications to relieve epigastric pain, intravenous fluids, and subtotal pancreatectomy if necessary.

viral hepatitis

Inflammation of the liver caused by a virus.

> **Hepatitis A** is viral hepatitis caused by the hepatitis A virus (HAV). It is a benign disorder spread by contaminated food or water and characterized by slow onset of symptoms. Complete recovery is expected. **Hepatitis B** is caused by the hepatitis B virus (HBV) and is transmitted by blood transfusion, sexual contact, or

A
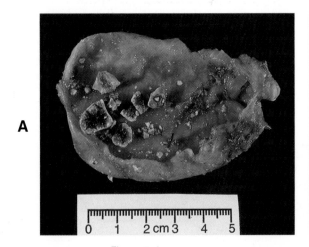

B
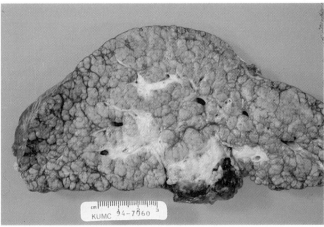

Figure 5-24

(A) Gallstones. Mechanical manipulation during laparoscopic cholecystectomy has caused fragmentation of several cholesterol gallstones, revealing interiors that are pigmented because of entrapped bile pigments. The gallbladder mucosa is reddened and irregular as result of coexistent acute and chronic cholecystitis. **(B) Liver with alcoholic cirrhosis.** The normal liver cells (hepatocytes) have been replaced by nodules that are yellow because of their high fat content. (Part **A** from Kumar V, Cotran RS, Robbins S: Basic Pathology, 7th ed. Philadelphia, WB Saunders, 2003, p. 629; Part **B** from Damjanov I: Pathology for the Health-Related Professions, 2nd ed. Philadelphia, WB Saunders, 2000, p. 290.)

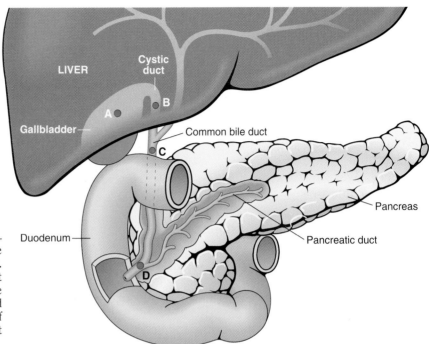

Figure 5–25

Gallstone positions. (A) Stone in the gallbladder causing mild or no symptoms. **(B)** Stone obstructing the cystic duct causing pain. **(C)** Stone obstructing the common bile duct causing pain and jaundice. **(D)** Stone at the lower end of the common bile duct and pancreatic duct causing pain, jaundice, and pancreatitis.

the use of contaminated needles or instruments. Severe infection can cause destruction of liver cells, cirrhosis, or death. A vaccine that provides immunity is available and recommended for persons at risk for exposure. **Hepatitis C** is caused by the hepatitis C virus (HCV) and is transmitted by blood transfusions or needle inoculation (such as intravenous drug users sharing needles). The acute illness may progress to chronic hepatitis.

In all types, liver enzymes may be elevated, indicating damage to liver cells. Symptoms include malaise, anorexia, hepatomegaly, jaundice, and abdominal pain.

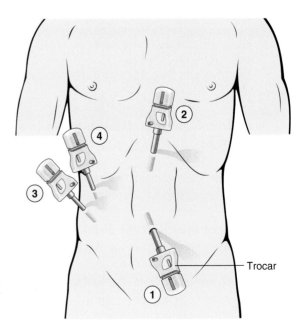

Figure 5–26

Trocars in place for laparoscopic cholecystectomy. Trocars are used to puncture and enter the abdomen. They are metal sleeves consisting of a hollow metal tube (cannula) into which fits an obturator (a solid, removable metal instrument with a sharp, three-cornered tip) used to puncture the wall of a body cavity. Once the obturator is removed, an endoscope and other instruments can be introduced through the trocar to perform laparoscopic surgery. **(1)** is an umbilical 10/11-mm trocar (the largest trocar diameter is 15). **(2)** is a 10/11-mm trocar at the midline. **(3)** and **(4)** are 5-mm trocars at the axillary line.

VI. Exercises

Remember to check your answers carefully with those given in Section VII, Answers to Exercises.

A. Match the following digestive system structures with their meanings below.

anus	esophagus	liver
cecum	gallbladder	pancreas
colon	ileum	pharynx
duodenum	jejunum	sigmoid colon

1. large intestine _____

2. small sac under the liver; stores bile _____

3. first part of the large intestine _____

4. opening of the digestive tract to the outside of the body _____

5. second part of the small intestine _____

6. tube connecting the throat to the stomach _____

7. third part of the small intestine _____

8. large organ located in the RUQ; secretes bile, stores sugar, produces blood proteins _____

9. throat _____

10. lower part of the colon _____

11. first part of the small intestine _____

12. organ under the stomach; produces insulin and digestive enzymes _____

B. Circle the term that correctly fits the definition given. You should be able to define the other terms as well!

1. **microscopic projections in the walls of the small intestine:**
   papillae   villi   rugae

2. **salivary gland near the ear:**
   submandibular   sublingual   parotid

3. **ring of muscle at the distal end of the stomach:**
   pyloric sphincter   uvula lower   esophageal sphincter

4. **soft, inner section of a tooth:**
   dentin   enamel   pulp

5. **chemical that speeds up reactions and helps digest foods:**
   triglyceride   amino acid   enzyme

6. **pigment released with bile:**
   glycogen   bilirubin   melena

7. **hormone produced by endocrine cells of the pancreas:**
   insulin   amylase   lipase

8. **rhythm-like movement of the muscles in the walls of the gastrointestinal tract:**
   deglutition   mastication   peristalsis

9. **breakdown of large fat globules:**
   absorption   emulsification   anabolism

10. **pointed, dog-like tooth medial to premolars:**
    incisor   canine   molar

C. Complete the following.

1. labi/o and cheil/o both mean _____

2. gloss/o and lingu/o both mean _____

3. or/o and stomat/o both mean _____

4. dent/i and odont/o both mean _____

5. lapar/o and celi/o both mean _____

6. gluc/o and glyc/o both mean _____

7. lip/o, steat/o, and adip/o all mean _____

8. -iasis and -osis both mean _____

9. chol/e and bil/i both mean _____

10. -ectomy and resection both mean _____

D. Build medical terms.

1. removal of a salivary gland _____

2. pertaining to the throat _____

3. hernia of the rectum _____

4. enlargement of the liver _____

5. surgical repair of the roof of the mouth _____

6. after meals _____

7. visual examination of the anal and rectal region _____

8. study of the cause (of disease) _____

9. incision of the common bile duct _____

10. pertaining to tooth and cheek (the surface of tooth against the cheek) _____

11. disease condition of the small intestine _____

12. new opening between the common bile duct and the jejunum _____

13. pertaining to surrounding the anus _____

14. new opening from the colon to the outside of the body _____

15. pertaining to under the lower jaw _____

16. pertaining to the face _____

E. Match the following doctors or dentists with their specialties.

colorectal surgeon	nephrologist	periodontist
endodontist	oral surgeon	proctologist
gastroenterologist	orthodontist	urologist

1. diagnoses and treats disorders of the anus and rectum _____

2. operates on the organs of the urinary tract _____

3. straightens teeth _____

4. performs root canal therapy _____

5. operates on the mouth and teeth _____

6. diagnoses and uses drugs to treat kidney disorders _____

7. diagnoses and treats gastrointestinal tract disorders _____

8. treats gum disease _____

9. operates on the intestinal tract _____

F. Build medical terms to describe the following inflammations.

1. inflammation of the appendix _____

2. inflammation of the large intestine _____

3. inflammation of the tube from the throat to the stomach _____

4. inflammation of the membrane around the abdomen _____

5. inflammation of the gallbladder _____

6. inflammation of the third part of the small intestine _____

7. inflammation of the pancreas _____

8. inflammation of the gums _____

9. inflammation of the liver _____

10. inflammation of the mouth _____

11. inflammation of the salivary gland _____

12. inflammation of the small and large intestine _____

G. *Match the following terms with their meanings below.*

anastomosis	gluconeogenesis	mesentery
biliary	glycogenolysis	mucosa
defecation	hyperbilirubinemia	parenteral
dysphagia	hyperglycemia	portal vein

1. high level of blood sugar _____

2. difficulty in swallowing _____

3. pertaining to administration other than through the intestinal tract _____

4. a mucous membrane _____

5. expulsion of feces from the body through the anus _____

6. breakdown (conversion) of animal starch to sugar _____

7. membrane that connects the small intestine to the abdominal wall _____

8. large vessel that takes blood to the liver from the intestines _____

9. new surgical connection between two previously unconnected organs _____

10. pertaining to bile ducts and organs _____

11. process of forming new sugar from proteins and fats _____

12. high levels of a bile pigment in the bloodstream _____

H. Give the names of the following gastrointestinal symptoms based on their descriptions.

1. passage of bright red blood from the rectum _____

2. lack of appetite _____

3. fat in the feces _____

4. black, tarry stools; feces containing digested blood _____

5. abnormal accumulation of fluid in the abdomen _____

6. rumbling noise produced by gas in the GI tract _____

7. gas expelled through the anus _____

8. an unpleasant sensation in the stomach and a tendency to vomit _____

9. loose, watery stools _____

10. difficulty in passing stools (feces) _____

I. Give short answers for the following.

1. What is jaundice? _____

2. Give three ways in which a patient can become jaundiced:

   a. _____

   b. _____

   c. _____

3. What does it mean when a disease is described as *idiopathic?* _____

J. Use the pathological terminology listed below to make your diagnosis.

achalasia   colorectal cancer   herpetic stomatitis
anal fistula   Crohn disease   oral leukoplakia
aphthous stomatitis   dental caries   periodontal disease
colonic polyposis

1. Ms. Jones complained of pain during swallowing. Her physician described her condition as caused by a failure of muscles in her lower esophagus to relax during swallowing. Diagnosis: _____.

2. An abnormal tube-like passageway near his anus caused Mr. Rosen's proctalgia. His doctor performed surgery to close off the abnormality. Diagnosis: _____.

3. Bebe's dentist informed her that the enamel of three teeth was damaged by bacteria-producing acid. Diagnosis: _____.

4. Paola's symptoms of chronic diarrhea, abdominal cramps, and fever led her doctor to suspect that she suffered from an inflammatory bowel disease affecting the distal portion of her ileum. The doctor prescribed steroid drugs to heal her condition. Diagnosis: _____.

5. Mr. Hart learned that the results of his colonoscopy showed the presence of small benign growths protruding from the mucous membrane of his large intestine. Diagnosis: _____.

6. During a routine dental checkup, Dr. Friedman discovered white plaques on Mr. Longo's buccal mucosa. He advised Mr. Longo, who was a chronic smoker and alcoholic, to have these precancerous lesions removed. Diagnosis: _____.

7. Every time Carl had a stressful time at work he developed a fever blister (cold sore) on his lip, resulting from reactivation of a previous viral infection. His doctor told him that there was no preventable treatment. Diagnosis: _____.

8. Mr. Green had a biopsy of a neoplastic lesion in his ascending colon. The pathology report indicated a malignancy. Radical (complete) colectomy followed by colostomy was necessary. Diagnosis: _____.

9. After irritating her mouth with vigorous tooth brushing, small ulcers (canker sores) appeared on Diane's gums. They were painful and annoying. Diagnosis: _____.

10. Failure to floss her teeth and remove dental plaque regularly led to Sharon's gingivitis and pyorrhea. Her dentist advised consulting a periodontist who could treat her condition. Diagnosis: _____.

K. Match the following pathological diagnoses with their definitions.

cholecystolithiasis	hemorrhoids	irritable bowel syndrome
cirrhosis	hepatitis	pancreatitis
diverticulosis	hiatal hernia	peptic ulcer
dysentery	ileus	ulcerative colitis
esophageal varices	intussusception	volvulus

1. protrusion of the upper part of the stomach through the diaphragm _____

2. painful, inflamed intestines caused by bacterial infection _____

3. swollen, twisted veins in the rectal region _____

4. open sore or lesion of the mucous membrane of the stomach or duodenum _____

5. failure of peristalsis with obstruction of intestines _____

6. twisting of the intestine upon itself _____

7. swollen, varicose veins in the distal portion of the esophagus _____

8. abnormal side-pockets (outpouchings) in the intestinal wall _____

9. chronic inflammation of the colon with ulcers _____

10. telescoping of the intestines _____

11. inflammation of the liver caused by type A, type B, or type C virus _____

12. inflammation of the pancreas _____

13. calculi in the sac that stores bile _____

14. chronic degenerative liver disease resulting from alcoholism and malnutrition _____

15. a group of symptoms (diarrhea and constipation, abdominal pain, bloating) associated with stress

    and tension, but without inflammation of the intestine _____

L. Complete the following terms from their meanings given below.

1. membrane (peritoneal fold) that holds the intestines together: mes _____

2. removal of the gallbladder: _____ ectomy

3. black or dark brown, tarry stools containing blood: mel _____

4. high levels of pigment in the blood (jaundice): hyper _____

5. pertaining to under the tongue: sub _____

6. twisting of the intestine upon itself: vol _____

7. organ under the stomach that produces insulin and digestive enzymes: pan _____

8. lack of appetite: an _____

9. swollen, twisted veins in the rectal region: _____ oids

10. new connection between two previously unconnected tubes: ana _____

11. absence of acid in the stomach: a _____

12. solid and fluids return to the mouth from the stomach: gastro _____

    re _____ disease

VII. Answers to Exercises

A

1. colon
2. gallbladder
3. cecum
4. anus
5. jejunum
6. esophagus
7. ileum
8. liver
9. pharynx
10. sigmoid colon
11. duodenum
12. pancreas

B

1. Villi. Papillae are nipple-like projections in the tongue where taste buds are located, and rugae are folds in the mucous membrane of the stomach and hard palate.
2. Parotid. The submandibular gland is under the lower jaw, and the sublingual gland is under the tongue.
3. Pyloric sphincter. The uvula is soft tissue hanging from the soft palate, and the lower esophageal sphincter is a ring of muscle between the esophagus and stomach.
4. Pulp. Dentin is the hard part of the tooth directly under the enamel and in the root, and enamel is the hard, outermost part of the tooth composing the crown.
5. Enzyme. A triglyceride is a large fat molecule, and an amino acid is substance produced when proteins are digested.
6. Bilirubin. Glycogen is animal starch that is produced in liver cells from sugar, and melena is dark, tarry stools.
7. Insulin. Amylase and lipase are digestive enzymes produced by the exocrine cells of the pancreas.
8. Peristalis. Deglutition is swallowing, and mastication is chewing.
9. Emulsification. Absorption is the passage of materials through the walls of the small intestine into the bloodstream, and anabolism is the process of building up proteins in a cell (protein synthesis).
10. Canine. An incisor is one of the four front teeth in the dental arch (not pointed or dog-like), and a molar is one of three large teeth just behind (distal to) the two premolar teeth.

C

1. lip
2. tongue
3. mouth
4. tooth
5. abdomen
6. sugar
7. fat
8. abnormal condition
9. gall, bile
10. removal, excision

Continued on following page

D

1. sialadenectomy
2. pharyngeal
3. rectocele
4. hepatomegaly
5. palatoplasty
6. postprandial (post cibum—cib/o means meals)
7. proctoscopy
8. etiology
9. choledochotomy
10. dentibuccal
11. enteropathy
12. choledochojejunostomy
13. perianal
14. colostomy
15. submandibular
16. facial

E

1. proctologist
2. urologist
3. orthodontist
4. endodontist
5. oral surgeon
6. nephrologist
7. gastroenterologist
8. periodontist
9. colorectal surgeon

F

1. appendicitis
2. colitis
3. esophagitis
4. peritonitis (note that the e is dropped)
5. cholecystitis
6. ileitis
7. pancreatitis
8. gingivitis
9. hepatitis
10. stomatitis
11. sialadenitis
12. enterocolitis (when two combining forms for gastrointestinal organs are in a term, use the one that is closest to the mouth first)

G

1. hyperglycemia
2. dysphagia
3. parenteral
4. mucosa
5. defecation
6. glycogenolysis
7. mesentery
8. portal vein
9. anastomosis
10. biliary
11. gluconeogenesis
12. hyperbilirubinemia

H

1. hematochezia
2. anorexia
3. steatorrhea
4. melena
5. ascites
6. borborygmus
7. flatus
8. nausea
9. diarrhea
10. constipation

I

1. yellow-orange coloration of the skin and other tissues (hyperbilirubinemia)
2. **a** any liver disease (hepatopathy—such as cirrhosis, hepatoma, or hepatitis), so that bilirubin is not processed into bile and cannot be excreted in feces
   b obstruction of bile flow, so that bile and bilirubin are not excreted and accumulate in the bloodstream
   c excessive hemolysis leading to overproduction of bilirubin and high levels in the bloodstream
3. its cause is not known

J

1. achalasia
2. anal fistula
3. dental caries
4. Crohn disease
5. colonic polyposis
6. oral leukoplakia
7. herpetic stomatitis
8. colorectal cancer
9. aphthous stomatitis
10. periodontal disease

K

1. hiatal hernia
2. dysentery
3. hemorrhoids
4. peptic ulcer
5. ileus
6. volvulus
7. esophageal varices
8. diverticulosis
9. ulcerative colitis
10. intussusception
11. viral hepatitis
12. pancreatitis
13. cholecystolithiasis (gallstones)
14. cirrhosis
15. irritable bowel syndrome

L

1. mesentery
2. cholecystectomy
3. melena
4. hyperbilirubinemia
5. sublingual
6. volvulus
7. pancreas
8. anorexia
9. hemorrhoids
10. anastomosis
11. achlorhydria
12. gastroesophageal reflux disease

VIII. Pronunciation of Terms

Pronunciation Guide

ā as in āpe   ă as in ăpple
ē as in ēven   ĕ as in ĕvery
ī as in īce   ĭ as in ĭnterest
ō as in ōpen   ŏ as in pŏt
ū as in ūnit   ŭ as in ŭnder

To test your understanding of the terminology in this chapter, write the meaning of each term in the space provided. In addition, you may wish to cover the terms and write them by looking at your definitions. Make sure your spelling is correct. The page number after each term indicates where it is defined or used in the text so you can easily check your responses.

Vocabulary and Terminology Sections

Term	Pronunciation	Meaning
absorption (151)	ăb-SŌRP-shŭn	
achlorhydria (159)	ā-chlōr-HĪ-drē-ă	
amino acids (151)	ă-MĒ-nō ĂS-ĭdz	
amylase (151)	ĂM-ĭ-lās	
anastomosis (156)	ă-năs-tō-MŌ-sĭs	
anus (151)	Ā-nŭs	
appendectomy (154)	ăp-ĕn-DĔK-tō-mē	
appendicitis (154)	ă-pĕn-dĭ-SĪ-tĭs	
appendix (151)	ă-PĔN-dĭks	
bile (151)	BĪL	
biliary (158)	BĬL-ē-ăr-ē	
bilirubin (151)	bĭl-ĭ-ROO-bĭn	
bowel (151)	BŎW-ĕl	
buccal mucosa (154)	BŬK-ăl mū-KŌ-să	
canine teeth (151)	KĀ-nīn tēth	
cecal (154)	SĒ-kăl	
cecum (151)	SĒ-kŭm	
celiac (154)	SĒ-lē-ăk	
cheilosis (155)	kī-LŌ-sĭs	
cholecystectomy (155)	kō-lĕ-sĭs-TĔK-tō-mē	
choledocholithiasis (159)	kō-lĕd-ō-kō-lĭ-THĪ-ă-sĭs	

choledochojejunostomy (157)	kō-lĕd-ō-kō-jĭ-jū-NŎS-tō-mē	
choledochotomy (155)	kō-lĕd-ō-KŎT-ō-mē	
cholelithiasis (158)	kō-lē-lĭ-THĪ-ă-sĭs	
colon (151)	KŌ-lĕn	
colonic (155)	kō-LŎN-ĭk	
colonoscopy (155)	kō-lŏn-ŎS-kō-pē	
colostomy (155)	kŏ-LŎS-tō-mē	
common bile duct (151)	KŎM-ĭn bīl dŭkt	
defecation (151)	dĕf-ĕ-KĀ-shŭn	
deglutition (151)	dē-gloo-TĬSH-ŭn	
dentibuccal (155)	dĕn-tē-BŬK-ăl	
dentin (151)	DĔN-tĭn	
digestion (151)	dī-JĔST-yŭn	
duodenal (155)	dū-ō-DĒ-năl or dū-ŎD-dĕ-năl	
duodenum (151)	dū-ō-DĒ-nŭm or dū-ŎD-dĕ-ŭm	
elimination (151)	ē-lĭm-ĭ-NĀ-shŭn	
emulsification (152)	ē-mŭl-sĭ-fĭ-KĀ-shŭn	
enamel (152)	ē-NĂM-ĕl	
endodontist (157)	ĕn-dō-DŎN-tĭst	
enterocolitis (155)	ĕn-tĕr-ō-kō-LĪ-tĭs	
enterocolostomy (156)	ĕn-tĕr-ō-kō-LŎS-tō-mē	
enzyme (156)	ĔN-zīm	
esophageal (156)	ĕ-sŏf-ă-JĒ-ăl	
esophagus (152)	ĕ-SŎF-ă-gŭs	
fatty acid (152)	FĂT-tē Ă-sĭd	
facial (157)	FĀ-shŭl	
feces (152)	FĒ-sēz	
gallbladder (152)	găwl-BLĂ-dĕr	
gastrointestinal tract (139)	găs-trō-ĭn-TĔS-tĭn-ăl trăct	

gastrojejunostomy (157)	găs-trō-jĭ-jū-NŎS-tō-mē	_____
gastrostomy (157)	găs-TRŎS-tō-mē	_____
gingivitis (157)	jĭn-jĭ-VĪ-tĭs	_____
gluconeogenesis (159)	gloo-kō-nē-ō-JĔN-ĕ-sĭs	_____
glucose (152)	GLOO-kōs	_____
glycogen (152)	GLĪ-kō-jĕn	_____
glycogenolysis (159)	glī-kō-jĕ-NŎL-ĭ-sĭs	_____
hepatoma (157)	hĕ-pă-TŌ-mă	_____
hepatomegaly (157)	hĕ-pă-tō-MĔG-ă-lē	_____
hydrochloric acid (152)	hī-drō-KLŎR-ĭk Ă-sĭd	_____
hyperbilirubinemia (158)	hī-pĕr-bĭl-ĭ-roo-bĭ-NĒ-mē-ă	_____
hyperglycemia (159)	hī-pĕr-glī-SĒ-mē-ă	_____
hypoglossal (157)	hī-pō-GLŎ-săl	_____
ileitis (157)	ĭl-ē-Ī-tĭs	_____
ileocecal sphincter (157)	ĭl-ē-ō-SĒ-kăl SFĬNGK-tĕr	_____
ileostomy (157)	ĭl-ē-ŎS-tō-mē	_____
ileum (152)	ĬL-ē-ŭm	_____
incisor (152)	ĭn-SĪ-zŏr	_____
insulin (152)	ĬN-sŭ-lĭn	_____
jejunum (152)	jĕ-JOO-nŭm	_____
labial (157)	LĀ-bē-ăl	_____
laparoscopy (157)	lă-pă-RŎS-kō-pē	_____
lipase (152)	LĪ-pās	_____
liver (152)	LĬ-vĕr	_____
lower esophageal sphincter (152)	LŌW-ĕr ĕ-sŏf-ă-JĒ-ăl SFĬNGK-tĕr	_____
mastication (152)	măs-tĭ-KĀ-shŭn	_____
mesentery (156)	MĔS-ĕn-tĕr-ē	_____
molar teeth (152)	MŌ-lăr tēth	_____
oral (158)	ŎR-ăl	_____
orthodontist (157)	ŏr-thō-DŎN-tĭst	_____

palate (153)	PĂL-ăt	_____
palatoplasty (158)	PĂL-ă-tō-plăs-tē	_____
pancreas (153)	PĂN-krē-ăs	_____
pancreatitis (158)	păn-krē-ă-TĪ-tĭs	_____
papillae (153)	pă-PĬL-ē	_____
parenteral (156)	pă-RĔN-tĕr-ăl	_____
parotid gland (153)	pă-RŎT-ĭd gland	_____
perianal (154)	pĕ-rē-Ā-năl	_____
periodontist (157)	pĕr-ē-ō-DŎN-tĭst	_____
peritonitis (158)	pĕr-ē-tō-NĪ-tĭs	_____
peristalsis (153)	pĕr-ĭ-STĂL-sĭs	_____
pharyngeal (158)	făr-ăn-JĒ-ăl or fă-RĬN-jē-ăl	_____
pharynx (153)	FĂR-ĭnks	_____
portal vein (153)	PŎR-tăl vān	_____
postprandial (159)	pōst-PRĂN-dē-ăl	_____
premolar teeth (140)	prē-MŌ-lăr tēth	_____
proctologist (158)	prŏk-TŎL-ō-jĭst	_____
protease (153)	PRŌ-tē-āse	_____
pulp (153)	pŭlp	_____
pyloric sphincter (153)	pī-LŎR-ĭk SFĬNGK-tĕr	_____
pyloroplasty (158)	pī-LŎR-ō-plăs-tē	_____
rectocele (158)	RĔK-tō-sēl	_____
rectum (153)	RĔK-tŭm	_____
rugae (153)	ROO-gē	_____
saliva (153)	să-LĪ-vă	_____
salivary glands (153)	SĂL-ĭ-vĕr-ē glăndz	_____
sialadenitis (158)	sī-ăl-ă-dĕ-NĪ-tĭs	_____
sialolith (159)	sī-ĂL-ō-lĭth	_____
sigmoid colon (153)	SĬG-moyd KŌ-lŏn	_____
sigmoidoscopy (158)	sĭg-moy-DŎS-kō-pē	_____

sphincter (153)	SFĬNGK-tĕr	
steatorrhea (161)	stē-ă-tō-RĒ-ă	
stomatitis (158)	stō-mă-TĪ-tĭs	
sublingual (157)	sŭb-LĬNG-wăl	
submandibular (157)	sŭb-măn-DĬB-ū-lăr	
triglycerides (153)	trī-GLĬ-sĕ-rīdz	
uvula (153)	Ū-vū-lă	
villi (153)	VĬL-ī	

Pathological Terminology

Term	Pronunciation	Meaning
achalasia (162)	ăk-ăh-LĀ-zē-ă	
anal fistula (164)	Ā-năl FĬS-tū-lă	
anorexia (160)	ăn-ō-RĔK-sē-ă	
aphthous stomatitis (161)	ĂF-thŭs stō-mă-TĪ-tĭs	
ascites (160)	ă-SĪ-tēz	
borborygmus (160)	bŏr-bō-RĬG-mŭs	
cholelithiasis (168)	kō-lĕ-lĭ-THĪ-ă-sĭs	
cirrhosis (168)	sĭr-RŌ-sĭs	
colonic polyposis (165)	kō-LŎN-ĭk pŏl-ĭ-PŌ-sĭs	
colorectal cancer (165)	kō-lō-RĔK-tăl KĂN-sĕr	
constipation (160)	cŏn-stĭ-PĀ-shŭn	
Crohn disease (166)	krōn dĭ-ZĒZ	
dental caries (162)	DĔN-tăl KĂR-ēz	
diarrhea (161)	dī-ăh-RĒ-ă	
diverticula (166)	dī-vĕr-TĬK-ū-lă	
diverticulosis (166)	dī-vĕr-tĭk-ū-LŌ-sĭs	
dysentery (166)	DĬS-ĕn-tĕr-ē	
dysphagia (161)	dĭs-PHĀ-jē-ă	
eructation (161)	ē-rŭk-TĀ-shŭn	
esophageal varices (162)	ĕ-sŏf-ă-JĒ-ăl VĂR-ĭ-sēz	

etiology (160)	ē-tē-ŎL-ō-jē	_____
flatus (161)	FLĀ-tŭs	_____
gastric carcinoma (162)	GĂS-trĭk kăr-sĭ-NŌ-mă	_____
gastroesophageal reflux disease (164)	găs-trō-ĕ-sŏf-ă-JĒ-ăl RĒ-flŭx dĭ-ZĒZ	_____
hematochezia (161)	hē-mă-tō-KĒ-zē-ă	_____
hemorrhoids (166)	HĔM-ō-roydz	_____
herpetic stomatitis (162)	hĕr-PĔT-ĭk stō-mă-TĪ-tĭs	_____
hiatal hernia (164)	hī-Ā-tăl HĔR-nē-ă	_____
icterus (161)	ĬK-tĕr-ŭs	_____
idiopathic (160)	ĭd-ē-ō-PĂTH-ĭk	_____
ileus (166)	ĬL-ē-ŭs	_____
inflammatory bowel disease (166)	ĭn-FLĂ-mă-tō-rē BŎW-ĕl dĭ-ZĒZ	_____
inguinal hernia (164)	ĬNG-wă-năl HĔR-nē-ă	_____
intussusception (167)	ĭn-tŭs-sŭs-SĔP-shŭn	_____
irritable bowel syndrome (167)	ĬR-ĭ-tă-b'l BŎW-ĕl SĬN-drōm	_____
jaundice (161)	JĂWN-dĭs	_____
melena (161)	MĔl-ĕ-nă or mĕ-LĒ-nă	_____
nausea (161)	NĂW-zē-ă	_____
oral leukoplakia (162)	ŎR-ăl lū-kō-PLĀ-kē-ă	_____
pancreatitis (168)	păn-krē-ă-TĪ-tĭs	_____
periodontal disease (162)	pĕr-ē-ō-DŎN-tăl dĭ-ZĒZ	_____
ulcer (164)	ŬL-sĕr	_____
ulcerative colitis (167)	ŬL-sĕr-ă-tĭv kō-LĪ-tĭs	_____
viral hepatitis (168)	VĪ-răl hĕp-ă-TĪ-tĭs	_____
volvulus (167)	VŎL-vū-lŭs	_____

NOTE: The review sheet for this chapter is combined with the review sheet for Chapter 6 on page 209.

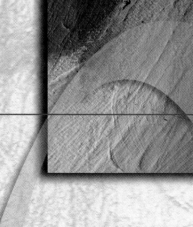

chapter

Additional Suffixes and Digestive System Terminology

This chapter is divided into the following sections

In this chapter you will

- Define new suffixes and use them with digestive system combining forms.
- List and explain laboratory tests, clinical procedures, and abbreviations common to the digestive system.
- Apply your new knowledge to understanding medical terms in their proper context, such as in medical reports and records.

I. Introduction

This chapter gives you practice in word building, while not introducing a large number of new terms. It uses many familiar terms from Chapter 5, which should give you a breather after your hard work.

Study the new suffixes in Section II first and complete the meanings of the terms in Sections II and III. Checking the meanings of the terms with a dictionary may prove helpful and add additional understanding.

The information included in Section IV (Laboratory Tests, Clinical Procedures, and Abbreviations) relates to the gastrointestinal system and will be useful for work in clinical or laboratory medical settings.

Section V (Practical Applications) gives you examples of medical language in context. Congratulate yourself as you decipher medical sentences, operation reports, case studies, and other material.

II. Suffixes

Write the meaning of the medical term in the space provided.

Suffix	Meaning	Terminology	Meaning
-ectasis, -ectasia	stretching, dilation, dilatation	bronchiectasis	*bronchial tubes stretching*
		Bronchi/o means bronchial tubes.	
		lymphangiectasia	
-emesis	vomiting	hematemesis	*vomiting blood*
		Bright red blood is vomited, often associated with esophageal varices or peptic ulcer.	
-lysis	destruction, breakdown, separation	hemolysis	
		Red blood cells are destroyed.	
-pepsia	digestion	dyspepsia	
-phagia	eating, swallowing	polyphagia	
		Excessive appetite and uncontrolled eating.	
		dysphagia	
		Difficult swallowing.	
		odynophagia	
		Pain (odyn/o) caused by swallowing.	

-plasty   surgical repair   rhino<u>plasty</u> _____

The structure of the nose is changed.

blepharo<u>plasty</u> _____

-ptosis   prolapse, fall, sag   pro<u>ptosis</u> _____

Pro- means before, forward. This term refers to the forward protrusion of the eye (exophthalmos).

-ptysis   spitting   hemo<u>ptysis</u> _____

From the respiratory tract and lungs.

-rrhage,   bursting forth   hemo<u>rrhage</u> _____
-rrhagia
                                         Loss of a large amount of blood in a short period.

meno<u>rrhagia</u> _____

Excessive bleeding at the time of menstruation. Men/o means menstrual flow or menstruation.

-rrhaphy   suture   hernio<u>rrhaphy</u> _____

Repair of a hernia. Herni/o means hernia.

-rrhea   flow, discharge   dysmeno<u>rrhea</u> _____

Pain associated with menstruation.

-spasm   sudden,   pyloro<u>spasm</u> _____
                     involuntary
                     contraction   broncho<u>spasm</u> _____
                     of muscles
                                         A chief characteristic of bronchitis and asthma.

-stasis   to stop; control   chole<u>stasis</u> _____

Flow of bile from the liver to the duodenum is interrupted.

hemo<u>stasis</u> _____

Bleeding is stopped by mechanical or chemical means, or by the coagulation process of the body.

-stenosis   tightening,   pyloric <u>stenosis</u> _____
                     stricture,
                     narrowing   *This is a congenital defect in newborns blocking the flow of food into the small intestine. Pyloromyotomy can correct the condition.*

-tresia   opening   a<u>tresia</u> _____

The closure of a normal body structure that should be open.

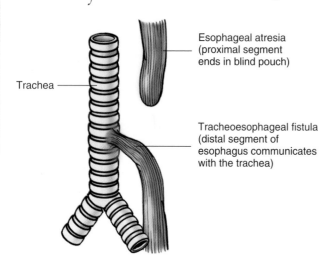

Trachea

Esophageal atresia
(proximal segment
ends in blind pouch)

Tracheoesophageal fistula
(distal segment of
esophagus communicates
with the trachea)

Figure 6–1

Esophageal atresia with tracheoesophageal fistula. (From Cotran RS, Kumar V, Collins T: Robbins Pathologic Basis of Disease, 6th ed., Philadelphia, WB Saunders, 1999, p. 777.)

esophageal atresia _____

A congenital anomaly in which the esophagus does not connect with the stomach. A tracheoesophageal fistula often accompanies this abnormality (Figure 6–1).

biliary atresia _____

Congenital hypoplasia or nonformation of bile ducts causes neonatal cholestasis and jaundice.

Many of the suffixes listed on pages 186-187 are also used alone as separate terms. Here are examples of how each term is used in a sentence.

ectasia	Mammary duct **ectasia** may cause mastitis.
lysis	The disease caused **lysis** of liver cells.
emesis (emetic)	If a child swallows poison, physicians prescribe a drug to induce **emesis**. An example of an emetic is a strong solution of salt or ipecac syrup.
ptosis	Mr. Smith's weakened eyelid muscles caused **ptosis** of his lids.
spasm	Eating spicy foods can lead to **spasm** of gastric sphincters.
stasis	Overgrowth of bacteria within the small intestine causes **stasis** of the intestinal contents.
stenosis	Projectile vomiting in an infant during feeding is a symptom of pyloric **stenosis.**

III. Combining Forms and Terminology

Write the meaning of the combining form and then the meaning of the term that includes that combining form in the spaces provided.

Combining Form	Meaning	Terminology	Meaning
bucc/o	*check*	buccal	
cec/o	*cecum*	cecal volvulus	
celi/o		celiac artery	
		Carries blood from the aorta to the abdomen.	
cheil/o		cheilosis	
		Characterized by scales and fissures on the lips and resulting from a deficiency of vitamin B_2 in the diet.	
chol/e		cholelithiasis	
cholangi/o		cholangiectasis	
cholecyst/o		cholecystectomy	
choledoch/o	*common in bile duct*	choledochal	
col/o	*colon*	colectomy	
		Surgeons perform laparoscopic-assisted colectomy (LAC) as an alternative to open colectomy to remove nonmetastatic colorectal carcinomas.	
colon/o	*colon*	colonoscopy	
dent/i	*tooth*	dentalgia	
duoden/o	*duodenum*	gastroduodenal anastomosis	
enter/o	*intestines, usually S.I.*	gastroenteritis	
esophag/o	*esophagus*	esophageal atresia	
		This congenital anomaly must be corrected surgically.	
gastr/o	*stomach*	gastrojejunostomy	

Term	Meaning	Term	Definition
gingiv/o	_____	gingivectomy	_____
gloss/o	_____	glossopharyngeal	_____
glyc/o	sugur	glycolysis	_____
hepat/o	liver	hepatomegaly	_____
herni/o	_____	herniorrhaphy	_____
ile/o	ileum	ileostomy	_____
jejun/o	jejunum	cholecystojejunostomy	_____
labi/o	_____	labioglossopharyngeal	_____
lingu/o	tongue	sublingual	_____
lip/o	_____	lipase	_____
lith/o	_____	cholecystolithiasis	_____
odont/o	tooth	periodontal membrane	_____
or/o	moth	oropharynx	_____

The tonsils are located in the oropharynx.

palat/o	palate	palatoplasty	_____

Also called palatorrhaphy, this procedure corrects cleft (split) palate, a congenital anomaly.

pancreat/o	pancreas	pancreatic	_____
proct/o	_____	proctosigmoidoscopy	_____
pylor/o	_____	pyloric stenosis	_____
rect/o	rectum	rectosigmoidoscopy	_____
sialaden/o	_____	sialadenectomy	_____
splen/o	_____	splenic flexure	_____

The bend in the transverse colon downward near the spleen.

steat/o	_____	steatorrhea	_____
stomat/o	mouth	aphthous stomatitis	_____

IV. Laboratory Tests, Clinical Procedures, and Abbreviations

Laboratory Tests

liver function tests (LFTs)

Tests for the presence of enzymes and bilirubin in serum (clear fluid that remains after blood has clotted)

Examples are **ALT** (*al*anine amino *t*ransaminase) or **SGPT** (*s*erum *g*lutamic-*p*yruvic *t*ransaminase) and **AST** (*as*partate amino *t*ransaminase) or **SGOT** (*s*erum *g*lutamic-*o*xaloacetic *t*ransaminase). ALT and AST are transaminases (enzymes) present in many tissues and elevated in the serum of patients with liver disease. High ALT and AST levels indicate damage to liver cells (as in hepatitis).

Alkaline phosphatase (alk phos) is another enzyme that may be elevated in patients with liver, bone, and other diseases.

Serum bilirubin levels are elevated in patients with liver disease and jaundice. A **direct bilirubin** test measures conjugated bilirubin (combined with a substance in the liver). High levels indicate liver disease or biliary obstruction. An **indirect bilirubin** test measures unconjugated bilirubin. Increased levels mean excessive hemolysis, as may occur in a newborn.

stool culture

Test for microorganisms present in stool.

Feces are placed in a growth medium and examined microscopically.

stool guaiac or **Hemoccult test**

Detection of blood in feces.

This is an important screening test for colon cancer. **Guaiac** (GWĪ-ăk) is a chemical from the wood of trees. When added to a stool sample, it reacts with occult (hidden) blood.

computed tomography; also called **CT, CT scan,** or **CAT scan**	**X-ray series showing cross-sectional images of internal organs allows visualization.**

A circular array of x-ray beams produces the cross-sectional image based on differences in tissue densities. Contrast material allows visualization of the GI tract, blood vessels, and organs (Fig. 6–4A, B, and C). **Tomography** (tom/o means to cut) produces a *series* of x-ray pictures showing multiple views of an organ.

Ultrasound

abdominal ultrasonography (ultrasound or **sonography)**	**Sound waves beamed into the abdomen, produce an image of abdominal viscera.**

Ultrasonography is especially useful for examination of fluid-filled structures such as the gallbladder.

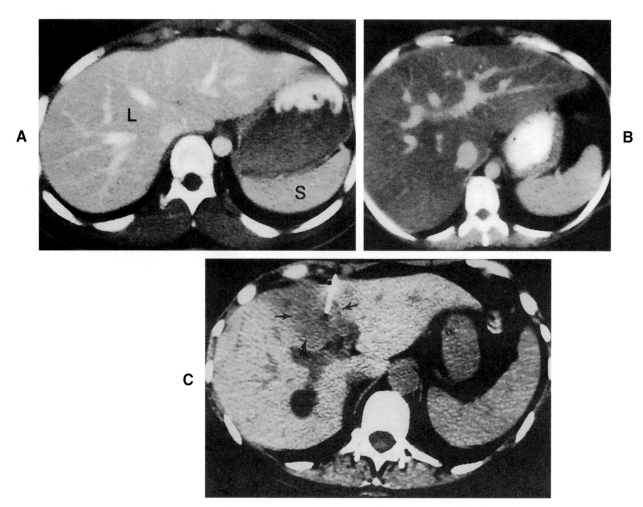

Figure 6-4

Computed tomographic images of normal and diseased liver. **(A) Normal liver.** Contrast material has been injected intravenously, making blood vessels appear bright. The liver (L) and spleen (S) are the same density. **(B) Fatty liver.** The radiodensity of the liver tissue is reduced because of the large volume of fat contained in the tissue, making it appear darker than normal. Compare to the spleen. **(C) CT-guided needle aspiration biopsy of a liver lesion.** The lesion (arrows) has a lower density than the surrounding liver. A needle has been placed into the liver tissue and its tip can be seen in the center of the lesion. Microscopic examination of material aspirated from the lesion revealed it to be a hepatocellular carcinoma. CT-guided needle placement can also be used to inset a catheter for drainage of a liver abscess (a collection of infection and pus). (From Heuman DM, Mills AS, McGuire HH: Gastroenterology, Philadelphia, WB Saunders, 1997, p. 166.)

magnetic resonance imaging (MRI)	**Magnetic and radio waves produce images of organs and tissues in all three planes of the body.**

This technique does not use x-rays and shows subtle differences in tissue composition.

Radioactive

liver scan	**Image of the liver after injecting radioactive material into the blood stream.**

Radioactive material (radioisotope) is injected intravenously and taken up by the liver cells. An image of the liver (scintiscan) is made using a special scanner (gamma camera) that records the radioisotope uptake by the liver cells.

Other Procedures

gastric bypass	**Reducing the size of the stomach and diverting food to the jejunum (gastrojejunostomy).**

This is bariatric (bar/o = weight) surgery for severe obesity. The Roux-en-Y gastric bypass procedure reduces the size of the stomach to a volume of 2 tablespoons and bypasses a large section of the small intestine.

gastrointestinal endoscopy	**Visual examination of the gastrointestinal tract using an endoscope.**

A physician places a flexible fiberoptic tube through the mouth or the anus to view parts of the gastrointestinal tract. Examples are **esophagogastroduodenoscopy, colonoscopy** (Fig. 6–5), **sigmoidoscopy, proctoscopy,** and **anoscopy.**

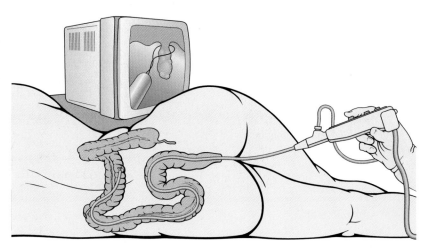

Figure 6–5

Colonoscopy and polypectomy. Prior to this procedure, a patient ingests agents to clean the bowel of feces. The patient is sedated and the gastroenterologist advances the instrument retrograde, guided by images from a video camera on the tip of the colonoscope. When a polyp is located, a wire snare is passed through the endoscope and looped around the stalk. After the loop is gently tightened, an electric current is applied to cut through the stalk. The polyp is removed for microscopic examination (biopsy).

liver biopsy	**Removal of liver tissue followed by microscopic visualization.**
	A physician inserts a needle through the skin to remove a small piece of tissue for microscopic examination. The average sample is less than 1 inch long. The procedure helps doctors diagnose cirrhosis, chronic hepatitis, and tumors of the liver.
nasogastric intubation	**Insertion of a tube through the nose into the stomach.**
	Physicians use a nasogastric (NG) tube to remove fluid postoperatively and to obtain gastric or intestinal contents for analysis.
paracentesis (abdominocentesis)	**Surgical puncture to remove fluid from the abdomen.**
	This procedure is necessary to drain fluid (ascites) from the peritoneal (abdominal) cavity.

Abbreviations

alk phos	alkaline phosphatase	**MRI**	magnetic resonance imaging
ALT, AST	alanine transaminase, aspartate transaminase (enzyme tests of liver function)	**NG tube**	nasogastric tube
		NPO	nothing by mouth *(nulla per os)*
BE	barium enema	**PEG tube**	percutaneous endoscopic gastrostomy tube (feeding tube)
BRBPR	bright red blood per (through) rectum; hematochezia	**PEJ tube**	percutaneous endoscopic jejunostomy tube (feeding tube)
BM	bowel movement	**PTHC**	percutaneous transhepatic cholangiography
CT scan	computed tomography		
EGD	esophagogastroduodenoscopy	**PUD**	peptic ulcer disease
ERCP	endoscopic retrograde cholangiopancreatography	**SGOT, SGPT**	enzyme tests of liver function; SGOT = AST, SGPT = ALT
GB	gallbladder	**TPN**	total parenteral nutrition
GERD	gastroesophageal reflux disease		This intravenous (IV) solution contains sugar (dextrose), proteins (amino acids), electrolytes (sodium, potassium, chloride), and vitamins
GI	gastrointestinal		
HBV	hepatitis B virus	**T tube**	tube placed in the biliary tract for drainage
IBD	inflammatory bowel disease		
LFTs	liver function tests; alk phos, bilirubin, AST (SGOT), ALT (SGPT)		

V. Practical Applications

This section contains an actual medical report using terms that you have studied in this and previous chapters. Explanations of more difficult terms are added in brackets. Questions based on your reading of the report follow. Check your answers on page 206, Answers to Practical Applications.

Colonoscopy Report

The patient is a 73-year-old female who underwent colonoscopy and polypectomy on June 10, 1997. Biopsy revealed an invasive carcinoma, and on June 12, 1997, she underwent a low anterior resection and coloproctostomy. Sixteen months later, on August 2, 1998, she was seen in the office for flexible sigmoidoscopy, and a polyp was detected. Colonoscopy was scheduled.

Description of Procedure. The fiberoptic colonoscope was introduced, and I could pass it to about 15 cm, at which point there appeared to be an anastomosis. The colonoscope passed easily through a wide-open anastomosis to 30 cm, at which point a very friable [easily crumbled] polyp, irregular, on a short little stalk, was encountered. This was snared, the coagulating [blood clotting] current was applied, and the pedicle [stalk of the polyp] was severed and recovered and sent to pathology for histological identification. The colonoscope was then reintroduced and passed through the rectum to the sigmoid colon. Again the anastomosis was seen, and proximal to this, the fulgurated [destroyed by high-frequency electric current] base of the removed polyp could be seen. No bleeding was encountered, and I continued to advance the colonoscope through the descending colon. I proceeded to advance the colonoscope through the splenic flexure in the transverse colon. Despite vigorous mechanical bowel preparation and the shortened colon from the previous resection, she had a considerable amount of stool, and it became progressively more difficult to visualize as I approached the hepatic flexure. Finally, at the hepatic flexure, I abandoned further evaluation and began to withdraw the colonoscope. The colonoscope passed through the transverse colon, splenic flexure, descending colon, sigmoid colon, rectum, and anus and was withdrawn. She tolerated the procedure well, but had some nausea. I will await the results of pathology, and in the event that it is not an invasive carcinoma, I would recommend a repeat colonoscopy in 6 months, at which time we will use a 48-hour, more vigorous mechanical bowel preparation.

Questions about the Colonoscopy Report

1. **On June 10, the initial procedure that the patient underwent was**
   (A) Anastomosis of two parts of the colon
   (B) Visual examination of the rectum and anus
   (C) Visual examination of the large bowel and removal of a growth
   (D) Resection of a portion of the colon
2. **On June 12 the patient had additional surgery to**
   (A) Remove a portion of the colon and reattach the cut end to the rectum
   (B) Join two parts of the small intestine
   (C) Reconnect the colon to the small intestine
   (D) Remove a portion of the distal end of the small intestine

Continued on following page

3. **Which term in the report refers to an anastomosis?**
   (A) Sigmoidoscopy
   (B) Colonoscopy
   (C) Low anterior resection
   (D) Coloproctostomy
4. **Why was it impossible to visualize the entire colon?**
   (A) The patient experienced nausea
   (B) Feces were blocking the colon
   (C) Tumor was blocking the colon
   (D) The hepatic flexure was twisted

VI. Exercises

Remember to check your answers carefully with those given in Section VII, Answers to Exercises.

A. Give the meanings of the following suffixes.

1. -pepsia _____

2. -ptysis _____

3. -emesis _____

4. -phagia _____

5. -ptosis _____

6. -rrhea _____

7. -rrhagia _____

8. -rrhaphy _____

9. -plasty _____

10. -lysis _____

11. -ectasis _____

12. -stenosis _____

13. -stasis _____

14. -spasm _____

15. -ectasia _____

B. Using the suffixes listed in exercise A and the following combining forms, build medical terms.

blephar/o   hemat/o   men/o
bronch/o   herni/o   pylor/o
chol/e   lymphangi/o   rhin/o
hem/o

1. painful menstrual flow _____

2. stoppage of bile (flow) _____

3. suture of a hernia _____

4. dilation of lymph vessels _____

5. spitting up blood (from the respiratory tract) _____

6. vomiting blood (from the digestive tract) _____

7. dilation of tubes leading from the windpipe into the lungs _____

8. surgical repair of eyelids _____

9. stopping blood flow _____

10. surgical repair of the nose _____

11. destruction of blood (red blood cells) _____

12. sudden, involuntary contraction of muscles at the distal region of the stomach _____

13. excessive bleeding (bursting forth of blood) during menstruation _____

14. sudden, involuntary contraction of muscles within the bronchial tubes _____

C. Give the meanings of the following terms.

1. dysphagia _____

2. polyphagia _____

3. dyspepsia _____

4. biliary atresia _____

5. proptosis _____

6. cholestasis _____

7. esophageal atresia _____

8. odynophagia _____

9. emesis _____

10. stenosis _____

D. Match the following surgical procedures with their meanings below.

blepharoplasty   colectomy   ileostomy
cecostomy   gastroduodenal anastomosis   paracentesis
cholecystectomy   gingivectomy   rectosigmoidoscopy
cholecystojejunostomy   herniorrhaphy   sphincterotomy

1. removal of the gallbladder _____

2. large bowel resection _____

3. suture of a weakened muscular wall (hernia) _____

4. new opening of the first part of the colon to the outside of the body _____

5. surgical repair of the eyelid _____

6. incision of a ring of muscles _____

7. new surgical connection between the stomach and the first part of the small intestine

   _____

8. opening of the third part of the small intestine to the outside of the body _____

9. removal of gum tissue _____

10. new surgical connection between the gallbladder and the second part of the small intestine

    _____

11. surgical puncture of the abdomen for withdrawal of fluid _____

12. visual examination of the rectum and sigmoid colon _____

E. Complete the following terms based on their meanings.

1. discharge of fat: steat _____

2. difficulty in swallowing: dys _____

3. abnormal condition of gallstones: chole _____

4. pertaining to the cheek: _____ al

5. pain in a tooth: dent _____

6. prolapse of an eyelid: blepharo _____

7. enlargement of the liver: hepato _____

8. pertaining to under the tongue: sub _____

9. removal of the gallbladder: _____ ectomy

10. pertaining to the common bile duct: chole _____

F. Give the meanings of the following terms.

1. cecal volvulus _____

2. aphthous stomatitis _____

3. celiac artery _____

4. lipase _____

5. cheilosis _____

6. oropharynx _____

7. glycolysis _____

8. glossopharyngeal _____

9. sialadenectomy _____

10. periodontal membrane _____

G. Match the name of the laboratory test or clinical procedure with its description.

abdominal ultrasonography   liver biopsy   serum bilirubin
barium enema   liver scan   small bowel follow-through
CT of the abdomen   nasogastric intubation   stool culture
endoscopic retrograde   percutaneous transhepatic   stool guaiac (Hemoccult)
   cholangiopancreatography   cholangiography
gastric bypass

1. measurement of bile pigment in the blood _____

2. placement of feces in a growth medium for bacterial analysis _____

3. x-ray examination of the lower gastrointestinal tract _____

4. imaging of abdominal viscera via sound waves _____

5. test to reveal hidden blood in feces _____

6. sequential x-ray images of the small intestine _____

7. injection of contrast material through the skin into the liver, to obtain x-ray images of bile vessels

_____

8. insertion of a tube through the nose into the stomach _____

9. transverse x-ray pictures of the abdominal organs _____

10. injection of contrast material via endoscope to obtain x-ray images of the pancreas and bile ducts

_____

11. reduction of stomach size and gastrojejunostomy _____

12. injection of radioactive material intravenously, and produces an image of liver cells as they take up

the radioactivity _____

13. percutaneous removal of liver tissue followed by microscopic examination _____

H. Give the meanings of the following abbreviations in column I. Then select the letter from the sentences in column II that makes the best association for each.

Column I

1. TPN _____ ____

2. PUD _____ ____

3. EGD _____ ____

4. IBD _____ ____

5. BE _____ ____

6. BRBPR _____ ____

7. LFTs _____ ____

8. GERD _____ ____

9. HBV _____ ____

10. CT _____ ____

Column II

A. Tests such as ALT, AST, alk phos, and serum bilirubin.

B. Heartburn is a symptom of this condition.

C. This general condition includes Crohn disease and ulcerative colitis.

D. *H. pylori* causes this condition.

E. Nothing by mouth (NPO), but intravenous feeding is allowed.

F. This is a lower gastrointestinal series.

G. X-ray procedure that produces a series of cross-sectional images.

H. This infectious agent causes chronic inflammation of the liver.

I. Hematochezia describes this gastrointestinal symptom.

J. Endoscopic visualization of the upper gastrointestinal tract.

I. Give the suffixes for the following terms.

1. bursting forth _____

2. flow, discharge _____

3. suture _____

4. dilation _____

5. narrowing, stricture _____

6. vomiting _____

7. spitting _____

8. prolapse _____

9. excision _____

10. digestion _____

11. eating, swallowing _____

12. hardening _____

13. to stop; control _____

14. surgical repair _____

15. opening _____

16. surgical puncture _____

17. involuntary contraction _____

18. new opening _____

19. incision _____

20. destruction, breakdown _____

J. Circle the correct term in parentheses to complete each sentence.

1. When Mrs. Smith developed diarrhea and crampy abdominal pain, she consulted a **(urologist, nephrologist, gastroenterologist)** and worried that she might have **(inflammatory bowel disease, esophageal varices, achalasia).**

2. After taking a careful history and physical, Dr. Blakemore diagnosed Mr. Bean, a long-time drinker, with **(hemorrhoids, pancreatitis, appendicitis).** Mr. Bean had complained of sharp midepigastric pain and a change in bowel habits.

3. Many pregnant women cannot lie flat after eating because of a burning sensation in their chest and throat. Doctors call this condition **(volvulus, dysentery, gastroesophageal reflux).**

4. Pediatric surgeons must be wary of **(inguinal hernia, pyloric stenosis, oral leukoplakia)** in young infants who display projectile vomiting.

5. Boris had terrible problems with his teeth. He needed not only a periodontist for his **(anorexia, ascites, gingivitis)** but also an **(endodontist, oral surgeon, orthodontist)** to straighten his teeth.

6. After six weeks of radiation therapy to her throat, Betty experienced severe esophageal irritation and inflammation. She complained to her doctor about her **(dyspepsia, odynophagia, hematemesis).**

7. Barbara had cramping and bloating before otherwise normal menstrual periods. Her physician prescribed pain medication to alleviate her **(dyspepsia, dysmenorrhea, menorrhagia).**

8. Chris had been a heavy alcohol drinker all of his adult life. His wife gradually noticed yellow discoloration of the whites of his eyes and skin. After a physical examination and blood tests, his family physician told him his **(colon, skin, liver)** was diseased. The yellow discoloration was **(jaundice, exophthalmos, proptosis)** and his condition was **(cheilosis, cirrhosis, hemostasis).**

9. When Carol had been a phlebotomist, she accidentally cut her finger while drawing a patient's blood. Unfortunately, the patient had **(pancreatitis, hemoptysis, hepatitis)** and the HBV was transmitted to Carol. Blood tests and **(liver biopsy, gastrointestinal endoscopy, stool culture)** confirmed Carol's unfortunate diagnosis. Her doctor told her that her condition was chronic and that she might be a candidate for a **(bone marrow, liver, kidney)** transplant in the future.

10. Operation Smile is a rescue project that performs **(herniorrhaphy, oral leukopenia, palatoplasty)** on children with a congenital cleft in the roof of their mouth.

VII. Answers to Exercises

A

1. digestion
2. spitting (from the respiratory tract)
3. vomiting
4. eating, swallowing
5. prolapse, falling, sagging
6. flow, discharge
7. bursting forth of blood
8. suture
9. surgical repair
10. destruction, breakdown, separation
11. stretching, dilation, dilatation
12. tightening, narrowed lumen, stricture
13. to stop; control
14. sudden, involuntary contraction of muscles
15. dilation, stretching, dilatation

B

1. dysmenorrhea
2. cholestasis
3. herniorrhaphy
4. lymphangiectasis
5. hemoptysis
6. hematemesis
7. bronchiectasis
8. blepharoplasty
9. hemostasis
10. rhinoplasty
11. hemolysis
12. pylorospasm
13. menorrhagia
14. bronchospasm

C

1. difficulty in swallowing
2. excessive (much) eating
3. difficult digestion
4. biliary ducts are not open (congenital anomaly)
5. forward prolapse (bulging) of the eyes (exophthalmos)
6. stoppage of flow of bile
7. esophagus is not open (closed off) at birth (congenital anomaly)
8. pain caused by swallowing
9. vomiting
10. tightening, stricture, narrowing

D

1. cholecystectomy
2. colectomy
3. herniorrhaphy
4. cecostomy
5. blepharoplasty
6. sphincterotomy
7. gastroduodenal anastomosis (gastroduodenostomy)— both are acceptable
8. ileostomy
9. gingivectomy
10. cholecystojejunostomy (cholecystojejunal anastomosis)
11. paracentesis (abdominocentesis)
12. rectosigmoidoscopy

E

1. steatorrhea
2. dysphagia
3. cholelithiasis
4. buccal
5. dentalgia
6. ptosis
7. hepatomegaly
8. sublingual
9. cholecystectomy
10. choledochal

F

1. twisted intestine in the area of the cecum
2. inflammation of the mouth with small ulcers
3. blood vessel bringing blood to the abdomen
4. enzyme to digest fat
5. abnormal condition of lips
6. the part of the throat near the mouth
7. breakdown of sugar
8. pertaining to the tongue and the throat
9. removal of a salivary gland
10. membrane surrounding a tooth

G

1. serum bilirubin
2. stool culture
3. barium enema
4. abdominal ultrasonography
5. stool guaiac (Hemoccult)
6. small bowel follow-through
7. percutaneous transhepatic cholangiography
8. nasogastric intubation
9. CT scan of the abdomen
10. endoscopic retrograde cholangiopancreatography (ERCP)
11. gastric bypass
12. liver scan
13. liver biopsy

H

1. total parenteral nutrition. E
2. peptic ulcer disease. D
3. esophagoduodenoscopy. J
4. inflammatory bowel disease. C
5. barium enema. F
6. bright red blood per rectum. I
7. liver function tests. A
8. gastroesophageal reflux disease. B
9. hepatitis B virus. H
10. computed tomography. G

I

1. -rrhagia, -rrhage
2. -rrhea
3. -rrhaphy
4. -ectasis, -ectasia
5. -stenosis
6. -emesis
7. -ptysis
8. -ptosis
9. -ectomy
10. -pepsia
11. -phagia
12. -sclerosis
13. -stasis
14. -plasty
15. -tresia
16. -centesis
17. -spasm
18. -stomy
19. -tomy
20. -lysis

Continued on following page

J

1. gastroenterologist; inflammatory bowel disease
2. pancreatitis
3. gastroesophageal reflux
4. pyloric stenosis
5. gingivitis; orthodontist
6. odynophagia
7. dysmenorrhea
8. liver; jaundice; cirrhosis
9. hepatitis; liver biopsy; liver
10. palatoplasty

Answers to Practical Applications

1. C
2. A
3. D
4. B

VIII. Pronunciation of Terms

Pronunciation Guide

ā as in āpe   ă as in ăpple
ē as in ēven   ě as in ěvery
ī as in īce   ĭ as in ĭnterest
ō as in ōpen   ŏ as in pŏt
ū as in ūnit   ŭ as in ŭnder

To test your understanding of the terminology in this chapter, define each term in the space provided. Then cover the term and write it while looking at your definition. Check your spelling! The page number after each term indicates where it is defined in the text, so you can easily check your responses.

Term	Pronunciation	Meaning
abdominal ultrasonography (194)	ăb-DŎM-ĭn-ăl ŭl-tră-sō-NŎG-ră-fē	
aphthous stomatitis (190)	ĂF-thŭs stō-mă-TĪ-tĭs	
atresia (181)	ā-TRĒ-zē-ă	
biliary atresia (188)	BĬL-ē-ăr-ē ā-TRĒ-zē-ă	
bronchiectasis (186)	brŏng-kē-ĔK-tă-sĭs	
bronchospasm (187)	BRŎNG-kō-spăsm	
buccal (189)	BŬK-ăl	
cecal volvulus (189)	SĒ-kăl VŎL-vū-lŭs	
celiac artery (189)	SĒ-lē-ăk ĂR-tĕr-ē	
cheilosis (189)	kī-LŌ-sis	
cholangiectasis (189)	kōl-ăn-jē-ĔK-tă-sĭs	
cholangiography (193)	kōl-ăn-jē-ŎG-ră-fē	

cholangiopancreatography (193)   kŏl-ăn-jē-ō-păn-krē-ă-TŎG-ră-fē   _____

cholecystectomy (189)   kō-lē-sĭs-TĔK-tō-mē   _____

cholecystojejunostomy (190)   kō-lē-sĭs-tō-jĕ-jŭ-NŎS-tō-mē   _____

cholecystolithiasis (190)   kō-lē-sĭs-tō-lĭ-THĪ-ă-sĭs   _____

choledochal (189)   kō-lē-DŎK-ăl   _____

cholelithiasis (189)   kō-lē-lĭ-THĬ-ă-sĭs   _____

cholestasis (187)   kō-lē-STĀ-sĭs   _____

colectomy (189)   kō-LĔK-tō-mē   _____

colonoscopy (189)   kō-lŏn-ŎS-kō-pē   _____

dentalgia (189)   dĕn-TĂL-jă   _____

dysmenorrhea (187)   dĭs-mĕn-ŏr-RĒ-ă   _____

dyspepsia (186)   dĭs-PĔP-sē-ă   _____

dysphagia (186)   dĭs-FĀ-jē-ă   _____

esophageal atresia (188)   ĕ-sŏf-ă-JĒ-ăl ā-TRĒ-zē-ă   _____

gastric bypass (195)   GĂS-trĭk- BĪ-păs   _____

gastroduodenal anastomosis (189)   găs-trō-dū-ō-DĒ-năl ă-nă-stō-MŌ-sĭs   _____

gastroenteritis (189)   găs-trō-ĕn-tĕ-RĪ-tĭs   _____

gastrointestinal endoscopy (195)   găs-trō-ĭn-TĔS-tĭn-ăl ĕn-DŎS-kō-pē   _____

gastrojejunostomy (189)   găs-trō-jĕ-jū-NŎS-tō-mē   _____

gingivectomy (190)   gĭn-gĭ-VĔK-tō-mē   _____

glossopharyngeal (190)   glŏs-ō-fă-rĭn-GĒ-al   _____

glycolysis (190)   glī-KŎL-ĭ-sĭs   _____

hematemesis (186)   hē-mă-TĔM-ĕ-sĭs   _____

hemolysis (186)   hē-MŎL-ĭ-sĭs   _____

hemoptysis (187)   hē-MŎP-tĭ-sĭs   _____

hemorrhage (187)   HĔM-ŏr-ĭj   _____

hemostasis (187)	hē-mō-STĀ-sĭs	_____
hepatomegaly (190)	hĕp-ă-tō-MĔG-ă-lē	_____
herniorrhaphy (187)	hĕr-nē-ŎR-ă-fē	_____
ileostomy (190)	ĭl-ē-ŎS-tō-mē	_____
labioglossopharyngeal (190)	lā-bē-ō-glŏs-ō-fă-RĬN-jē-ăl	_____
lipase (190)	LĪ-pās	_____
liver biopsy (196)	LĬ-vĕr BĪ-ŏp-sē	_____
liver scan (195)	LĬ-vĕr scăn	_____
lower gastrointestinal series (192)	LŎW-ĕr găs-trō-ĭn-TĔS-tĭ-năl SĔR-ēz	_____
lymphangiectasia (186)	lĭm-făn-jē-ĕk-TĀ-zē-ă	_____
menorrhagia (187)	mĕn-ŏr-RĀ-jă	_____
nasogastric intubation (196)	nā-zō-GĂS-trĭk ĭn-tū-BĀ-shŭn	_____
odynophagia (186)	ō-dĭn-ō-FĀ-jē-ă	_____
oropharynx (190)	ŏr-ō-FĂR-ĭnks	_____
palatoplasty (190)	PĂL-ă-tō-plăs-tē	_____
pancreatic (190)	păn-krē-ĂH-tĭk	_____
paracentesis (196)	păr-ă-sēn-TĒ-sĭs	_____
periodontal membrane (190)	pĕr-ē-ō-DŎN-tăl MĔM-brān	_____
polyphagia (186)	pŏl-ē-FĀ-jē-ă	_____
proctosigmoidoscopy (190)	prŏk-tō-sĭg-mŏyd-ŎS-kō-pē	_____
proptosis (187)	prŏp-TŌ-sĭs	_____
pyloric stenosis (187)	pī-LŎR-ĭk stĕ-NŌ-sĭs	_____
pylorospasm (187)	pī-LŎR-ō-spăsm	_____
rectosigmoidoscopy (190)	rĕk-tō-sĭg-mŏy-DŎS-kō-pē	_____
rhinoplasty (187)	rī-nō-PLĂS-tē	_____
sialadenectomy (190)	sī-ăl-ă-dĕ-NĔK-tō-mē	_____
splenic flexure (190)	SPLĔ-nĭk FLĔK-shŭr	_____
steatorrhea (190)	stē-ă-tō-RĒ-ă	_____
sublingual (190)	sŭb-LĬNG-wăl	_____

IX. Review Sheet

Write meanings for combining forms and suffixes in the space provided. Check your answers with information in Chapters 5 and 6 or in the Glossary (Medical Terms—English) at the end of the book.

COMBINING FORMS

Combining Form	Meaning	Combining Form	Meaning
amyl/o		col/o	
an/o		colon/o	
append/o		dent/i	
appendic/o		duoden/o	
bil/i		enter/o	
bilirubin/o		esophag/o	
bronch/o		eti/o	
bucc/o		gastr/o	
cec/o		gingiv/o	
celi/o		gloss/o	
cervic/o		gluc/o	
cheil/o		glyc/o	
chlorhydr/o		glycogen/o	
chol/e		hem/o	
cholangi/o		hemat/o	
cholecyst/o		hepat/o	
choledoch/o		herni/o	
cib/o		idi/o	
cirrh/o		ile/o	

Continued on following page

jejun/o	_____	pancreat/o	_____
labi/o	_____	peritone/o	_____
lapar/o	_____	pharyng/o	_____
lingu/o	_____	proct/o	_____
lip/o	_____	prote/o	_____
lith/o	_____	pylor/o	_____
lymphangi/o	_____	rect/o	_____
mandibul/o	_____	sialaden/o	_____
men/o	_____	sigmoid/o	_____
necr/o	_____	splen/o	_____
odont/o	_____	steat/o	_____
odyn/o	_____	stomat/o	_____
or/o	_____	tonsill/o	_____
palat/o	_____		

SUFFIXES

Suffix	Meaning	Suffix	Meaning
-ase	_____	-emia	_____
-centesis	_____	-genesis	_____
-chezia	_____	-graphy	_____
-ectasia	_____	-iasis	_____
-ectasis	_____	-lysis	_____
-ectomy	_____	-megaly	_____
-emesis	_____	-orexia	_____

-pathy _____   -rrhaphy _____

-pepsia _____   -rrhea _____

-phagia _____   -scopy _____

-plasty _____   -spasm _____

-prandial _____   -stasis _____

-ptosis _____   -stenosis _____

-ptysis _____   -stomy _____

-rrhage _____   -tomy _____

-rrhagia _____   -tresia _____

chapter

7

Urinary System

This chapter is divided into the following sections

In this chapter you will:

- Name the organs of the urinary system and describe their locations and functions.
- Give the meaning of various pathological conditions affecting the system.
- Recognize the use and interpretation of urinalysis as a diagnostic test.
- Define combining forms, prefixes, and suffixes of the system's terminology.
- List and explain some clinical procedures, laboratory tests, and abbreviations that pertain to the urinary system.
- Apply your new knowledge to understanding medical terms in their proper contexts, such as medical reports and records.

I. Introduction

You have just learned how food passes into the bloodstream through the digestive system. In a future chapter, you will learn how oxygen travels to the bloodstream through the respiratory system. Food and oxygen combine (during the process of catabolism) in body cells to produce energy. The small particles that compose the food and oxygen are rearranged into new combinations, called waste products. Because foods such as sugars and fats contain the elements carbon, hydrogen, and oxygen, waste products produced during their catabolism are the gas, carbon dioxide (carbon and oxygen), and water vapor (hydrogen and oxygen).

Protein foods, however, contain carbon, hydrogen, and oxygen plus **nitrogen**, and other elements. Thus, when proteins combine with oxygen, they produce **nitrogenous waste**. This waste product is more difficult to remove from the body.

The body cannot put nitrogenous waste efficiently into a gaseous form and exhale it, so it excretes it as a soluble (dissolved in water) waste substance called **urea.** The urinary system removes urea from the bloodstream so that it does not accumulate in the body and become toxic.

Urea is formed in the liver and travels via the bloodstream to the kidneys. There, urea passes out of the bloodstream as the kidneys produce **urine** (composed also of water, salts, and acids). Urine then travels down the ureters into the bladder and out of the body.

Besides removing urea from the blood, another important function of the kidneys is to maintain the proper balance of water, salts, and acids in the body fluids. Salts, such as **sodium** and **potassium,** and some acids are known as **electrolytes** (small molecules that conduct an electrical charge). Electrolytes are necessary for the proper functioning of muscle and nerve cells. The kidney adjusts the amounts of water and electrolytes by secreting some substances into the urine and holding back others in the bloodstream for use in the body.

In addition to forming urine and eliminating it from the body, the kidneys secrete substances such as **renin** (RĒ-nĭn) and erythropoietin. Renin is an enzymatic hormone important in the control of blood pressure. **Erythropoietin** (-poietin = substance that forms) is a hormone that stimulates the production of red blood cells in the bone marrow. The kidneys also secrete an active form of vitamin D, necessary for the absorption of calcium from the intestine. In addition, hormones such as insulin and parathyroid hormone are degraded and extracted from the bloodstream by the kidney.

II. Anatomy of the Major Organs

The following paragraphs describe the organs of the urinary system. Label Figure 7–1 as you identify each organ.

A **kidney** [1] is one of two bean-shaped organs behind the abdominal cavity (retroperitoneal) on either side of the spine in the lumbar region. The kidneys are embedded in a cushion of adipose tissue and surrounded by fibrous connective tissue for protection. These fist-sized organs weigh about 4 to 6 ounces each.

The kidneys consist of an outer **cortex** region (cortex means bark, as the bark of a tree) and an inner **medulla** region (medulla means marrow). The **hilum** is a depression on the medial border of the kidney. Blood vessels and nerves pass through the hilum.

A **ureter** [2] is one of two muscular tubes (16 to 18 inches long) lined with mucous membranes. Ureters carry urine in peristaltic waves from the kidneys to the urinary bladder.

The **urinary bladder** [3] is a hollow, muscular, sac in the pelvic cavity. It is a temporary reservoir for urine. The **trigone** is a triangular space at the base of the bladder where the ureters enter and the urethra exits.

The **urethra** [4] is a membranous tube that carries urine from the urinary bladder to the outside of the body. The process of expelling **(voiding)** urine through the urethra is

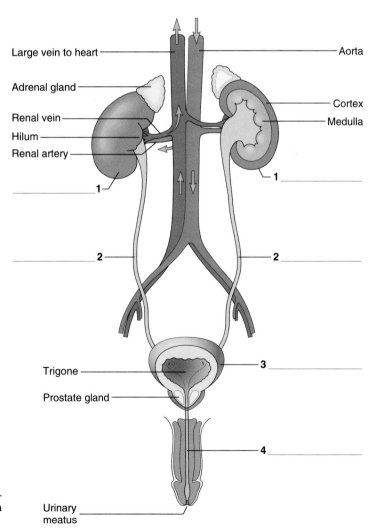

Figure 7-1

Organs of the urinary system in a male.

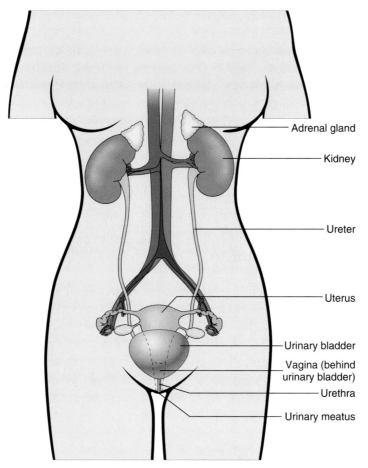

Figure 7-2

Female urinary system.

urination or **micturition.** The external opening of the urethra is the urinary **meatus.** The female urethra, about 1½ inches long, lies anterior to the vagina and vaginal meatus. The male urethra, about 8 inches long, extends downward through the prostate gland to the meatus at the tip of the penis. Figure 7–2 illustrates the female urinary system. Compare it with Figure 7–1, which shows the male urinary system.

III. How the Kidneys Produce Urine

Blood enters each kidney from the aorta by way of the right and left **renal arteries.** After the renal artery enters the kidney (at the hilum), the artery branches into smaller and smaller arteries. The smallest arteries, called **arterioles,** are located throughout the cortex of the kidney (Fig. 7–3A).

Because the arterioles are small, blood passes through them slowly but constantly. Blood flow through the kidney is so essential that the kidneys have their own special device for maintaining blood flow. If blood pressure falls in the vessels of the kidney, so that blood flow diminishes, the kidney produces **renin** and discharges it into the blood. Renin leads to the formation of a substance that stimulates the contraction of arterioles. This increases blood pressure and restores blood flow in the kidneys to normal.

Each arteriole in the cortex of the kidney leads into a mass of very tiny, coiled, and intertwined smaller blood vessels called **capillaries.** The collection of capillaries, shaped in the form of a tiny ball, is a **glomerulus.** There are about 1 million glomeruli in the cortex region of each kidney.

The kidneys produce urine by **filtration.** As blood passes through the many glomeruli, the thin walls of each glomerulus (the filter) permit water, salts, sugar, and **urea** (with other nitrogenous wastes such as **creatinine** and **uric acid**) to leave the bloodstream. These materials collect in a tiny, cup-like structure, a **Bowman capsule,** which surrounds each glomerulus (Fig. 7–3B). The walls of the glomeruli prevent large substances, such as proteins and blood cells, from filtering into the Bowman capsule. These substances remain in the blood and normally do not appear in urine.

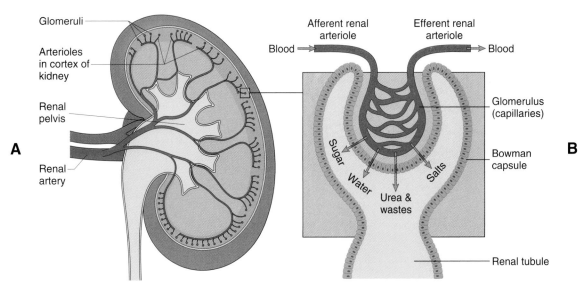

Figure 7–3

(A) Renal artery branching to form smaller arteries, arterioles, and glomeruli. **(B) Glomerulus** and **Bowman capsule.** Afferent arteriole carries blood toward (af-) the glomerulus. Efferent arteriole carries blood away (ef-) from the glomerulus.

Attached to each Bowman capsule is a long, twisted tube called a **renal tubule** (Figs. 7–3B and 7–4). As water, sugar, salts, urea, and other wastes pass through the renal tubule, most of the water, all of the sugar, and some salts (such as sodium) return to the bloodstream through tiny capillaries surrounding each tubule. This active process of **reabsorption** ensures that the body retains essential substances such as sugar, water, and salts. The final process in the formation of urine is **secretion** of some substances from the bloodstream into the renal tubule. These waste products of metabolism become toxic if allowed to accumulate in the body. Thus, acids, drugs (such as penicillin), and potassium (a salt) leave the body in urine.

Only wastes, water, salts, acids, and some drugs remain in the renal tubule. Each renal tubule, now containing urine (95 percent water, 5 percent urea, creatinine, salts, acids, and drugs), ends in a larger collecting tubule. See Figure 7–4, which reviews the steps involved in urine formation. The combination of a glomerulus and a renal tubule is called a **nephron**. There are more than 1 million nephrons in a kidney.

All collecting tubules lead to the **renal pelvis,** a basin-like area in the central part of the kidney. Small, cup-like regions of the renal pelvis are called **calyces** or **calices** (singular: **calyx** or **calix**). Figure 7–5 illustrates a section of the kidney and shows the renal pelvis and calyces.

The renal pelvis narrows into the **ureter,** which carries the urine to the **urinary bladder** where the urine is temporarily stored. Sphincters control the exit area of the bladder to the **urethra.** These muscular rings do not permit urine to leave the bladder. As the bladder fills up and pressure increases at the base of the bladder, a person notices a need to urinate and voluntarily relaxes the sphincter muscles.

Study the flow diagram in Figure 7–6 to trace the process of forming urine and expelling it from the body.

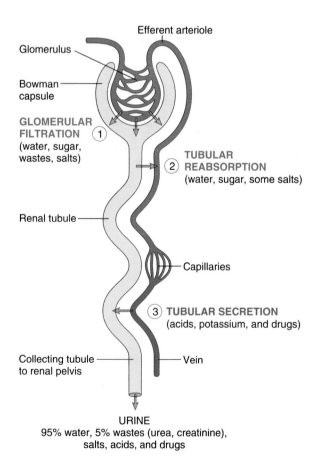

Efferent arteriole

Glomerulus

Bowman capsule

GLOMERULAR FILTRATION ① (water, sugar, wastes, salts)

TUBULAR REABSORPTION ② (water, sugar, some salts)

Renal tubule

Capillaries

③ **TUBULAR SECRETION** (acids, potassium, and drugs)

Collecting tubule to renal pelvis — Vein

URINE
95% water, 5% wastes (urea, creatinine), salts, acids, and drugs

Figure 7–4

Three steps in the formation of urine. (1) Glomerular filtration of water, sugar, wastes (urea and creatinine), and salts. **(2) Tubular reabsorption** of water, sugar, and some salts. **(3) Tubular secretion** of acids, potassium, and drugs.

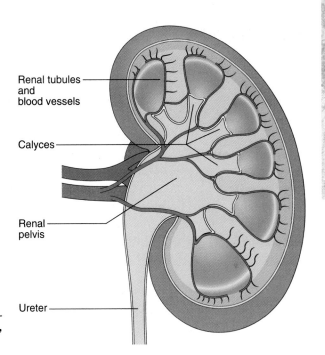

Renal tubules
and
blood vessels

Calyces

Renal
pelvis

Ureter

Figure 7–5

Section of the kidney showing renal pelvis, calyces, and ureter.

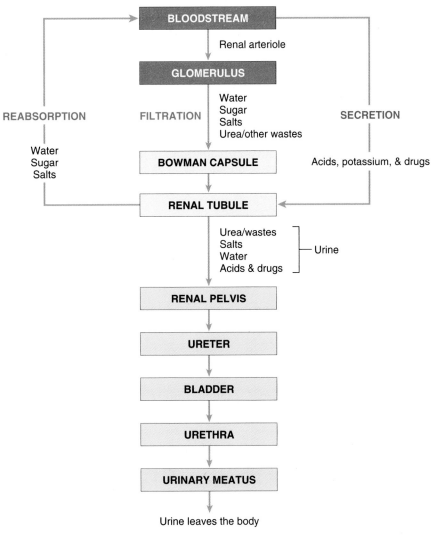

Figure 7–6

Flow diagram illustrating the process of forming and expelling urine.

IV. Vocabulary

arteriole	Small artery.
Bowman capsule	Cup-shaped capsule surrounding each glomerulus.
calyx or **calix** (plural: **calyces** or **calices**)	Cup-like collecting region of the renal pelvis.
catheter	Tube for injecting or removing fluids.
cortex	Outer region; the renal cortex is the outer region of the kidney (**cortical** means pertaining to the cortex).
creatinine	A waste product of muscle metabolism; nitrogenous waste excreted in urine.
electrolyte	A chemical that carries an electrical charge in a solution. Examples are potassium (K^+) and sodium (Na^+).
erythropoietin (EPO)	A hormone secreted by the kidney to stimulate the production of red blood cells.
filtration	Passive process whereby some substances, but not all, pass through a filter or other material. Blood pressure forces materials through the filter. About 180 quarts of fluid are filtered from the blood daily, but the kidney returns 98 to 99 percent of the water and salts. Only about $1\frac{1}{2}$ quarts (1500 mL) of urine are excreted daily.
glomerulus (plural: **glomeruli**)	Tiny ball of capillaries (microscopic blood vessels) in cortex of kidney.
hilum	Depression or pit in that part of an organ where blood vessels and nerves enter and leave.
kidney	One of two bean-shaped organs located behind the abdominal cavity on either side of the backbone in the lumbar region.
meatus	Opening or canal.
medulla	Inner region; the renal medulla is the inner region of the kidney (**medullary** means pertaining to the medulla).
micturition	Urination; the act of voiding.
nephron	The combination of glomerulus and renal tubule where filtration, reabsorption, and secretion take place in the kidney.
nitrogenous waste	Substance containing nitrogen and excreted in urine.
potassium (K^+)	A salt (electrolyte) secreted from the bloodstream into the renal tubules to leave the body in urine.

reabsorption	In this process, the renal tubules return materials necessary to the body back into the bloodstream.
renal artery	Carries blood to the kidney.
renal pelvis	Central collecting region in the kidney.
renal tubule	Microscopic tube in the kidney where urine is formed after filtration. In the renal tubule, the composition of urine is altered by the processes of reabsorption and secretion.
renal vein	Carries blood away from the kidney.
renin	An enzymatic hormone synthesized, stored, and secreted by the kidney; it raises blood pressure by influencing vasoconstriction (narrowing of blood vessels).
sodium (Na$^+$)	A salt (electrolyte) regulated in the blood and urine by the kidneys.
trigone	Triangular area in the bladder where the ureters enter and the urethra exits.
urea	Major nitrogenous waste product excreted in urine.
ureter	Tube leading from each kidney to the bladder.
urethra	Tube leading from the bladder to the outside of the body.
uric acid	Nitrogenous waste excreted in the urine.
urinary bladder	Sac that holds urine.
urination	Process of expelling urine; also called micturition.
voiding	Emptying of urine from the urinary bladder; urination or micturition.

V. Terminology: Structures, Substances, and Urinary Symptoms

Write the meanings of the medical terms in the spaces provided.

Structures			
Combining Form	Meaning	Terminology	Meaning
cali/o **calic/o**	calyx (calix)	caliectasis _____	
		caliceal _____	

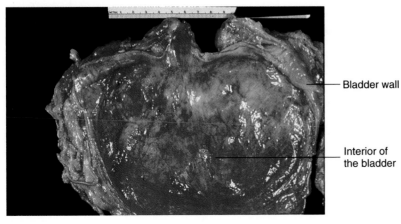

— Bladder wall

— Interior of
the bladder

Figure 7–7

Acute cystitis. Notice that the mucosa of the bladder is red and swollen. Bladder and urinary tract infections are more common in women because of the shorter urethra, which allows easier bacterial colonization of the urinary bladder. They usually occur without a known cause, but may be acquired during sexual intercourse ("honeymoon cystitis") or following surgical procedures and urinary catheterization. (From Damjanov I: Pathology for the Health-Related Professions, 2nd ed. Philadelphia, WB Saunders, 2000, p. 335.)

cyst/o	urinary bladder	cystitis _____

Bacterial infections often cause acute or chronic cystitis. In acute cystitis, the bladder (contains blood) as a result of mucosal hemorrhages (Fig. 7–7).

cystectomy _____

cystostomy _____

An opening is made into the urinary bladder from the outside of the body. A catheter is placed into the bladder for drainage.

glomerul/o	glomerulus (collection of capillaries)	glomerular _____

meat/o	meatus	meatal stenosis _____

meatotomy _____

nephr/o	kidney	paranephric _____

nephropathy _____
(ně-FRŎ-pă-thē)

nephroptosis _____

nephrolithotomy _____

Incision (percutaneous) into the kidney to remove a stone.

nephrosclerosis _____

Arterioles in the kidney are affected.

hydronephrosis _____

Obstruction of urine flow may be caused by renal calculi (Fig. 7–8), compression of the ureter by tumor, or hyperplasia of the prostate gland at the base of the bladder in males.

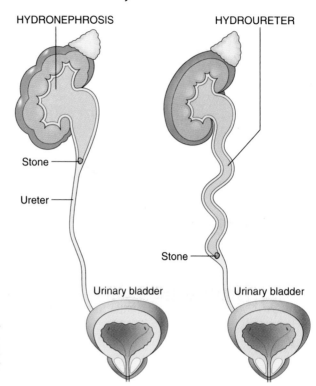

HYDRONEPHROSIS   HYDROURETER

Stone

Ureter

Stone

Urinary bladder   Urinary bladder

Figure 7–8

Hydronephrosis caused by a stone (obstruction) in the proximal part of a ureter and **hydroureter** with hydronephrosis caused by a stone in the distal part of the ureter.

		nephrostomy _____
		Temporary opening to the outside of the body (from the renal pelvis). This is necessary when a ureter becomes obstructed and the renal pelvis becomes distended with urine (hydronephrosis).
pyel/o	renal pelvis	pyelolithotomy _____
		Removal of a large calculus (stone) that contributes to blockage of urine flow and development of infection.
		pyelogram _____
		See discussion of intravenous (IVP) and retrograde pyelograms (RP) on pages 230 and 231, Section VIII, under Clinical Procedures.
ren/o	kidney	renal ischemia _____
		renal colic _____
		Colic is intermittent spasms of pain caused by inflammation and distention of a hollow organ. In renal colic, pain results from calculi in the kidney or ureter.
trigon/o	trigone (region of the bladder)	trigonitis _____

ureter/o	ureter	ureteroplasty _____
		ureterolithotomy _____
		ureteroileostomy _____

*After cystectomy, urologists form a pouch from a segment of the ileum and use it in place of the bladder to carry urine from the ureters out of the body. It is an **ileal conduit**.*

urethr/o	urethra	urethritis _____
		urethroplasty _____
		urethral stricture _____

*A **stricture** is an abnormal narrowing of an opening or passageway.*

| vesic/o | urinary bladder | perivesical _____ |

Do not confuse the term vesical with the term vesicle, which is a small blister on the skin.

vesicoureteral reflux _____

Substances and Symptoms

Combining Form or Suffix	Meaning	Terminology	Meaning
albumin/o	albumin (a protein in the blood)	albuminuria _____	

-uria means urine condition. This finding can indicate malfunction of the kidney as protein leaks out of damaged glomeruli.

| azot/o | nitrogen | azotemia _____ | |

This is reflected in an elevated BUN (blood urea nitrogen) test.

| bacteri/o | bacteria | bacteriuria _____ | |

Usually a sign of infection.

| dips/o | thirst | polydipsia _____ | |

A sign of diabetes insipidus or diabetes mellitus (see pages 229 and 230, Section VII, Pathological Terminology).

| ket/o keton/o | ketone bodies (ketoacids and acetone) | ketosis _____ | |

Often called ketoacidosis because acids accumulate in the blood and tissues. See page 226, ketone bodies, Section VI, Urinalysis.

ketonuria _____

lith/o	stone	nephrolithiasis _____

noct/i — night — nocturia _____

Noctiphobia is an irrational fear of night or darkness.

olig/o — scanty — oliguria _____

-poietin — substance that forms — erythropoietin _____

py/o — pus — pyuria _____

-tripsy — to crush — lithotripsy _____

See page 234, Section VIII, Clinical Procedures.

ur/o — urine (urea) — uremia _____

This toxic state results when nitrogenous waste products accumulate greatly in the blood.

enuresis _____

Literally, a condition of being in urine, and also called bedwetting.

diuresis _____

di- (from dia-) means complete. Caffeine and alcohol can produce diuresis, acting as diuretics to produce a diluted urine.

antidiuretic hormone _____

This substance (a hormone from the pituitary gland, and literally meaning against diuresis) normally acts on the renal tubules to cause water to be reabsorbed into the bloodstream. Also called ADH.

urin/o — urine — urinary incontinence _____

Incontinence literally means not (in-) able to hold (tin) together (con-). This is loss of control of the passage of urine from the bladder. Stress incontinence occurs with strain on the bladder opening when coughing or sneezing. Urgency incontinence occurs with inability to hold back urination when feeling the urge to void.

urinary retention _____

This symptom results with blockage to the outflow of urine from the bladder.

-uria — urination, urine condition — dysuria _____

anuria _____

hematuria _____

glycosuria _____

A symptom of diabetes mellitus.

polyuria _____

A symptom of both diabetes insipidus and diabetes mellitus. See pages 229 and 230, Section VII, Pathological Terminology.

VI. Urinalysis

Urinalysis is an examination of urine to determine the presence of abnormal elements that may indicate various pathological conditions.

The following are some of the tests made in a urinalysis:

1. **Color**—Normal urine color is yellow (amber) or straw-colored. A colorless, pale urine indicates a large amount of water in the urine, whereas a smoky-red or brown color of urine indicates the presence of large amounts of blood. Foods such as beets and certain drugs can also produce red hues in urine.

2. **pH**—This test reveals the chemical nature of urine. It indicates to what degree a solution (such as urine or blood) is **acidic** or **alkaline (basic).** The pH range is between 0 (very acid) and 14 (very alkaline). Normal urine is slightly acidic (6.5). However, in infections of the bladder, the urine pH may be alkaline, owing to the actions of bacteria in the urine that break down the urea and release an alkaline substance called ammonia.

3. **Protein**—Small amounts of protein are normally found in the urine but not in sufficient quantity to produce a positive result by ordinary methods of testing. When urinary tests for protein become positive, **albumin** is usually responsible. Albumin is the major protein in blood plasma. If it is detected in urine **(albuminuria),** it may indicate a leak in the glomerular membrane, which allows albumin to enter the renal tubule and pass into the urine.

   Through more sensitive testing, abnormal amounts of albumin may be detected **(microalbuminuria)** when ordinary tests are negative. Microalbuminuria is recognized as the earliest sign of renal involvement in diabetes mellitus (see page 230) and essential hypertension (see page 229).

4. **Glucose**—Sugar is not normally found in the urine. In most cases, when it does appear **(glycosuria),** it indicates **diabetes mellitus.** In diabetes mellitus, there is an excess of sugar in the bloodstream (hyperglycemia), which leads to the "spilling over" of sugar into the urine. The renal tubules cannot reabsorb all the sugar that filters out through the glomerular membrane.

5. **Specific gravity**—The specific gravity of urine reflects the amounts of wastes, minerals, and solids in the urine. It is a comparison of the density of urine with that of water. The urine of patients with diabetes mellitus has a higher-than-normal specific gravity because of the presence of sugar.

6. **Ketone bodies**—Ketones (sometimes referred to as **acetones,** which are a type of ketone body) are breakdown products resulting from fat catabolism in cells. Ketones accumulate in large quantities in blood and urine when the body breaks down fat,

instead of sugar, for fuel. Ketonuria occurs in diabetes mellitus when cells deprived of sugar must use up their available fat for energy. In starvation, when sugar is not available, ketonuria and ketosis (ketones in the blood) occur as fat is catabolized abnormally.

The presence of ketones in the blood is quite dangerous because ketones increase the acidity of the blood **(acidosis).** This can lead to coma (unconsciousness) and death.

7. **Sediment**—Abnormal particles are present in the urine as a sign of a pathological condition. Included are cells (epithelial cells, white blood cells, or red blood cells), bacteria, crystals, or **casts** (cylindrical structures of protein often containing cellular elements).

8. **Pus—Pyuria** gives a **turbid** (cloudy) appearance to urine. Large numbers of leukocytes (polymorphonuclears) are present because of infection or inflammation in the kidney or bladder.

9. **Phenylketonuria (PKU)**—Phenylketones are substances that accumulate in the urine of infants born lacking an important enzyme. The enzyme (phenylalanine hydroxylase) is necessary in cells to change one amino acid (phenylalanine) to another amino acid (tyrosine). Lack of the enzyme causes phenylalanine to reach high levels in the infant's bloodstream, which will eventually lead to mental retardation. The PKU test, done just after birth, can detect the phenylketonuria or phenylalanine in the blood. When it is detected, the infant is fed a low-protein diet that excludes phenylalanine to prevent mental retardation. The child must remain on this diet until adulthood.

10. **Bilirubin**—This pigment substance, which results from hemoglobin breakdown, may appear in the urine, darkening it, as an indication of liver or gallbladder disease. The diseased liver has difficulty removing bilirubin from the blood **(hyperbilirubinemia),** which causes excessive bilirubin to appear in the urine **(bilirubinuria).**

VII. Pathological Terminology: Kidney, Bladder, and Associated Conditions

Your expanding knowledge of medical terminology should help you understand the terminology in the following paragraphs.

Kidney

glomerulonephritis

Inflammation of the kidney glomerulus.

Acute glomerulonephritis may develop as part of a systemic disorder (a condition that affects many organs in the body) or may be idiopathic. It can also occur after an acute infection, as in poststreptococcal glomerulonephritis. In this condition, which appears 10 to 14 days after a streptococcal infection, no bacteria are actually found in the kidney, but inflammation results from an immune (antigen and antibody) reaction in the glomerulus. Most patients recover spontaneously, but in some cases the disease becomes chronic. Chronic glomerulonephritis can result in hypertension (high blood pressure), albuminuria (protein seeps through damaged glomerular walls), renal failure, and uremia. Drugs may be useful to control inflammation, and dialysis or transplant may be necessary if uremia occurs.

interstitial nephritis

Inflammation of the renal interstitium (connective tissue that lies between the renal tubules).

Acute interstitial nephritis, an increasingly common disorder, may develop after the administration of drugs. Characterized by fever, skin rash, eosinophils in the blood and urine, and poor renal function, recovery may occur when the patient discontinues using the offending agent. Recovery is helped with *corticosteroids* (anti-inflammatory agents).

nephrolithiasis

Kidney stones (renal calculi).

Kidney stones are usually composed of uric acid or calcium salts. Although the etiology is often unknown, conditions associated with an increase in the concentration of calcium (parathyroid gland tumors) or high levels of uric acid in the blood (**hyperuricemia**—associated with gouty arthritis) may contribute to the formation of calculi. Stones often lodge in the ureter or bladder as well as in the renal pelvis and may require removal by extracorporeal shock wave **lithotripsy** (see page 234, Section VIII, under Clinical Procedures) or surgery.

nephrotic syndrome

A group of symptoms caused by excessive protein loss in the urine (also called **nephrosis**).

In addition to marked proteinuria, symptoms include **edema** (swelling caused by fluid in tissue spaces), **hypoalbuminemia,** hypercholesterolemia, hypercoagulability (tendency of the blood to clot more than normal), and susceptibility to infections. Nephrotic syndrome may follow glomerulonephritis, exposure to toxins or drugs, and other pathological conditions, such as diabetes mellitus and malignant disease. Drugs may be useful to heal the leaky glomerulus.

polycystic kidneys

Multiple fluid-filled sacs (cysts) within and upon the kidney.

This hereditary condition usually remains **asymptomatic** (without symptoms) until adult life. Cysts progressively develop in both kidneys, leading to nephromegaly, hematuria, urinary tract infection, hypertension, and uremia. Figure 7–9A shows polycystic kidney disease.

A 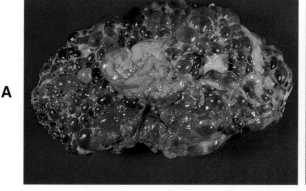 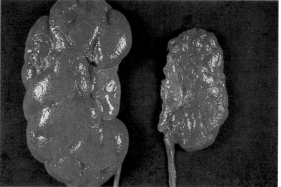 B

Figure 7–9

(A) Polycystic kidney disease. The kidneys contain masses of cysts. Typically, polycystic kidneys weigh 20 times more than their usual weight (150-200 grams). **(B) Chronic pyelonephritis.** Notice that one kidney is small, shrunken, and irregularly scarred. The other kidney is of normal size but also shows scarring. (From Damjanov I: Pathology for Health-Related Professions, 2nd ed. Philadelphia, WB Saunders, 2000, pp. 327 and 335.)

pyelonephritis	**Inflammation of the renal pelvis and renal medulla.**

Bacterial infection causes this common type of kidney disease. In acute pyelonephritis, many small **abscesses** (collections of pus) form in the renal pelvis and adjacent medulla. Urinalysis reveals pyuria. Treatment consists of antibiotics and surgical correction of any obstruction to urine flow. Chronic pyelonephritis (Figure 7–9B) may evolve from acute pyelonephritis. Recurrent infections lead to destruction of renal tissue and to scar formation.

renal cell carcinoma (hypernephroma)	**Cancerous tumor of the kidney in adulthood.**

This tumor accounts for 2 percent of all cancers in adults. Hematuria is the primary symptom, and the tumor often metastasizes to bones and lungs. Likelihood of survival depends on the extent of spread of the tumor. Nephrectomy is the treatment of choice.

renal failure	**Failure of the kidney to excrete wastes and maintain its filtration function.**

The kidney stops excreting nitrogenous waste products and acids derived from diet and body metabolism. Renal failure may be acute or chronic, reversible or progressive, mild or severe. The final phase of chronic renal failure is end-stage renal disease (ESRD), or currently called **chronic kidney disease (CKD).** Erythropoietin is used to treat patients with CKD. It increases red blood cells and results in marked improvement in energy levels. Hemodialysis, peritoneal dialysis, and renal transplantation are advised when medical measures have been exhausted.

renal hypertension	**High blood pressure resulting from kidney disease.**

Renal hypertension is the most common type of **secondary hypertension** (high blood pressure caused by an abnormal condition, such as glomerulonephritis or renal artery stenosis). If the cause of high blood pressure is not known, it is called **essential hypertension.** Chronic essential hypertension can cause arteriole walls in the kidney to become narrowed and thickened (nephrosclerosis), and this can produce glomerular ischemia, atrophy, and scarring of kidney tissue.

Wilms tumor	**Malignant tumor of the kidney occurring in childhood.**

This tumor may be treated with surgery, radiation, and chemotherapy.

Urinary Bladder

bladder cancer	**Malignant tumor of the urinary bladder.**

The bladder is the most common site of malignancy of the urinary system. It occurs more frequently in men (often smokers) and in persons over the age of 50, especially industrial workers exposed to dyes and leather. Symptoms include gross (visible to the naked eye) or microscopic hematuria and dysuria and increased urinary frequency. Cystoscopy with biopsy is the most common diagnostic procedure. Staging of the tumor is based on the depth to which the bladder wall (urothelium) has been penetrated and the extent of metastasis. Superficial tumors are removed by electrocauterization (burning). Cystectomy, chemotherapy, and radiation therapy are helpful for more invasive disease.

Associated Conditions

diabetes insipidus	**Inadequate secretion or resistance of the kidney to the action of antidiuretic hormone (ADH).**

Two major symptoms of this condition are polydipsia and polyuria. Lack of ADH prevents water from being reabsorbed into the blood through the renal tubules. Insipidus means tasteless, reflecting very dilute and watery urine, not sweet as in diabetes mellitus. The term **diabetes** comes from the Greek *diabainen,* meaning "to pass through." Both types of diabetes (insipidus and mellitus) are marked by excessive excretion of urine.

diabetes mellitus	**Inadequate secretion or improper utilization of insulin.**

Major symptoms of diabetes mellitus are glycosuria, hyperglycemia, polyuria, and polydipsia. Without insulin, sugar cannot leave the bloodstream and be available to body cells for energy. Sugar remains in the blood (hyperglycemia) and spills over into the urine (glycosuria) when the kidney cannot reabsorb it through the renal tubules. Mellitus means sweet, reflecting the content of the urine. The term diabetes, when used by itself, usually refers to the more common condition, diabetes mellitus, rather than diabetes insipidus.

VIII. Laboratory Tests, Clinical Procedures, and Abbreviations

Laboratory Tests

blood urea nitrogen (BUN) **Measurement of urea levels in blood.**

Normally, the blood urea level is low because urea is excreted in the urine continuously. However, when the kidney is diseased or fails, urea accumulates in the blood (uremia), leading to unconsciousness and death.

creatinine clearance test **Measures the rate at which creatinine is cleared from the blood by the kidney.**

A blood sample is drawn and the amount of creatinine concentration is compared with the amount of creatinine excreted in the urine during a 24-hour period. If the kidney is not functioning well in its job of clearing creatinine from the blood, there will be a disproportionate amount of creatinine in the blood compared with the amount in the urine.

Clinical Procedures

X-Rays

CT scan **X-ray image with detailed cross-sectional views of organs and tissues.**

Transverse x-ray views of the kidney, taken with or without contrast material, are useful in the diagnosis of tumors, cysts, abscesses, and hydronephrosis.

intravenous pyelogram (IVP) **X-ray image of the kidneys and uterus after injection of contrast into a vein.**

Also called an **excretory urogram**, this x-ray provides a test of renal function and shows cysts, tumors, infections, hydronephrosis, and calculi. An IVP **tomogram** shows a series of images of the kidney and may be required to see details.

kidneys, ureters, and bladder (KUB) **X-ray examination (without contrast) of the kidneys, ureters, and bladder.**

A KUB demonstrates the size and location of the kidneys in relation to other organs in the abdominopelvic region.

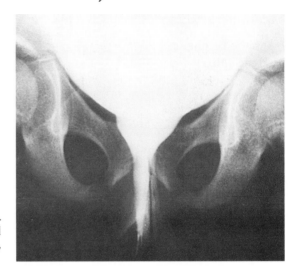

Figure 7–10

Voiding cystourethrogram showing a normal female urethra. (Courtesy William H. Bush, Jr., MD, University of Washington, Seattle.)

renal angiography	**X-ray examination (with contrast) of the vascular system (blood vessels) of the kidney.**
	This procedure helps diagnose kidney tumors and outline renal vessels in hypertensive patients.
retrograde pyelogram (RP)	**X-ray images of the kidneys, ureters, and bladder after injecting contrast through a urinary catheter into the ureters.**
	This technique, useful in locating urinary stones and obstructions, is helpful when poor renal function makes it impossible to visualize the urinary tract with intravenous contrast agents as in an IVP. It is a substitute for an IVP when a patient is allergic to intravenous contrast material.
voiding cystourethrogram (VCUG)	**X-ray record (with contrast) of the urinary bladder, ureters, and urethra while the patient is expelling urine.**
	The bladder is filled with contrast material as in a retrograde pyelogram, and x-rays are taken. See Figure 7–10.

Ultrasound

ultrasonography	**Process of imaging urinary tract structures using high frequency sound waves.**
	Kidney size, tumors, hydronephrosis, polycystic kidney, and ureteral and bladder obstruction can be diagnosed using sound waves.

Radioactive

radioisotope scan	**Image of the kidney after injecting into the bloodstream a radioactive substance (isotope) that concentrates in the kidney.**
	Pictures show the size and shape of the kidney **(renal scan)** and its function **(renogram).** These studies can indicate size of blood vessels, diagnose obstruction, and determine the individual functioning of each kidney.

Magnetic Imaging

magnetic resonance imaging (MRI)

A magnetic field and radio waves produce images of the kidney and surrounding structures in all three planes of the body.

The patient lies surrounded by a cylindrical magnetic resonance machine, and images are made of the pelvic and retroperitoneal regions using magnetic waves. This high-technology machine produces an image of internal organs based on the movement of small particles called protons.

Other Procedures

cystoscopy

Direct visual examination of urinary bladder with an endoscope (cystoscope).

A urologist introduces a hollow metal tube into the urinary meatus and passes it through the urethra into the bladder. Using a light source, special lenses, and mirrors, the bladder mucosa is examined for tumors, calculi, or inflammation. When a catheter is placed through the cystoscope, urine samples are withdrawn and contrast material injected into the bladder. See Figure 7–11. A **panendoscope** is a cystoscope that gives a wide-angle view of the bladder.

dialysis

Process of separating nitrogenous waste materials from the bloodstream when the kidneys no longer function.

There are two methods:
hemodialysis (HD) uses an artificial kidney machine that receives waste-filled blood from the patient's bloodstream, filters it, and returns the dialysed blood to the patient's body. See Figure 7–12.

peritoneal dialysis (PD) using a peritoneal **catheter** (tube), fluid is introduced into the peritoneal (abdominal) cavity. The fluid causes wastes in the capillaries of the peritoneum to pass out of the bloodstream and into the fluid. Fluid (with wastes) is then removed by catheter. When used to treat patients with chronic kidney disease, PD may be performed continuously by the patient without artificial support (CAPD, continuous ambulatory PD) or with the aid of a mechanical apparatus at night during sleep (CCPD, continuous cycling PD). Figure 7–13 illustrates CAPD.

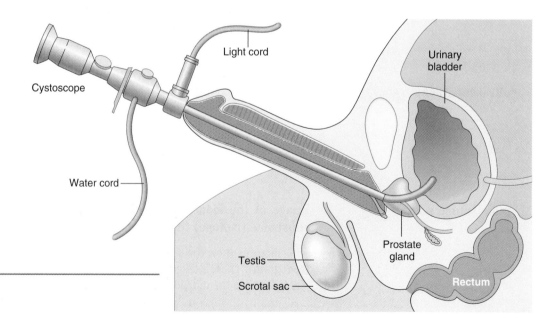

Figure 7–11

Cystoscopy.

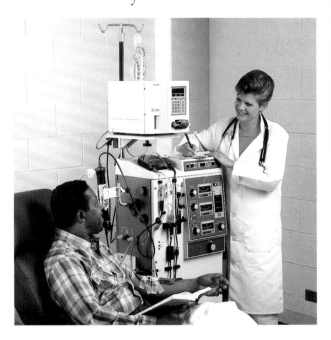

Figure 7–12

Patient receiving hemodialysis. (From Lewis SM, Heitkemper MM, Dirksen SR: Medical-Surgical Nursing: Assessment and Management of Clinical Problems, 5th ed. St. Louis, Mosby, 2000, p. 1328.)

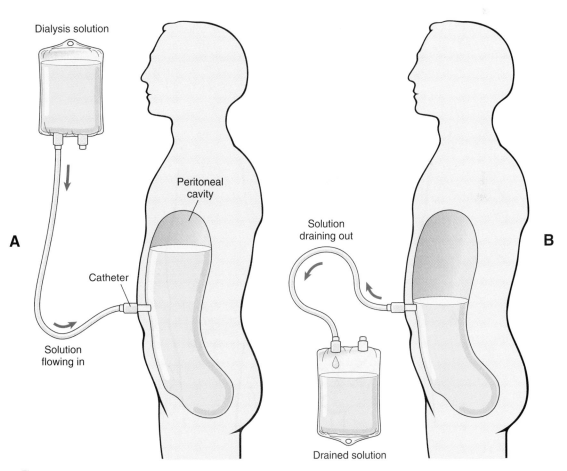

Figure 7–13

Continuous ambulatory peritoneal dialysis (CAPD). (A) The dialysis solution (dialysate) flows from a collapsible plastic bag through a catheter (a Tenckhoff peritoneal catheter) into the patient's peritoneal cavity. The empty bag is folded and inserted into undergarments. **(B)** After 4-8 hours, the bag is unfolded, and the fluid is allowed to drain into it by gravity. The full bag is discarded, and a new bag of fresh dialysate is attached.

extracorporeal shock wave lithotripsy (ESWL)

Shock waves crush urinary tract stones, which then pass from the body in urine.

After receiving anesthesia, the patient is immersed in a tank of water and shock waves are generated electrically. Using an x-ray image intensifier (fluoroscopy), the physician positions the patient so that the stone receives shock waves properly.

renal angioplasty

Dilation of narrowed areas in renal arteries.

An inflatable balloon attached to a catheter is inserted into the artery. Afterward, **stents** (metal meshed tubes) may be inserted to keep the vessel open.

renal biopsy

Removal of kidney tissue with microscopic examination by a pathologist.

Biopsy may be performed at the time of surgery (open) or through the skin (percutaneous, or closed). When the latter technique is used, the patient lies in the prone position and, following administration of local anesthesia to the overlying skin and muscles of the back, the physician inserts a biopsy needle.

renal transplantation

Surgical transfer of a complete kidney from a donor to a recipient.

Patients with renal failure may receive a kidney from a living donor, such as an identical twin (isograft) or other individual (allograft), or from a cadaver (dead body). Best results occur when the donor is closely related to the recipient, and better than 90 percent of the kidneys survive for one year or longer (Fig. 7–14).

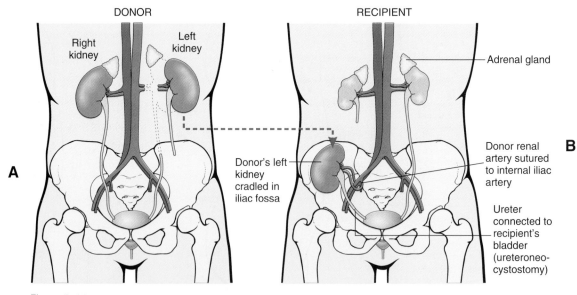

Figure 7–14

Renal (kidney) transplantation. (A) Left kidney of donor is removed for transplant. **(B)** Kidney is transplanted to right pelvis of the recipient. The renal artery and vein of the donor kidney are joined to the recipient's artery and vein, and the lower end of the donor ureter is connected to the recipient's bladder **(ureteroneocystostomy).** The health of the donor is not affected by losing one kidney. In fact, the remaining kidney enlarges (hypertrophies) to take over almost full function.

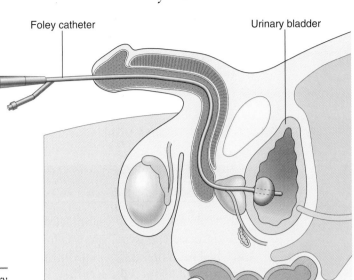

Foley catheter   Urinary bladder

Figure 7–15

A **Foley catheter** in place in the urinary bladder.

urinary catheterization

Passage of a flexible, tubular instrument through the urethra into the urinary bladder.

Catheters are used primarily for short- or long-term drainage of urine. A **Foley catheter** is an indwelling (left in the bladder) catheter held in place by a balloon inflated with air or liquid (Fig. 7–15).

Abbreviations

ADH	antidiuretic hormone; vasopressin
ARF	acute renal failure
BILI	bilirubin
BUN	blood urea nitrogen
CAPD	continuous ambulatory peritoneal dialysis
Cath	catheter, catheterization
CCPD	continuous cycling peritoneal dialysis
CKD	chronic kidney disease; a condition during which serum creatinine and BUN levels rise and may result in impairment of all body systems
CL⁻	chloride; an electrolyte excreted by the kidney
CRF	chronic renal failure; progressive loss of kidney function
cysto	cystoscopic examination
ESRD	end-stage renal disease; see CKD
ESWL	extracorporeal shock wave lithotripsy

HCO₃⁻	bicarbonate; an electrolyte conserved by the kidney
HD	hemodialysis
IC	interstitial cystitis; chronic inflammation of the bladder wall; not caused by bacterial infection and not responsive to conventional antibiotic therapy.
IVP	intravenous pyelogram
K⁺	potassium; an electrolyte
KUB	kidney, ureter, and bladder
Na⁺	sodium; an electrolyte
PD	peritoneal dialysis
pH	symbol for degree of acidity or alkalinity
PKU	phenylketonuria
sp gr	specific gravity
UA	urinalysis
UTI	urinary tract infection
VCUG	voiding cystourethrogram

IX. Practical Applications

This section contains an actual medical report using terms that you have studied in this and previous chapters. Questions are included to test your understanding. Answers to the questions are on page 244 after Answers to Exercises.

Case Report

The patient, a 50-year-old woman, presented herself at the clinic complaining of dysuria. This symptom was followed by sudden onset of hematuria and clots. There had been no history of urolithiasis, pyuria, or previous hematuria. Nocturia had been present about 5 years earlier. Panendoscopy revealed a carcinoma located about 2 cm from the left ureteral orifice. A partial cystectomy was carried out and the lesion cleared. No ileal conduit was necessary. A metastatic workup was negative. Bilateral pelvic lymphadenectomy revealed no positive nodes.

Questions on the Case Report

1. **Urological refers to which system of the body?**
   (A) Digestive
   (B) Reproductive
   (C) Excretory
2. **What was the patient's reason for appearing at the clinic?**
   (A) Scanty urination
   (B) Inability to urinate
   (C) Painful urination
3. **What acute symptom followed?**
   (A) Blood in the feces
   (B) Blood in the urine
   (C) Excessive urea in the blood
4. **Which of the following was a previous symptom?**
   (A) Pus in the urine
   (B) Blood in the urine
   (C) Excessive urination at night
5. **What diagnostic procedure was carried out?**
   (A) Lithotripsy
   (B) Cystoscopy using a wide-angle view of the bladder
   (C) Urinalysis
6. **The patient's diagnosis was**
   (A) Malignant tumor of the bladder
   (B) Tumor in the proximal ureter
   (C) Lymph nodes were affected by tumor
7. **Treatment was**
   (A) Ureteroileostomy
   (B) Removal of tumor and subtotal removal of the bladder
   (C) Not necessary because of negative lymph nodes

X. Exercises

Remember to check your answers carefully with those given in Section XI, Answers to Exercises.

A. *Using the following terms, trace the path of urine formation from afferent renal arterioles to the point at which urine leaves the body.*

Bowman capsule   renal pelvis   ureter   urinary bladder
glomerulus   renal tubule   urethra   urinary meatus

1. _____   5. _____

2. _____   6. _____

3. _____   7. _____

4. _____   8. _____

B. *Match the term in column I with the letter of a definition or term of similar meaning in column II.*

Column I

1. voiding   _____
2. trigone   _____
3. renal cortex   _____
4. renal medulla   _____
5. urea   _____
6. erythropoietin   _____
7. renin   _____
8. electrolyte   _____
9. hilum   _____
10. calyx (calix)   _____

Column II

A. a hormone secreted by the kidney that stimulates formation of red blood cells
B. notch on the surface of the kidney where blood vessels and nerve enter
C. micturition; urination
D. nitrogenous waste
E. cup-like collecting region of the renal pelvis
F. a small molecule that carries an electric charge in solution
G. inner region of the kidney
H. hormone made by the kidney that causes blood pressure to rise
I. triangular area in the bladder
J. outer section of the kidney

C. *Give the meanings of the following medical terms.*

1. caliceal _____

2. uric acid _____

3. urinary meatal stenosis _____

4. cystocele _____

5. pyelolithotomy _____

6. trigonitis _____

7. ureteroileostomy _____

8. urethrostenosis _____

9. vesicoureteral reflux _____

10. creatinine _____

11. medullary _____

12. cortical _____

D. Give the meanings of the following terms that relate to urinary symptoms.

1. azotemia _____

2. polydipsia _____

3. nocturia _____

4. urinary incontinence _____

5. oliguria _____

6. bacteriuria _____

7. albuminuria _____

8. enuresis _____

9. urinary retention _____

10. dysuria _____

11. polyuria _____

12. glycosuria _____

13. ketosis _____

14. anuria _____

E. Give short answers for the following.

1. What is the difference between hematuria and uremia? _____

2. What is diuresis? _____

3. What is a diuretic? _____

4. What is antidiuretic hormone? _____

F. Match the following terms that pertain to urinalysis with their meanings below.

albuminuria   hematuria   phenylketonuria   sediment
bilirubinuria   ketonuria   pyuria   specific gravity
glycosuria   pH

1. Abnormal particles present in the urine—cells, bacteria, casts, and crystals.

   _____

2. High levels of a substance appear in urine when a baby is born with a deficiency of an enzyme.
   The infant can become mentally retarded if she or he is not put on a strict diet that prevents the

   substance from accumulating in the blood and urine. _____

3. Smoky-red color of urine caused by the presence of blood. _____

4. Turbid (cloudy) urine caused by the presence of polymorphonuclear leukocytes and pus.

   _____

5. Sugar in the urine; a symptom of diabetes mellitus and a result of hyperglycemia.

   _____

6. This urine test reflects the acidity or alkalinity of the urine. _____

7. High levels of acids and acetones accumulate in the urine as a result of abnormal fat catabolism.

   _____

8. Dark pigment accumulates in urine as a result of liver or gallbladder disease.

   _____

9. This urine test reflects the concentration of the urine. _____

10. Leaky glomeruli can produce accumulation of protein in the urine. _____

G. Describe the following abnormal conditions that affect the kidney.

1. renal failure _____

2. polycystic kidney _____

3. interstitial nephritis _____

4. glomerulonephritis _____

5. nephrolithiasis _____

6. renal cell carcinoma _____

7. pyelonephritis _____

8. Wilms tumor _____

9. nephrotic syndrome _____

10. renal hypertension _____

H. Match the following terms with their meanings below.

abscess   edema   renal colic
catheter   essential hypertension   secondary hypertension
diabetes insipidus   nephroptosis   stricture
diabetes mellitus

1. idiopathic high blood pressure _____

2. swelling, fluid in tissues _____

3. narrowed area in a tube _____

4. collection of pus _____

5. inadequate secretion of insulin or improper utilization of insulin leads to this condition

_____

6. high blood pressure caused by kidney disease or another disease _____

7. tube for withdrawing or giving fluid _____

8. inadequate secretion or resistance of the kidney to the action of antidiuretic hormone

   _____

9. prolapse of a kidney _____

10. severe pain resulting from a stone that is blocking a ureter or a kidney

   _____

I. Give the meanings of the following abbreviations and then select the letter of the sentence that is the best association for each.

Column I	*Column II*
1. CAPD _____ ____	A. Bacterial invasion leads to this condition; acute cystitis is an example.
2. BUN _____ ____	B. This electrolyte is secreted by renal tubules into the urine.
3. IVP _____ ____	C. A machine removes nitrogenous wastes from a patient's blood.
4. cysto _____ ____	D. High levels of this test lead to the suspicion of renal disease.
5. UA _____ ____	E. This endoscopic procedure is used to examine the interior of the urinary bladder.
6. UTI _____ ____	F. Dialysate (fluid) is injected into the peritoneal cavity and then drained out.
7. CKD _____ ____	G. Contrast is injected into veins and x-rays are taken of the kidneys and urinary tract.
8. K⁺ _____ ____	H. X-rays are taken of the urinary bladder and urethra while a patient urinates.
9. VCUG _____ ____	I. The parts of this test include specific gravity, color, protein, glucose, and pH.
10. HD _____ ____	J. This condition includes mild to severe kidney failure.

F

1. sediment
2. phenylketonuria (phenylketones in the urine)
3. hematuria (blood in the urine)
4. pyuria (pus in the urine)
5. glycosuria (sugar in the urine)
6. pH
7. ketonuria (ketone bodies in the urine)
8. bilirubinuria (high levels of bilirubin in the urine)
9. specific gravity
10. albuminuria

G

1. kidney does not excrete wastes
2. multiple fluid-filled sacs form in and on the kidney
3. inflammation of the connective tissue (interstitium) lying between the renal tubules
4. inflammation of the glomerulus of the kidney (may be a complication following a streptococcal infection)
5. condition of kidney stones (renal calculi)
6. malignant tumor of the kidney in adults
7. inflammation of the kidney and renal pelvis (caused by a bacterial infection, such as *Escherichia coli*, that enters the urinary tract from the gastrointestinal tract)
8. malignant tumor of the kidney in children
9. group of symptoms (proteinuria, edema, hypoalbuminemia) that appears when the kidney is damaged by disease; also called nephrosis
10. high blood pressure caused by kidney disease

H

1. essential hypertension
2. edema
3. stricture
4. abscess
5. diabetes mellitus
6. secondary hypertension
7. catheter
8. diabetes insipidus
9. nephroptosis
10. renal colic

I

1. continuous ambulatory peritoneal dialysis. F
2. blood, urea, nitrogen. D
3. intravenous pyelogram. G
4. cystoscopy. E
5. urinalysis. I
6. urinary tract infection. A
7. chronic kidney disease. J
8. potassium. B
9. voiding cystourethrogram. H
10. hemodialysis. C

J

1. nephrectomy
2. nephrolithotomy
3. meatotomy
4. extracorporeal shock wave lithotripsy
5. ureteroileostomy
6. urethroplasty
7. nephrostomy
8. cystostomy
9. cystectomy
10. ureterolithotomy

K

1. nephrectomy
2. renal calculi
3. hydronephrosis
4. nephrosclerosis
5. enuresis
6. nephropathy
7. renal transplantation
8. hypertrophied
9. ketones
10. edema, nephrologist, nephrotic syndrome

Answers to Practical Applications

1. C
2. C
3. B
4. C
5. B
6. A
7. B

XII. Pronunciation of Terms

Pronunciation Guide

ā as in āpe   ă as in ăpple
ē as in ēven   ĕ as in ĕvery
ī as in īce   ĭ as in ĭnterest
ō as in ōpen   ŏ as in pŏt
ū as in ūnit   ŭ as in ŭnder

To test your understanding of the terminology in this chapter, write the meaning of each term in the space provided. In addition, you may wish to cover the terms and write them by looking at your definitions. Make sure your spelling is correct. The page number after each term indicates where it is defined or used in the text so you can easily check your responses.

Term	Pronunciation	Meaning
abscess (229)	ĂB-sĕs	
acetone (226)	ĂS-ĕ-tōn	
albuminuria (224)	ăl-bū-mĭ-NŪ-rē-ă	
antidiuretic hormone (225)	ăn-tĭ-dī-ū-RĔ-tĭk HŎR-mōn	
anuria (225)	ăn-Ū-rē-ă	
azotemia (224)	ă-zō-TĒ-mē-ă	
bacteriuria (224)	băk-tē-rē-Ū-rē-ă	
Bowman capsule (220)	BŌ-măn KĂP-sŭl	
caliceal (221)	kā-lĭ-SĒ-ăl	
caliectasis (221)	kā-lē-ĔK-tă-sĭs	
calyx (calix); calyces (calices) (220)	KĀ-lĭks; KĀ-lĭ-sēz	
catheter (220)	KĂ-thĕ-tĕr	
cortex (220)	KŎR-tĕks	
cortical (220)	KŎR-tĭ-kăl	
creatinine (220)	krē-ĂT-ĭ-nēn	
cystectomy (222)	sĭs-TĔK-tō-mē	
cystitis (222)	sĭs-TĪ-tĭs	
cystoscopy (232)	sĭs-TŎS-kō-pē	
cystostomy (222)	sĭs-TŎS-tō-mē	
diabetes insipidus (229)	dī-ă-BĒ-tēz ĭn-SĬP-ĭ-dŭs	

diabetes mellitus (230)	dī-ă-BĒ-tēz MĔL-ĭ-tŭs	
diuresis (225)	dī-ūr-RĒ-sĭs	
dysuria (225)	dĭs-Ū-rē-ă	
edema (228)	ĕ-DĒ-mă	
electrolyte (220)	ē-LĔK-trō-līt	
enuresis (225)	ĕn-ū-RĒ-sĭs	
erythropoietin (220)	ĕ-rĭth-rō-PŌ-ĭ-tĭn	
essential hypertension (229)	ĕ-SĔN-shŭl hī-pĕr-TĒN-shŭn	
filtration (220)	fĭl-TRĀ-shŭn	
glomerular (222)	glō-MĔR-ū-lăr	
glomerulonephritis (227)	glō-mĕr-ū-lō-nĕ-FRĪ-tĭs	
glomerulus; glomeruli (220)	glō-MĔR-ū-lŭs; glō-MĔR-ū-lī	
glycosuria (226)	glī-kōs-Ū-rē-ă	
hematuria (225)	hēm-ă-TŪ-rē-ă	
hemodialysis (232)	hē-mō-dī-ĂL-ĭ-sĭs	
hilum (220)	HĪ-lŭm	
hydronephrosis (222)	hī-drō-nĕ-FRŌ-sĭs	
interstitial nephritis (228)	ĭn-tĕr-STĬ-shŭl nĕ-FRĪ-tĭs	
intravenous pyelogram (230)	ĭn-tră-VĒ-nŭs PĪ-ĕl-ō-grăm	
ketonuria (224)	kē-tōn-Ū-rē-ă	
ketosis (224)	kē-TŌ-sĭs	
lithotripsy (225)	LĬTH-ō-trĭp-sē	
meatal stenosis (222)	mē-Ā-tăl stĕ-NŌ-sĭs	
meatotomy (222)	mē-ā-TŎT-ō-mē	
meatus (220)	mē-Ā-tŭs	
medulla (220)	mĕ-DŪL-ă or mĕ-DŬL-ă	
medullary (220)	MĔD-ū-lăr-ē	

micturition (220)	mĭk-tū-RĬSH-ŭn	_____
nephrolithiasis (228)	nĕf-rō-lĭ-THĪ-ă-sĭs	_____
nephrolithotomy (222)	nĕf-rō-lĭ-THŎT-ō-mē	_____
nephron (220)	NĔF-rŏn	_____
nephropathy (222)	nĕ-FRŎ-pă-thē	_____
nephroptosis (222)	nĕf-rŏp-TŌ-sĭs	_____
nephrosclerosis (222)	nĕf-rō-sklĕ-RŌ-sĭs	_____
nephrostomy (223)	nĕ-FRŎS-tō-mē	_____
nephrotic syndrome (228)	nĕ-FRŎT-ĭk SĬN-drōm	_____
nitrogenous waste (220)	nĭ-TRŎJ-ĕ-nŭs wāst	_____
nocturia (225)	nŏk-TŪ-rē-ă	_____
oliguria (225)	ŏl-ĭ-GŪ-rē-ă	_____
paranephric (222)	pă-ră-NĔF-rĭk	_____
peritoneal dialysis (232)	pĕr-ĭ-tō-NĒ-ăl dī-ĂL-ĭ-sĭs	_____
perivesical (224)	pĕ-rē-VĔS-ĭ-kăl	_____
phenylketonuria (227)	fē-nĭl-kē-tō-NŪ-rē-ă or fĕn-ĭl-kē-tō-NŪ-rē-ă	_____
polycystic kidneys (228)	pŏl-ē-SĬS-tĭk KĬD-nēz	_____
polydipsia (224)	pŏl-ē-DĬP-sē-ā	_____
polyuria (226)	pŏl-ē-Ū-rē-ă	_____
potassium (220)	pō-TĂ-sē-ŭm	_____
pyelogram (223)	PĪ-ĕ-lo-grăm	_____
pyelolithotomy (223)	pī-ĕ-lō-lĭ-THŎT-ō-mē	_____
pyelonephritis (229)	pī-ĕ-lō-nĕf-RĪ-tĭs	_____
pyuria (225)	pī-Ū-rē-ă	_____
reabsorption (221)	rē-ăb-SŎRP-shŭn	_____
renal angiography (231)	RĒ-năl ăn-jē-ŎG-ră-fē	_____
renal angioplasty (234)	RĒ-năl ĂN-jē-ō-plăs-tē	_____

renal artery (221)	RĒ-năl ĂR-tĕ-rē	
renal calculi (228)	RĒ-năl KĂL-kū-lī	
renal cell carcinoma (229)	RĒ-năl sĕl kăr-sĭ-NŌ-mă	
renal colic (223)	RĒ-năl KŎL-ĭk	
renal failure (229)	RĒ-năl FĀL-ŭr	
renal hypertension (229)	RĒ-năl hī-pĕr-TĔN-shŭn	
renal ischemia (223)	RĒ-năl ĭs-KĒ-mē-ă	
renal pelvis (221)	RĒ-năl PĔL-vĭs	
renal transplantation (234)	RĒ-năl trăns-plăn-TĀ-shŭn	
renal tubule (221)	RĒ-năl TŪ-būl	
renin (221)	RĒ-nĭn	
retrograde pyelogram (231)	RĔ-trō-grād PĪ-ĕ-lō-grăm	
secondary hypertension (229)	SĔ-kŏn-dă-rē hī-pĕr-TĔN-shŭn	
sodium (221)	SŌ-dē-ŭm	
stricture (224)	STRĬK-shŭr	
trigone (221)	TRĪ-gōn	
trigonitis (223)	trī-gō-NĪ-tĭs	
urea (221)	ū-RĒ-ă	
uremia (225)	ū-RĒ-mē-ă	
ureter (221)	ū-RĒ-tĕr or ŪR-ĕ-tĕr	
ureteroileostomy (224)	ū-rē-tĕr-ō-ĭl-ē-ŎS-tō-mē	
ureterolithotomy (224)	ū-rē-tĕr-ō-lĭ-THŎT-ō-mē	
ureteroneocystostomy (234)	ū-rē-tĕr-ō-nē-ō-sĭs-TŎS-tō-mē	
ureteroplasty (224)	ū-rē-tĕr-ō-PLĂS-tē	
urethra (221)	ū-RĒ-thră	
urethral stricture (224)	ū-RĒ-thrăl STRĬK-shŭr	
urethritis (224)	ū-rē-THRĪ-tĭs	

urethroplasty (224)   ū-rē-thrō-PLĂS-tē   _____

uric acid (221)   Ū-rĭk ĀS-ĭd   _____

urinalysis (226)   ū-rĭn-ĂL-ĭ-sĭs   _____

urinary bladder (221)   ŬR-ĭ-năr-ē BLĂ-dĕr   _____

urinary catheterization (235)   ŬR-ĭ-năr-ē kă-thĕ-tĕr-ĭ-ZĀ-shŭn   _____

urinary incontinence (225)   ŬR-ĭ-năr-ē ĭn-KŎN-tĭ-nĕns   _____

urinary retention (225)   ŬR-ĭ-năr-ē rē-TĔN-shŭn   _____

urination (221)   ŭr-ĭ-NĀ-shŭn   _____

vesicoureteral reflux (224)   vĕs-ĭ-kō-ū-RĒ-tĕr-ăl RĒ-flŭks   _____

voiding (221)   VOY-dĭng   _____

voiding
cystourethrogram (231)   VOY-dĭng
sĭs-tō-ū-RĒ-thrō-grăm   _____

Wilms tumor (229)   wĭlmz TŪ-mŭr   _____

XIII. Review Sheet

Write the meanings of the combining forms, suffixes, and prefixes in the spaces provided. Check your answers with the information in the chapter or in the glossary (Medical Terms—English) at the end of the book.

COMBINING FORMS

Combining Form	Meaning	Combining Form	Meaning
albumin/o		meat/o	
angi/o		necr/o	
arteri/o		nephr/o	
azot/o		noct/i	
bacteri/o		olig/o	
cali/o		py/o	
calic/o		pyel/o	
cyst/o		ren/o	
dips/o		tom/o	
glomerul/o		tox/o	
glyc/o		trigon/o	
glycos/o		ur/o	
hydr/o		ureter/o	
isch/o		urethr/o	
ket/o		urin/o	
keton/o		vesic/o	
lith/o			

SUFFIXES

Suffix	Meaning	Suffix	Meaning
-ectasis		-rrhea	
-emia		-sclerosis	
-lithiasis		-spasm	
-lithotomy		-stenosis	
-lysis		-stomy	
-megaly		-tomy	
-ole		-tripsy	
-plasty		-trophy	
-poietin		-ule	
-ptosis		-uria	
-rrhaphy			

PREFIXES

Prefix	Meaning	Prefix	Meaning
a-, an-		en-	
anti-		peri-	
dia-		poly-	
dys-		retro-	

Continued on following page

REVIEW OF ANATOMICAL TERMS

Match the number of the urinary system structure in column I with its location or function in column II.

Column I

Tiny structure surrounding each glomerulus; receives filtered _____ materials from blood.

Tubes carrying urine from kidney to urinary bladder. _____

Tubules leading from the Bowman capsule. Urine is formed _____ there as water, sugar, and salts are reabsorbed into the bloodstream.

Inner (middle) region of the kidney. _____

Muscular sac that serves as a reservoir for urine. _____

Cup-like divisions of the renal pelvis that receive urine from _____ the renal tubules.

Tube carrying urine from the bladder to the outside of the _____ body.

Central urine-collecting basin in the kidney that narrows into _____ the ureter.

Collection of capillaries through which materials from the _____ blood are filtered into the Bowman capsule.

Outer region of the kidney. _____

Column II

1. urethra
2. cortex
3. Bowman capsule
4. calices
5. renal pelvis
6. glomerulus
7. medulla
8. renal tubules
9. urinary bladder
10. ureters

chapter

Female Reproductive System

This chapter is divided into the following sections

In this chapter you will

- Name the organs of the female reproductive system, their locations, and combining forms.
- Explain how these organs and their hormones function in the processes of menstruation and pregnancy.
- Identify abnormal conditions of the female reproductive system and of the newborn child.
- Explain important laboratory tests, clinical procedures, and abbreviations related to gynecology and obstetrics.
- Apply your new knowledge to understanding medical terms in their proper contexts, such as medical reports and records.

I. Introduction

Sexual reproduction is the union of the nuclei of the female sex cell **(ovum)** and the male sex cell **(sperm cell)** that results in the creation of a new individual. The ovum and sperm cell are specialized cells differing primarily from normal body cells in one important way. Each sex cell (also called a **gamete**) contains exactly half the number of chromosomes of a normal body cell. When the nuclei of ovum and sperm cell unite, the cell produced receives half of its genetic material from its female parent and half from its male parent; thus it contains a full, normal complement of hereditary material.

Gametes are produced in special organs called **gonads** in both males and females. The female gonads are the **ovaries,** and the male gonads are the **testes.** After an ovum leaves the ovary, it travels down a duct **(fallopian tube)** leading to the **uterus** (womb). If **coitus** (copulation, sexual intercourse) has occurred, and sperm cells are present in the fallopian tube, union of the ovum and sperm may take place. The union is called **fertilization.** The **embryo** (called the **fetus** after the 2nd month) then begins a 40-week (approximately 9 month) period of development **(gestation, pregnancy)** within the uterus.

The female reproductive system consists of organs that produce **ova** and provide a place for the growth of the embryo. In addition, the female reproductive organs supply important hormones that contribute to the development of female secondary sex characteristics (body hair, breast development, structural changes in bones and fat).

Ova mature and are released from the ovary from the onset of **puberty** (beginning of the fertile period when secondary sex characteristics develop) to **menopause** (cessation of fertility and diminishing of hormone production). Women are born with all the eggs that they will possibly release. However, it is not until the onset of puberty that the eggs mature and start to leave the ovary. If fertilization occurs at any time during the years between puberty and menopause, the fertilized egg may grow and develop within the uterus. Various hormones are secreted from the ovary and from a blood-vessel–filled organ **(placenta)** that grows in the wall of the uterus during pregnancy. The placenta provides nutrition and oxygen to the growing embryo. If fertilization does not occur, hormone changes result in shedding of the uterine lining, and bleeding, or **menstruation,** occurs.

The hormones of the ovaries, **estrogen** and **progesterone**, play important roles in the processes of menstruation and pregnancy, and in the development of secondary sex characteristics. The **pituitary gland**, located at the base of the brain, secretes other hormones that govern the functions of the ovaries, breasts, and uterus.

Gynecology is the study of the female reproductive system (organs, hormones, and diseases); **obstetrics** (*obstetrix* means "midwife") is a specialty concerned with pregnancy and the delivery of the fetus; and **neonatology** is the study and treatment of the newborn child.

II. Organs of the Female Reproductive System

Uterus, Ovaries, and Associated Organs

Label Figures 8–1 and 8–3 as you read the following text.

Figure 8–1 is a side view of the female reproductive organs and shows their relationship to the other organs in the pelvic cavity. The **ovaries** [1] (only one ovary shown in this lateral view) are a pair of small, almond-shaped organs located in the pelvis. The **fallopian tubes** [2] (only one shown in this view) lead from each ovary to the **uterus** [3], which is a muscular organ situated between the urinary bladder and the rectum. The uterus normally rests in a bent-forward position and about 3 inches long in a nonpregnant woman. Midway between the uterus and the rectum is a region in the abdominal cavity known as the **cul-de-sac** [4]. Physicians often examine this region for the presence of cancerous growths.

The **vagina** [5] is a tube extending from the uterus to the exterior of the body. **Bartholin glands** [6] are two small, rounded glands on either side of the vaginal orifice. These glands produce a mucous secretion that lubricates the vagina. The **clitoris** [7] is an organ of sensitive, erectile tissue located anterior to the vaginal orifice and in front of the urethral meatus.

The region between the vaginal orifice and the anus is the **perineum** [8]. The perineum can be torn in childbirth and cause injury to the anal sphincter. To avoid a perineal tear, the obstetrician often deliberately cuts the perineum obliquely (on a slant) before delivery. This incision is an **episiotomy.** The perineum can be easily sewn together (repaired) after childbirth.

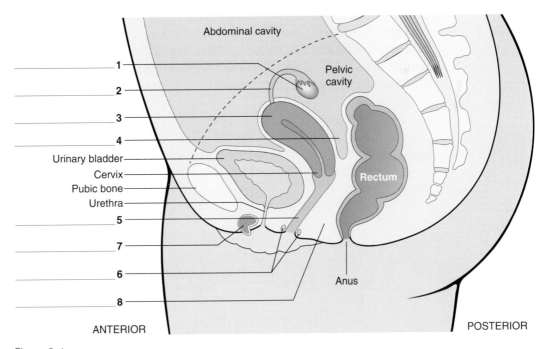

Figure 8–1

Organs of the female reproductive system, lateral view.

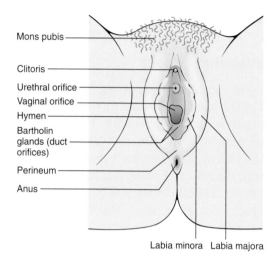

Figure 8–2

Female external genitalia (vulva). The *mons* pubis (L. *mons*, mountain) is a pad of tissue overlying the pubic symphysis. After puberty it is covered with pubic hair.

The external genitalia (organs of reproduction) of the female are collectively called the **vulva.** Figure 8–2 shows the various structures that are part of the vulva. The **labia majora,** the outer lips of the vagina, surround the smaller, inner lips, which are the **labia minora.** The **hymen** is a mucous membrane partially covering the entrance to the vagina. The clitoris and Bartholin glands are also parts of the vulva.

Figure 8–3 is an anterior view of the female reproductive system. Each **ovary** [1] is held in place on either side of the uterus by a **utero-ovarian ligament** [2].

There are thousands of small sacs called **graafian follicles** [3] within each ovary. Each graafian follicle contains an **ovum** [4]. When an ovum matures, its graafian follicle ruptures through the surface and releases the ovum from the ovary. This is **ovulation.** A ruptured follicle fills first with blood and then with a yellow, fat-like material. It is then the **corpus luteum** [5] meaning yellow body. The corpus luteum secretes hormones to maintain the very first stages of pregnancy.

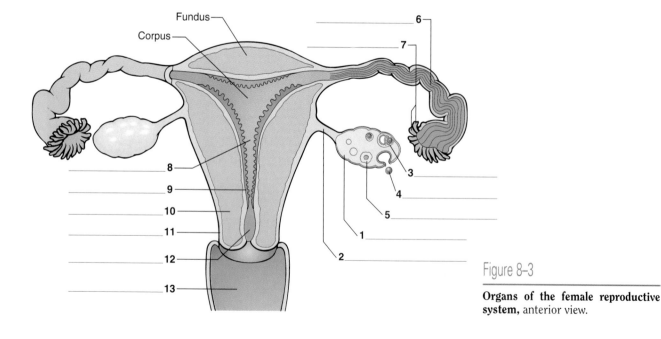

Figure 8–3

Organs of the female reproductive system, anterior view.

A fallopian tube [6], is about 5½ inches long and lies near each ovary. Collectively, the fallopian tubes, ovaries, and supporting ligaments are the **adnexa** (accessory structures) of the uterus. The egg, after its release from the ovary, is caught up by the finger-like ends of the fallopian tube. These ends are the **fimbriae** [7]. The tube itself is lined with cilia (small hairs) that, through their motion, sweep the ovum along. It usually takes the ovum about 5 days to pass through the fallopian tube.

If sperm cells are present in the fallopian tube, fertilization may occur. If sperm cells are not present, the ovum remains unfertilized and eventually disintegrates.

The fallopian tubes, one on either side, lead into the **uterus** [8], a pear-shaped organ with muscular walls and a mucous membrane lining filled with a rich supply of blood vessels. The rounded upper portion of the uterus is the **fundus,** and the larger, central section is the **corpus** (body of the organ). The specialized epithelial mucosa of the uterus is the **endometrium** [9]; the middle, muscular layer is the **myometrium** [10]; and the outer, membranous tissue layer is the **uterine serosa** [11]. The outermost layer of an organ in the abdomen or thorax is known as a serosa.

The narrow, lower portion of the uterus is the **cervix** [12], which means neck. The cervical opening leads into a 3-inch-long tube called the **vagina** [13], which opens to the outside of the body.

The Breast (Accessory Organ of Reproduction)

Label Figure 8–4 as you read the following description of breast structures.

The breasts are two **mammary glands** located in the upper anterior region of the chest. The **glandular tissue** [1] contains milk glands that develop in response to hormones from the ovaries during puberty. The breasts also contain **fibrous** and **fatty tissue** [2], special **lactiferous** (milk-carrying) **ducts** [3], and **sinuses** (cavities) [4] that carry milk to the opening, or nipple. The breast nipple is the **mammary papilla** [5], and the dark-pigmented area around the mammary papilla is the **areola** [6].

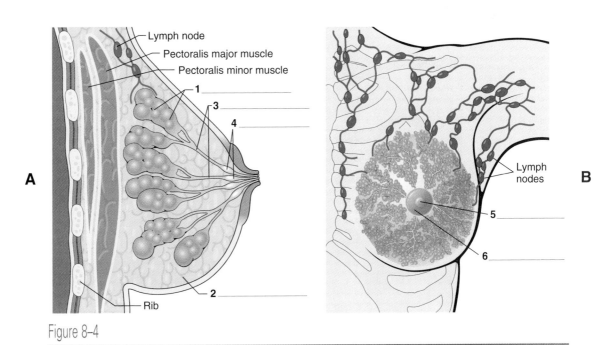

Figure 8–4

Views of the breast. (A) Sagittal. **(B)** Frontal. Notice the numerous lymph nodes.

During pregnancy, the hormones from the ovaries and the placenta stimulate glandular tissues in the breasts to their full development. After **parturition** (giving birth), hormones from the pituitary gland stimulate the production of milk **(lactation).**

III. Menstruation and Pregnancy

Menstrual Cycle (Fig. 8–5)

Menarche, or the first menstrual cycle, occurs at the onset of puberty. Each menstrual cycle lasts for 28 days. These days can be divided into four time periods, useful in describing the events of the cycle. The approximate time periods are:

Days 1-5 (menstrual period)   Discharge of bloody fluid containing disintegrated endometrial cells, glandular secretions, and blood cells.

Days 6-12   After bleeding ceases, the endometrium begins to repair itself. The maturing graafian follicle in the ovaries releases **estrogen,** which aids in the repair. The ovum grows in the graafian follicle during this period.

Days 13-14 (ovulatory period)   On about the 14th day of the cycle, the graafian follicle ruptures **(ovulation)** and the egg leaves the ovary, passing through the fallopian tube.

Days 15-28   The empty graafian follicle fills with a yellow material and is now the **corpus luteum.** The corpus luteum functions as an endocrine organ and secretes two hormones, **estrogen** and **progesterone,** into the bloodstream. These hormones

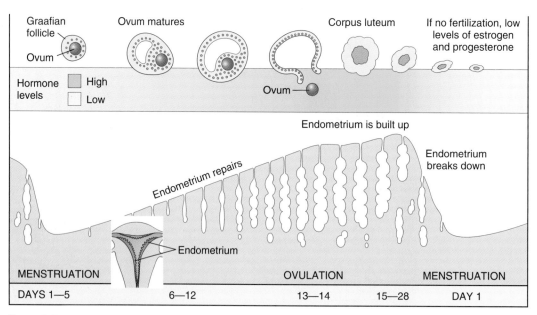

Figure 8–5

The menstrual cycle.

stimulate the building up of the lining of the uterus in anticipation of fertilization of the egg and pregnancy.

If fertilization does *not* occur, the corpus luteum in the ovary stops producing progesterone and estrogen and regresses. At this time, because of the lowered levels of progesterone and estrogen, some women have symptoms of depression, breast tenderness, and irritability before menstruation. These symptoms are known as **premenstrual syndrome (PMS).** About 5 days after the decrease in hormones, the uterine endometrium breaks down and the menstrual period begins (days 1-5).

Note: Cycles vary from 21 days to as long as 42 or longer. Ovulation occurs exactly 14 days before the end of the cycle. So, a person with a 42-day cycle ovulates on day 28, while a woman with a 21-day cycle ovulates on day 7.

Pregnancy

If fertilization does occur in the fallopian tube, the fertilized egg travels to the uterus and implants in the uterine endometrium. The corpus luteum in the ovary continues to produce progesterone and estrogen. This supports the vascular and muscular development of the uterine lining.

The **placenta,** a vascular organ, now forms within the uterine wall. The placenta is derived from maternal endometrium and from the **chorion,** the outermost membrane that surrounds the developing embryo. The **amnion,** the innermost of the embryonic membranes, holds the fetus suspended in an amniotic cavity surrounded by a fluid called the **amniotic fluid.** The amnion and fluid are sometimes known as the "bag or sac of water," which ruptures (breaks) during labor.

The maternal blood and the fetal blood never mix during pregnancy, but important nutrients, oxygen, and wastes are exchanged as the blood vessels of the baby (coming from the umbilical cord) lie side by side with the mother's blood vessels in the placenta. Figure 8–6A and B shows the embryo's implantation in the uterus and its relationship to the placenta and enveloping membranes (chorion and amnion).

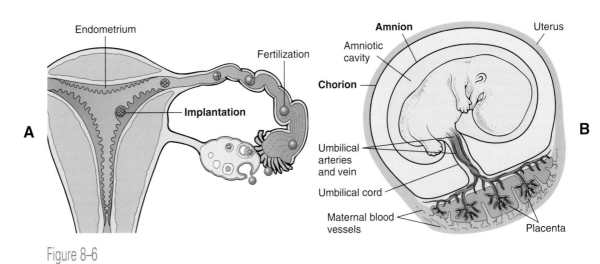

Figure 8–6

(A) Implantation of the embryo in the endometrium. (B) The placenta and membranes (**chorion** and **amnion**).

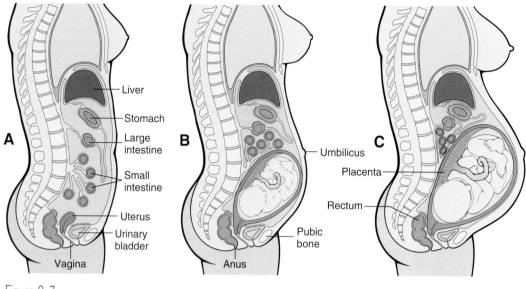

Figure 8–7

Sagittal sections of pregnancy. (A) Nonpregnant woman. **(B)** Woman 20 weeks pregnant. **(C)** Woman 30 weeks pregnant.

As the placenta develops in the uterus, it produces its own hormone, **human chorionic gonadotropin (HCG).** When women test their urine with a pregnancy test, HCG confirms or denies that they are pregnant. HCG stimulates the corpus luteum to continue producing hormones until about the third month of pregnancy, when the placenta takes over the endocrine function and releases estrogen and progesterone. Progesterone maintains the development of the placenta. Low levels of progesterone can lead to spontaneous abortion in pregnant women and menstrual irregularities in nonpregnant women.

The uterus normally lies in the pelvis. During pregnancy, the uterus expands as the fetus grows, and the superior part rises out of the pelvic cavity. By about 28 to 30 weeks, it occupies a large part of the abdominopelvic cavity and reaches the epigastric region (Fig. 8–7).

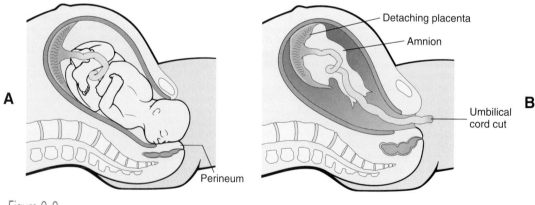

Figure 8–8

(A) Cephalic presentation ("crowning") of the fetus during delivery from the vaginal (birth) canal. **(B)** Between 10 and 15 minutes after the parturition (birth), the placenta separates from the uterine wall. Forceful contractions expel the placenta and attached membranes, also called the afterbirth. The three phases of labor are: (I) dilation of the cervix, (II) expulsion or birth of the infant, and (III) delivery of the placenta.

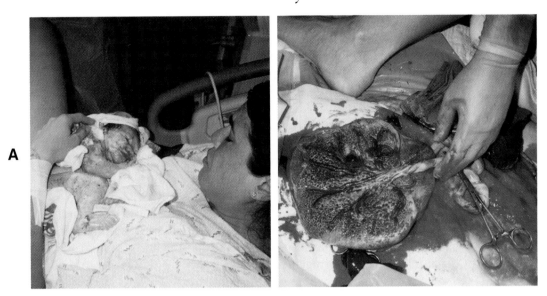

Figure 8-9

(A) My newborn grandaughter, Beatrix Bess (Bebe) Thompson, and her mother, Dr. Elizabeth Chabner Thompson, minutes after Bebe's birth. Notice that Bebe's skin is covered with vernix caseosa, a mixture of a fatty secretion from fetal sebaceous (oil) glands and dead skin. The vernix protects the fetus' delicate skin from abrasions, chapping, and hardening as a result of being bathed in amniotic fluid. **(B)** The placenta and umbilical cord just after expulsion from the uterus.

The onset of true labor is marked by rhythmic contractions, dilation of the cervix, and a discharge of bloody mucus from the cervix and vagina ("show"). In a normal delivery position, the head appears first (cephalic presentation) and helps to dilate the cervix. After vaginal delivery of the baby, the placenta follows and the physician (or family member) cuts the umbilical cord (Fig. 8–8). Figure 8–9A and B shows photographs of a newborn and its placenta with attached cord, minutes after birth. The expelled placenta is the **afterbirth.**

IV. Hormonal Interactions

The events of menstruation and pregnancy depend not only on hormones from the ovaries (estrogen and progesterone) but also on hormones from the **pituitary gland.** The pituitary gland secretes **follicle-stimulating hormone (FSH)** and **luteinizing hormone (LH)** after the onset of menstruation. As their levels rise in the bloodstream, FSH and LH stimulate maturation of the ovum and ovulation. After ovulation, LH in particular influences the maintenance of the corpus luteum and its production of estrogen and progesterone.

During pregnancy, the high levels of estrogen and progesterone cause the pituitary gland to stop producing FSH and LH. Therefore, while a woman is pregnant, additional eggs do not mature and ovulation cannot occur. This hormonal interaction wherein a high level of hormones (estrogen and progesterone) shuts off production of another set of hormones (FSH and LH) is **negative feedback.** Oral contraceptive (birth control pills) work by negative feedback. The pills contain varying amounts of estrogen and progesterone. When taken, the level of hormones rises in the blood. Negative feedback occurs, and the pituitary does not release FSH or LH. Without FSH or LH, ovulation and pregnancy do not occur. Subdermal implants containing estrogen and progesterone are effective for up to 5 years. The most common device is called Norplant.

Other female contraceptive measures include the **IUD (intrauterine device)** and the **diaphragm.** A physician inserts the IUD, a small coil inside the uterus. It prevents implantation of the fertilized egg. Use of the IUD carries risks, including ectopic uterine pregnancy, infection, uterine perforation, and painful menstrual flow. The diaphragm, a rubber, cup-shaped device inserted, before coitus, covers the cervix to prevent the entrance of sperm into the uterus.

When all the ova are used up and secretion of estrogen from the ovaries lessens, **menopause** begins. Menopause signals the gradual ending of the menstrual cycle. Premature menopause occurs before age 35, whereas delayed menopause occurs after age 58. Artificial menopause occurs if the ovaries are removed by surgery or made nonfunctional by radiation therapy or by forms of chemotherapy.

During menopause, when estrogen levels fall, the most common symptoms are hot flashes (temperature regulation in the brain is disturbed), insomnia, and vaginal atrophy (lining of the vagina dries and thins, predisposing it to irritation and discomfort during sexual intercourse). **Estrogen replacement therapy (ERT),** given orally or as a transdermal patch, relieves the symptoms of menopause and delays the development of weak bones (osteoporosis). ERT use is associated with an increased risk of breast cancer, stroke, or heart attack. It should be used only after careful consideration of potential risks and benefits.

V. Vocabulary

This list reviews many of the new terms introduced in the text. Short definitions reinforce your understanding of the terms. See Section XII of this chapter for pronunciation of more difficult terms.

adnexa uteri	Fallopian tubes, ovaries, and supporting ligaments.
amnion	Innermost membrane around the developing embryo.
areola	Dark-pigmented area around the breast nipple.
Bartholin glands	Small exocrine glands at the vaginal orifice.
cervix	Lower, neck-like portion of the uterus.
chorion	Outermost layer of the two membranes surrounding the embryo; it is part of the placenta.
clitoris	Organ of sensitive erectile tissue anterior to the urinary meatus.
coitus	Sexual intercourse; copulation. Pronunciation is KŌ-ĭ-tus.
corpus luteum	Empty graafian follicle that secretes estrogen and progesterone after release of the egg cell; literally means yellow (luteum) body (corpus).
cul-de-sac	Region within the pelvis, midway between the rectum and the uterus.
embryo	Stage in prenatal development from implantation of the fertilized ovum until the second month of pregnancy.

endometrium	Inner mucous membrane lining the uterus.
estrogen	Hormone produced by the ovaries; responsible for promoting female secondary sex characteristics.
fallopian tube	One of a pair of ducts through which the ovum travels to the uterus.
fertilization	Union of the sperm cell and ovum from which the embryo develops.
fetus	Embryo from the eighth week after fertilization until birth.
fimbriae (plural)	Finger-like projections at the end of the fallopian tubes.
follicle-stimulating hormone (FSH)	Hormone produced by the pituitary gland; stimulates maturation of the ovum.
gamete	Male or female sexual reproductive cell; sperm cell or ovum.
genitalia	Reproductive organs; also called genitals.
gestation	Period from fertilization of the ovum to birth; pregnancy.
gonad	Organ in the male (testis) and female (ovary) that produces gametes.
graafian follicle	Developing sac enclosing each ovum within the ovary. Only about 400 of these sacs mature in a woman's lifetime.
gynecology	Study of the female reproductive organs including the breasts.
human chorionic gonadotropin (HCG)	Hormone produced by the placenta to sustain pregnancy by stimulating (-tropin) the mother's ovaries to produce estrogen and progesterone.
hymen	Mucous membrane partially or completely covering the vaginal orifice.
labia	Lips of the vagina; labia majora are the larger, outermost lips, and labia minora are the smaller, innermost lips.
lactiferous ducts	Tubes that carry milk within the breast.
luteinizing hormone (LH)	Hormone produced by the pituitary gland; promotes ovulation.
mammary papilla	Nipple of the breast. A papilla is any small nipple-shaped projection.
menarche	Beginning of the first menstrual period during puberty.
menopause	Gradual ending of menstruation.
menstruation	Monthly shedding of the uterine lining. Menses (Latin, *mens,* month) is the normal flow of blood and tissue that occurs during menstruation.
myometrium	Muscle layer lining the uterus.

neonatology	Branch of medicine that concentrates on the care of the newborn (neonate).
obstetrics	Branch of medicine concerned with pregnancy and childbirth.
orifice	An opening.
ovary	One of a pair of female organs (gonads) on each side of the pelvis. Ovaries are almond-shaped, about the size of large walnuts, and produce egg cells (ova) and hormones.
ovulation	Release of the ovum from the ovary.
ovum (plural: **ova**)	Egg cell; female gamete.
parturition	Act of giving birth.
perineum	In females, the area between the anus and the vagina.
pituitary gland	Endocrine gland at the base of the brain. It produces hormones to stimulate the ovaries.
placenta	Vascular organ that develops during pregnancy in the uterine wall. It is a communication between maternal and fetal bloodstreams.
pregnancy	Growth and developmental process in a woman from fertilization through embryonic and fetal periods to birth; gestation.
progesterone	Hormone produced by the corpus luteum in the ovary and the placenta of pregnant women.
puberty	Period of life when the ability to reproduce begins; secondary sex characteristics appear and gametes are produced.
uterine serosa	Outermost layer surrounding the uterus.
uterus	Hollow, pear-shaped muscular female organ in which the embryo develops and from which menstruation occurs. The upper portion is the fundus; the middle portion is the corpus; and the lower, neck portion is the cervix (see Fig. 8–3).
vagina	Tube extending from the uterus to the exterior of the body.
vulva	External genitalia of the female; includes the labia, hymen, and clitoris.

VI. Terminology: Combining Forms, Suffixes, and Prefixes

Write the meanings of the medical terms in the spaces provided.

Combining Forms

Combining Form	Meaning	Terminology	Meaning
amni/o	amnion	amniocentesis	
		amniotic fluid	
		Produced by fetal membranes and the fetus.	
cervic/o	cervix, neck	endocervicitis	
chori/o **chorion/o**	chorion	choriogenesis	
		chorionic	
colp/o	vagina	colporrhaphy	
		colposcopy	
culd/o	cul-de-sac	culdocentesis	
		Placement of a needle through the posterior wall of the vagina, with withdrawal of fluid for diagnostic purposes.	
episi/o	vulva	episiotomy	
		An incision through the skin of the perineum enlarges the vaginal orifice for delivery.	
galact/o	milk	galactorrhea	
		Abnormal, persistent discharge of milk, commonly seen with pituitary gland tumors.	
gynec/o	woman, female	gynecomastia	
		Enlargement of one or both breasts in a male. It often occurs with puberty, aging, or can be drug related.	

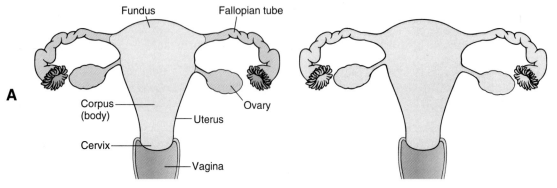

Figure 8–10

(A) Total hysterectomy. The entire uterus (fundus, corpus, and cervix) is removed, but the ovaries and fallopian tubes remain. In a **laparoscopic assisted vaginal hysterectomy**, the abdominal wall remains intact and the surgeon removes the uterus through an incision in the vagina with the aid of a laparoscope. This is called "keyhole surgery." **(B) Total hysterectomy with bilateral salpingo-oophorectomy** (fallopian tubes and ovaries are removed). A radical hysterectomy is removal of the entire uterus, ovaries, fallopian tubes, lymph nodes, and the top half of the vagina.

hyster/o	uterus, womb	hysterectomy _____
		Abdominal: removal through the abdominal wall; vaginal: removal through the vagina. A total abdominal hysterectomy (TAH) is removal of the entire uterus (including the cervix) through an abdominal incision (Fig. 8–10).
		hysteroscopy _____
		A gynecologist uses an endoscope (passed through the vagina) to view the uterine cavity.
lact/o	milk	lactogenesis _____
		lactation _____
		The normal secretion of milk.
mamm/o	breast	mammary _____
		mammoplasty _____
		Includes reduction and augmentation (enlargement) operations.
mast/o	breast	mastitis _____
		Usually caused by streptococcal or staphylococcal infection.
		mastectomy _____
		Mastectomy procedures are discussed under carcinoma of the breast (see page 273, Section VII, Pathology).
men/o	menses, menstruation	amenorrhea _____
		Absence of menses for 6 months or for longer than 3 of the patient's normal menstrual cycles.

dysmenorrhea _____

oligomenorrhea _____

Infrequent or scanty menstrual periods.

menorrhagia _____

Abnormally heavy or long menstrual periods. Fibroids (see page 271, Section VII, Pathology) are a leading cause of menorrhagia.

metr/o   uterus   metrorrhagia _____
metri/o

Uterine bleeding other than caused by menstruation. Possible causes of metrorrhagia include ectopic pregnancy, cervical polyps, and ovarian and uterine tumors.

menometrorrhagia _____

Excessive uterine bleeding at and between menstrual periods.

endometriosis _____

See Section VII, Pathology.

my/o   muscle   myometrium _____

myom/o   muscle tumor myomectomy _____

Removal of fibroids from the uterus.

nat/i   birth   neonatal _____

The first 4 weeks of life after birth.

obstetr/o midwife   obstetric _____

o/o   egg   oogenesis _____

oophor/o ovary   bilateral oophorectomy _____

Oophor/o means to bear (phor/o) eggs (o/o).

ov/o   egg   ovum _____

ovari/o   ovary   ovarian _____

ovul/o   egg   anovulatory _____

perine/o perineum   perineorrhaphy _____

phor/o   to bear   oophoritis _____

salping/o fallopian tubes salpingectomy _____

Figure 8–10B shows a total hysterectomy with bilateral salpingo-oophorectomy.

uter/o	uterus	uterine prolapse _____
vagin/o	vagina	vaginal orifice _____

Orifice means opening.

vaginitis _____

Bacteria and yeast (Candida) commonly cause this infection. Use of antibiotics can change the internal environment (pH) of the vagina and destroy normally occurring bacteria, allowing yeast to grow.

vulv/o	vulva	vulvovaginitis _____

Suffixes

Suffix	Meaning	Terminology	Meaning
-arche	beginning	menarche _____	
-cyesis	pregnancy	pseudocyesis _____	

Pseudo- means false. No pregnancy exists, but symptoms such as weight gain and amenorrhea occur.

-gravida	pregnancy	primigravida _____	

A woman during her first pregnancy (primi- means first). Gravida is also used as a noun to describe a pregnant woman, and it may be followed by numbers to indicate the number of pregnancies (gravida 1, 2, 3).

-parous	to bear, bring forth	primiparous _____	

An adjective describing a woman who has borne (delivered) at least one child. Para is also used as a noun and may be followed by numbers to indicate the number of deliveries after the 20th week of gestation (para 1, 2, 3). When a woman arrives on the labor and delivery floor, her gravidity and parity are important facts to include in her medical and surgical history. For example, a G2 P2 is a woman who has had 2 pregnancies and 2 deliveries.

-rrhea	discharge	leukorrhea _____	

This nonbloody vaginal discharge may be mucoid or purulent (containing pus) and a sign of infection or cervicitis.

menorrhea _____

-salpinx	uterine tube	pyosalpinx _____	
-tocia	labor, birth	dystocia _____	

oxytocia _____

*Oxy- means rapid. The pituitary gland releases **oxytocin,** which stimulates the pregnant uterus to contract (labor begins). It also stimulates milk secretion from mammary glands.*

-version	act of turning	cephalic <u>version</u> _____	

The fetal head turns or is turned toward the cervix. **Fetal presentation** *is the manner in which the fetus appears to the examiner during delivery. A breech presentation is buttocks first or feet first in a footling breech; a cephalic presentation is head first.*

Prefixes			
Prefix	**Meaning**	**Terminology**	**Meaning**
dys-	painful	<u>dys</u>pareunia _____	
		Dĭs-pă-ROO-nē-ă. Pareunia means sexual intercourse.	
endo-	within	<u>endo</u>metritis _____	
		Usually caused by a bacterial infection.	
in-	in	<u>in</u>volution of the uterus _____	
		Vol- means to roll. The uterus returns to its normal nonpregnant size.	
intra-	within	<u>intra</u>uterine device _____	
		Figure 8–11A shows an IUD in place in the uterus.	
multi-	many	<u>multi</u>para _____	
		<u>multi</u>gravida _____	
		A woman who has been pregnant more than once.	
nulli-	no, not, none	<u>nulli</u>gravida _____	
		<u>nulli</u>para _____	

Para 0. Figure 8–11B shows the cervix of a nulliparous woman and the cervix of a parous woman (who has had a vaginal delivery).

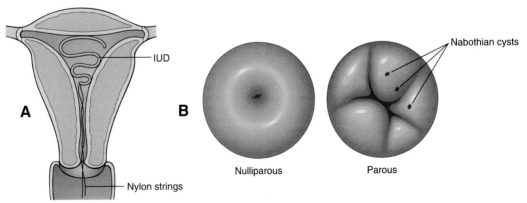

Figure 8–11

(A) Intrauterine device (IUD) to prevent implantation of the fertilized egg. **(B)** The **cervix** of a **nulliparous woman** (the os, or opening, is small and perfectly round) and the **cervix** of a **parous woman** (the os is wide and irregular). Nabothian cysts are normal plugged glands of the cervix, common in women who have borne children. These views would be visible under colposcopic examination.

pre-	before	prenatal _____
primi-	first	primipara _____
retro-	backward	retroversion _____

The uterus is abnormally turned backward.

VII. Pathology: Gynecological/Breast, Pregnancy, Neonatal

Gynecological and Breast

Uterus

carcinoma of the cervix

Malignant cells within the cervix (cervical cancer).

Cervical carcinoma occurs more commonly in women who have sexual intercourse at an early age, multiple sexual partners, a history of sexually transmitted diseases, and evidence of a **human papilloma virus (HPV)** infection. Early neoplastic changes in the cervix vary from **dysplasia** (abnormal cell growth) to **carcinoma *in situ*** (CIS) (localized cancer growth). Pathologists grade these preinvasive neoplastic lesions **cervical intraepithelial neoplasia (CIN)** from I to III as viewed on a **Pap smear** (microscopic examination of cells scraped off the cervical epithelium). Pap smears give important screening information because CIN may be curable with resection. Further biopsy and resection **(conization)** may be necessary to diagnose and treat CIS. Surgery (hysterectomy) and radiation therapy combined with chemotherapy treat more extensive and metastatic disease.

cervicitis

Inflammation of the cervix.

This condition can become chronic because the lining of the cervix is not renewed each month as is the uterine lining during menstruation.

Bacteria, such as *Chlamydia trachomatis* and *Neisseria gonorrhoeae* commonly affect the cervix. Acute cervicitis, marked by **cervical erosions,** or ulcers, appears as raw, red patches on the cervical mucosa. **Leukorrhea** (clear, white, or yellow pus-filled vaginal discharge) is also a symptom of cervical erosion.

After excluding the presence of malignancy (by Pap smear or biopsy), **cryocauterization** (destroying tissue by freezing) of the eroded area and treatment with antibiotics may be indicated.

carcinoma of the endometrium (endometrial cancer)

Malignant tumor of the uterus (adenocarcinoma).

The major symptom of endometrial cancer (the most common gynecological tumor) is postmenopausal bleeding. The malignancy occurs more often in women exposed to high levels of estrogen from exogenous estrogen (pills), estrogen-producing tumors, or obesity (estrogen is produced by fat tissue) and in nulliparous women. Physicians perform **dilation** (opening the cervical canal) and **curettage** (scraping the inner lining of the uterus) to diagnose the disease. When confined to the uterus, surgery (hysterectomy) can cure the disease. Radiation oncologists administer radiation therapy for patients with more advanced disease.

endometriosis

Endometrial tissue is found in abnormal locations, including the ovaries, fallopian tubes, supporting ligaments, or small intestine.

Abnormal growth of the endometrium produces scar tissue, which causes dysmenorrhea, pelvic pain, infertility (inability to become pregnant), and dyspareunia. Most cases develop as a result of bits of menstrual endometrium that pass backward through the **lumen** (opening) of the fallopian tube and into the peritoneal cavity. Often, when disease affects the ovaries, large blood-filled cysts, called chocolate cysts, develop. Treatment ranges from symptomatic relief of pain and drugs that suppress the menstrual cycle to surgical removal of ectopic endometrial tissue and hysterectomy.

fibroids

Benign tumors in the uterus.

Fibroids, also called **leiomyomata** or **leiomyomas** (lei/o = smooth, my/o = muscle, and -oma = tumor), are composed of fibrous tissue and muscle. If fibroids grow too large and cause symptoms such as metrorrhagia, pelvic pain, or menorrhagia, hysterectomy or myomectomy is indicated. Figure 8–12 shows the location of uterine fibroids.

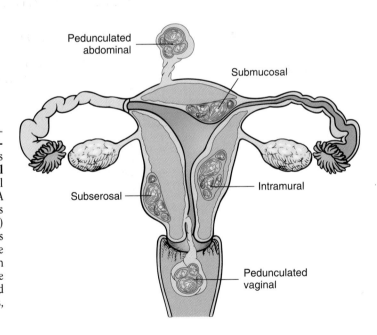

Figure 8–12

Location of uterine fibroids (leiomyomas). Pedunculated growths protrude on stalks. A **subserosal** mass lies under the serosal (outermost) layer of the uterus. A **submucosal** leiomyoma grows under the mucosal (innermost) layer. **Intramural** (mural means wall) masses arise within the muscular uterine wall. (From Damjanov I: Pathology for the Health-Related Professions, 2nd ed. Philadelphia, WB Saunders, 2000, p. 376.)

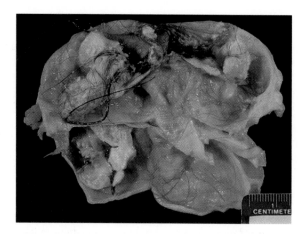

Figure 8-13

Dermoid cyst of the ovary with hair, skin, and teeth. (Courtesy Dr. Elizabeth Chabner Thompson.)

Ovaries

ovarian carcinoma

Malignant tumor of the ovary (adenocarcinoma).

Carcinomas of the ovary account for more deaths than those of cancers of the cervix or the uterus together. The tumor, which may be cystic or solid in consistency, is usually discovered in an advanced stage as an abdominal mass and may produce few symptoms in its early stages. In most patients, the disease metastasizes within or beyond the pelvic region before diagnosis. Surgery (oophorectomy and salpingectomy), and chemotherapy are used as therapeutic measures.

ovarian cysts

Collections of fluid within a sac (cyst) in the ovary.

Some cysts are lined by cells that are typical, normal lining cells of the ovary. These cysts originate in unruptured graafian follicles (follicle cysts) or in follicles that have ruptured and have immediately been sealed (luteal cysts). Other cysts may be lined with tumor cells (**cystadenomas** and **cystadenocarcinomas**). Physicians decide to remove these cysts to distinguish between benign and malignant tumors.

Dermoid cysts are lined with a variety of cell types, including skin, hair, teeth, and cartilage, and arise from immature egg cells in the ovary. Because of the strange assortment of tissue in the tumor (Fig. 8–13), these cysts are often called benign cystic teratomas (terat/o = monster). Surgical removal cures this condition.

Fallopian Tubes

pelvic inflammatory disease (PID)

Inflammation in the pelvic region; salpingitis.

The leading causes of PID are gonorrhea and chlamydia (sexually transmitted infections or STIs). They often occur at the same time, and repetitive episodes of these infections can lead to adhesions and scarring within the fallopian tubes. After PID, women have increased risk of ectopic pregnancies and difficulty getting pregnant. Symptoms include vaginal discharge, pain in the abdomen (LLQ and RLQ), fever, and tenderness on **palpation** (examining by touch) of the cervix. Antibiotics are used as treatment. More information on STIs in women and men can be found in Chapter 9 (page 314).

Breast

carcinoma of the breast   **Malignant tumor of the breast (arising from milk glands and ducts).**

The most common type of breast cancer is **invasive ductal carcinoma**. Figure 8–14A shows the tumor on a mammogram. Figure 8–14B is a cut section of an invasive ductal carcinoma. Other pathologic types are medullary carcinoma and lobular carcinoma.

Breast cancer first spreads to lymph nodes in the axilla (armpit) adjacent to the affected breast and then to the skin and chest wall. From the lymph nodes it may also metastasize to other body organs, including bone, liver, lung, or brain. The diagnosis is first established by a biopsy, using either a needle core, a needle aspiration, or surgical specimen.

For small primary tumors, the lump and immediately surrounding tissue is removed (**lumpectomy**). In order to determine whether the tumor has spread to lymph nodes, a **sentinel node biopsy (SNB)** is performed. In this procedure a blue dye or a radioisotope is injected into the tumor site and tracks to the axillary lymph nodes. By visualizing the path of the dye or radioactivity, it is possible to identify the lymph nodes most likely to contain tumor. These lymph nodes, the sentinel nodes, are removed first, and if negative, the procedure can be stopped at this point. Radiation to the breast and to any involved lymph nodes then follows to kill remaining tumor cells.

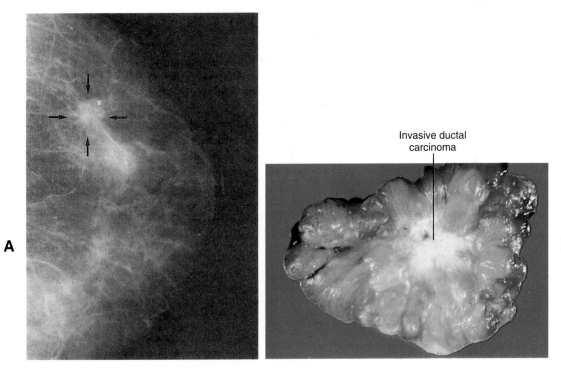

A

Invasive ductal
carcinoma

B

Figure 8–14

(A) Arrows in mammogram point to invasive carcinoma of the breast. **(B)** Cut section of invasive ductal carcinoma of the breast. (From Cotran RS, Kumar V, Collins T: Robbins Pathologic Basis of Disease, 6th ed. Philadelphia, WB Saunders, 1999, pp. 1113 and 1110.)

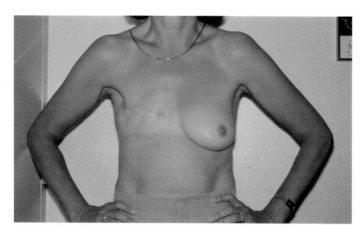

Figure 8–15

Surgical scar, modified radical mastectomy, right breast. (Courtesy Dr. Elizabeth Chabner Thompson.)

An alternative surgical procedure is a **modified radical mastectomy** (Figure 8–15), which is removal of the whole breast, lymph nodes, and adjacent chest wall muscle. After either lumpectomy or mastectomy if lymph nodes are involved with cancer, **adjuvant chemotherapy** may be given to prevent recurrence of the tumor.

Following mastectomy, a surgical procedure called a trans-rectus abdominis musculocutaneous flap **(TRAM flap)** can be used to reconstruct the breast. A muscle from the lower abdomen is tunneled under the abdominal and thoracic wall to its new location at the mastectomy scar (Fig. 8–16).

It is also important to test the breast cancer tumor for the presence of **estrogen receptors (ER).** These receptor proteins indicate that the tumor will respond to hormonal therapy. If metastases should subsequently develop, this information will be valuable in selecting further treatment. Selective estrogen receptor modulators **(SERMs)** function like estrogen in some tissues but block estrogen's effect in others. Examples of SERMs are **tamoxifen** and **raloxifene (Evista).** These drugs block the potentially harmful action of estrogen on breast tissue but preserve estrogen's benefits for bone maintenance and cardiovascular effects. An alternative drug, **Arimidex**, blocks the formation of estrogen and is equally in treating breast cancer positive for estrogen receptors.

A second receptor protein, her-2/neu, is found on some breast cancers and signals a more aggressive clinical course. **Herceptin**, an antibody that binds to and blocks her-2/neu, is effective in stopping growth when used with chemotherapy.

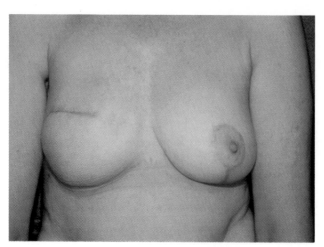

Figure 8–16

TRAM flap breast reconstruction. Right breast shows the results of TRAM flap reconstruction. Notice that the nipple reconstruction has not yet been performed. The left breast shows a lumpectomy scar. (Courtesy Dr. Elizabeth Chabner Thompson.)

fibrocystic disease

Small sacs of tissue and fluid in the breast.

Women with this common benign condition notice a nodular (lumpy) consistency of the breast, often associated with premenstrual tenderness and fullness. Mammography and surgical biopsy are indicated to differentiate fibrocystic changes from carcinoma of the breast.

Pregnancy

abruptio placentae

Premature separation of the implanted placenta.

Abruptio placentae (Latin, *ab*, "away from," *rumpere*, "to rupture") occurs secondary to trauma, such as a fall, or because of vascular insufficiency resulting from hypertension or preeclampsia (see page 276). Symptoms include a sudden searing (burning) abdominal pain and bleeding. It is an obstetrical emergency.

choriocarcinoma

Malignant tumor of the pregnant uterus.

The tumor may appear following pregnancy or abortion. Cure is possible with surgery and chemotherapy.

ectopic pregnancy

Implantation of the fertilized egg in any site other than the normal uterine location.

The condition occurs in up to 1 percent of pregnancies, and 90 percent of these occur in the fallopian tubes **(tubal pregnancy).** Rupture of the ectopic pregnancy within the fallopian tube can lead to massive hematosalpinx. Surgeons remove the implant and preserve the fallopian tube before rupture occurs. Other sites of ectopic pregnancies include the ovaries and abdominal cavity, and all are surgical emergencies.

placenta previa

Placental implantation over the cervical os (opening) or in the lower region of the uterine wall (Fig. 8–17).

This condition can result in less oxygen supply to the fetus and increased risk of hemorrhage and infection for the mother. Maternal symptoms include painless bleeding, hemorrhage, and premature labor. Cesarean delivery is usually recommended.

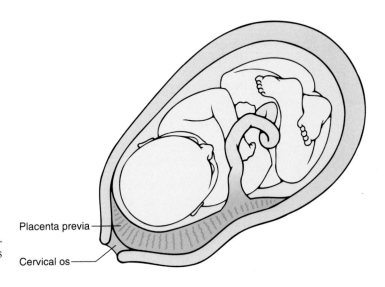

Figure 8–17
_____

Placenta previa. Previa means before or in the front of.

Placenta previa

Cervical os

preeclampsia

Abnormal condition of pregnancy characterized by the triad of high blood pressure, proteinuria, and edema.

Mild preeclampsia can be managed by bed rest and close monitoring of blood pressure. Women with severe preeclampsia are treated with medications such as magnesium sulfate to prevent seizures, and the baby is delivered as quickly as possible.

Neonatal

The following terms describe conditions or symptoms that can affect the newborn. The **Apgar score** is a system of scoring an infant's physical condition 1 and 5 minutes after birth. **Heart rate, respiration, color, muscle tone,** and **response to stimuli** are rated 0, 1, or 2. The maximum total score is 10. Infants with low Apgar scores require prompt medical attention (Fig. 8–18).

Down syndrome

Chromosomal abnormality (trisomy-21) results in mental retardation, retarded growth, a flat face with a short nose, low-set ears, and slanted eyes.

erythroblastosis fetalis

Hemolytic disease in the newborn caused by a blood group (Rh factor) incompatibility between the mother and the fetus.

hyaline membrane disease

Acute lung disease commonly seen in the premature newborn.

This condition, also called **respiratory distress syndrome of the newborn,** is caused by deficiency of **surfactant,** a protein necessary for proper lung function. Surfactant can be administered to the newborn to cure the condition. Hyaline refers to the shiny (hyaline means glassy) membrane that forms in the lung sacs.

APGAR SCORING CHART

SIGN	0	1	2
Heart rate	Absent	Below 100	Over 100
Respiratory effort	Absent	Slow, irregular	Good, crying
Muscle tone	Limp	Some flexion of extremities	Active motion
Response to catheter in nostril (tested after oropharynx is clear)	No response	Grimace	Cough or sneeze
Color	Blue, pale	Body pink, extremities blue	Completely pink

Figure 8–18

Apgar scoring chart. (Modified from O'Toole M [ed]: Miller-Keane Encyclopedia of Medicine, Nursing and Allied Health, 6th ed. Philadelphia, WB Saunders, 1997, p. 116.)

hydrocephalus	**Accumulation of fluid in the spaces of the brain.**

In an infant, the entire head can enlarge because the bones of the skull do not completely fuse together at birth. The soft spot, normally present between the cranial bones of the fetus, is called a **fontanelle.** Hydrocephalus occurs because of a problem in the circulation of fluid within the brain and spinal cord.

pyloric stenosis	**Narrowing of the opening of the stomach to the duodenum.**

Surgical repair of the pyloric opening may be necessary.

VIII. Clinical Tests, Procedures, and Abbreviations

Clinical Tests

Pap smear (test)	**Microsurgery examination of stained cells from the vagina and cervix.**

The physician, after inserting a vaginal **speculum** (instrument to hold apart the vaginal walls), uses a wooden spatula and a cotton swab to take secretions from the cervix and vagina (Fig. 8–19). Microscopic analysis of the cell smear (spread on a glass slide) detects cervical or vaginal carcinoma.

pregnancy test	**Blood or urine test to detect the presence of HCG.**

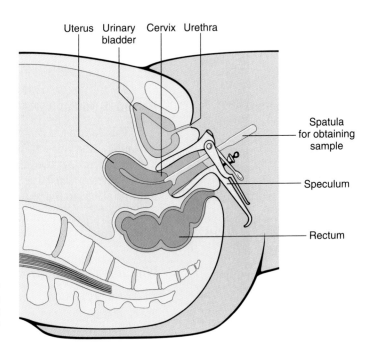

Figure 8–19

Method of obtaining a sample for a **Pap smear.** The test is 95 percent accurate in diagnosing early carcinoma of the cervix.

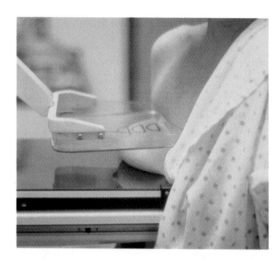

Figure 8–20

Mammography. The machine compresses the breast and x-rays (top to bottom and lateral) are taken. (Courtesy Dr. Elizabeth Chabner Thompson.)

Procedures

X-Rays

hysterosalpingography

X-ray imaging of the uterus and fallopian tubes after injection of contrast material.

mammography

X-ray imaging of the breast.

Women at 50 years of age are advised to have a baseline mammogram for later comparison if needed. Every 1 to 2 years a mammogram is recommended for women over the age of 50 to screen for breast cancer. Figure 8–20 illustrates a mammography. Physicians now use MRI of the breast to monitor high-risk women, in conjunction with mammography.

Ultrasound

pelvic ultrasonography

Record of sound waves as they bounce off organs in the pelvic region.

This technique can evaluate fetal size, maturity, and organ development as well as fetal and placental position. Uterine tumors and other pelvic masses, including abscesses, are also diagnosed by ultrasonography. **Transvaginal ultrasound** allows the radiologist a closer, sharper look at organs within the pelvis. The sound probe is placed in the vagina instead of across the pelvis or abdomen.

Gynecological Procedures

aspiration

Withdrawal of fluid from a cavity or sac.

Aspiration needle biopsy is a valuable technique for evaluating a patient with breast disease.

cauterization

Process of burning a part of the body.

Destruction of abnormal tissue with chemicals (silver nitrate), dry ice, or an electrically heated instrument. Cauterization is used to treat cervical dysplasia or cervical erosion. The loop electrocautery excision procedure (**LEEP**) is used to biopsy abnormal cervical tissue.

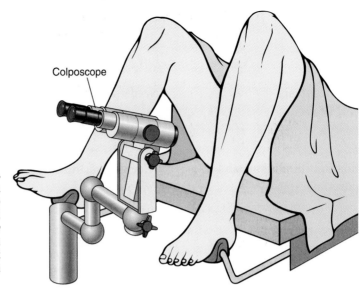

Colposcope

Figure 8–21

Colposcopy is used to evaluate a patient with an abnormal Pap smear. The female being examined lies in the **dorsal lithotomy position.** This is the same position used to remove a urinary tract stone (lithotomy means incision to remove a stone).

colposcopy

Visual examination of the vagina and cervix using a colposcope.

A colposcope is a lighted, magnifying instrument resembling a small, mounted pair of binoculars. Physicians prefer this procedure when cervical dysplasia is present because it identifies the specific areas of abnormal cells. A biopsy can then be taken for more accurate diagnosis (Fig. 8–21).

conization

Removal of a cone-shaped section of the cervix.

The physician removes the section with a **cold knife** (blade) or **laser** (a device that produces a very thin beam of concentrated high-energy light) so as not to distort the tissue for biopsy (Fig. 8–22).

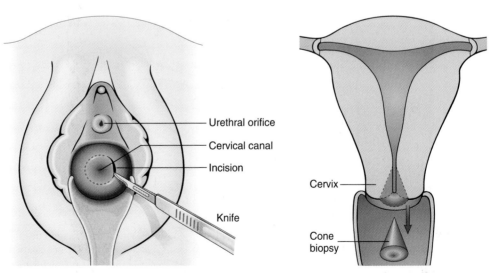

Urethral orifice
Cervical canal
Incision
Knife
Cervix
Cone biopsy

Figure 8–22

Two views of **conization of the cervix.**

cryosurgery

Use of cold temperatures to destroy tissue.

A liquid nitrogen probe produces the freezing (cry/o means cold) temperature. Also called **cryocauterization**.

culdocentesis

Needle aspiration of fluid from the cul-de-sac.

The physician inserts a needle through the vagina into the cul-de-sac. The presence of blood may indicate a ruptured ectopic pregnancy.

dilation (dilatation) and curettage (D&C)

Widening of the cervix and scraping the endometrium of the uterus.

Dilation is accomplished by inserting a series of probes of increasing size. A curet (metal loop at the end of a long, thin handle) is then used to remove the uterine lining. This procedure helps diagnose uterine disease and halt prolonged or heavy uterine bleeding. When necessary, a D&C is used to remove the tissue during a spontaneous or therapeutic abortion (Fig. 8–23).

exenteration

Removal of internal organs.

Pelvic exenteration is removal of the organs and adjacent structures of the pelvis.

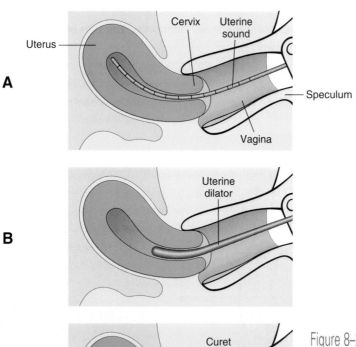

Figure 8–23

Dilation and curettage (D&C) of the uterus. **(A)** The uterine cavity is explored with a uterine sound (a slender instrument to measure the depth of the uterus to prevent perforation during dilation. **(B)** Uterine dilators (Hanks or Hagar) in graduated sizes are used to slowly dilate the cervix. **(C)** The uterus is gently curetted and specimens are collected.

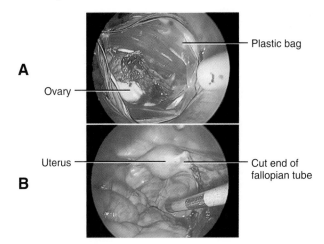

A

Ovary ———— Plastic bag

B

Uterus ———— Cut end of fallopian tube

Figure 8–24

Laparoscopic oophorectomy. (A) Notice the ovary placed in a plastic bag. The bag was inserted through the laparoscope, then opened and the ovary placed inside. Both are extracted through the laparoscope, leaving the uterus and cut end of the fallopian tube **(B)**.

laparoscopy   **Visual examination of the abdominal cavity.**

This procedure, also known as minimally invasive surgery, involves small incisions near a woman's navel with introduction of a laparoscope and other instruments. Uses of laparoscopy include inspection and removal of ovaries and fallopian tubes, diagnosis of endometriosis, and removal of fibroids. See Figure 8–24.

tubal ligation   **Blocking the fallopian tubes to prevent fertilization from occurring.**

This **sterilization** procedure (making an individual incapable of reproduction) is performed using laparoscopy.

Procedures During Pregnancy

abortion   **Spontaneous or induced termination of pregnancy before the fetus can exist on its own.**

Major methods for abortion include vaginal evacuation by D&C or vacuum aspiration (suction) and stimulation of uterine contractions by injection of saline (salt) into the amniotic cavity (second trimester).

amniocentesis   **Surgical puncture of the amniotic sac to withdraw amniotic fluid for analysis** (Figure 8-25).

The cells of the fetus, found in the fluid, are cultured (grown), and cytological and biochemical studies are performed.

Figure 8–25

Amniocentesis. The obstetrician places a long needle through the patient's abdominal wall into the amniotic cavity. His placement (avoiding the fetus and the placenta) is guided by concurrent ultrasound images produced by the transducer in the hand of the radiologist. The yellow amniotic fluid is aspirated into the syringe attached to the needle. This procedure took place in the 16th week of pregnancy. The indication for the amniocentesis was a low AFP (alpha-fetoprotein) level. This suggested a higher risk that the baby had Down syndrome. Karyotype analysis (received 10 days later) showed normal chromosome configuration.

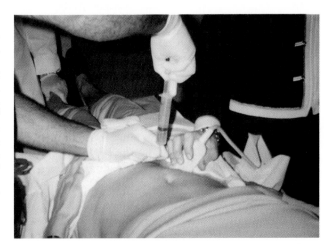

cesarean section	**Surgical incision of the abdominal wall and uterus to deliver a fetus.**
	Indications for cesarean section include cephalopelvic disproportion, abruptio placentae or placenta previa, fetal distress (fetal hypoxia), and breech or shoulder presentation. The name comes from the traditional belief that Julius Caesar was delivered by this operation.
chorionic villus sampling	**Sampling of placental tissues (chorionic villi) for prenatal diagnosis.**
	The sample of tissue is removed with a catheter inserted into the uterus. The procedure can be performed earlier than amniocentesis, at about 9 to 12 weeks of gestation.
fetal monitoring	**Use of ultrasonography to record the fetal heart rate and maternal uterine contractions during labor.**
pelvimetry	**Measurement of the dimensions of the maternal pelvis.**
	Pelvimetry helps determine if the mother's pelvis will allow passage of the fetus through the birth canal. This examination is important during protracted labor or with breech presentation.

Abbreviations

AB	abortion
AFP	alpha-fetoprotein; high levels in amniotic fluid of fetus or maternal serum indicate increased risk of neurological birth defects in the infant.
ASCUS	atypical squamous cells of unknown significance; abnormal Pap smear but does not meet the criteria for a lesion
BSE	breast self-examination
C-section	cesarean section
CIN	cervical intraepithelial neoplasia
CIS	carcinoma *in situ*
CS	cesarean section
CVS	chorionic villus sampling
Cx	cervix
D & C	dilation (dilatation) and curettage
DCIS	ductal carcinoma *in situ;* a precancerous breast lesion that indicates a higher risk for invasive ductal breast cancer

DES	diethylstilbestrol; an estrogen compound used in the treatment of menopausal problems involving estrogen deficiency; if administered during pregnancy, it has been found to be related to subsequent tumors in the daughters (rarely in sons) of mothers so treated.
DUB	dysfunctional uterine bleeding
ECC	endocervical curettage
EDC	estimated date of confinement
EMB	endometrial biopsy
ERT	estrogen replacement therapy
FHR	fetal heart rate
FSH	follicle-stimulating hormone
G	gravida (pregnant)
GYN	gynecology
HCG; hCG	human chorionic gonadotropin
HDN	hemolytic disease of the newborn
HPV	human papilloma virus

HSG	hysterosalpingography	**Path**	pathology
IUD	intrauterine device; contraceptive	**PID**	pelvic inflammatory disease
LEEP	loop electrocautery excision procedure	**PMS**	premenstrual syndrome
LH	luteinizing hormone	**primip**	primipara; primiparous
LMP	last menstrual period	**RDS**	respiratory distress syndrome
multip	multipara; multiparous	**SERMs**	selective estrogen receptor modulators
OB	obstetrics	**SLN biopsy**	sentinel node biopsy; blue dye or radioisotopes (or both) identifies the first lymph node draining the breast lymphatics
OCPs	oral contraceptive pills		
Para 2-0-1-2	woman's reproductive history: 2 full-term infants, 0 preterm, 1 abortion, and 2 living children	**TAH-BSO**	total abdominal hysterectomy with bilateral salpingo-oophorectomy
Pap smear	Papanicolaou smear (test for cervical or vaginal cancer)	**TRAM flap**	trans-rectus abdominis musculocutaneous flap; breast reconstruction

IX. Practical Applications

This section contains medical terms that you have studied in this and previous chapters. Explanations of more difficult terms are added in brackets. Answers to the questions are on page 296 after Answers to Exercises.

Operative Report. Preoperative Diagnosis: Menorrhagia, Leiomyomata

Anesthetic: General
Material forwarded to laboratory for examination:

A. Endocervical curettings
B. Endometrial curettings

Operation performed: Dilation and curettage of the uterus
With the patient in the dorsal lithotomy position [legs are flexed on the thighs, thighs flexed on the abdomen and abducted] and sterilely prepped and draped, manual examination of the uterus revealed it to be 6- to 8-week size, retroflexed; no adnexal masses noted. The anterior lip of the cervix was then grasped with a tenaculum

Continued on following page

[a hook-like surgical instrument for grasping and holding parts]. The cervix was dilated up to a #20 Hank's dilator. The uterus was sounded [depth measured] up to 4 inches. A sharp curettage of the endocervix showed only a scant amount of tissue. With a sharp curettage, the uterus was curetted in a clockwise fashion with an irregularity noted in the posterior floor. A large amount of hyperplastic endometrial tissue was removed. The patient tolerated the procedure well.

    Operative diagnosis: Leiomyomata uteri

Sentences Using Medical Terminology

1. Mammogram report: The breast parenchyma [essential tissue] is symmetrical bilaterally. There are no abnormal masses or calcifications in either breast. The axillae are normal.
2. This is a 43-year-old G3P2 with premature ovarian failure and now on ERT. She has history of endocervical atypia [cells are not normal or typical] secondary to chlamydial infection, which is now being treated.
3. The patient is a 40-year-old gravida II, para II, white female admitted for exploratory celiotomy [laparotomy] to remove and evaluate 10-cm left adnexal mass. Discharge diagnosis: (1) endometriosis, left ovary; (2) benign cystic teratoma [dermoid cyst], left ovary.

Operating Schedule: General Hospital

Match the surgery list in column I with an indication for surgery in column II.

Column I—Surgery

1 Conization of the cervix   _____

2. Vaginal hysterectomy with colporrhaphy   _____

3. TAH-BSO, pelvic and periaortic lymphadenectomy   _____

4. Exploratory laparotomy for uterine myomectomy   _____

5. Excision of bilateral gynecomastia   _____

6. Modified radical mastectomy   _____

Column II—Indications

A. Persistent, excessive breast tissue in a male

B. Fibroids

C. Endometrial carcinoma

D. Adenocarcinoma of the breast

E. Suspected cervical cancer

F. Uterine prolapse

X. Exercises

Remember to check your answers carefully with those given in Section XI, Answers to Exercises.

A. *Match the following terms for structures or tissues with their meanings below.*

amnion	clitoris	labia	placenta
areola	endometrium	mammary papilla	uterine serosa
cervix	fallopian tubes	ovaries	vagina
chorion	fimbriae	perineum	vulva

1. inner lining of the uterus _____

2. area between the anus and the vagina in females _____

3. dark-pigmented area around the breast nipple _____

4. finger-like ends of the fallopian tube _____

5. ducts through which the egg travels into the uterus from the ovary _____

6. organ of sensitive erectile tissue in females; anterior to urethral orifice _____

7. nipple of the breast _____

8. blood-vessel–filled organ that develops during pregnancy in the uterine wall and serves as a

   communication between maternal and fetal bloodstreams _____

9. lower, neck-like portion of the uterus _____

10. innermost membrane around the developing embryo _____

11. outermost layer of the membranes around the developing embryo and forming part of the placenta

   _____

12. membrane surrounding the uterus _____

13. lips of the vagina _____

14. female gonads; producing ova and hormones _____

15. includes the perineum, labia, clitoris, and hymen; external genitalia _____

16. muscular tube extending from the uterus to the exterior of the body _____

B. Identify the following terms.

1. fetus _____

2. lactiferous ducts _____

3. gametes _____

4. gonads _____

5. adnexa uteri _____

6. cul-de-sac _____

7. genitalia _____

8. Bartholin glands _____

9. graafian follicle _____

10. corpus luteum _____

C. Match the terms below with their descriptions.

coitus   human chorionic gonadotropin   myometrium
estrogen   luteinizing hormone   prenatal
fertilization   menarche   progesterone
follicle-stimulating hormone

1. a hormone produced by the ovaries; responsible for femaleness and buildup of the uterine lining

   during the menstrual cycle _____

2. a hormone produced by the pituitary gland to stimulate the maturation of the graafian follicle and

   ovum in the ovary _____

3. sexual intercourse _____

4. before birth _____

5. beginning of the first menstrual period during puberty _____

6. hormone produced by the placenta to sustain pregnancy by stimulating the ovaries to produce

   estrogen and progesterone _____

7. muscle layer lining the uterus _____

8. hormone produced by the corpus luteum in the ovary and also by the placenta of a pregnant

   woman _____

9. hormone produced by the pituitary gland to promote ovulation _____

10. fusion of the nuclei of the sperm and ovum _____

D. Give the meanings of the following.

1. galact/o and lact/o both mean _____

2. colp/o and vagin/o both mean _____

3. mamm/o and mast/o both mean _____

4. metr/o, uter/o, and hyster/o all mean _____

5. oophor/o and ovari/o both mean _____

6. o/o, ov/o, and ovul/o all mean _____

7. in- and endo- both mean _____

8. -cyesis and -gravida both mean _____

9. salping/o and -salpinx both mean _____

10. episi/o and vulv/o both mean _____

E. Complete the terms based on the meanings given.

1. inflammation of the cervix: _____ itis

2. suture of the vagina: colp _____

3. surgical puncture to remove fluid from the cul-de-sac: _____ centesis

4. surgical repair of the breast: mammo _____

5. removal of both fallopian tubes: bi _____ ectomy

6. pertaining to newborn: neo _____

7. difficult labor: dys _____

8. first menstrual period: men _____

9. rapid labor: _____ tocia

10. production of milk: lacto _____

F. Give the meanings of the following symptoms.

1. amenorrhea _____

2. dysmenorrhea _____

3. leukorrhea _____

4. metrorrhagia _____

5. galactorrhea _____

6. menorrhagia _____

7. pyosalpinx _____

8. dyspareunia _____

9. menometrorrhagia _____

10. oligomenorrhea _____

G. State whether the following sentences are true or false and explain your answers.

1. After a total (complete) hysterectomy, a woman still has regular menstrual periods.

   _____

2. After a total hysterectomy, a woman may still produce estrogen and progesterone.

   _____

3. Birth control pills prevent pregnancy by reducing the levels of FSH and LH in the bloodstream.

   _____

4. After a total hysterectomy with bilateral salpingo-oophorectomy, a doctor may advise estrogen

   replacement therapy. _____

5. A modified radical mastectomy involves removal of the entire breast, axillary lymph nodes, and chest

   wall muscle. _____

6. An episiotomy is an incision of the cervix and is part of a Pap smear. _____

7. Human chorionic gonadotropin is produced by the ovaries during pregnancy.

_____

8. Gynecomastia is a common condition in pregnant women. _____

9. Treatment for endometriosis is uterine myomectomy. _____

10. A gravida 3, para 2 is a woman who has given birth 3 times. _____

11. A nulligravida is a woman who has had several pregnancies. _____

12. Pseudocyesis is the same condition as a tubal pregnancy. _____

13. Fibrocystic changes in the breast are a malignant condition. _____

14. Cystadenomas occur in the ovaries. _____

15. FSH and LH are ovarian hormones. _____

H. Give the meanings of the following terms.

1. parturition _____

2. menopause _____

3. menarche _____

4. ovulation _____

5. gestation _____

6. anovulatory _____

7. dilatation _____

8. lactation _____

9. nulliparous _____

10. oophoritis _____

I. Match the following terms with their meanings as given below.

abruptio placentae   choriocarcinoma   leiomyomas
carcinoma *in situ*   cystadenocarcinoma   placenta previa
cervical carcinoma   endometrial carcinoma   preeclampsia
cervicitis   endometriosis

1. malignant tumor of the ovary _____

2. chlamydial infection causing inflammation in the lower, neck-like portion of the uterus

   _____

3. cancerous tumor cells are localized in a small area _____

4. condition during pregnancy or shortly thereafter, marked by hypertension, proteinuria, and

   edema _____

5. uterine tissue located outside the uterus (in the ovaries or cul-de-sac or attached to the

   peritoneum) _____

6. premature separation of a normally implanted placenta _____

7. placenta implantation over the cervical opening _____

8. malignant tumor of the pregnant uterus _____

9. malignant condition that can be diagnosed by a Pap smear, revealing dysplastic changes in cells

   _____

10. malignant condition of the inner lining of the uterus _____

11. benign muscle tumors in the uterus _____

J. Give the name of the test or procedure described below.

1. burning of abnormal tissue with chemicals or an electrically heated instrument:

   _____

2. contrast material is injected into the uterus and fallopian tubes, and x-rays are taken:

   _____

3. cold temperature is used to destroy tissue:

   _____

4. visual examination of the vagina and cervix:

_____

5. widening the cervical opening and scraping the lining of the uterus:

_____

6. withdrawal of fluid by suction with a needle:

_____

7. process of recording x-ray images of the breast:

_____

8. a cone-shaped section of the cervix is removed for diagnosis or treatment of cervical dysplasia:

_____

9. surgical puncture to remove fluid from the cul-de-sac:

_____

10. echoes from sound waves create an image of structures in the region of the hip:

_____

11. blocking the fallopian tubes to prevent fertilization from occurring:

_____

12. visual examination of the abdominal cavity:

_____

13. HCG is measured in the urine or blood:

_____

14. cells are taken from the cervix or vagina for microscopic analysis:

_____

15. removal of internal organs and adjacent structures the pelvis:

_____

K. Match the obstetrical and neonatal terms with the descriptions given below.

abortion	erythroblastosis fetalis	hydrocephalus
Apgar score	fetal monitoring	pelvimetry
cephalic version	fetal presentation	pyloric stenosis
cesarean section	fontanelle	respiratory distress syndrome

1. Turning the fetus so that the head presents during birth _____.

2. Measurement of the dimensions of the maternal pelvic bone _____.

3. The soft spot between the newborn's cranial bones _____.

4. The evaluation of the newborn's physical condition _____.

5. Premature termination of pregnancy is known as _____.

6. Removal of the fetus by abdominal incision of the uterus _____.

7. Acute lung disease in the premature newborn: surfactant deficiency _____.

8. Use of a machine to electronically record fetal heart rate during labor _____.

9. Narrowing of the opening of the stomach to the small intestine in the infant

_____.

10. Hemolytic disease of the newborn _____.

11. Accumulation of fluid in the spaces of a neonate's brain _____.

12. Manner in which the fetus appears to the examiner during delivery _____.

L. Give medical terms for the following meanings. Pay careful attention to spelling.

1. benign muscle tumors in the uterus: _____

2. no menstrual discharge: _____

3. accessory organs of the uterus: _____

4. suture of the vagina: _____

5. removal of an ovary: _____

6. condition of female breasts (in a male): _____

7. reproductive organs: _____

8. widening: _____

9. scraping: _____

10. ovarian hormone that sustains pregnancy: _____

11. nipple-shaped elevation on the breast: _____

12. inflammation of the vulva and vagina: _____

M. Give the meanings of the following abbreviations and then select the letter of the sentence that is the best association for each.

Column I

1. CIN_____ ____

2. FSH _____ ____

3. D&C _____ ____

4. multip _____ ____

5. C-section _____ ____

6. AFP_____ ____

7. DCIS_____ ____

8. TAH-BSO _____ ____

9. primip _____ ____

10. SERMs _____ ____

Column II

A. This woman has given birth to three infants.

B. Elevated levels of the protein may induce, fetal spinal cord abnormalities.

C. This woman has given birth for the first time.

D. Secretion from the pituitary gland stimulates the ovaries.

E. This procedure stops abnormal uterine bleeding.

F. Preinvasive changes in the lining of the neck of the uterus.

G. Surgical procedure to remove the uterus, fallopian tubes, and ovaries.

H. Surgical delivery of an infant through an abdominal incision.

I. Drugs that block estrogen's effect on breast tissue; tamoxifen is an example.

J. Precancerous breast lesion.

N. Circle the term in parentheses that best completes the meaning of each sentence.

1. Dr. Hanson felt that it was important to do a **(culdocentesis, Pap smear, amniocentesis)** once yearly on each of her GYN patients to screen for abnormal cells.

2. When Doris missed her period, her doctor checked for the presence of **(LH, IUD, HCG)** in Doris' urine to see if she was pregnant.

3. Ellen was 34 weeks pregnant, experiencing bad headaches, a 10-pound weight gain in 2 days, and blurry vision. Dr. Murphy told her to go to the obstetrical emergency room because she suspected **(preeclampsia, pelvic inflammatory disease, fibroids).**

4. Dr. Harris felt a breast mass when examining Mrs. Clark. She immediately ordered a **(dilation and curettage, hysterosalpingogram, mammogram)** for her 35-year-old patient.

5. Clara knew that she should not ignore her fevers and yellow vaginal discharge and the pain in her side. She had previous episodes of **(PMS, PID, DES)** treated with IV antibiotics. She worried that she might have a recurrence.

6. After years of trying to become pregnant, Jill decided to speak to her **(hematologist, gynecologist, urologist)** about *in vitro* **(gestation, parturition, fertilization)**.

7. To harvest her ova, Jill's physician prescribed hormones to stimulate egg maturation and **(coitus, lactation, ovulation)**. Ova were surgically removed and fertilized with sperm cells in a petri dish.

8. Next, multiple embryos were implanted into Jill's **(fallopian tube, vagina, uterus)** and she received hormones to ensure the survival of at least one embryo.

9. The IVF was successful and after **(abdominal CT, ultrasound, pelvimetry)**, Jill was told that she would have twins in 8½ months.

10. At 37 weeks, Jill went into labor. Under continuous **(chorionic villus sampling, culdocentesis, fetal monitoring)**, two healthy infants were delivered vaginally.

XI. Answers to Exercises

A

1. endometrium
2. perineum
3. areola
4. fimbriae
5. fallopian tubes
6. clitoris
7. mammary papilla
8. placenta
9. cervix
10. amnion
11. chorion
12. uterine serosa
13. labia
14. ovaries
15. vulva
16. vagina

B

1. the embryo from the third month (after 8 weeks) to birth
2. tubes that carry milk within the breast
3. sex cells; the egg and sperm cells
4. organs (ovaries and testes) in the female and male that produce gametes
5. ovaries, fallopian tubes, and supporting ligaments (accessory parts of the uterus)
6. the region of the abdomen between the rectum and the uterus
7. reproductive organs (genitals)
8. small exocrine glands at the vaginal orifice that secrete a lubricating fluid
9. the developing sac in the ovary that encloses the ovum
10. empty graafian follicle that secretes estrogen and progesterone after ovulation

C

1. estrogen
2. follicle-stimulating hormone
3. coitus
4. prenatal
5. menarche
6. human chorionic gonadotropin
7. myometrium
8. progesterone
9. luteinizing hormone
10. fertilization

D

1. milk
2. vagina
3. breast
4. uterus
5. ovary
6. egg
7. in, within
8. pregnancy
9. fallopian tube
10. vulva (external female genitalia)

E

1. cervicitis
2. colporrhaphy
3. culdocentesis
4. mammoplasty
5. bilateral salpingectomy
6. neonatal
7. dystocia
8. menarche
9. oxytocia
10. lactogenesis

F

1. no menstrual flow
2. painful menstrual flow
3. white discharge (from the vagina and associated with cervicitis)
4. bleeding from the uterus at irregular intervals
5. abnormal discharge of milk from the breasts
6. profuse or prolonged menstrual bleeding occurring at regular intervals
7. pus in the uterine tubes
8. painful sexual intercourse
9. heavy bleeding at and between menstrual periods
10. scanty menstrual flow

G

1. False. Total hysterectomy means removal of the entire uterus so that menstruation does not occur.
2. True. Total hysterectomy does not mean that the ovaries have been removed.
3. True. Most birth control pills contain estrogen and progesterone, which cause negative feedback to the pituitary gland, lowering FSH and LH in the bloodstream and preventing ovulation.
4. True. This may be necessary to treat symptoms of estrogen loss (vaginal atrophy, hot flashes) and to prevent bone deterioration (osteoporosis).
5. True. A modified radical mastectomy involves removal of the breast, axillary nodes, and chest wall muscle.
6. False. An episiotomy is an incision of the perineum and is performed during delivery to prevent the tearing of the perineum.
7. False. HCG is produced by the *placenta* during pregnancy.
8. False. Gynecomastia is a condition of increased breast development in *males*.
9. False. Myomectomy means removal of muscle tumors (fibroids). Endometriosis is abnormal location of uterine tissue outside the uterine lining.
10. False. A gravida 3, para 2 is a woman who has had two children but is pregnant with her third.
11. False. A nulligravida has had no pregnancies. A multigravida has had many pregnancies.
12. False. A pseudocyesis is a false pregnancy (no pregnancy occurs), and a tubal pregnancy is an example of ectopic pregnancy (pregnancy occurs in the fallopian tube, not in the uterus).
13. False. Fibrocystic changes in the breast are a benign condition.
14. True. Cystadenomas are glandular sacs lined with tumor cells; they occur in the ovaries.
15. False. FSH and LH are pituitary gland hormones. Estrogen and progesterone are secreted by the ovaries.

H

1. act of giving birth
2. gradual ending of menstrual function
3. beginning of the first menstrual period at puberty
4. release of the ovum from the ovary
5. pregnancy
6. pertaining to no ovulation (egg is not released from the ovary)
7. widening
8. production of milk
9. a woman who has never given birth
10. inflammation of the ovaries

I

1. cystadenocarcinoma
2. cervicitis
3. carcinoma *in situ*
4. preeclampsia
5. endometriosis
6. abruptio placentae
7. placenta previa
8. choriocarcinoma
9. cervical carcinoma
10. endometrial carcinoma
11. leiomyomas

J

1. cauterization
2. hysterosalpingography
3. cryosurgery or cryocauterization
4. colposcopy
5. dilation (dilatation) and curettage
6. aspiration
7. mammography
8. conization
9. culdocentesis
10. pelvic ultrasonography
11. tubal ligation
12. laparoscopy
13. pregnancy test
14. Pap smear
15. pelvic exenteration

K

1. cephalic version
2. pelvimetry
3. fontanelle
4. Apgar score
5. abortion
6. cesarean section
7. hyaline membrane disease
8. fetal monitoring
9. pyloric stenosis
10. erythroblastosis fetalis
11. hydrocephalus
12. fetal presentation

L

1. fibroids or leiomyomata
2. amenorrhea
3. adnexa
4. colporrhaphy
5. oophorectomy
6. gynecomastia
7. genitalia
8. dilation
9. curettage
10. progesterone
11. mammary papilla
12. vulvovaginitis

Continued on following page

M

1. cervical intraepithelial neoplasia. F
2. follicle-stimulating hormone. D
3. dilation (dilatation) and curettage. E
4. multipara. A
5. cesarean section. H

6. alpha-fetoprotein. B
7. ductal carcinoma *in situ*. J
8. total abdominal hysterectomy with bilateral salpingo-oophorectomy. G

9. primipara. C
10. selective estrogen receptor modulators. I

N

1. Pap smear
2. HCG
3. preeclampsia
4. mammogram

5. PID
6. gynecologist; fertilization
7. ovulation

8. uterus
9. ultrasound
10. fetal monitoring

Answers to Practical Applications

1. E
2. F
3. C

4. B
5. A
6. D

XII. Pronunciation of Terms

Pronunciation Guide

ā as in āpe   ă as in ăpple
ē as in ēven   ĕ as in ĕvery
ī as in īce   ĭ as in ĭnterest
ō as in ōpen   ŏ as in pŏt
ū as in ūnit   ŭ as in ŭnder

To test your understanding of the terminology in this chapter, write the meaning of each term in the space provided. In addition, you may wish to cover the terms and write them by looking at your definitions. Make sure your spelling is correct. The page number after each term indicates where it is defined or used in the text so you can easily check your responses.

Vocabulary and Terminology

Term	Pronunciation	Meaning
adnexa uteri (262)	ăd-NĔK-să Ū-tĕ-rī	_____
amenorrhea (266)	āmĕn-ō-RĒ-ă	_____
amniocentesis (265)	ăm-nē-ō-sĕn-TĒ-sĭs	_____
amnion (262)	ĂM-nē-ŏn	_____
amniotic fluid (265)	ăm-nē-ŎT-ĭk FLOO-ĭd	_____
anovulatory (267)	ăn-ŎV-ū-lă-tōr-ē	_____
areola (262)	ă-RĒ-ō-lă	_____

Bartholin glands (262)	BĂR-thō-lĭn glandz	_____
bilateral oophorectomy (267)	bī-LĂ-tĕr-ăl ō-ŏf-ō-RĔK-tō-mē or oo-fō-RĔK-tō-mē	_____
cephalic version (269)	sĕ-FĂL-lĭk VĔR-shŭn	_____
cervix (262)	SĔR-vĭkz	_____
choriogenesis (265)	kŏr-ē-ō-JĔN-ĕ-sĭs	_____
chorion (262)	KŌ-rē-ŏn	_____
chorionic (265)	kō-rē-ŎN-ĭk	_____
clitoris (262)	KLĬ-tō-rĭs	_____
coitus (262)	KŌ-ĭ-tŭs	_____
colporrhaphy (265)	kŏl-PŎR-ă-fē	_____
colposcopy (265)	kŏl-PŎS-kō-pē	_____
corpus luteum (262)	KŎR-pŭs LŪ-tē-ŭm	_____
cul-de-sac (262)	KŬL-dĕ-săk	_____
culdocentesis (265)	kŭl-dō-sĕn-TĒ-sĭs	_____
dysmenorrhea (267)	dĭs-mĕn-ō-RĒ-ă	_____
dyspareunia (269)	dĭs-pă-ROO-nē-ă	_____
dystocia (268)	dĭs-TŌ-sē-ă	_____
embryo (262)	ĔM-brē-ō	_____
endocervicitis (265)	ĕn-dō-sĕr-vĭs-SĪ-tĭs	_____
endometritis (269)	ēn-dō-mē-TRĪ-tis	_____
endometrium (263)	ĕn-dō-MĒ-trē-ŭm	_____
episiotomy (265)	ĕ-pĭs-ē-ŎT-ō-mē	_____
estrogen (263)	ĔS-trō-jĕn	_____
fallopian tube (263)	fă-LŌ-pē-ăn tūb	_____
fertilization (263)	fĕr-tĭl-ĭ-ZĀ-shŭn	_____
fetal presentation (269)	FĒ-tăl prĕ-sĕn-TĀ-shŭn	_____

fetus (263)	FĒ-tŭs	
fimbriae (263)	FĬM-brē-ē	
follicle-stimulating hormone (263)	FŎL-lĭ-k'l STĬM-ū-lā-tĭng HŌR-mōn	
galactorrhea (265)	gă-lăk-tō-RĒ-ă	
gamete (263)	GĂM-ēt	
genitalia (263)	jĕn-ĭ-TĀ-lē-ă	
gestation (263)	jĕs-TĀ-shŭn	
gonad (263)	GŌ-năd	
graafian follicle (263)	GRĂF-ē-ăn FŎL-lĭ-k'l	
gynecology (263)	gī-nĕ-KŎL-ō-jē	
gynecomastia (265)	gī-nĕ-kō-MĂS-tē-ă	
human chorionic gonadotropin (263)	HŪ-măn kō-rē-ŎN-ĭk gō-nă-dō-TRŌ-pĭn	
hymen (263)	HĪ-mĕn	
hysterectomy (266)	hĭs-tĕr-ĔK-tō-mē	
hysteroscopy (266)	hĭs-tĕr-ŎS-kō-pē	
intrauterine device (269)	ĭn-tră-Ū-tĕ-rĭn dĕ-VĪS	
involution (269)	ĭn-vō-LŪ-shŭn	
labia (263)	LĀ-bē-ă	
lactation (266)	lăk-TĀ-shŭn	
lactiferous ducts (263)	lăk-TĬ-fĕ-rŭs dŭkts	
lactogenesis (266)	lăk-tō-JĔN-ĕ-sĭs	
leukorrhea (268)	loo-kō-RĒ-ă	
luteinizing hormone (263)	LŪ-tĕ-nī-zĭng HŎR-mōn	
mammary (266)	MĂM-ŏr-ē	
mammary papilla (263)	MĂM-ŏr-ē pă-PĬL-ă	
mammoplasty (266)	MĂM-ō-plăs-tē	

mastectomy (266)	măs-TĔK-tō-mē	_____
mastitis (266)	măs-TĪ-tĭs	_____
menarche (263)	mĕ-NĂR-kē	_____
menometrorrhagia (267)	mĕn-ō-mĕt-rō-RĀ-jă	_____
menopause (263)	MĒN-ō-păwz	_____
menorrhea (268)	mĕn-ō-RĒ-ă	_____
menorrhagia (267)	mĕn-ō-RĀ-jă	_____
menstruation (263)	mĕn-strū-Ā-shŭn	_____
metrorrhagia (267)	mĕ-trō-RĀ-jă	_____
multigravida (269)	mŭl-tē-GRĂV-ĭ-dă	_____
multipara (269)	mŭl-TĬP-ă-ră	_____
myomectomy (267)	mī-ō-MĔK-tō-mē	_____
myometrium (263)	mī-ō-MĒ-trē-ŭm	_____
neonatal (267)	nē-ō-NĀ-tăl	_____
neonatology (264)	nē-ō-nā-TŎL-ō-jē	_____
nullipara (269)	nŭl-LĬP-ă-ră	_____
obstetrics (264)	ŏb-STĔT-rĭkz	_____
oligomenorrhea (267)	ŏl-ĭ-gō-mĕn-ō-RĒ-ă	_____
oogenesis (267)	ō-ō-JĔN-ĕ-sĭs	_____
oophoritis (267)	ō-ōf-ōr-Ī-tĭs	_____
orifice (264)	ŎR-ĭ-fĭs	_____
ovarian (267)	ō-VĂ-rē-an	_____
ovary (264)	Ō-vă-rē	_____
ovulation (264)	ŏv-ū-LĀ-shŭn	_____
ovum; ova (264)	Ō-vŭm; Ō-vă	_____
oxytocia (268)	ŏks-ē-TŌ-sē-ă	_____
oxytocin (268)	ŏks-ē-TŌ-sĭn	_____

parturition (264)	păr-tū-RĬSH-ŭn	
perineorrhaphy (267)	pĕ-rĭ-nē-ŎR-ră-fē	
perineum (264)	pĕ-rĭ-NĒ-ŭm	
pituitary gland (264)	pĭ-TŪ-ĭ-tăr-ē glănd	
placenta (264)	plă-SĔN-tă	
prenatal (270)	prē-NĀ-tăl	
primigravida (268)	prī-mĭ-GRĂV-ĭ-dă	
primipara (270)	prī-MĬ-pă-ră	
primiparous (268)	prī-MĬP-ă-rŭs	
progesterone (264)	prō-JĔS-tĕ-rōn	
pseudocyesis (268)	sū-dō-sī-Ē-sĭs	
puberty (264)	PŪ-bĕr-tē	
pyosalpinx (268)	pī-ō-SĂL-pĭnks	
retroversion (270)	rĕ-trō V_R-j_n	
salpingectomy (267)	săl-pĭng-JĔK-tō-mē	
salpingitis (272)	săl-pĭng-JĪ-tĭs	
uterine serosa (264)	Ū-tĕr-ĭn sĕ-RŌ-să	
uterus (264)	Ū-tĕr-ŭs	
vagina (264)	vă-JĪ-nă	
vaginal orifice (268)	vā-jī-năl ŎR-ĭ-fĭs	
vaginitis (268)	vă-jĭ-NĪ-tĭs	
vulva (264)	VŬL-vă	
vulvovaginitis (268)	vŭl-vō-vă-jĭ-NĪ-tĭs	

Pathological Conditions, Clinical Tests, and Procedures

Term	Pronunciation	Meaning
abortion (281)	ă-BŎR-shŭn	
abruptio placentae (275)	ă-BRŬP-shē-ō plă-SĔN-tē	
Apgar score (276)	ĂP-găr skōr	

aspiration (278)	ăs-pĕ-RĀ-shŭn	_____
carcinoma *in situ* (270)	kăr-sĭ-NŌ-mă ĭn SĪ-tū	_____
carcinoma of the breast (273)	kăr-sĭ-NŌ-mă of the brĕst	_____
carcinoma of the cervix (270)	kăr-sĭ-NŌ-mă of the SĔR-vĭkz	_____
carcinoma of the endometrium (271)	kăr-sĭ-NŌ-mă of the ĕn-dō-MĒ-trē-ŭm	_____
cauterization (278)	kăw-tĕr-ĭ-ZĀ-shŭn	_____
cervical dysplasia (270)	SĔR-vĭ-kăl dĭs-PLĀ-zē-ă	_____
cervicitis (270)	sĕr-vĭ-SĪ-tĭs	_____
cesarean section (282)	sĕ-SĀ-rē-ăn SĔK-shŭn	_____
Chlamydia (270)	klă-MĬD-ē-ă	_____
choriocarcinoma (275)	kō-rē-ō-kăr-sĭ-NŌ-mă	_____
chorionic villus sampling (282)	kō-rē-ŎN-ik VĬL-us SĂMP-lĭng	_____
colposcopy (279)	kōl-PŎS-kō-pē	_____
conization (279)	kō-nĭ-ZĀ-shŭn	_____
cryocauterization (280)	krī-ō-kăw-tĕr-ĭ-ZĀ-shŭn	_____
culdocentesis (280)	kŭl-dō-sĕn-TĒ-sĭs	_____
cystadenocarcinoma (272)	sĭs-tăd-ĕ-nō-kăr-sĭ-NŌ-mă	_____
cystadenoma (272)	sĭs-tăd-ĕ-NŌ-mă	_____
dermoid cyst (272)	DĔR-moyd sĭst	_____
dilatation (280)	dĭ-lă-TĀ-shŭn	_____
dilation and curettage (280)	dī-LĀ-shŭn and kŭr-ĕ-TĂZH	_____
ectopic pregnancy (275)	ĕk-TŎP-ĭk PRĔG-năn-sē	_____
endometriosis (271)	ĕn-dō-mē-trē-Ō-sĭs	_____
erythroblastosis fetalis (276)	ĕ-rĭth-rō-blăs-TŌ-sĭs fĕ-TĂ-lĭs	_____
exenteration (280)	ĕks-ĕn-tĕ-RĀ-shŭn	_____
fetal monitoring (282)	FĒ-tăl MŎN-ĭ-tĕ-rĭng	_____
fibrocystic disease (275)	fī-brō-SĬS-tĭk dĭ-ZĒZ	_____

fibroids (271)	FĪ-broydz	
hyaline membrane disease (276)	HĪ-ă-lĭn MĔM-brān dĭ-ZĒZ	
hydrocephalus (277)	hī-drō-SĔF-ă-lŭs	
hysterosalpingography (278)	hĭs-tĕr-ō-săl-pĭng-ŎG-ră-fē	
laparoscopy (281)	lă-pă-RŎS-kō-pē	
leiomyomas (271)	lī-ō-mī-Ō-măz	
mammography (278)	măm-MŎG-ră-fē	
ovarian carcinoma (272)	ō-VĂR-ē-an kăr-sĭ-NŌ-mă	
ovarian cyst (272)	ō-VĂR-ē-an sĭst	
palpation (272)	păl-PĀ-shŭn	
Pap smear (277)	Păp smēr	
pelvic inflammatory disease (272)	PĔL-vĭk ĭn-FLĂM-mă-tō-rē dĭ-ZĒZ	
pelvic ultrasonography (278)	PĔL-vĭk ŭl-tră-sŏn-ŎG-ră-fē	
pelvimetry (282)	pĕl-VĬM-ĭ-trē	
placenta previa (275)	plă-SĔN-tă PRĒ-vē-ă	
preeclampsia (276)	prē-ĕ-KLĂMP-sē-ă	
pyloric stenosis (277)	pī-LŎR-ĭk stĕ-NŌ-sĭs	
respiratory distress syndrome (276)	RĔS-pĭr-ă-tō-rē dĭs-STRĔS SĬN-drōm	
tubal ligation (281)	TOO-băl lī-GĀ-shŭn	

XIII. Review Sheet

Write the meanings of the word parts in the spaces provided and test yourself. Check your answers with the information in the chapter or in the glossary (Medical Terms—English) at the end of the book.

COMBINING FORMS

Combining Form	Meaning	Combining Form	Meaning
amni/o	_____	my/o	_____
cephal/o	_____	myom/o	_____
cervic/o	_____	nat/i	_____
chori/o	_____	obstetr/o	_____
chorion/o	_____	olig/o	_____
colp/o	_____	o/o	_____
culd/o	_____	oophor/o	_____
episi/o	_____	ov/o	_____
galact/o	_____	ovari/o	_____
gynec/o	_____	ovul/o	_____
hyster/o	_____	perine/o	_____
lact/o	_____	phor/o	_____
mamm/o	_____	py/o	_____
mast/o	_____	salping/o	_____
men/o	_____	uter/o	_____
metr/o	_____	vagin/o	_____
metri/o	_____	vulv/o	_____

Continued on following page

SUFFIXES

Suffix	Meaning	Suffix	Meaning
-arche		-ptosis	
-cele		-rrhagia	
-cyesis		-rrhaphy	
-ectasis		-rrhea	
-ectomy		-salpinx	
-flexion		-scopy	
-genesis		-stenosis	
-gravida		-stomy	
-itis		-tocia	
-pareunia		-tomy	
-parous		-tresia	
-plasia		-version	
-plasty			

PREFIXES

Prefix	Meaning	Prefix	Meaning
bi-		oxy-	
dys-		peri-	
endo-		pre-	
in-		primi-	
intra-		pseudo-	
multi-		retro-	
nulli-		uni-	

chapter

Male Reproductive System

This chapter is divided into the following sections

In this chapter you will

- Name, locate, and describe the functions of the organs of the male reproductive system.
- Define some abnormal and pathological conditions that affect the male system.
- Differentiate among several types of sexually transmitted infections.
- Define many combining forms used to describe the structures of this system.
- Explain various laboratory tests, clinical procedures, and abbreviations that are pertinent to the system.
- Apply your new knowledge to understanding medical terms in their proper contexts, such as medical reports and records.

I. Introduction

The male sex cell, the **spermatozoon** (sperm cell), is microscopic—in volume, only one third the size of a red blood cell, and less than 1/100,000th the size of the female ovum. A relatively uncomplicated cell, the sperm is composed of a head region, containing nuclear hereditary material (chromosomes), and a tail region, consisting of a **flagellum** (hair-like process). The flagellum makes the sperm motile, somewhat resembling a tadpole. The spermatozoon cell contains relatively little food and cytoplasm, as it lives only long enough to travel from its point of release from the male to where the egg cell lies within the female (fallopian tube). Only one spermatozoon out of approximately 300 million sperm cells released during a single **ejaculation** (ejection of sperm and fluid from the male urethra) can penetrate a single ovum and result in fertilization of the ovum.

If more than one egg is passing down the fallopian tube when sperm are present, multiple fertilizations are possible, and twins, triplets, quadruplets, and so forth may occur. Twins resulting from the fertilization of separate ova by separate sperm cells are called **fraternal twins.** Fraternal twins, developing *in utero* with separate placentas, can be of the same sex or different sexes and resemble each other no more than ordinary brothers and sisters. Fraternal twinning is hereditary; the daughters of mothers of twins can carry the gene.

Identical twins result from fertilization of a single egg cell by a single sperm. As the fertilized egg cell divides and forms many cells, it somehow splits and each part continues separately to undergo further division, each producing an embryo. Depending on when the embryo splits (day 1, 2, or 3), the fetuses will share the same gestational sac and/or placenta. Identical twins are always of the same sex and are very similar in form and feature.

The organs of the male reproductive system are designed to produce and release billions of spermatozoa throughout the lifetime of a male from puberty onward. In addition, the male reproductive system secretes a hormone called **testosterone.** Testosterone is responsible for the production of the bodily characteristics of the male (such as beard, pubic hair, and deeper voice) and for the proper development of male gonads **(testes)** and accessory organs **(prostate gland** and **seminal vesicles)** that secrete fluids to ensure the lubrication and viability of sperm.

II. Anatomy

Label Figure 9–1 as you study the following description of the anatomy of the male reproductive system.

The male gonads consist of a pair (only one is pictured here) of **testes** (singular: **testis**), also called **testicles** [1], which develop in the abdomen at about the level of the kidneys before descending during embryonic development into the **scrotum** [2], a sac enclosing the testes on the outside of the body.

The scrotum, lying between the thighs, exposes the testes to a lower temperature than that of the rest of the body. This lower temperature is necessary for the adequate maturation and development of sperm **(spermatogenesis).** Lying between the anus and the scrotum, at the floor of the pelvic cavity in the male, the **perineum** [3] is analogous to the perineal region in the female.

The interior of a testis is composed of a large mass of narrow, coiled tubules called the **seminiferous tubules** [4]. These tubules contain cells that manufacture spermatozoa. The seminiferous tubules are the **parenchymal tissue** of the testis, which means that they perform the essential work of the organ (formation of sperm). Other cells in the testis, called **interstitial cells,** manufacture an important male hormone, **testosterone.**

All body organs contain **parenchyma** (parenchymal cells or tissue), which perform the essential functions of the organ. Organs also contain supportive, connective, and framework

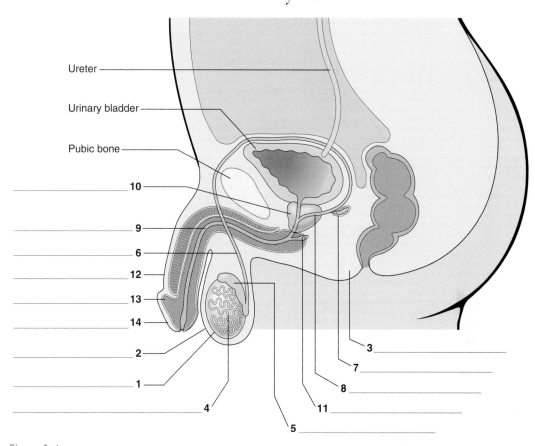

Ureter

Urinary bladder

Pubic bone

10

9

6

12

13

14

2

1

4

3

7

8

11

5

Figure 9–1

Male reproductive system, sagittal view.

tissue, such as blood vessels, connective tissues, and sometimes muscle as well. This supportive tissue is called **stroma (stromal tissue).**

After formation, sperm cells move through the seminiferous tubules and collect in ducts that lead to a large tube, the **epididymis** [5], at the upper part of each testis. The spermatozoa mature, become motile in the epididymis, and are temporarily stored there. An epididymis runs down the length of each testicle (the coiled tube is about 16 feet long) and then turns upward again and becomes a narrow, straight tube called the **vas deferens** [6] or **ductus deferens.** Figure 9–2 shows the internal structure of a testis and the epididymis. The vas deferens is about 2 feet long and carries the sperm up into the pelvic region, at the level of the urinary bladder, merging with ducts from the **seminal vesicles** [7] to form the **ejaculatory duct** [8] leading toward the urethra. During a **vasectomy** or **sterilization** procedure, the urologist cuts and ties off each vas deferens.

The seminal vesicles, two glands (only one is shown in Figure 9–1) located at the base of the bladder, open into the ejaculatory duct as it joins the **urethra** [9]. They secrete a thick, sugary, yellowish substance that nourishes the sperm cells and forms much of the volume of ejaculated semen. **Semen** is a combination of fluid and spermatozoa (sperm cells account for less than 1 percent of the semen volume) that is ejected from the body through the urethra. In the male, as opposed to in the female, the genital orifice combines with the urinary (urethral) opening.

The **prostate gland** [10] lies at the region where the vas deferens enters the urethra, almost encircling the upper end of the urethra. It secretes a thick fluid that, as part of semen, aids the motility of the sperm. The muscular tissue of the prostate aids in the expulsion of

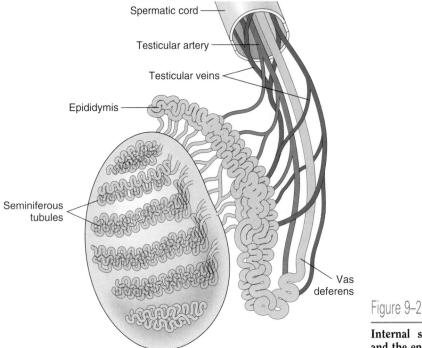

Spermatic cord

Testicular artery

Testicular veins

Epididymis

Seminiferous tubules

Vas deferens

Figure 9–2

Internal structure of a testis and the epididymis.

sperm during ejaculation. **Cowper (bulbourethral) glands** [11], lying below the prostate gland, also secrete fluid into the urethra.

The urethra passes through the **penis** [12] to the outside of the body. The penis is composed of erectile tissue and at its tip expands to form a soft, sensitive region called the **glans penis** [13]. Ordinarily, a fold of skin called the **prepuce,** or **foreskin** [14], covers the glans penis. During a circumcision the foreskin is removed, leaving the glans penis visible at all times.

Erectile dysfunction (impotence) is the inability of the adult male to achieve an erection. Viagra (sildenafil citrate) is a drug that increases blood flow to the penis, enhancing ability to have an erection.

The flow diagram in Figure 9–3 traces the path of spermatozoa from their formation in the seminiferous tubules of the testes to the outside of the body.

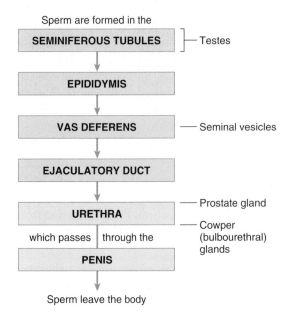

Sperm are formed in the

SEMINIFEROUS TUBULES — Testes

EPIDIDYMIS

VAS DEFERENS — Seminal vesicles

EJACULATORY DUCT

URETHRA — Prostate gland
— Cowper (bulbourethral) glands

which passes | through the

PENIS

Sperm leave the body

Figure 9–3

The **passage of sperm** from the seminiferous tubules in the testes to the outside of the body.

III. Vocabulary

This list reviews new terms introduced in the text. Short definitions reinforce your understanding, and Section X of this chapter gives pronunciation of the terms.

bulbourethral gland	One of a pair of exocrine glands near the male urethra.
Cowper gland	Bulbourethral gland.
ejaculation	Ejection of sperm and fluid from the male urethra.
ejaculatory duct	Tube through which semen enters the urethra.
epididymis (plural: **epididymides**)	One of a pair of long, tightly coiled tubes lying on top of each testis. It carries sperm from the seminiferous tubules to the vas deferens.
erectile dysfunction	Inability of an adult male to achieve an erection; impotence.
flagellum	Hair-like projection on a sperm cell that makes it motile (able to move).
fraternal twins	Two infants born of the same pregnancy from two separate ova fertilized by two different sperm. See Figure 9–4.
glans penis	Sensitive tip of the penis.
identical twins	Two infants resulting from division of one fertilized egg into two distinct embryos. Conjoined ("Siamese") twins are incompletely separated identical twins.

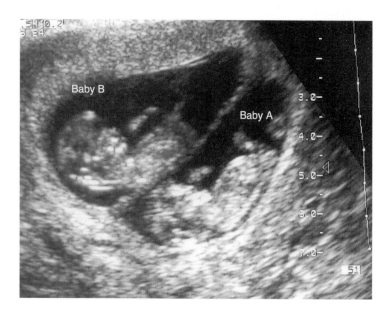

Figure 9-4

Fraternal twins (Marcos and Matheus Carmo). Notice the 6-week-old embryos in two separate amniotic sacs. (Courtesy Julianna Carmo.)

impotence	See erectile dysfunction. From Latin *im*, "hot" and *potentia*, "power."
interstitial cells of the testis	Cells that lie between the seminiferous tubules and produce the hormone testosterone. A pituitary gland hormone (luteinizing hormone [LH]) stimulates the interstitial cells to produce testosterone.
parenchyma	Tissue composed of the essential cells of any organ. In the testes, parenchymal tissue includes seminiferous tubules that produce sperm.
perineum	Area between the anus and scrotum in the male.
prepuce (foreskin)	Skin covering the tip of the penis.
prostate gland	Gland, in men, at the base of the urinary bladder that secretes a fluid into the urethra during ejaculation.
scrotum	External sac that contains the testes in men.
semen	Spermatozoa and fluid (prostatic and other glandular secretions).
seminal vesicle	Either of paired sac-like male glands that secrete a fluid into the vas deferens.
seminiferous tubules	Narrow, coiled tubules that produce sperm in the testes.
spermatozoon (plural: **spermatozoa**)	Sperm cell.
sterilization	Any procedure rendering an individual incapable of reproduction; for example, vasectomy and tubal ligation.
stroma	Supportive, connective tissue of an organ, as distinguished from its parenchyma.
testis (plural: **testes**)	Male gonad that produces spermatozoa and the hormone testosterone; testicle.
testosterone	Hormone secreted by the interstitial tissue of the testes; responsible for male sex characteristics.
vas deferens	Narrow tube (one on each side) that carries sperm from the epididymis into the body and toward the urethra. Also called ductus deferens.

IV. Combining Forms and Terminology

Write the meanings of the medical terms in the spaces provided.

Combining Form	Meaning	Terminology	Meaning
andr/o	male	androgen _____	
		Testosterone is an androgen. The testes in males and the adrenal glands in both men and women produce androgens.	
balan/o	glans penis (Greek, *balanos*, acorn)	balanitis _____	
		Bacteria or viruses often cause inflammation and infections of the male reproductive system (Fig. 9–5A).	
cry/o	cold	cryogenic surgery _____	
		A method used to remove portions of the prostate gland during a transurethral resection of the prostate.	
crypt/o	hidden	cryptorchism _____	
		In this congenital condition, one or both testicles do not descend, by the time of birth, into the scrotal sac from the abdominal cavity (Fig. 9–5B).	

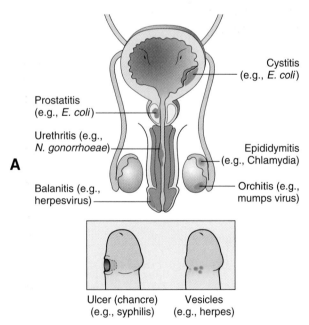
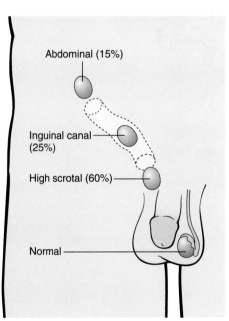

A **B**

Figure 9–5

(A) Infections of the male reproductive system. *E. coli (Escherichia coli)* are bacteria commonly found in the large intestine; they are a common cause of urinary tract infections such as cystitis. **Chlamydia** are bacteria that invade the urethra and travel to the epididymis. **Gonococci *(Neisseria gonorrhoeae)*** are bacteria that affect the mucous membranes of genital and urinary organs. **Herpesvirus** affects the external genetalia, causing vesicles (blisters). **(B) Cryptorchism.** (From Damjanov I: Pathology for Health-Related Professions, 2nd ed., Philadelphia, WB Saunders, 2000, p. 347.)

epididym/o   epididymis   epididymitis _____

Symptoms are fever, chills, pain in the groin, tender, swollen epididymis.

gon/o   seed (Greek,   gonorrhea _____
                   gone, seed)
                                       See Sexually Transmitted Infections, page 317.

hydr/o   water, fluid   hydrocele _____

See Abnormal and Pathological Conditions, page 314.

orch/o, orchi/o,   testis, testicle (the   orchiectomy _____
orchid/o   botanical name for
                       orchid, the flower,   *Orchidectomy. Castration in males.*
                       is derived from the
                       Greek word *orchis,*   anorchism _____
                       meaning testicle; it
                       describes the fleshy   orchitis _____
                       tubers on the root-
                       stocks of the plant)   *Caused by injury or by the mumps virus, which also infects the salivary glands.*

prostat/o   prostate gland   prostatitis _____

Bacterial (E. coli) prostatitis is often associated with urethritis and infection of the lower urinary tract.

                                       prostatectomy _____

semin/i   semen, seed   seminiferous tubules _____

-ferous means pertaining to bearing or carrying.

                                       seminal vesicles _____

sperm/o   spermatozoa, semen   spermolytic _____
spermat/o
                                       Noun suffixes ending in -sis, like -lysis, form adjectives by dropping the -sis and adding -tic.

                                       oligospermia _____

                                       aspermia _____

Lack of formation or ejaculation of semen (sperm and fluid).

terat/o	monster (Greek, *teras*, "monster")	terato<u>ma</u> _____	

A tumor occurring in the testes composed of different types of tissue, such as bone, hair, cartilage, and skin cells. See page 314, Section V, under Pathological Conditions (carcinoma of the testes).

test/o   testis, testicle   <u>test</u>icular _____

The term testis originates from a Latin term meaning "witness." In ancient times men would take an oath with one hand on their testes, swearing by their manhood to tell the truth.

varic/o   varicose veins   <u>varic</u>ocele _____

A collection of varicose (swollen, twisted) veins above the testes. See page 315.

vas/o   vessel, duct (referring to the vas deferens)   <u>vas</u>ectomy _____

See page 319, Section VI, under Clinical Procedures.

zo/o   animal life   a<u>zo</u>ospermia _____

Lack of spermatozoa in the semen. Causes include testicular dysfunction, chemotherapy, blockage of the epididymis, or vasectomy.

Suffixes

Suffix	Meaning	Terminology	Meaning
-genesis	formation	spermato<u>genesis</u> _____	
-one	hormone	testoster<u>one</u> _____	

ster/o indicates that this is a type of steroid compound.

Suffix	Meaning	Terminology	Meaning
-pexy	fixation, put in place	orchio<u>pexy</u> _____	

An operation to correct cryptorchism.

Suffix	Meaning	Terminology	Meaning
-stomy	new opening	vasovaso<u>stomy</u> _____	

Reversal of vasectomy; a urologist rejoins the cut ends of the vas deferens.

V. Pathological Conditions; Sexually Transmitted Infections

Abnormal and Pathological Conditions

Testes

carcinoma of the testes   **Malignant tumor of the testicles.**

Testicular tumors are rare except in the 15- to 35-year-old age group. The most common tumor, a **seminoma,** arises from embryonic cells in the testes. Non-seminomatous tumors are **embryonal carcinoma, teratoma,** and **teratocarcinoma** (combination of embryonal carcinoma and teratoma). Teratomas are composed of tissue such as bone, hair, cartilage, and skin cells (terat/o means "monster").

Tumors of the testes can be treated and cured with surgery (orchiectomy), radiotherapy, and chemotherapy.

cryptorchism; cryptorchidism   **Undescended testicles.**

Orchiopexy is performed to bring the testes into the scrotum, if they do not descend on their own before the boy is 2 years old. Undescended testicles put the male at high risk of sterility and testicular cancer.

hydrocele   **Sac of clear fluid in the scrotum.**

Hydroceles may be congenital or occur as a response to infection or tumors. Often idiopathic, they can be differentiated from testicular masses by *transillumination* (shining a light source to the side of a scrotal enlargement). If the hydrocele does not resolve on its own, hydrocelectomy may be necessary. The sac is aspirated via needle and syringe or surgically removed through an incision in the scrotum (Fig. 9–6).

testicular torsion   **Twisting of the spermatic cord** (Fig. 9–6).

The rotation of the spermatic cord cuts off blood supply to the testis. It is most frequent in the 1st year of life and during puberty. Surgical correction within 5 hours of onset of symptoms can save the testis.

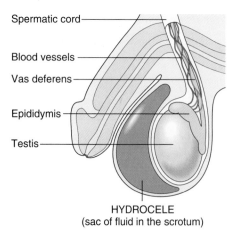 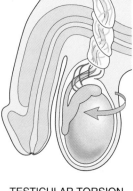 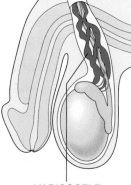

Spermatic cord
Blood vessels
Vas deferens
Epididymis
Testis

HYDROCELE
(sac of fluid in the scrotum)

TESTICULAR TORSION
(twisted spermatic cord)

VARICOCELE
(dilated spermatic veins)

Figure 9–6

Hydrocele, testicular torsion, and **varicocele.**

varicocele

Enlarged, dilated veins near the testicle.

This condition is associated with oligospermia and azoospermia. Oligospermic men with varicoceles and scrotal pain should have a varicocelectomy. In this procedure, the internal spermatic vein is ligated (a segment is cut out and the ends are tied off), leading to a marked increase in fertility (Fig. 9–6).

Prostate Gland

carcinoma of the prostate

Malignant tumor of the prostate gland.

This cancer commonly occurs in men who are older than 50 years of age. **Digital rectal examination** (Fig. 9–7) can detect the tumor at a later stage, but early detection depends on a **prostate-specific antigen** (**PSA**) **test**. PSA is a protein tumor marker that is elevated in prostate cancer. The normal PSA level is 4.0 ng/mL or less.

Diagnosis requires identification by a pathologist of abnormal prostate tissue in a prostate biopsy. **Transrectal ultrasound (TRUS)** guides the precise placement of the biopsy needle. Computed tomography (CT) detects lymph node metastases.

Treatment consists of surgery (prostatectomy), radiation therapy, and/or hormonal chemotherapy. Because prostatic cells are stimulated to grow in the presence of androgens, antiandrogen hormones are used to slow tumor growth by depriving the cells of testosterone. Prostate cancer can also be treated with leupron, a hormone that blocks pituitary stimulation of the testes. Radioactive seeds implanted in the prostate are also used to destroy tumor cells.

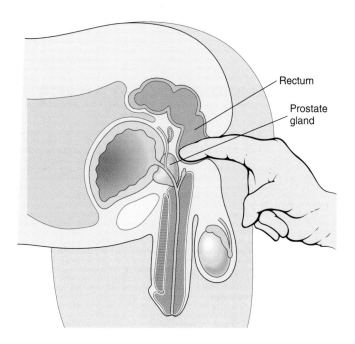

Figure 9–7

Digital rectal examination (DRE) of the prostate gland.

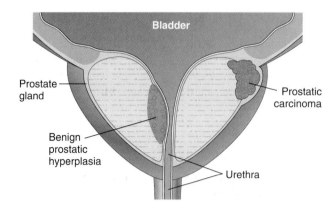

Bladder

Prostate gland

Prostatic carcinoma

Benign prostatic hyperplasia

Urethra

Figure 9–8

The prostate gland with carcinoma and benign prostatic hyperplasia (BPH). Carcinoma usually arises around the sides of the gland, whereas BPH occurs in the center of the gland. Because prostate cancers are located more peripherally, they can be palpated on digital rectal exam (DRE).

prostatic hyperplasia	**Benign growth of cells within the prostate gland; benign prostatic hyperplasia (BPH).**

BPH is a common occurrence in men older than 60 years of age. Urinary obstruction and inability to empty the bladder completely are symptoms. Figure 9–8 shows the prostate gland with BPH and with carcinoma. Surgical treatment by **transurethral resection (TURP)** is curative. An endoscope (resectoscope) is inserted into the penis and through the urethra. Prostatic tissue is removed by an electrical hot-loop attached to the resectoscope.

Several drugs to relieve BPH symptoms have been approved by the FDA. Finasteride (Proscar) inhibits production of a potent testosterone that is involved in the enlargement of the prostate. Other drugs, alpha-blockers such as tamsulosin (Flomax), act by relaxing the smooth muscle of the prostate and the neck of the bladder.

Penis

hypospadias; hypospadia	**Congenital opening of the male urethra on the undersurface of the penis** (Fig. 9–9A).

Hypospadias (-spadias means the condition of tearing or cutting) occurs in 1 of every 300 live male births and can be corrected surgically.

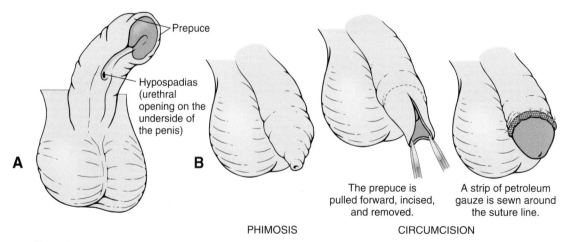

Prepuce

Hypospadias (urethral opening on the underside of the penis)

A

B

The prepuce is pulled forward, incised, and removed.

A strip of petroleum gauze is sewn around the suture line.

PHIMOSIS

CIRCUMCISION

Figure 9–9

(A) Hypospadias. Surgical repair involves excising a portion of the prepuce, wrapping it (the graft) around a catheter, suturing it to the distal part of the urethra, and bringing it to the exit at the tip of the penis. **(B) Phimosis** and **circumcision** to correct the condition.

phimosis
: **Narrowing (stricture) of the opening of the prepuce over the glans penis; phim/o means to muzzle.**

  This condition can interfere with urination and cause secretions to accumulate under the prepuce, leading to infection. Treatment is by circumcision (cutting around the prepuce to remove it) (Fig. 9–9B).

Sexually Transmitted Infections (STI)

The following conditions, previously called **venereal** (transmitted by sexual or genital contact) **diseases** or **sexually transmitted diseases**, occur in both men and women and are the most easily communicable diseases in the world. They are transmitted by sexual contact.

chlamydial infection
: **Bacteria *(Chlamydia trachomatis)* invade the urethra and reproductive tract of men and the vagina and cervix of women.**

  Within 3 weeks after becoming infected, men may experience dysuria and a white or clear discharge from the penis. The term **nonspecific urethritis** is used to describe this condition in men.

  Women may develop a yellowish endocervical discharge, but often the disease is asymptomatic. Tetracycline (an antibiotic) cures the infection.

gonorrhea
: **Inflammation of the genital tract mucous membranes, caused by infection with gonococci (berry-shaped bacteria).**

  Other areas of the body, such as the eye, oral mucosa, rectum, and joints, may be affected as well. Symptoms include dysuria and a yellow, mucopurulent (**purulent** means pus-filled) discharge from the urethra. The ancient Greeks mistakenly thought that this discharge was a leakage of semen; hence they named the condition **gonorrhea,** meaning "discharge of seed" (gon/o).

  Many women carry the disease asymptomatically, and others have pain, vaginal and urethral discharge, and salpingitis (pelvic inflammatory disease [PID]). As a result of sexual activity, men and women can acquire anorectal and pharyngeal gonococcal infections as well. Chlamydial infection and gonorrhea often occur together. When treating these infections, doctors give antibiotics for both and treat both partners.

herpes genitalis
: **Infection of the skin and mucosa of the genitals, caused by the herpes simplex virus (HSV).**

  Most cases of herpes genitalis are caused by HSV type II (although some are caused by HSV I, which is commonly associated with oral infections). Symptoms are reddening of skin with small, fluid-filled blisters and ulcers. Initial episodes may also involve inguinal lymphadenopathy, fever, headache, and malaise. Remissions and relapse periods occur; no drug is known to be effective as a cure. Neonatal herpes is a serious complication that affects infants born to women infected near the time of delivery. Gynecologists deliver infants by cesarean section to prevent herpes infection when the mother has an active case during labor. Studies suggest that women with herpes genitalis have a higher risk of developing vulvar and cervical cancer.

syphilis	**Chronic STI caused by a spirochete (spiral-shaped bacterium).**

A **chancre** (hard ulcer) usually appears on the external genitalia a few weeks after bacterial infection. Lymphadenopathy follows as the infection spreads to internal organs. Later stages include damage to the brain, spinal cord, and heart. Syphilis (named after a shepherd in an Italian poem) can be congenital in the fetus if it is transmitted from the mother during pregnancy. Penicillin is the treatment.

VI. Laboratory Tests, Clinical Procedures, and Abbreviations

Laboratory Tests

PSA test

Measures levels of prostate-specific antigen in the blood.

PSA is produced by cells within the prostate gland. Elevated levels of PSA are associated with enlargement of the prostate gland and prostate cancer.

semen analysis

Ejaculated fluid is examined microscopically.

Sperm cells are counted and examined for motility and shape. The test is part of fertility studies and is also required to establish the effectiveness of vasectomy. Men with less than 20 million sperm/mL of semen are usually sterile (not fertile). Sterility can result when adult males become ill with mumps, an infectious disease affecting the testes (inflammation and deterioration of spermatozoa).

Clinical Procedures

castration

Surgical excision of testicles or ovaries.

Castration may be performed to reduce production and secretion of hormones that stimulate growth of malignant cells (in breast cancer and prostate cancer). When a male is castrated before puberty, he becomes a **eunuch** (Greek, *eune*, "couch," *echein*, "to guard"). Male secondary sex characteristics fail to develop.

circumcision

Surgical procedure to remove the prepuce of the penis.

See Figure 9–9B.

digital rectal examination (DRE)

Finger palpation through the rectum to examine the prostate gland.

See Figure 9–7.

transurethral resection of the prostate (TURP)

Excision of parts of the prostate gland using a resectoscope through the urethra.

This procedure treats benign prostatic hyperplasia (BPH). An electrical hot-loop destroys the prostatic tissue, which is removed through the resectoscope (Fig. 9–10).

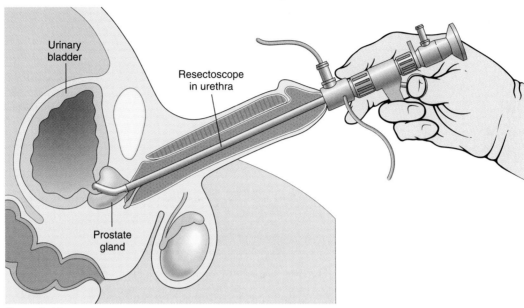

Figure 9–10

Transurethral resection of the prostate (TURP). The resectoscope contains a light, valves for controlling irrigating fluid, and an electrical loop that cuts tissue and seals blood vessels. The urologist uses a wire loop through the resectoscope to remove obstructing tissue one piece at a time. The pieces are carried by the fluid into the bladder and flushed out at the end of the operation.

vasectomy

Bilateral surgical removal of a part of the vas deferens.

A urologist cuts the vas deferens on each side, removes a piece, and performs a **ligation** (to tie and bind off) of the free ends with sutures (Fig. 9–11). The procedure is performed under local anesthesia and through an incision in the scrotal sac. Because spermatozoa cannot leave the body, the male is sterile, but not castrated. Normal hormone secretion, sex drive, and potency (ability to have an erection) are intact. The body reabsorbs unexpelled sperm. In a small number of cases, a vasovasostomy can successfully reverse vasectomy.

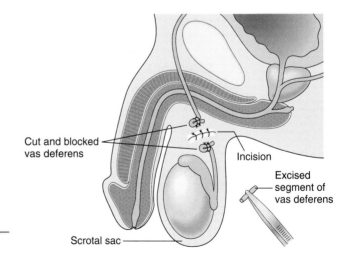

Figure 9–11

Vasectomy.

Abbreviations

BPH	benign prostatic hyperplasia (also called benign prostatic hypertrophy)	**STI**	sexually transmitted infections
DRE	digital rectal examination	**TRUS**	transrectal ultrasound (test to assess the prostate gland and to guide the precise placement of a biopsy needle)
GU	genitourinary		
HSV	herpes simplex virus	**TUIP**	transurethral incision of the prostate
PID	pelvic inflammatory disease	**TUMT**	transurethral microwave thermotherapy
		TUNA	transurethral needle ablation
PSA	prostate-specific antigen		
RPR	rapid plasma reagin (test for syphilis)	**TURP**	transurethral resection of the prostate

VII. Practical Applications

Answers to the questions are on page 328 after Answers to Exercises.

Case Report: A Man with Post-TURP Complaints

The patient is a 70-year-old man who underwent a TURP for BPH 5 years ago and now has severe obstructive urinary symptoms with a large postvoid residual.

On DRE, his prostate was found to be large, bulky, and nodular, with palpable extension to the left seminal vesicle. His PSA level was 120 ng/mL [normal is 0-4 ng/mL] and a bone scan was negative. A pelvic sonogram revealed bilateral external iliac adenopathy with lymph nodes measuring 1.5 cm on average [normal lymph node size is less than 1 cm]. A prostatic biopsy revealed a poorly differentiated adenocarcinoma.

This patient most likely has at least stage D1 disease [distant metastases with pelvic lymph node involvement]. Recommendation is hormonal drug treatment to suppress secretion of testosterone, which stimulates prostatic tumor growth.

Questions on the Case Report

1. **Five years previously, the patient had which type of surgery?**
   (A) Removal of testicles
   (B) Perineal prostatectomy
   (C) Partial prostatectomy (transurethral)
2. **What was the reason for the surgery then?**
   (A) Cryptorchism
   (B) Benign overgrowth of the prostate gland
   (C) Testicular cancer

3. **What symptom does he have now?**
   (A) Burning pain on urination
   (B) Urinary retention
   (C) Premature ejaculation
4. **What examination allowed the physician to feel the tumor?**
   (A) Finger inserted into rectum
   (B) Pelvic sonogram
   (C) Prostate-specific antigen test
5. **Where had the tumor spread?**
   (A) Pelvic lymph nodes
   (B) Pelvic lymph nodes and left seminal vesicle
   (C) Pelvic bone
6. **What is likely to stimulate prostatic adenocarcinoma growth?**
   (A) Hormonal drug treatment
   (B) Prostatic biopsy
   (C) Testosterone secretion
7. **Stage D1 means that the tumor**
   (A) Is localized in the hip area
   (B) Is confined to the prostate gland
   (C) Has spread to lymph nodes and other organs
8. **Why is staging of tumors important?**
   (A) To classify the extent of spread of the tumor and to plan treatment
   (B) To make the initial diagnosis
   (C) To make an adequate biopsy of the tumor

FYI: Anabolic Steroids

Anabolic steroids are male hormones (androgens) that increase body weight and muscle size and may be used by doctors to increase growth in boys who do not mature physically as expected for their age. Steroids are also used by athletes in an effort to increase strength and enhance performance; however, there are significant detrimental side effects to their use:

1. High levels of anabolic steroids cause acne, hepatic tumors, and sterility (testicular atrophy and oligospermia).
2. In women, the androgenic effect of anabolic steroids leads to male hair distribution, deepening of voice, amenorrhea, and clitoral enlargement.
3. Anabolic steroid use also causes hypercholesterolemia, hypertension, jaundice (liver abnormalities), and salt and water retention (edema).

VIII. Exercises

Remember to check your answers carefully with those given in Section IX, Answers to Exercises.

A. Build medical terms.

1. inflammation of the testes _____

2. inflammation of the tube that carries the spermatozoa to the vas deferens

_____

3. resection of the prostate gland _____

4. inflammation of the prostate gland _____

5. the process of producing (the formation of) sperm cells _____

6. fixation of undescended testicle _____

7. inflammation of the glans penis _____

8. condition of scanty sperm _____

9. no sperm or semen are produced _____

10. pertaining to a testicle _____

B. Give the meanings of the following medical terms.

1. hypospadias _____

2. parenchyma _____

3. stroma _____

4. cryogenic _____

5. interstitial cells of the testes _____

6. testosterone _____

7. phimosis _____

8. azoospermia _____

9. androgen _____

10. testicular seminoma _____

11. teratocarcinoma _____

C. Give medical terms for the descriptions below.

1. tube above each testis; carries and stores sperm _____

2. gland surrounding the urethra at the base of the urinary bladder _____

3. parenchymal tissue of the testes; produces spermatozoa _____

4. sperm cell _____

5. foreskin _____

6. male gonad; produces hormone and sperm cells _____

7. pair of sacs; secrete fluid into ejaculatory ducts _____

8. sac on outside of the body enclosing the testes _____

9. tube carrying sperm from the epididymis toward the urethra _____

10. pair of glands near the urethra; secrete fluid into the urethra _____

D. Match the term in column I with the letter of its meaning in column II.

Column I

1. castration _____

2. semen analysis _____

3. ejaculation _____

4. purulent _____

5. vasectomy _____

6. circumcision _____

7. ligation _____

8. cryosurgery _____

Column II

A. to tie off or bind
B. removal of a piece of the vas deferens
C. orchiectomy
D. removal of the prepuce
E. destruction of tissue by freezing
F. pus-filled
G. test of fertility (reproductive ability)
H. ejection of sperm and fluid from the urethra

E. Give medical terms for the following abnormal conditions.

1. prostatic enlargement, nonmalignant _____

2. opening of the urethra on the undersurface of the penis _____

3. sexually transmitted infection with herpes virus _____

4. malignant tumor of the prostate gland _____

5. enlarged, swollen veins near the testes _____

6. sexually transmitted infection; primary stage marked by chancre _____

7. malignant tumor of the testes (three types) _____,

_____ , and _____

8. STI etiologic agent is berry-shaped bacteria marked by inflammation of genital mucosa and

mucopurulent discharge _____

9. undescended testicles _____

10. sac of clear fluid in the scrotum _____

F. Give the meanings of the following abbreviations and then select the letter from the sentence that is the best association for each.

Column I

1. PSA_____ ____

2. BPH _____ ____

3. TURP _____ ____

4. TRUS _____ ____

5. DRE _____ ____

6. HSV _____ ____

7. STI _____ ____

Column II

A. Manual diagnostic procedure to examine the prostate gland.
B. Relieves symptoms of prostate gland enlargement.
C. Etiological agent of a sexually transmitted infection; characterized by blister formation.
D. Noncancerous enlargement of the prostate gland.
E. Chlamydia, gonorrhea, and syphilis are examples of this general condition.
F. Helpful procedure in guiding a prostatic biopsy needle.
G. High blood serum levels of this protein indicate prostatic carcinoma.

G. Review exercise. Give the meanings of the following.

1. -stasis _____

2. -sclerosis _____

3. -stenosis _____

4. -cele _____

5. -rrhagia _____

6. -ptosis _____

7. -plasia _____

8. -phagia _____

9. -rrhaphy _____

10. -pexy _____

11. -ectasis _____

12. -centesis _____

13. -genesis _____

14. balan/o _____

15. oophor/o _____

16. salping/o _____

17. hyster/o _____

18. metr/o _____

19. colp/o _____

20. mast/o _____

H. Match the following surgical procedures with the reasons they would be performed.

bilateral orchiectomy
circumcision
hydrocelectomy
orchiopexy

radical (complete)
   prostatectomy
TURP

varicocelectomy
vasectomy
vasovasostomy

1. carcinoma of the prostate gland _____

2. cryptorchism _____

3. sterilization (hormones remain and potency is not impaired) _____

4. benign prostatic hyperplasia _____

5. abnormal collection of fluid in a scrotal sac _____

6. reversal of sterilization procedure _____

7. teratocarcinoma of the testes _____

8. phimosis _____

9. swollen, twisted veins above the testes _____

I. Give the following medical terms based on their meanings and partial spellings. Check your answers carefully.

1. gland at the base of the urinary bladder in males: pro _____ gland

2. coiled tube on top of each testis: epi _____

3. essential cells of an organ: par _____

4. foreskin: pre _____

5. bacteria that is the major cause of nonspecific urethritis in males and cervicitis in females:

   Ch _____

6. ulcer that forms on genital organs after infection with syphilis: ch _____

7. androgen produced by the interstitial cells of the testis: test _____

8. fluid secreted by male reproductive glands and ejaculated with sperm: se _____

J. Circle the correct terminology to complete the following sentences.

1. Fred's doctors could feel only one testicle shortly after his birth and suggested close following of his condition of **(gonorrhea, cryptorchism, prostatic hyperplasia).**

2. Bob had many sexual partners, one of whom had been diagnosed with **(testosterone, phimosis, chlamydial infection),** a highly infectious STI.

3. At age 65, Mike had some difficulty with urgency and discomfort when urinating. His doctor did a digital rectal examination to examine his **(prostate gland, urinary bladder, vas deferens).**

4. Just after his birth, Nick's parents had a difficult time deciding whether to have the boy undergo **(TURP, castration, circumcision).**

5. Ted noticed a hard ulcer called a **(eunuch, chancre, seminoma)** on his penis and made an appointment with his doctor, a **(gastroenterologist, gynecologist, urologist).** The doctor viewed a specimen of the ulcer under the microscope and did a blood test, which revealed that Ted had contracted **(gonorrhea, herpes genitalis, syphilis).**

6. After his fifth child was born, Art decided to have a **(vasovasostomy, hydrocelectomy, vasectomy)** to prevent conception of another child. A (an) **(nephrologist, urologist, abdominal surgeon)** performed the procedure to cut and ligate the **(urethra, epididymis, vas deferens).**

7. Twenty-six-year-old Lance noticed a hard testicular mass. His physician prescribed a brief trial with **(antibodies, antibiotics, pain killers)** to rule out **(epididymitis, testicular cancer, varicocele).** The mass remained and Lance underwent **(epididymectomy, orchiectomy, prostatectomy)** and lymph node resection. The mass was a **(seminoma, prostate cancer, hydrocele).**

8. Sarah and Steve had been trying to conceive a child for 7 years. Steve had a **(digital rectal examination, TURP, semen analysis),** which revealed 25 percent normal sperm count with 10 percent motility. He was told he had **(anorchism, aspermia, oligospermia).**

9. To boost his sperm count, Steve was given **(estrogen, testosterone, progesterone).** As a side effect, this **(androgen, progestin, enzyme)** gave him a case of acne lasting several months.

10. Sarah eventually became pregnant. An ultrasound examination showed two embryos in separate **(peritoneal, scrotal, amniotic)** sacs. Sarah delivered two healthy **(identical, fraternal, perineal)** twin girls.

IX. Answers to Exercises

A

1. orchitis
2. epididymitis
3. prostatectomy
4. prostatitis
5. spermatogenesis
6. orchiopexy
7. balanitis
8. oligospermia
9. aspermia
10. testicular

B

1. Congenital anomaly in which the urethra opens on the underside of the penis.
2. The distinctive, essential tissue or cells of an organ, as for example, glomeruli and tubules of the kidney, seminiferous tubules of the testis.
3. The supportive and connective tissue of an organ.
4. Pertaining to producing cold or low temperatures.
5. The cells that produce the hormone testosterone. These cells are stimulated by luteinizing hormone from the pituitary gland.
6. A hormone made by the intestitial cells of the testes; responsible for secondary sex characteristics.
7. A narrowing, or stenosis, of the foreskin on the glans penis.
8. Lack of spermatozoa in the semen.
9. Hormone producing male characteristics.
10. Malignant tumor of the testes composed of germ or embryonic cells.
11. Malignant tumor of testes (composed of embryonic tissue forming bone, hair, skin, cartilage).

C

1. epididymis
2. prostate gland
3. seminiferous tubules (semin = semen, fer = to carry)
4. spermatozoon
5. prepuce
6. testis; testicle
7. seminal vesicles
8. scrotum; scrotal sac
9. vas deferens
10. bulbourethral or Cowper glands

D

1. C
2. G
3. H
4. F
5. B
6. D
7. A
8. E

E

1. benign prostatic hyperplasia
2. hypospadias
3. herpes genitalia
4. adenocarcinoma of the prostate
5. varicocele
6. syphilis
7. embryonal carcinoma; seminoma; teratoma or teratocarcinoma
8. gonorrhea
9. cryptorchism
10. hydrocele

F

1. prostate-specific antigen. G
2. benign prostatic hyperplasia. D
3. transurethral resection of the prostate. B
4. transrectal ultrasound. F
5. digital rectal examination. A
6. herpes simplex virus. C
7. sexually transmitted infection. E

G

1. to stop, control; place
2. hardening
3. narrowing
4. hernia, swelling
5. bursting forth (of blood)
6. prolapse
7. formation
8. eating, swallowing
9. suture
10. fixation
11. widening
12. surgical puncture to remove fluid
13. producing
14. glans penis
15. ovary
16. fallopian tube
17. uterus
18. uterus
19. vagina
20. breast

H

1. radical (complete) prostatectomy
2. orchiopexy
3. vasectomy
4. TURP
5. hydrocelectomy
6. vasovasostomy
7. bilateral orchiectomy
8. circumcision
9. varicocelectomy

Continued on following page

I

1. prostate
2. epididymis
3. parenchyma

4. prepuce
5. Chlamydia
6. chancre

7. testosterone
8. semen or seminal

J

1. cryptorchism
2. chlamydial infection
3. prostate gland
4. circumcision

5. chancre; urologist; syphilis
6. vasectomy; urologist; vas deferens
7. antibiotics; epididymitis; orchiectomy; seminoma

8. semen analysis; oligospermia
9. testosterone; androgen
10. amniotic; fraternal

Answers to Practical Applications

1. C
2. B
3. B

4. A
5. B
6. C

7. C
8. A

X. Pronunciation of Terms

Pronunciation Guide

ā as in āpe   ă as in ăpple
ē as in ēven   ĕ as in ĕvery
ī as in īce   ĭ as in ĭnterest
ō as in ōpen   ŏ as in pŏt
ū as in ūnit   ŭ as in ŭnder

To test your understanding of the terminology in this chapter, write the meaning of each term in the space provided. In addition, you may wish to cover the terms and write them by looking at your definitions. Make sure your spelling is correct. The page number after each term indicates where it is defined or used in the text so you can easily check your responses.

Term	Pronunciation	Meaning
androgen (311)	ĂN-drō-jĕn	_____
anorchism (312)	ăn-ŎR-kĭzm	_____
aspermia (312)	ā-SPĔR-mē-ă	_____
azoospermia (313)	ā-zō-ō-SPĔR-mē-ă	_____
balanitis (311)	băl-ă-NĪ-tĭs	_____
bulbourethral gland (309)	bŭl-bō-ū-RĒ-thrăl glănd	_____
castration (318)	kăs-TRĀ-shŭn	_____
chancre (318)	SHĂNG-kĕr	_____
chlamydial infection (317)	klă-MĬD-ē-al in-FĔK-shŭn	_____

circumcision (318)	sĕr-kŭm-SĬZH-ŭn
Cowper gland (309)	CŎW-pĕr glănd
cryogenic surgery (311)	krī-ō-GĔN-ik SŬR-jĕr-ē
cryptorchism (314)	krĭp-TŎR-kĭzm
ejaculation (309)	ē-jăk-ū-LĀ-shŭn
ejaculatory duct (309)	ē-JĂK-ū-lā-tŏr-ē dŭkt
embryonal carcinoma (314)	ĕm-brē-ŎN-ăl kăr-sĭ-NŌ-mă
epididymis (309)	ĕp-ĭ-DĬD-ĭ-mĭs
epididymitis (312)	ĕp-ĭ-dĭd-ĭ-MĪ-tĭs
erectile dysfunction (309)	ē-RĔK-tīl dĭs-FŬNG-shŭn
eunuch (318)	Ū-nŭk
flagellum (309)	flă-JĔL-ŭm
fraternal twins (309)	fră-TĔR-năl twĭnz
gonorrhea (317)	gŏn-ō-RĒ-ă
herpes genitalis (317)	HĔR-pēz jĕn-ĭ-TĂL-ĭs
hydrocele (314)	HĪ-drō-sēl
hypospadias (316)	hī-pō-SPĀ-dē-ăs
identical twins (309)	ī-DĔN-tĭ-kăl twĭnz
interstitial cells (310)	ĭn-tĕr-STĬSH-ăl sĕlz
impotence (310)	ĬM-pō-tĕns
ligation (319)	lī-GĀ-shun
oligospermia (312)	ŏl-ĭ-gō-SPĔR-mē-ă
orchiectomy (312)	ŏr-kē-ĔK-tō-mē
orchiopexy (313)	ŏr-kē-ō-PĔK-sē
orchitis (312)	ŏr-KĪ-tĭs
parenchyma (310)	pă-RĔNG-kĭ-mă
perineum (310)	pĕr-ĭ-NĒ-ŭm

phimosis (317)   fĭ-MŌ-sĭs   _____

prepuce (310)   PRĒ-pŭs   _____

prostatectomy (312)   prŏs-tă-TĔK-tō-mē   _____

prostate gland (310)   PRŎS-tāt glănd   _____

prostatic hyperplasia (316)   prŏs-TĂT-ĭk hĭ-pĕr-PLĀ-zē-ă   _____

prostatitis (312)   prŏs-tă-TĪ-tĭs   _____

purulent (317)   PŪR-ū-lent   _____

scrotum (310)   SKRŌ-tŭm   _____

semen (310)   SĒ-mĕn   _____

seminal vesicles (310)   SĔM-ĭn-ăl VĔS-ĭ-k'lz   _____

seminiferous tubules (310)   sĕ-mĭ-NĬF-ĕr-ŭs TŪB-ūlz   _____

seminoma (314)   sĕ-mĭ-NŌ-mă   _____

spermatogenesis (313)   spĕr-mă-tō-JĔN-ĕ-sĭs   _____

spermatozoa (310)   spĕr-mă-tō-ZŌ-ă   _____

spermatozoon (310)   spĕr-mă-tō-ZŌ-ōn   _____

spermolytic (312)   spĕr-mō-LĬT-ĭk   _____

sterilization (310)   stĕr-ĭ-lĭ-ZĀ-shŭn   _____

stroma (310)   STRŌ-mă   _____

syphilis (318)   SĬF-ĭ-lĭs   _____

teratoma (313)   tĕr-ă-TŌ-mă   _____

testicular (313)   tĕs-TĬK-ŭ-lăr   _____

testicular torsion (314)   tĕs-TĬK-ū-lăr TŎR-shŭn   _____

testis (310)   TĔS-tĭs   _____

testosterone (310)   tĕs-TŎS-tĕ-rōn   _____

varicocele (315)   VĀR-ĭ-kō-sēl   _____

vas deferens (310)   văs DĔF-ĕr-ĕnz   _____

vasectomy (319)   vă-SĔK-tō-mē   _____

vasovasostomy (313)   vă-zō-vă-ZŎS-tō-mē   _____

XI. Review Sheet

Write the meanings of the word parts in the spaces provided. Check your answers with the information in the chapter or in the glossary (Medical Terms—English) at the end of the book.

COMBINING FORMS

Combining Form	Meaning	Combining Form	Meaning
andr/o	_____	prostat/o	_____
balan/o	_____	semin/i	_____
cry/o	_____	sperm/o	_____
crypt/o	_____	spermat/o	_____
epididym/o	_____	terat/o	_____
gon/o	_____	test/o	_____
hydr/o	_____	varic/o	_____
orch/o	_____	vas/o	_____
orchi/o	_____	zo/o	_____
orchid/o	_____		

SUFFIXES

Suffix	Meaning	Suffix	Meaning
-cele	_____	-one	_____
-ectomy	_____	-pexy	_____
-gen	_____	-plasia	_____
-genesis	_____	-rrhea	_____
-genic	_____	-stomy	_____
-lysis	_____	-tomy	_____
-lytic	_____	-trophy	_____

Nervous System

This chapter is divided into the following sections

In this chapter you will

- Name, locate, and describe the functions of the major organs and parts of the nervous system.
- Recognize nervous system combining forms and make terms using them with new and familiar suffixes.
- Define several pathological conditions affecting the nervous system.
- Describe some laboratory tests, clinical procedures, and abbreviations that pertain to the system.
- Apply your new knowledge to understanding medical terms in their proper contexts, such as medical reports and records.

I. Introduction

The nervous system is one of the most complex of all human body systems. More than 10 billion nerve cells operate constantly all over the body to coordinate the activities we do consciously and voluntarily, as well as those that occur unconsciously or involuntarily. We speak; we move muscles; we hear; we taste; we see; we think; our glands secrete hormones; we respond to danger, pain, temperature, and touch; and we have memory, association, and discrimination. All of these functions compose only a small number of the many activities controlled by our nervous systems.

Microscopic **nerve cells** collected into macroscopic bundles called **nerves** carry electrical messages all over the body. External stimuli, as well as internal chemicals such as **acetylcholine,** activate the cell membranes of nerve cells in order to release stored electrical energy within the cells. This energy, when released and passed through the length of the nerve cell, is called the **nervous impulse.** External **receptors** (sense organs) as well as internal receptors in muscles and blood vessels receive these impulses and transmit them to the complex network of nerve cells in the brain and spinal cord. Within this central part of the nervous system, impulses are recognized, interpreted, and finally relayed to other nerve cells that extend out to all parts of the body, such as muscles, glands, and internal organs.

II. General Structure of the Nervous System

The nervous system is classified into two major divisions: the **central nervous system (CNS)** and the **peripheral nervous system.** The central nervous system consists of the **brain** and **spinal cord.** The peripheral nervous system consists of 12 pairs of **cranial nerves** and 31 pairs of **spinal nerves.** The cranial nerves carry impulses between the brain and the head and neck. The one exception is the 10th cranial nerve, called the vagus nerve. It carries messages to and from the chest and abdomen, as well as the head and neck regions. Table 10–1 lists the cranial nerves and the parts of the body they affect. The spinal nerves carry messages between the spinal cord and the chest, abdomen, and extremities.

Table 10–1. **CRANIAL NERVES AND THEIR FUNCTIONS**

A **sensory nerve** carries messages *toward the brain* from sense organs. A **motor nerve** carries messages *from the brain* to muscles and internal organs. Some nerves (mixed) carry both sensory and motor fibers.

Cranial Nerve	Function
I. Olfactory (sensory)	Smell
II. Optic (sensory)	Vision
III. Oculomotor (motor)	Eye movement and pupil size
IV. Trochlear (motor)	Eye movement
V. Trigeminal	
V.1 Ophthalmic (sensory)	Face and scalp sensation
V.2 Maxillary (sensory)	Mouth and nose sensation
V.3 Mandibular (mixed)	Chewing
VI. Abducens (motor)	Eye movement
VII. Facial (mixed)	Face and scalp movement
	Tongue taste sensation
	Ear pain and temperature
VIII. Vestibulocochlear (sensory)	Hearing and balance
IX. Glossopharyngeal (mixed)	Sensation in the ear
	Tongue and throat sensations
	Throat movement
X. Vagus (mixed)	Throat, voice box, chest, abdominal sensations
	Voice box and throat movement
	Chest movement
XI. Accessory (motor)	Neck muscle movement
XII. Hypoglossal (motor)	Tongue movement

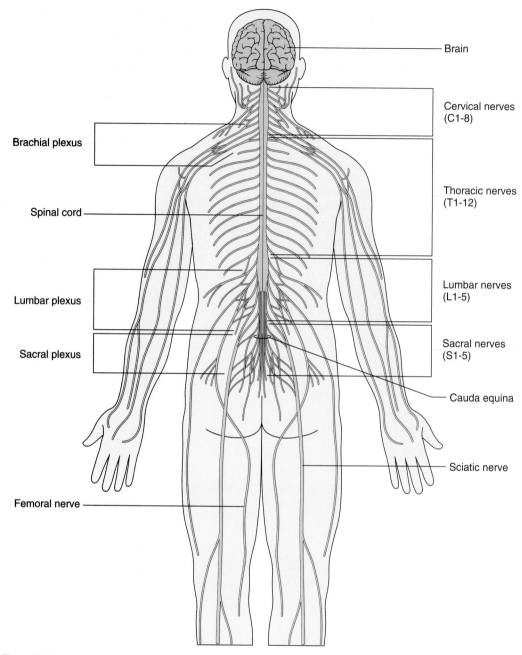

Brain

Cervical nerves
(C1-8)

Brachial plexus

Thoracic nerves
(T1-12)

Spinal cord

Lumbar nerves
(L1-5)

Lumbar plexus

Sacral nerves
(S1-5)

Sacral plexus

Cauda equina

Sciatic nerve

Femoral nerve

Figure 10–1

The brain and the spinal cord, spinal nerves, and spinal plexuses. The **femoral nerve** is a lumbar nerve leading to and from the thigh (femur). The **sciatic nerve** is a sacral nerve beginning in a region of the hip. The **cauda equina** ("horse's tail") is a bundle of spinal nerves below the end of the spinal cord.

The spinal and cranial nerves are composed of nerves that help the body respond to changes in the outside world. They include **sense receptors** for sight (eye), hearing and balance (ear), smell (olfactory), and **sensory nerves** that carry messages related to changes in the environment *toward the brain*. In addition, **motor nerves** travel *from the brain* to muscles of the body, telling them how to respond.

In addition to the spinal and cranial nerves (whose functions are mainly voluntary and involved with sensations of smell, taste, sight, hearing, and muscle movements), the peripheral nervous system also contains a large group of nerves that function involuntarily or automatically, without conscious control. These peripheral nerves belong to the **autonomic nervous system.** This system of nerve fibers carries impulses *from* the central nervous system to the glands, heart, blood vessels, and the involuntary muscles found in the walls of tubes like the intestines and hollow organs like the stomach and urinary bladder. The autonomic nerves carry impulses away from the central nervous system.

Some autonomic nerves are **sympathetic** nerves and others are **parasympathetic** nerves. The sympathetic nerves stimulate the body in times of stress and crisis; they increase heart rate and forcefulness, dilate (relax) airways so more oxygen can enter, increase blood pressure, stimulate the adrenal glands to secrete epinephrine (adrenaline), and inhibit intestinal contractions slowing digestion. The parasympathetic nerves normally act as a balance for the sympathetic nerves. Parasympathetic nerves slow down heart rate, contract the pupils of the eye, lower blood pressure, stimulate peristalsis to clear the rectum, and increase the quantity of secretions like saliva.

A **plexus** is a large network of nerves in the peripheral nervous system. The brachial (brachi/o means arm), and lumbar-sacral plexuses are examples. Figure 10–1 illustrates the relationship of the brain and spinal cord to the spinal nerves and plexuses.

Figure 10–2 summarizes the divisions of the central and peripheral nervous systems.

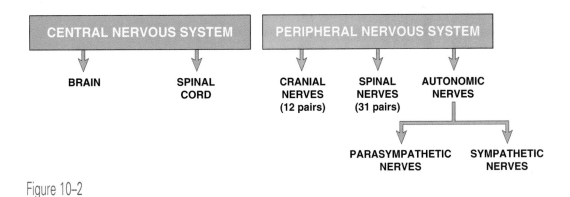

Figure 10–2

Divisions of the central nervous system (CNS) and peripheral nervous system (PNS). The autonomic nervous system is a part of the peripheral nervous system.

III. Neurons, Nerves, and Glia

A **neuron** is an individual nerve cell, a microscopic structure. Impulses pass along the parts of a nerve cell in a definite manner and direction. The parts of a neuron are pictured in Figure 10–3; label it as you study the following.

A **stimulus** begins an impulse in the branching fibers of the neuron, which are called **dendrites** [1]. A change in the electrical charge of the dendrite membranes is thus begun, and the nervous impulse moves along the dendrites like the movement of falling dominoes. The impulse, traveling in only one direction, next reaches the **cell body** [2], which contains the **cell nucleus** [3]. Small collections of nerve cell bodies outside the brain and spinal cord are called **ganglia** (singular: **ganglion**). Extending from the cell body is the **axon** [4], which carries the impulse away from the cell body. Axons are covered with a fatty tissue called a **myelin sheath** [5]. The myelin sheath gives a white appearance to the nerve fiber—hence the term white matter, as in parts of the spinal cord and the white matter of the brain and most peripheral nerves. The gray matter of the brain and spinal cord is composed of the cell bodies of neurons that appear gray because they are not covered by a myelin sheath.

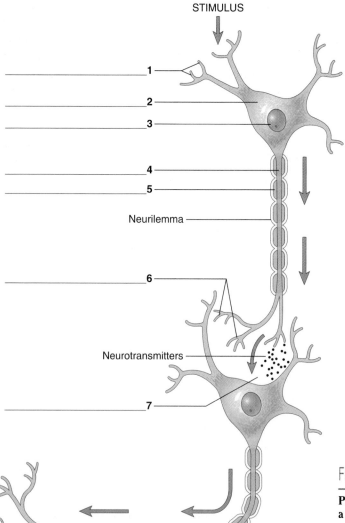

STIMULUS

1

2

3

4

5

Neurilemma

6

Neurotransmitters

7

Figure 10–3

Parts of a neuron and the pathway of a nervous impulse. Neurons are the **parenchymal** (essential) **cells** of the nervous system.

Another axon covering, called the **neurilemma,** is a membranous sheath outside the myelin sheath on the nerve cells of peripheral nerves. The nervous impulse passes through the axon to leave the cell via the **terminal end fibers** [6] of the neuron. The space where the nervous impulse jumps from one neuron to another is called the **synapse** [7]. The transfer of the impulse across the synapse depends on the release of a chemical substance, called a **neurotransmitter,** by the neuron that brings the impulse to the synapse. Tiny sacs containing the neurotransmitter are located at the ends of neurons, and they release the neurotransmitter into the synapse. **Acetylcholine, epinephrine (adrenaline), dopamine,** and **serotonin** are examples of neurotransmitters.

Whereas a neuron is a microscopic structure within the nervous system, a **nerve** is macroscopic, able to be seen with the naked eye. A nerve consists of a bundle of dendrites and axons that travel together like strands of rope. Peripheral nerves that carry impulses *to* the brain and spinal cord from stimulus receptors like the skin, eye, ear, and nose are **sensory nerves;** those that carry impulses *from* the CNS to organs that produce responses, (e.g., muscles and glands), are called **motor nerves.**

Neurons and nerves are the **parenchymal** tissue of the nervous system; they do the essential work of the system by conducting impulses throughout the body. The **stromal** tissue of the nervous system consists of other cells called **glia (neuroglia).** These cells hold the nervous system together and help the nervous system ward off infection and injury by phagocytosis (engulfing foreign material). Glia cells do not transmit impulses. They are far more numerous than neurons and can reproduce, whereas neurons cannot.

There are three types of supporting or glial (neuroglial) cells. **Astrocytes (astroglial cells)** are star-like (astr/o means star) and transport water and salts between capillaries and neurons. **Microglia (microglial cells)** are small cells with many branching processes. As phagocytes, they protect neurons in response to inflammation. **Oligodendroglia (oligodendroglial cells)** have few (olig/o means few or scanty) dendrites. These cells form the myelin sheath that protects axons in the CNS. Another cell, called an **ependymal cell** (*ependyma* in Greek means "upper garment") lines membranes within the brain and around the spinal cord and helps form the fluid that circulates within the brain and spinal cord.

Glial cells, particularly the astrocytes, are associated with blood vessels and regulate the passage of potentially harmful substances from the blood into the nerve cells of the brain. This protective barrier between the blood and brain cells is called the **blood–brain barrier.** Figure 10–4 illustrates glial cells.

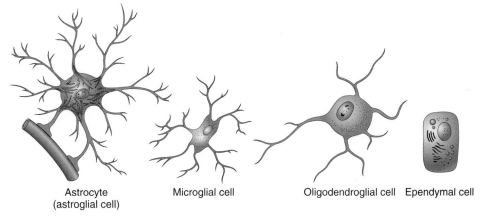

Astrocyte   Microglial cell   Oligodendroglial cell   Ependymal cell
(astroglial cell)

Figure 10–4

Glial cells (neuroglial cells). These are the supportive, protective, and connective cells of the CNS. Glial cells are **stromal** (framework) **tissue,** whereas neurons carry impulses and are parenchymal tissue.

IV. The Brain

The brain controls body activities. In the human adult, it weighs about 3 pounds and has many different parts, all of which control different aspects of body functions.

The largest part of the brain is the "thinking" area or **cerebrum**. On the surface of the cerebrum, nerve cells lie in sheets, called the **cerebral cortex**. These sheets, arranged in folds called **gyri** are separated from each other by grooves, known as **sulci**. The brain is divided in half, a right side and a left side, and each in a **cerebral hemisphere**. Each hemisphere is subdivided into four major lobes named for the cranial (skull) bones that overlie them. Figure 10–5 shows these lobes (frontal, parietal, occipital, and temporal) as well as gyri and sulci.

The cerebrum has many functions. All thought, judgment, memory, association, and discrimination take place within it. In addition, sensory impulses are received through afferent cranial nerves, and when registered in the cortex, they are the basis for perception. Cranial nerves carry motor impulses from the cerebrum to muscles and glands, and these produce movement and activity. Figure 10–5 shows the location of some of the centers in the cerebral cortex that control speech, vision, smell, movement, hearing, and thought processes.

In the middle of the cerebrum, there are spaces, or canals, called **ventricles** (pictured in Fig. 10–6). They contain a watery fluid that flows throughout the brain and around the spinal cord. This fluid is **cerebrospinal fluid (CSF)**, and it protects the brain and spinal cord from shock protein, and like a cushion. CSF is usually clear and colorless and contains lymphocytes, sugar, and chlorides. Spinal fluid can be withdrawn for diagnosis or relief of pressure on the brain; this is called a **lumbar puncture (LP)**. A hollow needle is

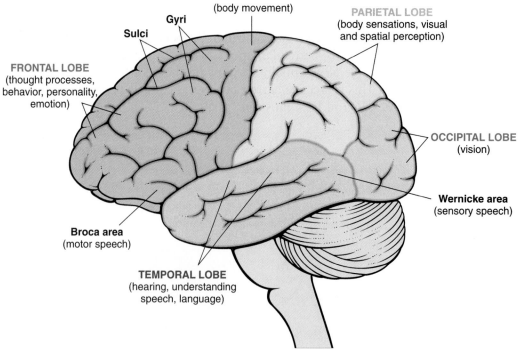

Figure 10-5

Left cerebral hemisphere (lateral view). Gyri (convolutions) and sulci (fissures) are indicated. Notice the lobes of the cerebrum and the functional centers that control speech, vision, movement, hearing, thinking, and other processes.

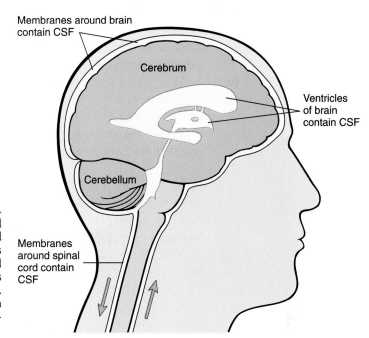

Figure 10–6

Circulation of cerebrospinal fluid (CSF) in the brain (ventricles) and around the spinal cord. CSF is formed within the ventricles and circulates between the membranes around the brain and spinal cord. CSF empties into the bloodstream through the membranes surrounding the brain and spinal cord.

Membranes around brain contain CSF

Cerebrum

Ventricles of brain contain CSF

Cerebellum

Membranes around spinal cord contain CSF

inserted in the lumbar region of the spinal column below the region where the nervous tissue of the spinal cord ends, and fluid is withdrawn.

Two other important parts of the brain, the **thalamus** and **hypothalamus**, are below the cerebrum (Fig. 10–7). The thalamus integrates and monitors sensory impulses from skin, suppressing some and magnifying others. Perception of pain is controlled by this area

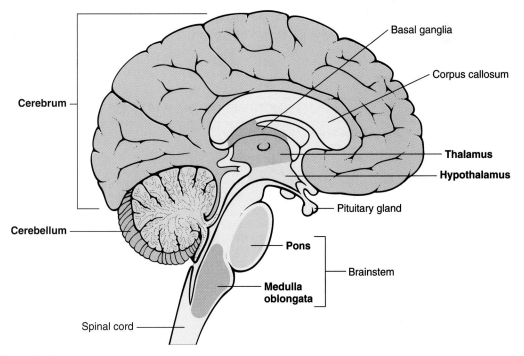

Basal ganglia

Corpus callosum

Cerebrum

Thalamus

Hypothalamus

Pituitary gland

Cerebellum

Pons

Brainstem

Medulla oblongata

Spinal cord

Figure 10–7

Parts of the brain: cerebrum, thalamus, hypothalamus, cerebellum, pons, and medulla oblongata. Note the location of the pituitary gland below the hypothalamus. The **basal ganglia** regulate how we move. The **corpus callosum** lies in the center of the brain and connects the two hemispheres.

of the brain. The hypothalamus (below the thalamus) contains neurons that control body temperature, sleep, appetite, sexual desire, and emotions such as fear and pleasure. The hypothalamus also regulates the release of hormones from the pituitary gland at the base of the brain and integrates the activities of the sympathetic and parasympathetic nervous systems.

The following structures within the brain lie in the back and below the cerebrum and connect the cerebrum with the spinal cord: the cerebellum, pons, and medulla oblongata. The pons and medulla are part of the **brainstem**.

The **cerebellum** functions to coordinate voluntary movements and maintain balance and posture.

The **pons** is a part of the brainstem that literally means "bridge." It contains nerve fiber tracts that connect the cerebellum and cerebrum with the rest of the brain. Nerves to the eyes and face lie here.

The **medulla oblongata**, also in the brainstem, connects the spinal cord with the rest of the brain. Nerve tracts cross from right to left and left to right in the medulla oblongata. For example, nerve cells that control movement of the left side of the body are found in the right half of the cerebrum. These cells send out axons that cross over (decussate) to the opposite side of the brain in the medulla oblongata and then travel down the spinal cord.

In addition, the medulla oblongata contains the following important vital centers that regulate internal activities of the body. These are:

1. Respiratory center controls muscles of respiration in response to chemicals or other stimuli.
2. Cardiac center slows the heart rate when the heart is beating too rapidly.
3. Vasomotor center affects (constricts or dilates) the muscles in the walls of blood vessels, thus influencing blood pressure.

Figure 10–7 shows the locations of the thalamus, hypothalamus, cerebellum, pons, and medulla oblongata. Table 10–2 reviews the functions of these parts of the brain.

Table 10–2. **FUNCTIONS OF THE PARTS OF THE BRAIN**

Part of the Brain	Functions
Cerebrum	Thinking, personality, sensations, movements, memory
Thalamus	Relay station for sensory impulses; pain
Hypothalamus	Body temperature, sleep, appetite, emotions, control of the pituitary gland
Cerebellum	Coordination of voluntary movements and balance
Pons	Connection of nerves (to the eyes and face)
Medulla oblongata	Nerve fibers cross over, left to right and right to left; contains centers to regulate heart, blood vessels, and respiratory system

V. The Spinal Cord and Meninges

Spinal Cord

The **spinal cord** is a column of nervous tissue extending from the medulla oblongata to the second lumbar vertebra within the vertebral column. Below the end of the spinal cord is the **cauda equina** (horse's tail), a fan of nerve fibers (see Fig. 10–1). The spinal cord carries all the nerves to and from the limbs and lower part of the body, and it is the pathway for impulses going to and from the brain. A cross-section of the spinal cord (Fig. 10–8) reveals an inner section of **gray matter** (containing cell bodies and dendrites of peripheral nerves) and an outer region of **white matter** (containing the nerve fiber tracts with myelin sheaths) conducting impulses to and from the brain.

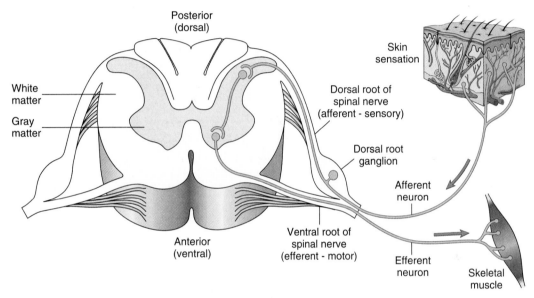

Figure 10–8

The spinal cord, showing gray and white matter (transverse view). Afferent neurons bring impulses from a sensory receptor (such as the skin) into the spinal cord. Efferent neurons carry impulses from the spinal cord to effector organs (such as skeletal muscle).

Meninges

The **meninges** are three layers of connective tissue membranes that surround the brain and spinal cord. Label Figure 10–9 as you study the following description of the meninges.

The outermost membrane of the meninges is the **dura mater** [1]. This thick, tough membrane contains channels through which blood can enter the brain tissue. The **subdural space** [2] is below the dura membrane, and contains blood vessels. The second layer around the brain and spinal cord is the **arachnoid membrane** [3]. The arachnoid (spider-like) membrane is loosely attached to the other meninges by web-like fibers so there is a space for fluid between the fibers and the third membrane. This is the **subarachnoid space** [4], containing CSF. The third layer of the meninges, closest to the brain and spinal cord, is the **pia mater** [5]. It contains delicate ("pia") connective tissue with a rich supply of blood vessels. Most physicians refer to the pia and arachnoid membranes together as pia-arachnoid.

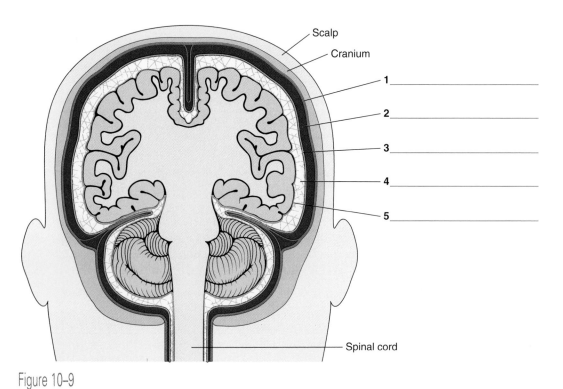

Figure 10–9

The meninges, frontal view.

VI. Vocabulary

This list reviews new terms introduced in the text. Short definitions reinforce your understanding of the terms. Section XIII gives help in pronouncing more difficult terms.

acetylcholine   Neurotransmitter chemical released at the ends of some nerve cells.

arachnoid membrane   Middle layer of the three membranes (meninges) that surround the brain and spinal cord. The Greek *arachne* means "spider."

astrocyte   A type of glial (neurological) cell; connective, supporting cell of the nervous system. Astrocytes transport water and salts from capillaries.

autonomic nervous system Nerves that control involuntary body functions of muscles, glands, and internal organs.

axon   Microscopic fiber that carries the nervous impulse along a nerve cell.

blood-brain barrier   Blood vessels (capillaries) that selectively let certain substances enter the brain tissue and keep other substances out.

brainstem   Lower portion of the brain that connects the cerebrum with the spinal cord. The pons and medulla oblongata are part of the brainstem.

cauda equina   Collection of spinal nerves below the end of the spinal cord.

cell body   Part of a nerve cell that contains the nucleus.

central nervous system (CNS) Brain and the spinal cord.

cerebellum   Part of the brain that coordinates muscle movements and maintains balance.

cerebral cortex   Outer region of the cerebrum; containing sheets of nerve cells; gray matter of the brain.

cerebrospinal fluid (CSF) Fluid that circulates throughout the brain and spinal cord.

cerebrum   Largest part of the brain; responsible for voluntary muscular activity, vision, speech, taste, hearing, thought, and memory.

dendrite	Microscopic branching fiber of a nerve cell that is the first part to receive the nervous impulse.
dura mater	Thick, outermost layer of the meninges surrounding and protecting the brain and spinal cord; from the Latin, meaning "hard mother."
ependymal cell	A cell that lines the fluid-filled sacs of the brain and spinal cord.
ganglion (plural: **ganglia**)	A collection of nerve cell bodies in the peripheral nervous system.
glial cells (neuroglia)	Cells in the nervous system that do not carry impulses but are supportive and connective in function. Examples are astrocytes, microglial cells, and oligodendroglia. There are about 100 billion glial cells.
gyrus (plural: **gyri**)	Sheets of nerve cells that produce elevation in the surface of the cerebral cortex; convolution.
hypothalamus	Portion of the brain beneath the thalamus; controls sleep, appetite, body temperature, and secretions from the pituitary gland.
medulla oblongata	The part of the brain just above the spinal cord; controls breathing, heartbeat, and the size of blood vessels; nerve fibers cross over here.
meninges	Three protective membranes that surround the brain and spinal cord.
microglial cell	One type of glial cell. A microglial cell is a phagocyte.
motor nerves	Carry messages away from the brain and spinal cord to muscles and organs; efferent (ef = away) nerves.
myelin sheath	Fatty tissue that surrounds, protects, and insulates the axon of a nerve cell. These sheaths are white in color (white matter).
nerve	Macroscopic structure consisting of axons and dendrites in bundles like strands of rope.
neuron	A nerve cell; carries impulses throughout the body. There are about 10 billion neurons.
neurotransmitter	Chemical messenger, released at the end of a nerve cell. It stimulates or inhibits another cell, which can be a nerve cell, muscle cell, or gland cell. Examples of neurotransmitters are acetylcholine, epinephrine, dopamine, and serotonin.
oligodendroglial cell	Glial cell that forms the myelin sheath covering axons.
parasympathetic nerves	Involuntary, autonomic nerves that help regulate body functions like heart rate and respiration.

parenchyma Essential, distinguishing cells of an organ. Neurons are the parenchymal tissue of the brain.

peripheral nervous system Nerves outside the brain and spinal cord; cranial, spinal, and autonomic nerves.

pia mater Thin, delicate inner membrane of the meninges.

plexus (plural: **plexuses**) Large, interlacing network of nerves. Examples are lumbar-sacral and brachial (brachi/o means arm) plexuses. The term originated from the Indo-European *plek* meaning "to weave together."

pons Part of the brain anterior to the cerebellum and between the medulla and the rest of the brain (Latin, *pons* means "bridge"). It is a bridge connecting various parts of the brain.

receptor Organ that receives a nervous stimulation and passes it on to nerves within the body. The skin, ears, eyes, and taste buds are receptors.

sensory nerves Carry messages to the brain and spinal cord from a receptor; afferent (af = toward) nerves.

stimulus (plural: **stimuli**) Change (light, sound, touch) in the internal or external environment that evokes a response.

stroma Connective and supporting tissue of an organ. Glial cells are the stromal tissue of the brain.

sulcus (plural: **sulci**) Depression or groove in the surface of the cerebral cortex; fissure.

sympathetic nerves Autonomic nerves that influence body functions involuntarily in times of stress.

synapse The space (juncture) through which a nervous impulse is transmitted from one neuron to another or from a neuron to another cell, such as a muscle or gland cell. From the Greek *synapsis*, "a point of contact."

thalamus Main relay center of the brain. It conducts impulses between the spinal cord and the cerebrum; incoming sensory messages are relayed through the thalamus to appropriate centers in the cerebrum. The Latin *thalamus*, meaning "room," comes from the Romans who thought this part of the brain was hollow—therefore resembling a room.

ventricles of the brain Reservoirs (canals) in the interior of the brain that contain cerebrospinal fluid.

VII. Combining Forms and Terminology

This section is divided into terms that describe organs and structures of the nervous system and those that relate to neurological symptoms. Write the meanings of the medical terms in the spaces provided.

Organs and Structures			
Combining Form	Meaning	Terminology	Meaning
cerebell/o	cerebellum	cerebellar	_____
cerebr/o	cerebrum	cerebrospinal fluid	_____
		cerebral cortex	_____

Cortical means pertaining to the cortex or outer area of an organ.

dur/o	dura mater	subdural hematoma	_____
		epidural hematoma	_____

Figure 10–10 shows subdural, epidural, and intracerebral hematomas.

encephal/o	brain	encephalitis	_____
		encephalopathy	_____
		anencephaly	_____

This is the most common congenital brain malformation; it is not compatible with life and may be detected with amniocentesis or ultrasonography of the fetus.

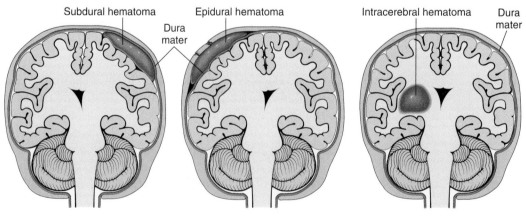

Figure 10–10

Hematomas. A **subdural hematoma** results from the tearing of veins between the dura and arachnoid membranes. It is often the result of blunt trauma, such as in boxing lesions and in elderly patients who have fallen out of bed. An **epidural hematoma** occurs between the skull and the dura as the result of a ruptured meningeal artery after a fracture of the skull. An **intracerebral hematoma** is caused by bleeding directly into brain tissue, such as can occur in the case of uncontrolled hypertension (high blood pressure).

gli/o	glue, parts of the nervous system that support and connect	glial cells _____ *Stromal or connective tissue of the nervous system.* glioblastoma _____ *This is a highly malignant tumor (-blast means immature).*
lept/o	thin, slender	leptomeningitis _____ *The pia and arachnoid membranes are known as the leptomeninges because of their thin, delicate structure.*
mening/o, meningi/o	membranes, meninges	meningeal _____ meningioma _____ *Slowly growing, benign tumor.* meningomyelocele _____ *Neural tube defect caused by failure of the neural tube to close during embryonic development. This abnormality occurs in infants born with spina bifida. See Section VIII, Pathological Conditions, page 353.*
my/o	muscle	myoneural _____
myel/o	spinal cord (means bone marrow in other contexts)	myelogram _____ poliomyelitis _____ *Polio means gray matter. This viral disease affects the gray matter of the spinal cord, leading to paralysis of muscles that rely on the damaged neurons. Effective vaccines developed in the 20th century have made "polio" relatively uncommon.*
neur/o	nerve	neuropathy _____ polyneuritis _____
pont/o	pons	cerebellopontine _____ *-ine means pertaining to.*
radicul/o	nerve root (of spinal nerves)	radiculopathy _____ radiculitis _____ *This results in pain and hyperesthesia.*
thalam/o	thalamus	thalamic _____
thec/o	sheath (refers to the meninges)	intrathecal injection _____ *Chemicals, such as chemotherapeutic drugs, can be delivered into the subarachnoid space.*

vag/o	vagus nerve (10th cranial nerve)	vagal _____
		This cranial nerve has branches to the head and neck as well as to the chest (larynx, trachea, bronchial tubes, lungs, and heart) and abdomen (esophagus, stomach, and intestines).

Symptoms Combining Form or Suffix	Meaning	Terminology	Meaning
alges/o **-algesia**	excessive sensitivity to pain	analgesia _____ hypalgesia _____ *Diminished sensation to pain.*	
-algia	pain	neuralgia _____ cephalgia _____ *Most headaches result from vasodilation (widening) of blood vessels in tissues surrounding the brain or from tension in neck and scalp muscles. A **migraine** is a severe headache often accompanied by nausea and vomiting. Prodromal symptoms sometimes include sensitivity to light and sound and an aura phase of flashes before the eyes and partial blindness.*	
caus/o	burning	causalgia _____ *Intense burning pain following injury to a sensory nerve.*	
comat/o	deep sleep (coma)	comatose _____ *A **coma** is a state of unconsciousness from which the patient cannot be aroused. Semicomatose refers to a stupor (unresponsiveness) from which a patient can be aroused. In an irreversible coma (brain death) there is complete unresponsivity to stimuli, no spontaneous breathing or movement, and a flat EEG.*	
esthesi/o **-esthesia**	feeling, nervous sensation	anesthesia _____ *Lack of normal sensation (e.g., absence of sense of touch or pain). Two common types of regional anesthesia are spinal and epidural (caudal) blocks (Fig. 10–11).* hyperesthesia _____ *A light touch with a pin may provoke increased sensation.* paresthesia _____ *Par- (from para-) means abnormal. Paresthesias include burning, prickling, tingling sensations, or numbness for no apparent reason.*	
kines/o **-kinesia**	movement	bradykinesia _____	

-kinesis	movement	hyperkinesis _____
-kinetic		*Amphetamines (CNA stimulants) are used to treat hyperkir*
		children, but the mechanism of their action is not understood.
		akinetic _____
-lepsy	seizure	epilepsy _____
		See page 354, Section VIII, Pathological Conditions.
		narcolepsy _____
		Sudden, uncontrollable compulsion to sleep (narc/o = stupor, sleep).
		Amphetamines and stimulant drugs are prescribed to prevent attacks.
lex/o	word, phrase	dyslexia _____
		Reading, writing, and learning disorders.
-paresis	slight paralysis (weakness)	hemiparesis _____
		Affects either right or left side (half) of the body. **Paresis** *is also used by itself to mean partial paralysis or weakness of muscles.*
-phasia	speech	aphasia _____
		Motor *(also called Broca or expressive)* **aphasia** *is present when a patient knows what she or he wants to say but cannot do so or is slow to do so. A patient with* **sensory aphasia** *articulates (pronounces) words easily but uses them inappropriately. This patient has difficulty understanding written and verbal commands and cannot repeat them.*

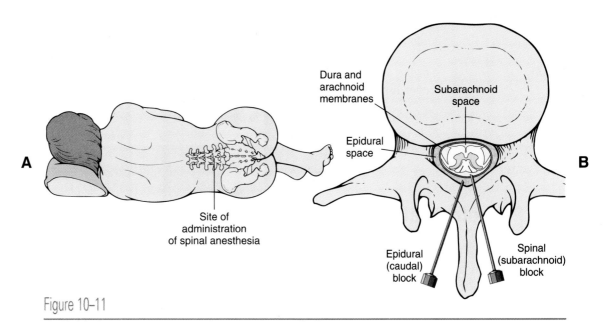

Figure 10–11

(A) Positioning of a patient for spinal anesthesia. (B) Cross-section of the spinal cord showing injection sites for **epidural** and **spinal blocks (anesthesia).** Epidural (caudal) anesthesia is achieved by injecting an agent into the epidural space in the sacral region and is commonly used in obstetrics. Spinal anesthesia is achieved by injecting local anesthetics into the subarachnoid space. Patients experience loss of sensation and paralysis of feet, legs, and abdomen.

-plegia	paralysis (loss or impairment of the ability to move parts of the body)	hemiplegia _____
		Affects right or left half of the body and results from a stroke or other brain injury. The hemiplegia is contralateral to the brain lesion because motor nerve fibers from the right half of the brain cross to the left side of the body (in the medulla oblongata).
		paraplegia _____
		Originally, the term paraplegia meant a stroke (paralysis) on one side (para-). Now, however, the term means paralysis of both legs and the lower part of the body caused by injury or disease of the spinal cord at the lumbar level.
		quadriplegia _____
		Quadri- means four. All four extremities are affected. Injury is at the cervical level of the spinal cord.
-praxia	action	apraxia _____
		Movements and behavior are not purposeful. A patient with motor apraxia cannot use an object or perform a task, although it is understood.
-sthenia	strength	neurasthenia _____
		Nervous exhaustion and fatigue often following depression.
syncop/o	to cut off, cut short	syncopal _____
		Syncope (SĬN-kō-pē) *is fainting; sudden and temporary loss of consciousness caused by inadequate flow of blood to the brain. The term syncope comes from a Greek word meaning cutting into pieces, implying that a fainting spell meant one's strength was "cut off."*
tax/o	order, coordination	ataxia _____
		Persistent unsteadiness on the feet can be caused by a disorder involving the cerebellum.

VIII. Pathological Conditions

The bones of the skull, the vertebral column, and the meninges containing CSF, provide a hard box with interior cushion around the brain and spinal cord. In addition, glial cells surrounding neurons form a blood–brain barrier that prevents many potentially harmful substances in the bloodstream from gaining access to neurons. However, these protective factors are counterbalanced by the sensitivity of nerve cells to oxygen deficiency (brain cells die in a few minutes when deprived of oxygen) and by inability of neurons to regenerate (adult nerve cells do not undergo cell division and cannot replace themselves).

Neurological diseases may be classified in the following categories of disorders:

1. Congenital
2. Degenerative, Movement, and Seizure
3. Infectious (meningitis and encephalitis)

4. Neoplastic (tumors)
5. Traumatic
6. Vascular (stroke)

Congenital Disorders

hydrocephalus

Abnormal accumulation of fluid (CSF) in the brain.

If circulation of CSF in the brain or spinal cord is impaired, it accumulates under pressure in the ventricles of the brain. To relieve pressure on the brain, a catheter (shunt) is placed from the ventricle of the brain into the peritoneal space (ventriculoperitoneal shunt) so that the CSF is continuously drained from the brain.

Hydrocephalus can also occur in an adult as a result of tumors and infections.

spina bifida

Congenital defect in the lumbar spinal column caused by imperfect union of vertebral parts (neural tube defect).

In **spina bifida occulta** the vertebral defect is covered over with skin and evident only on x-ray examination. **Spina bifida cystica** is a more severe form, involving protrusion of the meninges **(meningocele)** or protrusion of the meninges and spinal cord **(meningomyelocele)** (Fig. 10–12A and B.)

The etiology of neural tube defects is unknown. Prenatal diagnosis is helped by new imaging methods and testing maternal blood samples for alpha-fetoprotein.

MENINGOCELE

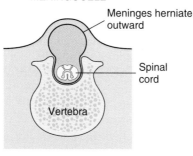

A

MYELOMENINGOCELE

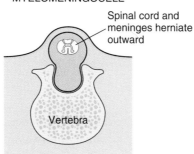

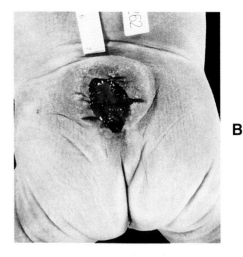

B

Figure 10–12

(A) Spina bifida with meningocele and with meningomyelocele. (B) Meningomyelocele. Both the meninges and spinal cord are included in a cystlike structure visible just above the buttocks. This condition is commonly associated with hydrocephalus. Because meningomyelocele exposes the CNS to the outside environment, infection is a common complication. (**A** modified from Damjanov I: Pathology for the Health-Related Professions, 2nd ed., Philadelphia, WB Saunders, 2000, p. 486; **B** from Kumar V, Cotran R, Robbins SL: Basic Pathology, 7th ed., Philadelphia, WB Saunders, 2003, p. 822.)

Degenerative, Movement, and Seizure Disorders

Alzheimer disease (AD)

Brain disorder marked by gradual deterioration of mental capacity (dementia) beginning in middle age.

An early sign is loss of memory for recent events, persons, and places, followed by impairment of judgment, comprehension, and intellect. Anxiety, depression, and emotional disturbances occur as well. On autopsy there is atrophy of the cerebral cortex and widening of the cerebral sulci, especially in the frontal and temporal regions (Fig. 10–13A). Microscopic examination shows **senile plaques** resulting from degeneration of neurons and **neurofibrillary tangles** (bundles of fibrils in the cytoplasm of a neuron) in the cerebral cortex. Deposits of **amyloid** (a protein) occur in neurofibrillary tangles, senile plaques and in blood vessels. The cause of AD remains unknown, although genetic factors may play a role. A mutation on chromosome 14 has been linked to familial cases. There is as yet no effective treatment.

amyotrophic lateral sclerosis (ALS)

Degenerative disease of motor neurons in the spinal cord and brainstem; motor neuron disease.

ALS presents in adulthood and affects men more often than women. Symptoms are weakness and atrophy of muscles in the hands, forearms, and legs, followed by difficulty in swallowing, talking, and dyspnea as the respiratory muscles become affected. Etiology (cause) and cure for ALS are both unknown.

A famous baseball player, Lou Gehrig, became a victim of this disease in the mid 1900s and thus the condition was known as Lou Gehrig disease.

epilepsy

Chronic brain disorder characterized by recurrent seizure activity.

A seizure is an abnormal, sudden excessive discharge of electrical activity within the brain. Seizures are often symptoms of underlying brain pathological conditions, such as brain tumors, meningitis, vascular disease, or scar tissue from a head injury. **Tonic-clonic seizures (ictal events)** are characterized by a sudden loss of consciousness, falling down, and then tonic contractions (stiffening of muscles) followed by clonic contractions (twitching and jerking movements of the limbs). These convulsions are often preceded by an **aura,** which is a peculiar sensation appearing before more definite symptoms. Dizziness, numbness, or visual disturbances are examples of an aura. **Absence seizures (petit mal seizures)** are a minor form of seizure consisting of momentary clouding of consciousness and loss of contact with the environment. Drug therapy (anticonvulsants) is used for control of epileptic seizures.

After seizures, there may be neurologic symptoms such as weakness; called **postictal events**. Epilepsy comes from the Greek *epilepsis,* meaning "a laying hold of." The Greeks thought a victim of a seizure was laid hold of by some mysterious force.

Huntington disease

Hereditary nervous disorder caused by degenerative changes in the cerebrum and involving bizarre, abrupt, involuntary, dance-like movements.

This condition begins in adulthood (between the ages of 30 and 45) and results in personality changes with choreic (meaning dance) movements (uncontrollable, irregular, jerking movements of the arms, legs, and face).

The genetic defect in patients with Huntington disease is located on chromosome 4. Patients can be tested for the gene; however, no cure exists and management is symptomatic.

multiple sclerosis (MS)

Destruction of the myelin sheath on neurons in the CNS and its replacement by plaques of sclerotic (hard) tissue (Fig. 10–13B).

One of the leading causes of neurological disability in persons 20 to 40 years of age, MS is a chronic disease often marked by long periods of stability (remission) and worsening (relapse). **Demyelination** (loss of myelin insulation) prevents the conduction of nerve impulses through the axon and causes paresthesias, muscle weakness, unsteady **gait** (manner of walking), and paralysis. There may be visual (blurred and double vision) and speech disturbances as well. Etiology is unknown, but it is likely to be an autoimmune or viral disease in which lymphocytes react against myelin. Immunosuppressive agents (interferon, steroids, or chemotherapy) are often given with benefit.

myasthenia gravis

Neuromuscular disorder characterized by weakness (-asthenia) of voluntary muscles (attached to bones).

Myasthenia gravis means "grave muscle weakness" and is a chronic autoimmune disorder. Antibodies block the ability of acetylcholine (neurotransmitter) to transmit the nervous impulse from nerve to muscle cell. Normal muscle contraction fails to occur. Onset of symptoms is usually gradual with ptosis of the upper eyelid, double vision (diplopia), and facial weakness. Therapy to reverse symptoms includes anticholinesterase drugs, which inhibit the enzyme that breaks down acetylcholine. Corticosteroids (prednisone) and immunosuppressive drugs (azathioprine, methotrexate, and cyclophosphamide) are also used in treatment. **Thymectomy** (removal of the thymus gland, the source of antibodies against nerve impulse transmission) is an alternative method of treatment and is beneficial to many patients.

A
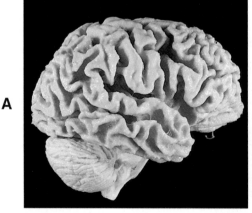

B
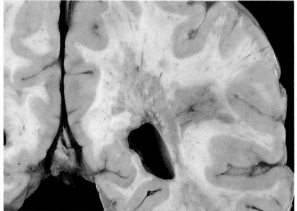

Figure 10–13

(A) Alzheimer disease. Generalized loss of brain parenchyma (neuronal tissue) results in the narrowing of the cerebral cortical gyri and the widening of the sulci. **(B) Multiple sclerosis (MS).** The typical MS plaque is a well-defined, gray-pink lesion that can occur anywhere in the brain or spinal cord. Common sites are the white matter around the ventricles of the brain, the optic nerves, and the white matter of the spinal cord. (From Kumar V, Cotran RS, Robbins SL: Basic Pathology, 7th ed., Philadelphia, WB Saunders, 2003, pp. 843 and 838.)

palsy	**Paralysis (partial or complete loss of motor function).**

Cerebral palsy is partial paralysis and lack of muscular coordination caused by loss of oxygen (hypoxia) or blood flow to the cerebrum during gestation or in the perinatal period. **Bell palsy** is paralysis on one side of the face. Etiology is likely infection with a virus, and therapy is directed against the virus (antivirals) and nerve swelling.

Parkinson disease (parkinsonism)	**Degeneration of nerves in the basal ganglia, occurring in later life and leading to tremors, weakness of muscles, and slowness of movement.**

This slowly progressive condition is caused by a deficiency of **dopamine** (neurotransmitter) made by cells in the basal ganglia (see Fig. 10–7). Motor disturbances include stooped posture, shuffling gait, muscle stiffness (rigidity), and often a tremor of the hands.

Drugs such as levodopa plus carbidopa (Sinemet) to increase dopamine levels in the brain are **palliative** (relieving symptoms but not curative) measures. Implantation of fetal brain tissue containing dopamine-producing cells is an experimental treatment but has produced uncertain results.

Tourette syndrome	**Involuntary, spasmodic, twitching movements; uncontrollable vocal sounds; and inappropriate words.**

These involuntary movements, usually beginning with twitching of the eyelid and muscles of the face with verbal outbursts, are called **tics.** Although the cause of Tourette syndrome is not known, it is associated with either an excess of dopamine or a hypersensitivity to dopamine. Psychological problems do not cause Tourette syndrome, but physicians have had some success in treating it with the antipsychotic drug haloperidol (Haldol), antidepressants, and mood stabilizers.

Infectious Disorders

herpes zoster (shingles)	**Viral infection affecting peripheral nerves.**

Blisters and pain spread along peripheral nerves and are caused by inflammation due to herpesvirus **(herpes zoster),** the same virus that causes chickenpox (varicella). Reactivation of the chickenpox virus (herpes varicella-zoster), which remained in the body after the person had chickenpox, occurs.

meningitis	**Inflammation of the meninges; leptomeningitis.**

This condition can be caused by bacteria **(pyogenic meningitis)** or viruses **(aseptic** or **viral meningitis).** Symptoms are fever and signs of meningeal irritation, such as headache, photophobia (sensitivity to light), and a stiff neck. Lumbar punctures are performed to examine CSF. Physicians use antibiotics to treat the more serious pyogenic form, and antivirals for the viral form.

human immunodeficiency virus (HIV) encephalopathy	**Brain disease and dementia occurring with AIDS.**

As many as 60 percent of patients with AIDS develop neurological dysfunction. In addition to encephalitis and dementia (loss of mental functioning), patients develop brain tumors and other infections as well.

Neoplastic Disorders

brain tumors

Abnormal growths of brain tissue and meninges.

Most of the primary brain tumors arise from glial cells **(gliomas)** or the meninges **(meningiomas).** Examples of gliomas are **astrocytoma** (Fig. 10–14A), **oligodendroglioma** and **ependymoma.** The most malignant form of the astrocytoma is **glioblastoma multiforme** (-blast means immature) (Fig. 10–14B). Tumors can cause swelling **(cerebral edema)** and hydrocephalus. If there is increased CSF pressure, swelling may also occur near the optic nerve (at the back of the eye). Gliomas are removed surgically, and radiotherapy is used for those that are not completely resected. Steroids are given to reduce swelling after surgery.

Meningiomas are usually benign and surrounded by a capsule, but they may cause compression and distortion of the brain.

About 15 percent of tumors in the brain are single or multiple metastatic growths. Most arise from the lung, breast, skin (melanoma), kidney, and gastrointestinal tract and spread to the brain.

Traumatic Disorders

cerebral concussion

Temporary brain dysfunction (brief loss of consciousness) after injury, usually clearing within 24 hours.

There is no evidence of structural damage to the brain tissue. Severe concussions may lead to coma.

cerebral contusion

Bruising of brain tissue as a result of direct trauma to the head; neurological deficits persist longer than 24 hours.

A contusion is usually associated with a fracture of the skull. Subdural and epidural hematomas occur, leading to permanent brain injury with altered memory, speech, or epilepsy.

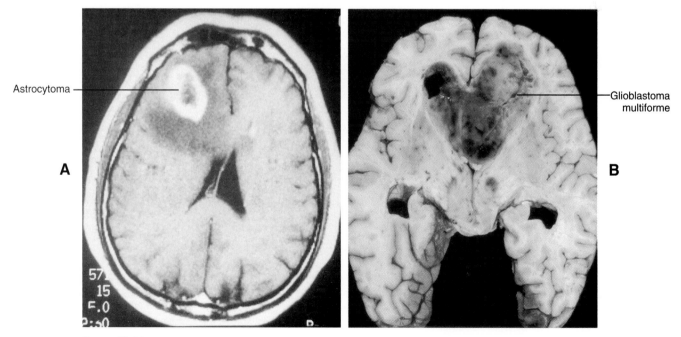

Figure 10–14

(A) Computed tomographic (CT) scan of **an astrocytoma. (B) Glioblastoma multiforme,** on autopsy, appearing as a necrotic, hemorrhagic, infiltrating mass. (From Cotran RS, Kumar V, Collins T: Robbins Pathologic Basis of Disease, 6th ed. Philadelphia, WB Saunders, 1999, p. 1344.)

Vascular Disorders

cerebrovascular accident (CVA)   **Disruption in the normal blood supply to the brain; stroke.**

This condition, also known as a **cerebral infarction,** is the result of a loss of oxygen to the brain. There are three types of strokes (Fig. 10–15):

1. **Thrombotic**—blood clot **(thrombus)** in the arteries leading to the brain, resulting in **occlusion** (blocking) of the vessel. Atherosclerosis leads to this common type of stroke as blood vessels become blocked over time. Before total occlusion occurs, a patient may experience symptoms that point to the gradual occlusion of blood vessels. These short episodes of neurological dysfunction are known as **TIAs (transient ischemic attacks).**
2. **Embolic**—an **embolus** (a dislodged thrombus) travels to cerebral arteries and occludes a small vessel. This type of stroke occurs very suddenly.
3. **Hemorrhagic**—a blood vessel, such as the cerebral artery, breaks and bleeding occurs. This type of stroke can be fatal and results from advancing age, atherosclerosis, or high blood pressure, all of which result in degeneration of cerebral blood vessels. With small hemorrhages, the body reabsorbs the blood and the patient makes good recovery with only slight disability. In a younger patient, cerebral hemorrhage is usually caused by mechanical injury associated with skull fracture or bursting of an arterial **aneurysm** (weakness in the vessel wall that balloons and eventually bursts).

The major risk factors for stroke are hypertension, diabetes, smoking and heart disease. Other risk factors include obesity, substance abuse (cocaine), and elevated cholesterol levels.

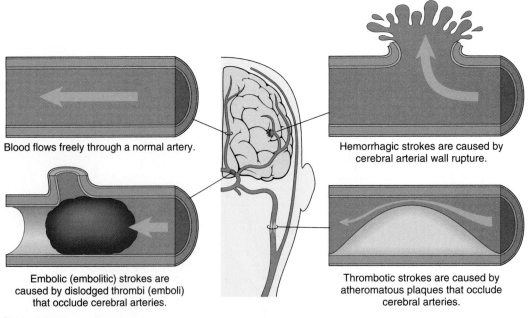

Blood flows freely through a normal artery.

Embolic (embolitic) strokes are caused by dislodged thrombi (emboli) that occlude cerebral arteries.

Hemorrhagic strokes are caused by cerebral arterial wall rupture.

Thrombotic strokes are caused by atheromatous plaques that occlude cerebral arteries.

Figure 10–15

Three types of strokes: thrombotic, embolic, and **hemorrhagic.** (Modified from Ignatavicius DD, Workman ML: Medical-Surgical Nursing: Critical Thinking for Collaborative Care, 4th ed., Philadelphia, WB Saunders, 2002, p. 975.)

Thrombotic strokes are treated medically with anticoagulant (clot-dissolving) drug therapy (tissue plasminogen activator, or tPA, is started within 3 hours after the onset of a stroke) and surgically with carotid endarterectomy (removal of the atherosclerotic plaque from the inner lining of an artery in the neck).

■ *Study Section*

The following is a review of new terms used in Section VIII, Pathological Conditions. Practice spelling each term and know its meaning.

absence seizure	Minor (petit mal) form of seizure, consisting of momentary clouding of consciousness and loss of contact with the environment.
aneurysm	Weakening of a blood vessel; can lead to hemorrhage and CVA (stroke).
astrocytoma	Malignant tumor of glial brain cells (astrocytes).
aura	Peculiar sensation appearing before more definite symptoms.
-blast	Immature cells (as in glio*blast*oma).
dementia	Mental decline and deterioration.
demyelination	Destruction of myelin on axons of nerves (as in multiple sclerosis).
dopamine	A neurotransmitter that is deficient in Parkinson disease.
embolus	A mass (clot) of material travels through the bloodstream and suddenly blocks a vessel.
gait	Manner of walking.
herpes zoster	Herpesvirus that causes shingles—eruption of blisters in a pattern that follows the path of peripheral nerves around the trunk of the body; zoster means "girdle."
ictal event	Pertaining to a sudden, acute onset, as the convulsions of an epileptic seizure.
occlusion	Blockage.
palliative	Relieving symptoms but not curing.
thymectomy	Removal of the thymus gland (a lymphocyte-producing gland in the chest); used as treatment for myasthenia gravis.
TIA	Transient ischemic attack; mini-stroke.
tonic-clonic seizure	Major convulsive seizure marked by sudden loss of consciousness, stiffening of muscles, and twitching and jerking movements.

IX. Laboratory Tests, Clinical Procedures, and Abbreviations

Laboratory Tests

cerebrospinal fluid analysis   **Samples of CSF are examined.**

Doctors measure water, glucose, sodium, chloride, and protein as well as the number of red (RBC) and white (WBC) blood cells. CSF analysis can also detect tumor cells (via cytology) and viruses. These studies are used to diagnose infection, tumors, or multiple sclerosis.

Clinical Procedures

X-Rays

cerebral angiography   **X-ray images of the blood vessel system in the brain after injection of contrast material.**

Contrast is injected into the femoral artery (in thigh) and motion picture x-rays are taken rapidly. These images diagnose vascular disease (aneurysm, occlusion, hemorrhage) in the brain.

computed tomography (CT) of the brain   **X-rays compose a computerized cross-sectional image of the brain and spinal cord.**

Contrast material may be injected intravenously to highlight abnormalities. The contrast leaks through the **blood-brain barrier** from blood vessels into the brain tissue and shows tumors, hemorrhage, and blood clots. Operations are performed using the CT scan as a road map.

myelography   **X-ray images of the spinal cord after injection of contrast medium into the subarachnoid space.**

CT scans and magnetic resonance imaging (MRI) are now replacing myelography, which is a more invasive technique.

Magnetic Imaging

magnetic resonance imaging (MRI) of the brain   **Magnetic and radio waves create an image of the brain in all three planes.**

MRI and CT complement each other in diagnosing brain and spinal cord lesions. MRI is excellent for viewing strokes and tumors and changes caused by trauma and Alzheimer disease. **Magnetic resonance angiography (MRA)** produces images of blood vessels using magnetic resonance techniques.

Radioactive Study

positron emission tomography (PET) scan   **Images produced after injection of radioactive glucose or oxygen.**

Active brain tissue uses radioactive glucose or oxygen so the images give information about brain function. PET scans provide valuable information about patients with Alzheimer disease, stroke, schizophrenia, and epilepsy (see Figure 10–16).

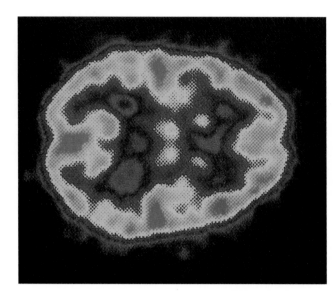

Figure 10–16

A **PET scan of the brain** showing decreased metabolic activity after a seizure (noted as green areas on the scan). (From Black JM, Hawks JH, Keene AM: Medical-Surgical Nursing: Clinical Management for Positive Outcomes, 6th ed., Philadelphia, WB Saunders, 2001, p. 197.)

Ultrasound

Doppler/ultrasound studies   **Using sound waves to detect blood flow in the carotid and intracranial arteries.**

The carotid artery carries blood to the brain. These studies can detect occlusion in blood vessels.

Other Procedures

electroencephalography (EEG)   **Recording of the electrical activity of the brain.**

EEG demonstrates seizure activity resulting from brain tumors, other diseases, and injury to the brain.

lumbar (spinal) puncture (LP)   **CSF is withdrawn from between two lumbar vertebrae** (Fig. 10–17).

A device to measure the pressure of CSF may be attached to the end of the needle after it has been inserted. Contrast medium for myelography or injection of intrathecal medicines may be administered as well. Some patients experience headache after LP.

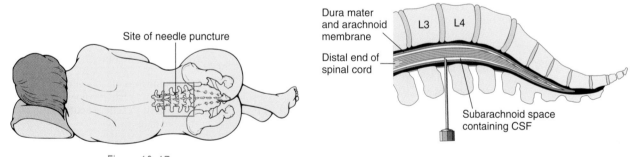

Figure 10–17

Lumbar (spinal) puncture. The patient lies laterally, with the knes drawn up to the abdomen and the chin brought down to the chest. This position increases the spaces between the vertebrae. The lumbar puncture needle is inserted between the 3rd and 4th (or 4th and 5th) lumbar vertebrae, and it enters the subarachnoid space.

A

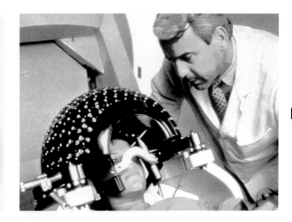

B

Figure 10-18

(A) The Leksell Gamma Knife Radiosurgery System. (B) Stereotactic frame in place to allow accurate focus of the radiotherapy beams. (Courtesy Elekta Instruments, Norcross, GA.)

stereotactic radiosurgery

Use of a specialized instrument to locate targets in the brain.

The stereotactic instrument is fixed onto the skull and guides the insertion of a needle by three-dimensional measurement. A **gamma knife** (high-energy radiation beams) can treat deep and often inaccessible intracranial brain tumors and abnormal blood vessel masses **(arteriovenous malformations)** without surgical incision (Fig. 10–18).

Abbreviations

AD	Alzheimer disease
AFP	alpha-fetoprotein (elevated levels in amniotic fluid and maternal blood are associated with congenital malformations of the nervous system, such as anencephaly and spina bifida)
ALS	amyotrophic lateral sclerosis
AVM	arteriovenous malformation (congenital tangle of arteries and veins in the cerebrum)
CNS	central nervous system
CSF	cerebrospinal fluid
CT	computed tomography
CVA	cerebrovascular accident
EEG	electroencephalogram
GABA	gamma-aminobutyric acid (neurotransmitter)
ICP	intracranial pressure; normal pressure is 5-15 mmHg
LP	lumbar puncture

MAC	monitored anesthetic care
MG	myasthenia gravis
MRA	magnetic resonance angiography
MRI	magnetic resonance imaging
MS	multiple sclerosis
½ P	hemiparesis
PET	positron emission tomography
Sz	seizure
TBI	traumatic brain injury
TENS	transcutaneous electrical nerve stimulation (a battery-powered device used to relieve acute and chronic pain)
TIA	transient ischemic attack (temporary interference with the blood supply to the brain)
tPA	tissue plasminogen activator (a clot-dissolving drug used as therapy for strokes)

X. Practical Applications

Answers to the questions are on page 374 after Answers to Exercises.

Case Report

This patient was admitted on January 14 with a history of progressive right hemi-paresis for the previous 1 to 2 months; fluctuating numbness of the right arm, thorax, and buttocks; jerking of the right leg; periods of speech arrest; diminished comprehension in reading; and recent development of a hemiplegic gait. He is suspected of having a left parietal tumor [the parietal lobes of the cerebrum are on either side under the roof of the skull].

Examinations done before hospitalization included skull films, EEG, and CSF analysis, which were all normal. After admission, an MRI was abnormal in the left parietal region, as was the EEG.

An MRA to assess cerebral blood vessels was attempted, but the patient became progressively more restless and agitated after sedation, so the procedure was stopped. During the recovery phase from the sedation, the patient was alternately somnolent [sleepy] and violent, but it was later apparent that he had developed almost a complete aphasia and right hemiplegia.

In the next few days, he became more alert, although he remained dysarthric [from *arthroun*, "to utter distinctly"] and hemiplegic.

MRI and MRA under general anesthesia on January 19 showed complete occlusion of the left internal carotid artery with cross-filling of the left anterior and middle cerebral arteries from the right internal carotid circulation.

Final diagnosis: Left cerebral infarction caused by left internal carotid artery occlusion.

[Fig. 10–19 shows the common carotid arteries and their branches within the head and brain.]

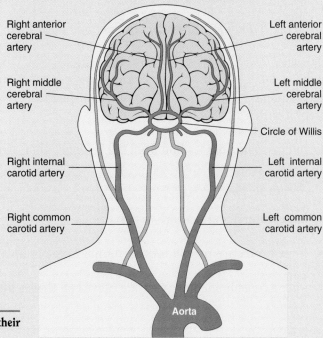

Right anterior cerebral artery

Right middle cerebral artery

Right internal carotid artery

Right common carotid artery

Left anterior cerebral artery

Left middle cerebral artery

Circle of Willis

Left internal carotid artery

Left common carotid artery

Aorta

Figure 10–19

Common carotid arteries and their branches.

Continued on following page

Questions on the Case Report
1. **The patient was admitted with a history of**
   (A) Right-sided paralysis caused by a previous stroke
   (B) Paralysis on the left side of his body
   (C) Increasing slight paralysis on the right side of his body
2. **The patient has also experienced periods of**
   (A) Aphasia and dyslexia
   (B) Dysplastic gait
   (C) Apraxia and aphasia
3. **After his admission, where did the MRI show an abnormality?**
   (A) Right posterior region of the brain
   (B) Left and right sides of the brain
   (C) Left side of the brain
4. **What test determined the final diagnosis?**
   (A) EEG for both sides of the brain
   (B) CSF analysis and cerebral angiography
   (C) Magnetic resonance imaging and magnetic resonance angiography
5. **What was the final diagnosis?**
   (A) A stroke; necrotic tissue in the left cerebrum caused by blockage of an artery
   (B) Cross-filling of blood vessels from the left to the right side of the brain
   (C) Cerebral palsy on the left side of the brain with cross-filling of two cerebral arteries

XI. Exercises

Remember to check your answers carefully with those given in Section XII, Answers to Exercises.

A. *Match the following neurological structures with their meanings as given below.*

astrocyte	dendrite	neuron
axon	meninges	oligodendroglial cell
cauda equina	myelin sheath	plexus
cerebral cortex		

1. microscopic fiber leading from the cell body that carries the nervous impulse along a nerve cell

_____

2. large, interlacing network of nerves _____

3. three protective membranes surrounding the brain and spinal cord _____

4. microscopic branching fiber of a nerve cell that is the first part to receive the nervous impulse

_____

5. outer region of the largest part of the brain; composed of gray matter _____

6. glial cell that transports water and salts between capillaries and nerve cells

   _____

7. glial cell that produces myelin _____

8. a nerve cell that transmits a nervous impulse _____

9. collection of spinal nerves below the end of the spinal cord at the level of the second lumbar

   vertebra _____

10. protective fatty tissue that surrounds the axon of a nerve cell _____

B. Give the meanings of the following terms.

1. dura mater _____

2. central nervous system _____

3. peripheral nervous system _____

4. arachnoid membrane _____

5. hypothalamus _____

6. synapse _____

7. sympathetic nerves _____

8. medulla oblongata _____

9. pons _____

10. cerebellum _____

11. thalamus _____

12. ventricles of the brain _____

13. brainstem _____

14. cerebrum _____

15. ganglion _____

C. Match the following terms with the meanings or associated terms below.

glia (neuroglia)   neurotransmitter   sensory nerves
gyri   parenchymal cell   subarachnoid space
motor nerves   pia mater   sulci

1. innermost meningeal membrane _____

2. carry messages away from (efferent) the brain and spinal cord to muscles and glands

   _____

3. carry messages toward (afferent) the brain and spinal cord from receptors

   _____

4. grooves in the cerebral cortex _____

5. contains cerebrospinal fluid _____

6. elevations in the cerebral cortex _____

7. acetylcholine is an example of this chemical that is released at the end of a nerve cell and stimulates

   or inhibits another cell _____

8. essential cell of the nervous system; a neuron _____

9. connective and supportive (stromal) tissue _____

D. Choose the correct term to fit the definition given.

1. disease of the brain **(encephalopathy, myelopathy)**

2. part of the brain that controls muscular coordination and balance **(cerebrum, cerebellum)**

3. collection of blood above the dura mater **(subdural hematoma, epidural hematoma)**

4. inflammation of the pia and arachnoid membranes **(leptomeningitis, causalgia)**

5. condition of absence of a brain **(hypalgesia, anencephaly)**

6. inflammation of the gray matter of the spinal cord **(poliomyelitis, polyneuritis)**

7. pertaining to the membranes around the brain and spinal cord **(cerebellopontine, meningeal)**

8. disease of nerve roots (of spinal nerves) **(neuropathy, radiculopathy)**

9. hernia of the meninges and the spinal cord **(meningomyelocele, meningioma)**

10. pertaining to a cranial nerve **(thalamic, vagal)**

E. Give the meanings of the following terms.

1. cerebral cortex _____

2. intrathecal _____

3. polyneuritis _____

4. thalamic _____

5. myelogram _____

6. meningioma _____

7. glioma _____

8. subdural hematoma _____

F. Match the following neurological symptoms with the meanings below.

aphasia	dyslexia	narcolepsy
ataxia	hemiparesis	neurasthenia
bradykinesia	hyperesthesia	paraplegia
causalgia	motor apraxia	syncope

1. reading, writing, or learning disorder _____

2. condition of no coordination _____

3. condition of slow movement _____

4. condition of increased nervous sensation _____

5. seizure of sleep; uncontrollable compulsion to sleep _____

6. inability to speak _____

7. inability to perform a task _____

8. slight paralysis in the right or left half of the body _____

9. burning pain _____

10. paralysis in the lower part of the body (damage to lower part of the spinal cord)

_____

11. fainting _____

12. nervous exhaustion (lack of strength) and fatigue _____

G. Give the meanings of the following terms.

1. analgesia _____

2. motor aphasia _____

3. paresis _____

4. quadriplegia _____

5. asthenia _____

6. comatose _____

7. paresthesia _____

8. hyperkinesis _____

9. anesthesia _____

10. causalgia _____

11. akinetic _____

12. hypalgesia _____

H. Match the following terms with their descriptions below. The terms in boldface should give you a clue to the pathological condition described.

Alzheimer disease	Huntington disease	myasthenia gravis
amyotrophic lateral sclerosis	hydrocephalus	Parkinson disease
Bell palsy	multiple sclerosis	spina bifida cystica
epilepsy		

1. Destruction of myelin sheaths (demyelination) and their replacement by plaques of **hard** tissue lead

   to this condition. _____

2. Sudden, transient disturbances of brain function cause **seizures** in this abnormal condition.

   _____

3. The **spinal** column is imperfectly joined (a **split** in a vertebra occurs), and part of the meninges and spinal cord can herniate out of the spinal cavity in this congenital condition.

   _____

4. This condition involves **atrophy** of muscles and paralysis caused by damage to motor neurons in the

   spinal cord and brainstem. _____

5. In this hereditary condition, the patient displays bizarre, abrupt, involuntary, **dance**-like

   movements, as well as decline in mental functions. _____

6. Cerebrospinal **fluid** accumulates in the **head** (in the ventricles of the brain) in this condition.

   _____

7. This neuromuscular disorder is marked by **loss of muscle strength** because of the inability of
   a neurotransmitter (acetylcholine) to transmit impulses from nerve cells to muscle cells.

   _____

8. Degeneration of nerves in the basal ganglia occur in later life, leading to tremors, shuffling
   gait, and muscle stiffness; **dopamine** (neurotransmitter) is deficient in the brain.

   _____

9. This condition begins in middle age and is marked by deterioration of mental capacity **(dementia)**;
   autopsy shows cerebral cortex atrophy, widening of cerebral sulci, and microscopic neurofibrillary

   tangles. _____

10. Unilateral facial **paralysis** characterizes this condition. _____

I. *Give the meanings of the following abnormal conditions.*

1. astrocytoma _____

2. pyogenic meningitis _____

3. Tourette syndrome _____

4. cerebral contusion _____

5. cerebrovascular accident _____

6. cerebral concussion _____

7. herpes zoster _____

8. cerebral embolus _____

9. cerebral thrombosis _____

10. cerebral hemorrhage _____

11. cerebral aneurysm _____

12. HIV encephalopathy _____

J. Match the term in column I with the letter of its associated term or meaning in column II.

Column I   *Column II*

  1. ataxia _____   A. relieving, but not curing
                                                B. virus that causes chickenpox and shingles
  2. aura _____   C. uncoordinated gait
                                                D. neurotransmitter
  3. transient ischemic attack _____   E. peculiar symptoms appearing before more definite
                                                   symptoms
  4. tonic-clonic seizure _____   F. malignant brain tumor of immature glial cells
                                                G. major epileptic seizure; ictal event
  5. herpes zoster _____   H. interruption of blood supply to the cerebrum;
                                                   mini-stroke
  6. palliative _____   I. minor epileptic seizure
                                                J. blockage
  7. dopamine _____

  8. occlusion _____

  9. absence seizure _____

  10. glioblastoma multiforme _____

K. Describe what happens in the following two procedures.

  1. MRI of the brain _____

  2. stereotactic radiosurgery with gamma knife _____

_____

L. Give the meanings of the following abbreviations and then select the letter of the best association for each.

Column I   *Column II*

  1. EEG _____ ____   A. Gradual dementia beginning in middle age.
                                                B. Stroke; embolus, hemorrhage, or thrombosis
  2. PET scan _____ ____   are etiological factors.
                                                C. Intrathecal medications can be administered
  3. AFP_____ ____   through this procedure.
                                                D. This fluid is analyzed for abnormal blood
  4. MS _____ ____   cells, chemicals, and protein.
                                                E. Procedure to diagnose abnormal electrical
  5. MRI_____ ____   activity in the brain.
                                                F. Mini-stroke; caused by temporary interference
  6. LP_____ ____   with the blood supply to the brain.
                                                G. High levels in amniotic fluid and maternal
  7. CVA_____ ____   blood are associated with spina bifida.

8. AD_____ ____

9. TIA _____ ____

10. CSF_____ ____

H. Diagnostic procedure allows excellent visualization of soft tissue in the brain.

I. Radioactive glucose is taken up by the brain, and images recorded.

J. Destruction of the myelin sheath in the CNS occurs with plaques of hard scar tissue.

M. *Select the terms that complete the meanings of the sentences.*

1. Suzy had such severe headaches that she could find relief only with strong analgesics. Her condition of **(spina bifida, migraine, epilepsy)** was debilitating.

2. Paul was in a coma after his high-speed car accident. His physicians were concerned that he had suffered a **(palsy, meningomyelocele, contusion and subdural hematoma)** as a result of the accident.

3. Dick went to the emergency department complaining of dizziness, nausea, and headache. The physician, suspecting ICP, prescribed corticosteroids, and Dick's symptoms disappeared. They returned, however, when the steroids were discontinued. A (an) **(MRI of the brain, electroencephalogram, CSF analysis)** revealed a large brain lesion. It was removed surgically and determined to be an **(embolus, glioblastoma multiforme, migraine)**.

4. Dorothy felt tingling sensations in her hands and noticed blurred vision and numbness in her arm, all signs of **(herpes zoster, meningitis, TIA)**. Her physician requested **(myelography, MRA, lumbar puncture)** to assess any damage to cerebral blood vessels and possible stroke.

5. When Bill noticed ptosis and muscle weakness in his face, he reported these symptoms to his doctor. The doctor diagnosed his condition as **(Tourette syndrome, Huntington disease, myasthenia gravis)** and prescribed **(dopamine, anticonvulsants, anticholinesterase drugs)**, which relieved his symptoms.

6. To rule out bacterial **(epilepsy, encephalomalacia, meningitis)**, Dr. Phillips, a pediatrician, requested an **(EEG, PET scan, LP)** be performed on the febrile (feverish) child.

7. Eight-year-old Barry reversed his letters and had difficulty learning to read and write words. His family physician diagnosed his problem as **(aphasia, dyslexia, ataxia)**.

8. After his head hit the steering wheel during a recent automobile accident, Clark noticed **(hemiparesis, paraplegia, hyperesthesia)** on the left side of his body. A head CT scan revealed **(narcolepsy, neurasthenia, subdural hematoma)**.

9. For her 35th birthday, Elizabeth's husband threw her a surprise party. She was so startled by the crowd that she experienced a weakness of muscles and loss of consciousness. Friends placed her on her back in a horizontal position with her head low to improve blood flow to her brain. She soon recovered from her **(myoneural, syncopal, hyperkinetic)** episode.

10. Near her 65th birthday, Estelle began having difficulty remembering recent events. Over the next five years, she developed age-related **(dyslexia, dementia, seizures)** and was diagnosed with **(multiple sclerosis, myasthenia gravis, Alzheimer disease)**.

N. Complete the spelling of the following terms based on their meanings.

1. part of the brain that controls sleep, appetite, temperature, and secretions of the pituitary gland:

   hypo _____

2. pertaining to fainting: syn _____

3. abnormal sensations: par _____

4. slight paralysis: par _____

5. inflammation of a spinal nerve root: _____ itis

6. inability to speak: a _____

7. movements and behavior that are not purposeful: a _____

8. lack of muscular coordination: a _____

9. reading, writing, and learning disorders: dys _____

10. excessive movement: hyper _____

11. paralysis in one half (right or left) of the body: _____ plegia

12. paralysis in the lower half of the body: _____ plegia

13. paralysis in all four limbs: _____ plegia

14. nervous exhaustion and fatigue: neur _____

XII. Answers to Exercises

A

1. axon
2. plexus
3. meninges
4. dendrite
5. cerebral cortex
6. astrocyte
7. oligodendroglial cell
8. neuron
9. cauda equina
10. myelin sheath

B

1. outermost meningeal layer surrounding the brain and spinal cord
2. the brain and the spinal cord
3. nerves outside the brain and spinal cord; cranial, spinal, and autonomic nerves
4. middle meningeal membrane surrounding the brain and spinal cord
5. the part of the brain below the thalamus; controls sleep, appetite, body temperature, and secretions from the pituitary gland
6. space through which a nervous impulse is transmitted from a nerve cell to another nerve cell or to a muscle or gland cell
7. autonomic nerves that influence body functions involuntarily in times of stress
8. part of the brain just above the spinal cord that controls breathing, heartbeat, and the size of blood vessels
9. part of the brain anterior to the cerebellum and between the medulla

and the upper parts of the brain; connects these parts of the brain
10. posterior part of the brain that coordinates voluntary muscle movements
11. part of the brain below the cerebrum; relay center that conducts impulses

between the spinal cord and the cerebrum
12. canals in the interior of the brain that are filled with CSF
13. lower portion of the brain that connects the cerebrum with the spinal cord (includes the pons and the medulla)

14. largest part of the brain; controls voluntary muscle movement, vision, speech, hearing, thought, memory
15. a collection of nerve cell bodies outside the brain and spinal cord

C

1. pia mater
2. motor nerves
3. sensory nerves

4. sulci
5. subarachnoid space
6. gyri

7. neurotransmitter
8. parenchymal cell
9. glia (neuroglia)

D

1. encephalopathy
2. cerebellum
3. epidural hematoma
4. leptomeningitis

5. anencephaly
6. poliomyelitis
7. meningeal

8. radiculopathy
9. meningomyelocele
10. vagal

E

1. the outer region of the cerebrum (contains gray matter)
2. pertaining to within a sheath through the meninges and into the subarachnoid space

3. inflammation of many nerves
4. pertaining to the thalamus
5. record (x-ray) of the spinal cord (after contrast is injected via lumbar puncture)

6. tumor of the meninges
7. tumor of neuroglial cells (a brain tumor)
8. mass of blood below the dura mater (outermost meningeal membrane)

F

1. dyslexia
2. ataxia
3. bradykinesia
4. hyperesthesia

5. narcolepsy
6. aphasia
7. motor apraxia
8. hemiparesis

9. causalgia
10. paraplegia
11. syncope
12. neurasthenia

G

1. lack of sensitivity to pain
2. inability to speak (cannot articulate words, but can understand speech and knows what she or he wants to say)
3. slight paralysis
4. paralysis in all four extremities (damage is to the cervical part of the spinal cord)

5. no strength (weakness)
6. pertaining to coma (loss of consciousness from which the patient cannot be aroused)
7. condition of abnormal sensations (prickling, tingling, numbness, burning) for no apparent reason

8. excessive movement
9. condition of no sensation or nervous feeling
10. intense burning pain
11. pertaining to without movement
12. diminished sensation to pain

H

1. multiple sclerosis
2. epilepsy
3. spina bifida cystica
4. amyotrophic lateral sclerosis

5. Huntington disease
6. hydrocephalus
7. myasthenia gravis

8. Parkinson disease
9. Alzheimer disease
10. Bell palsy

I

1. tumor of neuroglial brain cells (astrocytes)
2. inflammation of the meninges (bacterial infection with pus formation)
3. involuntary spasmodic, twitching movements (tics), uncontrollable vocal sounds, and inappropriate words
4. bruising of brain tissue as a result of direct trauma to the head
5. disruption of the normal blood supply to the brain; stroke or cerebral infarction

6. temporary brain dysfunction; loss of consciousness that usually clears within 24 hours
7. neurological condition caused by infection with herpes zoster virus; blisters form along the course of peripheral nerves
8. blockage of a blood vessel in the cerebrum caused by material from another part of the body that suddenly occludes the vessel

9. blockage of a blood vessel in the cerebrum caused by the formation of a clot within the vessel
10. bursting forth of blood from a cerebral artery (can cause a stroke)
11. a widening of a blood vessel (artery) in the cerebrum; the aneurysm can burst and lead to a CVA
12. brain disease (dementia and encephalitis) caused by infection with AIDS virus

Continued on following page

J

1. C	5. B	8. J
2. E	6. A	9. I
3. H	7. D	10. F
4. G		

K

1. Use of magnetic and radio waves to create an image (in frontal, transverse, or sagittal plane) of the brain.

2. an instrument (stereotactic) is fixed onto the skull and locates a target by three-dimensional measurement;

gamma radiation beams are used to treat deep brain lesions

L

1. electroencephalography. E
2. positron emission tomography. I
3. alpha-fetoprotein. G
4. multiple sclerosis. J
5. magnetic resonance imaging. H
6. lumbar puncture. C
7. cerebrovascular accident. B
8. Alzheimer disease. A
9. transient ischemic attack. F
10. cerebrospinal fluid. D

M

1. migraine
2. contusion and subdural hematoma
3. MRI of the brain; glioblastoma multiforme
4. TIA; MRA
5. myasthenia gravis; anticholinesterase drugs
6. meningitis; LP
7. dyslexia
8. hemiparesis; subdural hematoma
9. syncopal
10. dementia; Alzheimer disease

N

1. hypothalamus
2. syncopal
3. paresthesias
4. paresis
5. radiculitis
6. aphasia
7. apraxia
8. ataxia
9. dyslexia
10. hyperkinesis
11. hemiplegia
12. paraplegia
13. quadriplegia
14. neurasthenia

Answers to Practical Applications

1. C	4. C
2. A	5. A
3. C	

XIII. Pronunciation of Terms

Pronunciation Guide

ā as in āpe	ă as in ăpple
ē as in ēven	ĕ as in ĕvery
ī as in īce	ĭ as in ĭnterest
ō as in ōpen	ŏ as in pŏt
ū as in ūnit	ŭ as in ŭnder

To test your understanding of the terminology in this chapter, write the meaning of each term in the space provided. In addition, you may wish to cover the terms and write them by looking at your definitions. Make sure your spelling is correct. The page number after each term indicates where it is defined or used in the text so you can easily check your responses.

Vocabulary and Combining Forms and Terminology

Term	Pronunciation	Meaning
acetylcholine (345)	ăs-ĕ-tĭl-KŌ-lēn	_____
akinetic (351)	ă-kĭ-NĔT-ĭk	_____
analgesia (350)	ăn-ăl-JĒ-zē-ă	_____
anencephaly (348)	ăn-ĕn-SĔF-ă-lē	_____
anesthesia (350)	ăn-ĕs-THĒ-zē-ă	_____
aphasia (351)	ă-FĀ-zē-ă	_____
apraxia (352)	ā-PRĂK-sē-ă	_____
arachnoid membrane (345)	ă-RĂK-noyd MĔM-brān	_____
astrocyte (345)	ĂS-trō-sīt	_____
ataxia (352)	ă-TĂK-sē-ă	_____
autonomic nervous system (345)	ăw-tō-NŎM-ĭk NĔR-vŭs SĬS-tĕm	_____
axon (345)	ĂK-sŏn	_____
blood-brain barrier (345)	blŭd-brān BĂ-rē-ĕr	_____
bradykinesia (350)	brā-dē-kĭ-NĒ-zē-ă	_____
brainstem (345)	BRĀN-stĕm	_____
cauda equina (345)	KĂW-dă ĕ-QUĪ-nă	_____
causalgia (350)	kăw-ZĂL-jă	_____
cephalgia (350)	sĕ-FĂL-jă	_____
cerebellar (348)	sĕr-ĕ-BĔL-ăr	_____
cerebellopontine (349)	sĕr-ĕ-bĕl-ō-PŎN-tēn	_____
cerebellum (345)	sĕr-ĕ-BĔL-ŭm	_____
cerebral cortex (345)	sĕ-RĒ-brăl (or SĔR-ĕ-brăl) KŎR-tĕks	_____
cerebrospinal fluid (345)	sĕ-rē-brō-SPĪ-năl FLŪ-ĭd	_____
cerebrum (345)	sĕ-RĒ-brŭm	_____

coma (350)	KŌ-mă	_____
comatose (350)	KŌ-mă-tōs	_____
dendrite (346)	DĔN-drīt	_____
dura mater (346)	DŬR-ă MĂ-tĕr	_____
dyslexia (351)	dĭs-LĔK-sē-ă	_____
encephalitis (348)	ĕn-sĕf-ă-LĪ-tĭs	_____
encephalopathy (348)	ĕn-sĕf-ă-LŎP-ă-thē	_____
ependymal cell (346)	ĕp-ĔN-dĭ-măl sĕl	_____
epidural hematoma (348)	ĕp-ĕ-DŪ-răl hē-mă-TŌ-mă	_____
epilepsy (351)	ĔP-ĭ-lĕp-sē	_____
ganglion (346)	GĂNG-lē-ŏn	_____
glial cell (346)	GLĒ-ăl sĕl	_____
glioblastoma (349)	glē-ō-blă-STŌ-mă	_____
gyrus; gyri (346)	JĪ-rŭs; JĪ-rē	_____
hemiparesis (351)	hĕm-ē-pă-RĒ-sĭs	_____
hemiplegia (352)	hĕm-ē-PLĒ-jă	_____
hypalgesia (350)	hīp-ăl-GĒ-zē-ă	_____
hyperesthesia (350)	hī-pĕr-ĕs-THĒ-zē-ă	_____
hyperkinesis (351)	hī-pĕr-kĭ-NĒ-sĭs	_____
hypothalamus (346)	hī-pō-THĂL-ă-mŭs	_____
intrathecal (349)	ĭn-tră-THĒ-kăl	_____
leptomeningitis (349)	lĕp-tō-mĕn-ĭn-JĪ-tĭs	_____
medulla oblongata (346)	mĕ-DŪL-ă (or mĕ-DŬL-ă) ŏb-lŏn-GĂ-tă	_____
meningeal (349)	mĕ-NĬN-jē-ăl or mĕ-nĭn-JĒ-ăl	_____
meninges (346)	mĕ-NĬN-jēz	_____
meningioma (349)	mĕ-nĭn-jē-Ō-mă	_____
meningomyelocele (349)	mĕ-nĭng-gō-MĪ-ĕ-lō-sēl	_____

microglial cell (346)	mĭ-krō-GLĒ-ăl sĕl	_____
motor nerves (346)	MŌ-tĕr nĕrvz	_____
myelin sheath (346)	MĪ-ĕ-lĭn shēth	_____
myelogram (349)	MĪ-ĕ-lō-grăm	_____
myoneural (349)	mī-ō-NŬR-ăl	_____
narcolepsy (351)	NĂR-kō-lĕp-sē	_____
neuralgia (350)	nŭr-ĂL-jă	_____
neurasthenia (352)	nŭr-ăs-THĒ-nē-ă	_____
neuroglia (346)	nŭr-ō-GLĒ-ă	_____
neuron (346)	NŪ-rŏn	_____
neuropathy (349)	nū-RŎP-ă-thē	_____
neurotransmitter (346)	nū-rō-trănz-MĬT-ĕr	_____
oligodendroglial cell (346)	ŏl-ĭ-gō-dĕn-drō-GLĒ-ăl sĕl	_____
paraplegia (352)	păr-ă-PLĒ-jă	_____
parasympathetic nerves (346)	păr-ă-sĭm-pă-THĔT-ĭk nervz	_____
parenchyma (347)	păr-ĔN-kĭ-mă	_____
paresis (351)	pă-RĒ-sĭs	_____
paresthesia (350)	păr-ĕs-THĒ-zē-ă	_____
peripheral nervous system (347)	pĕ-RĬF-ĕr-ăl NĔR-vŭs SĬS-tĕm	_____
pia mater (347)	PĒ-ă MĂ-tĕr	_____
plexus (347)	PLĔK-sŭs	_____
poliomyelitis (349)	pō-lē-ō-mī-ĕ-LĪ-tĭs	_____
polyneuritis (349)	pŏl-ē-nū-RĪ-tĭs	_____
pons (347)	pŏnz	_____
quadriplegia (352)	kwŏd-rĭ-PLĒ-jă	_____
radiculopathy (349)	ră-dĭk-ū-LŎP-ă-thē	_____
radiculitis (349)	ră-dĭk-ū-LĪ-tĭs	_____

sensory nerves (347)	SĔN-sō-rē nĕrvz	_____
stimulus (347)	STĬM-ū-lŭs	_____
stroma (347)	STRŌ-mă	_____
subdural hematoma (348)	sŭb-DŪ-răl hē-mă-TŌ-mă	_____
sulcus; sulci (347)	SŬL-kŭs; SŬL-sī	_____
sympathetic nerves (347)	sĭm-pă-THĔT-ĭk nĕrvz	_____
synapse (347)	SĬN-ăps	_____
syncopal (352)	SĬN-kō-păl	_____
syncope (352)	SĬN-kō-pē	_____
thalamic (349)	THĂL-ă-mĭk or thă-LĂM-ĭk	_____
thalamus (347)	THĂL-ă-mŭs	_____
vagal (350)	VĀ-găl	_____
ventricles of the brain (347)	VĔN-trĭ-k'lz of the brān	_____

Pathological Conditions, Laboratory Tests, and Clinical Procedures

Term	Pronunciation	Meaning
absence seizures (359)	ĂB-sĕns SĒ-zhŭrz	_____
Alzheimer disease (354)	ĂLZ-hī-mĕr dĭ-ZĒZ	_____
amyotrophic lateral sclerosis (354)	ā-mī-ō-TRŌ-fĭk LĂ-tĕr-ăl sklĕ-RŌ-sis	_____
aneurysm (359)	ĂN-ūr-ĭ-zĭm	_____
astrocytoma (359)	ăs-trō-sī-TŌ-mă	_____
aura (359)	ĂW-ră	_____
Bell palsy (356)	bĕl PĂL-zē	_____
cerebral angiography (360)	sĕ-RĒ-brăl ăn-jē-ŎG-ră-fē	_____
cerebral concussion (357)	sĕ-RĒ-brăl kŏn-KŬS-shŭn	_____
cerebral contusion (357)	sĕ-RĒ-brăl kŏn-TŪ-shŭn	_____
cerebral hemorrhage (358)	sĕ-RĒ-brăl HĔM-ŏr-ĭj	_____

cerebral palsy (355)	sĕ-RĒ-brăl (or SĔR-ĕ-brăl) PĂL-zē	_____
cerebrospinal fluid analysis (360)	sĕ-rē-brō-SPĪ-năl FLOO-ĭd ă-NĂL-ĭ-sĭs	_____
cerebrovascular accident (358)	sĕ-rē-brō-VĂS-kū-lăr ĂK-sĭ-dĕnt	_____
computed tomography (360)	kŏm-PŪ-tĕd tō-MŎG-ră-fē	_____
dementia (359)	dĕ-MĔN-shē-ă	_____
demyelination (359)	dē-mī-ĕ-lĭ-NĀ-shun	_____
dopamine (359)	DŌ-pă-mēn	_____
Doppler/ultrasound studies (361)	DŎP-lĕr ŬL-tră-sound STŪ-dēz	_____
electroencephalography (361)	ĕ-lĕk-trō-ĕn-sĕf-ă-LŎG-ră-fē	_____
embolus (359)	ĔM-bō-lŭs	_____
epilepsy (354)	ĔP-ĭ-lĕp-sē	_____
gait (359)	GĀT	_____
glioblastoma multiforme (357)	glē-ō-blăs-TŌ-mă mŭl-tē-FŎR-mă	_____
herpes zoster (356)	HĔR-pēz ZŎS-tĕr	_____
HIV encephalopathy (356)	HIV ĕn-sĕf-ă-LŎP-ă-thē	_____
Huntington disease (354)	HŬN-ting-tŏn dĭ-ZĒZ	_____
hydrocephalus (353)	hī-drō-SĔF-ă-lŭs	_____
ictal event (359)	ĬK-tăl ē-VĔNT	_____
lumbar puncture (361)	LŬM-băr PŬNK-shŭr	_____
magnetic resonance imaging (360)	măg-NĔT-ĭk rĕ-zō-NĂNCE ĬM-ă-jĭng	_____
meningitis (356)	mĕn-ĭn-JĪ-tĭs	_____
migraine (350)	MĪ-grān	_____
multiple sclerosis (355)	mŭl-tĭ-p'l sklĕ-RŌ-sĭs	_____
myasthenia gravis (355)	mī-ăs-THĒ-nē-ă GRĂ-vĭs	_____

occlusion (359)   ō-KLŪ-jŭn   _____

palliative (359)   PĂ-lē-ă-tĭv   _____

palsy (356)   PĂWL-zē   _____

Parkinson disease (356)   PĂR-kĭn-sŭn dĭ-ZĒZ   _____

petit mal seizures (354)   pĕ-TĒ măl SĒ-zhŭrz   _____

positron emission tomography (360)   PŎS-ĭ-trŏn ē-MĬ-shŭn tō-MŎG-ră-fē   _____

shingles (356)   SHĬNG-ălz   _____

spina bifida (353)   SPĬ-nă BĬF-ĭ-dă   _____

stereotactic radiosurgery (362)   stĕ-rē-ō-TĂK-tĭk rā-dē-ō SŬR-gĕr-ē   _____

thrombosis (358)   thrŏm-BŌ-sĭs   _____

thymectomy (359)   thī-MĔK-tō-mē   _____

tonic-clonic seizures (359)   TŎN-ĭk-KLŌ-nĭk SĒ-zhŭrz   _____

Tourette syndrome (356)   tŭ-RĔT SĬN-drōm   _____

transient ischemic attack (358)   TRĂN-zē-ĕnt ĭs-KĒ-mĭk ă-TĂK   _____

XIV. Review Sheet

Write the meanings of the word parts in the spaces provided. Check your answers with the information in the chapter or in the glossary (Medical Terms—English) at the end of the book.

COMBINING FORMS

Combining Form	Meaning	Combining Form	Meaning
alges/o		lex/o	
angi/o		mening/o, meningi/o	
caus/o		my/o	
cephal/o		myel/o	
cerebell/o		narc/o	
cerebr/o		neur/o	
comat/o		pont/o	
crani/o		radicul/o	
cry/o		spin/o	
dur/o		syncop/o	
encephal/o		tax/o	
esthesi/o		thalam/o	
gli/o		thec/o	
hydr/o		troph/o	
kines/o		vag/o	
lept/o			

Continued on following page

PREFIXES

Prefix	Meaning	Prefix	Meaning
a-, an-	_____	micro-	_____
dys-	_____	para-	_____
epi-	_____	polio-	_____
hemi-	_____	poly-	_____
hyper-	_____	quadri-	_____
hypo-	_____	sub-	_____
intra-	_____		

SUFFIXES

Suffix	Meaning	Suffix	Meaning
-algesia	_____	-ose	_____
-algia	_____	-paresis	_____
-blast	_____	-pathy	_____
-cele	_____	-phagia	_____
-esthesia	_____	-phasia	_____
-gram	_____	-plegia	_____
-graphy	_____	-praxia	_____
-ine	_____	-ptosis	_____
-itis	_____	-sclerosis	_____
-kinesia, -kinesis	_____	-sthenia	_____
-kinetic	_____	-tomy	_____
-lepsy	_____	-trophy	_____
-oma	_____		

chapter

Cardiovascular System

This chapter is divided into the following sections

In this chapter you will

- Name the parts of the heart and associated blood vessels and their functions in the circulation of blood.
- Trace the pathway of blood through the heart.
- List the meanings of major pathological conditions affecting the heart and blood vessels.
- Define combining forms that relate to the cardiovascular system.
- Recognize the meaning of many laboratory tests, clinical procedures, and abbreviations pertaining to the cardiovascular system.
- Apply your new knowledge to understand medical terms in their proper context, such as in medical reports and records.

I. Introduction

In previous chapters we explored the terminology of the digestive, urinary, reproductive, and nervous systems and the function of organs in those systems. The cells of the organs are dependent on a constant supply of nutrients and oxygen. When the supplies are delivered, and chemically combined, they release energy necessary to do the work of each cell.

How does the body assure that oxygen and food will be delivered to all its cells? The cardiovascular system, consisting of the heart (a powerful muscular pump) and blood vessels (fuel line and transportation network), performs this important work. This chapter explores terminology related to the heart and blood vessels.

II. Blood Vessels and the Circulation of Blood

Blood Vessels

There are three types of blood vessels in the body: arteries, veins, and capillaries.

Arteries are the large blood vessels that lead away from the heart. Their walls are made of connective tissue, muscle tissue, elastic fibers, and an innermost layer of epithelial cells called **endothelium.** Endothelial cells, which line all blood vessels, secrete factors that affect the size of blood vessels, reduce blood clotting, and promote the growth of blood vessels. Because arteries carry blood away from the heart, they must be strong enough to withstand the high pressure of the pumping action of the heart. Their elastic walls allow them to expand as the heartbeat forces blood into the arterial system throughout the body. Smaller branches of arteries are called **arterioles.** Arterioles are thinner than arteries and carry the blood to the tiniest of blood vessels, the capillaries.

Capillaries have walls that are only one endothelial cell thick. These delicate, microscopic vessels carry nutrient-rich, oxygenated blood from the arteries and arterioles to the body cells. Their thin walls allow passage of oxygen and nutrients out of the bloodstream and into the cells. There, the nutrients are burned in the presence of oxygen (catabolism) to release needed energy. At the same time, waste products such as carbon dioxide and water pass out of cells and into the thin-walled capillaries. Waste-filled blood then flows back to the heart in small veins called **venules,** which branch to form larger vessels called veins.

Veins have thinner walls compared to arteries. They conduct blood (that has given up most of its oxygen) toward the heart from the tissues. Veins have little elastic tissue and less connective tissue than arteries, and blood pressure in veins is extremely low compared with pressure in arteries. In order to keep blood moving back toward the heart, veins have valves that prevent the backflow of blood and keep the blood moving in one direction. Muscular action also helps the movement of blood in veins. Figure 11–1 illustrates the differences in blood vessels.

ARTERY

Outer layer　Muscle layer　Elastic layer　Inner layer　Endothelium

VEIN

Outer layer　Muscle layer　Inner layer　Valve　Endothelium

CAPILLARY

Endothelium

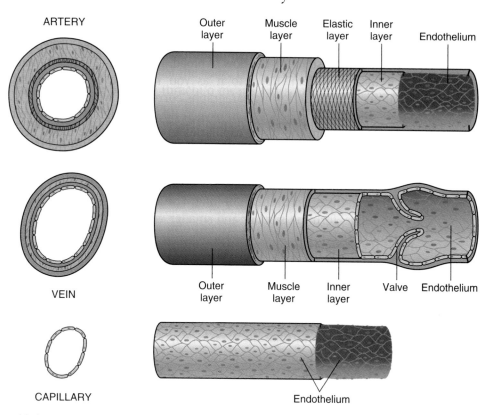

Figure 11–1

Blood vessels. Observe the differences in thickness of walls among an artery, vein, and capillary. All three vessels are lined with endothelium. Endothelial cells actively secrete substances that prevent clotting and regulate the tone of blood vessels. Examples of endothelial secretions are endothelium-derived relaxing factor (EDRF) and endothelin (a vasoconstrictor). (Some parts modified from Damjanov I: Pathology for the Health-Related Professions, 2nd ed. Philadelphia, WB Saunders, 2000, p. 143.)

III. Anatomy of the Heart

The human heart weighs less than a pound, is roughly the size of an adult fist, and lies in the thoracic cavity, just behind the breastbone in the mediastinum (between the lungs).

The heart is a pump, consisting of four chambers: two upper chambers called **atria** (singular: **atrium**) and two lower chambers called **ventricles.** It is actually a double pump, bound into one organ and synchronized very carefully. Blood passes through each pump in a definite pattern. Pump station number one, on the right side of the heart, sends oxygen-deficient blood to the lungs, where the blood picks up oxygen and releases its carbon dioxide. The newly oxygenated blood returns to the left side of the heart to pump station number two and does not mix with the oxygen-poor blood in pump station number one. Pump station number two then forces the oxygenated blood out to all parts of the body. At the body tissues, the blood loses its oxygen, and on returning to the heart, to pump station number one, blood poor in oxygen (rich in carbon dioxide) is sent out to the lungs to begin the cycle anew.

Label Figure 11–4 as you learn the names of the parts of the heart and the vessels that carry blood to and from it.

Oxygen-poor blood enters the heart through the two largest veins in the body, the **venae cavae.** The **superior vena cava** [1] drains blood from the upper portion of the body, and the **inferior vena cava** [2] carries blood from the lower part of the body.

The venae cavae bring oxygen-poor blood that has passed through all of the body to the **right atrium** [3], the thin-walled upper right chamber of the heart. The right atrium contracts to force blood through the **tricuspid valve** [4] (cusps are the flaps of the valves) into the **right ventricle** [5], the lower right chamber of the heart. The cusps of the tricuspid valve form a one-way passage designed to keep the blood flowing in only one direction. As the right ventricle contracts to pump oxygen-poor blood through the **pulmonary valve** [6] into the **pulmonary artery** [7], the tricuspid valve stays shut, thus preventing blood from pushing back into the right atrium. The pulmonary artery then branches to carry oxygen-deficient blood to each lung.

The blood that enters the lung capillaries from the pulmonary artery soon loses its large quantity of carbon dioxide into the lung tissue, and the carbon dioxide is expelled. At the same time, oxygen enters the capillaries of the lungs and is brought back to the heart via the **pulmonary veins** [8]. The newly oxygenated blood enters the **left atrium** [9] of the heart from the pulmonary veins. The walls of the left atrium contract to force blood through the **mitral valve** [10] into the **left ventricle** [11].

The left ventricle has the thickest walls of all four heart chambers (three times the thickness of the right ventricle). It must pump blood with great force so that the blood travels through arteries to all parts of the body. The left ventricle propels the blood through the **aortic valve** [12] into the **aorta** [13], which branches to carry blood all over the body. The aortic valve closes to prevent return of aortic blood to the left ventricle.

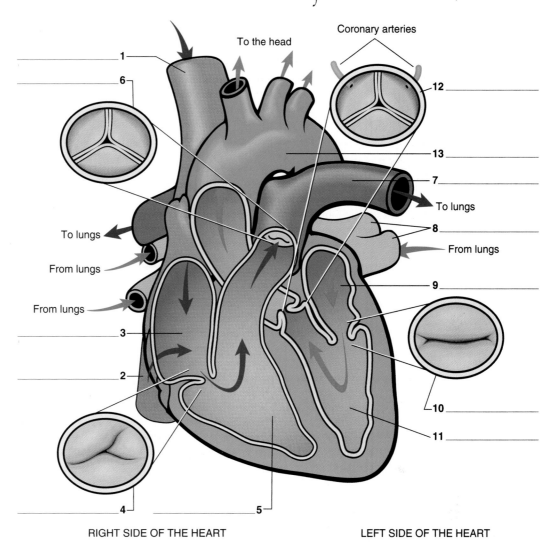

RIGHT SIDE OF THE HEART   LEFT SIDE OF THE HEART

Figure 11–4

Structure of the heart. Blue arrows indicate oxygen-poor blood flow. Red arrows show oxygenated blood flow. (Modified from Damjanov I: Pathology for the Health-Related Professions, 2nd ed. Philadelphia, WB Saunders, 2000, p. 142.)

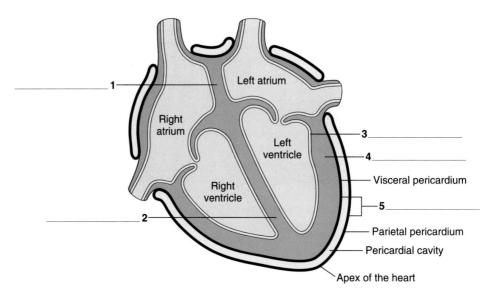

Figure 11–5

The walls of the heart and pericardium. Note that the apex of the heart is the conical (shaped like a cone) lower tip of the heart.

In Figure 11–5 notice that the four chambers of the heart are separated by partitions called **septa** (singular: **septum**). (Label Fig. 11–5 as you read these paragraphs.) The **interatrial septum** [1] separates the two upper chambers (atria), and the **interventricular septum** [2], a muscular wall, comes between the two lower chambers (ventricles).

Figure 11–5 shows the three layers of the heart. The **endocardium** [3], a smooth layer of endothelial cells, lines the interior of the heart and heart valves. The **myocardium** [4], the middle, muscular layer of the heart wall, is its thickest layer. The **pericardium** [5], a fibrous and membranous sac, surrounds the heart. It is composed of two layers, the **visceral pericardium,**

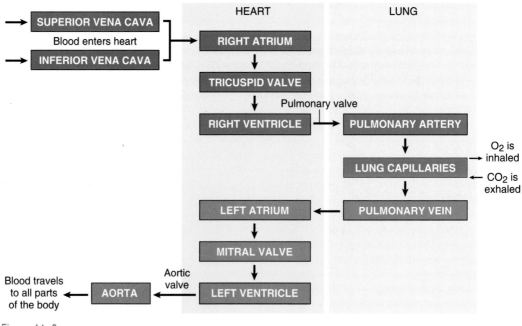

Figure 11–6

Pathway of blood through the heart.

adhering to the heart, and the **parietal** (parietal means wall) **pericardium,** lining the outer fibrous coat. The **pericardial cavity** (between the visceral and the parietal pericardia) normally contains 10 to 15 mL of fluid, which lubricates the membranes as the heart beats.

Figure 11–6 schematically traces the flow of blood through the heart.

IV. Physiology of the Heart

Heartbeat and Heart Sounds

There are two phases of the heartbeat: **diastole** (relaxation) and **systole** (contraction). Diastole occurs when the ventricle walls relax and blood flows into the heart from the venae cavae and the pulmonary veins. The tricuspid and mitral valves open in diastole, as blood passes from the right and left atria into the ventricles. The pulmonary and aortic valves close during diastole (Fig. 11–7).

Systole occurs next, as the walls of the right and left ventricles contract to pump blood into the pulmonary artery and the aorta. Both the tricuspid and the mitral valves are closed during systole, thus preventing the flow of blood back into the atria (see Fig. 11–7).

This diastole-systole cardiac cycle occurs between 70 and 80 times per minute (100,000 times a day). The heart pumps about 3 ounces of blood with each contraction. This means that about 5 quarts of blood are pumped by the heart in 1 minute (75 gallons an hour and about 2000 gallons a day).

Closure of the heart valves is associated with audible sounds, such as "lub, dub, lub, dub," which can be heard when listening to a normal heart with a stethoscope. The "lub" is associated with closure of the tricuspid and mitral valves at the beginning of systole and the "dub" with the closure of the aortic and pulmonary valves at the end of systole. The "lub" sound is called the first heart sound and the "dub" is the second heart sound because the normal cycle of the heartbeat starts with the beginning of systole. An abnormal heart sound is known as a **murmur.**

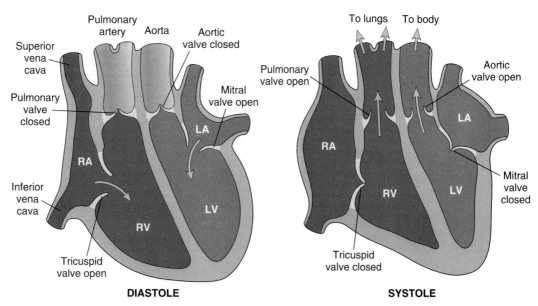

Figure 11–7

Phases of the heartbeat: diastole and systole. During diastole, the tricuspid and mitral valves are open as blood enters the ventricles. During systole, the pulmonary and aortic valves are open as blood is pumped to the pulmonary artery and aorta. RA = right atrium; RV = right ventricle; LA = left atrium; LV = left ventricle.

Conduction System of the Heart

What keeps the heart at its perfect rhythm? Although the heart does have nerves that can affect its rate, they are not primarily responsible for its beat. The heart starts beating in the embryo before the heart is supplied with nerves, and it will continue to beat in experimental animals even when the nerve supply is cut.

Primary responsibility for initiating the heartbeat rests with a small region of specialized muscle tissue in the posterior portion of the right atrium, where an electrical impulse originates. This region of the right atrium, the **sinoatrial node (SA node),** is the **pacemaker** of the heart. The current of electricity generated by the pacemaker causes the walls of the atria to contract and force blood into the ventricles (ending diastole).

Almost like ripples in a pond of water when a stone is thrown, the wave of electricity passes from the pacemaker to another region of the myocardium. This region is at the posterior portion of the interatrial septum and is called the **atrioventricular node (AV node).** The AV node immediately sends the excitation wave to a bundle of specialized muscle fibers called the **atrioventricular bundle** or **bundle of His** (pronounced hiss). Within the interventricular septum, the bundle of His divides into **right and left bundle branches,** which form the conduction myofibers that extend through the ventricle walls and stimulate them to contract. Thus systole occurs and blood is pumped away from the heart. A short rest period follows, and then the pacemaker begins the wave of excitation across the heart again. Figure 11–8 shows the conduction system of the heart.

The record used to detect these electrical changes in heart muscle as the heart beats is an **electrocardiogram** (ECG or EKG, from the Greek root *kardia*). The normal ECG shows five waves, or **deflections,** that represent the electrical changes as a wave of excitation spreads through the heart. The deflections are called P, QRS, and T waves. Figure 11–9 illustrates P, QRS, and T waves in a normal ECG. The ECG diagnoses electrical problems in the heart, such as arrhythmias.

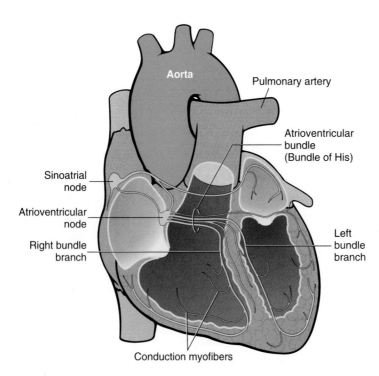

Figure 11–8

Conduction system of the heart.

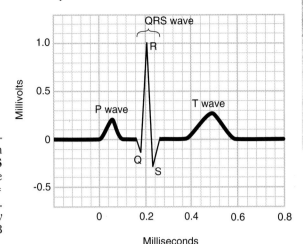

Figure 11-9

Electrocardiogram. P wave = spread of excitation wave over the atria just before contraction; **QRS wave** = spread of excitation wave over the ventricles as the ventricles contract; **T wave** = electrical recovery and relaxation of ventricles. (From Applegate MS: The Anatomy and Physiology Learning System, 2nd ed. Philadelphia, WB Saunders, 2000, p. 250.)

Normal heart rhythm (originating in the SA node and traveling through the heart) is called **sinus rhythm.** Sympathetic nerves speed up the heart rate during conditions of emotional stress or vigorous exercise. Parasympathetic nerves slow the heart rate when there is no need for extra pumping.

V. Blood Pressure

Blood pressure is the force that the blood exerts on the arterial walls. This pressure is measured by a device called a **sphygmomanometer.**

The sphygmomanometer consists of a rubber bag inside a cloth cuff that is wrapped around the upper arm, just above the elbow. The rubber bag is inflated with air by means of a rubber bulb. As the bag is pumped up, the pressure within it increases and is measured on a recording device attached to the cuff.

The vessels in the upper arm are compressed by the air pressure in the bag. When there is sufficient air pressure in the bag to stop the flow of blood in the main artery of the arm (brachial artery), the pulse in the lower arm (where the observer is listening with a stethoscope) obviously drops.

Air is then allowed to escape from the bag and the pressure is lowered slowly, allowing the blood to begin to make its way through the gradually opening artery. At the point when the person listening with the stethoscope first hears the sounds of the pulse beats, the reading on the device attached to the cuff shows the higher, systolic, blood pressure (pressure in the artery when the left ventricle is contracting to force the blood into the aorta and other arteries).

As air continues to escape, the sounds become progressively louder. Finally, when a change in sound from loud to soft occurs, the observer makes note of the pressure on the recording device. This is called the diastolic blood pressure (pressure in the artery when the ventricles are relaxing and the heart is filling, receiving blood from the venae cavae and pulmonary veins).

Blood pressure is usually expressed as a fraction: for example, 120/80, in which 120 represents the systolic pressure and 80 the diastolic pressure.

VI. Vocabulary

This list reviews new terms introduced in the text. Short definitions reinforce your understanding of the terms. See Section XIII of this chapter for pronunciation of terms.

aorta	Largest artery in the body.
arteriole	Small artery.
artery	Largest type of blood vessel; carries blood away from the heart to all parts of the body. Notice that artery and away begin with an "a."
atrioventricular bundle (bundle of His)	Specialized muscle fibers in the wall between the ventricles that carry the electric impulses to the ventricles.
atrioventricular node (AV node)	Specialized tissue at the base of the wall between the two upper heart chambers. Electrical impulses pass from the pacemaker (SA node) through the AV node to the bundle of His.
atrium (plural: **atria**)	One of two upper chambers of the heart.
capillary	Smallest blood vessel. Materials pass to and from the bloodstream through the thin capillary walls.
carbon dioxide (CO$_2$)	Gas (waste) released by body cells, transported via veins to the heart, and then to the lungs for exhalation.
coronary arteries	The blood vessels that branch from the aorta and carry oxygen-rich blood to the heart muscle.
deoxygenated blood	Blood that is oxygen-poor.
diastole	Relaxation phase of the heartbeat. From the Greek *diastole,* meaning "dilation."
endocardium	Inner lining of the heart.
endothelium	Innermost lining of blood vessels.
mitral valve	Valve between the left atrium and the left ventricle of the heart (Fig. 11–10); bicuspid valve.
murmur	Abnormal heart sound caused by improper closure of the heart valves.
myocardium	Muscle layer of the heart.
oxygen	Gas that enters the blood through the lungs and travels to the heart to be pumped via arteries to all body cells.
pacemaker	Specialized nervous tissue in the right atrium that begins the heartbeat; also called the **sinoatrial node.** A cardiac pacemaker is an electronic apparatus implanted in the chest to stimulate heart muscle.

pericardium
Sac-like membrane surrounding the heart.

pulmonary artery
Artery carrying oxygen-poor blood from the heart to the lungs.

pulmonary circulation
Flow of blood from the heart to the lungs and back to the heart.

pulmonary valve
Positioned between the right ventricle and the pulmonary artery.

pulmonary vein
One of two pairs of vessels carrying oxygenated blood from the lungs to the left atrium of the heart.

pulse
Beat of the heart as felt through the walls of the arteries.

septum (plural: **septa**)
Partition; in the cardiovascular system, between the right and left sides of the heart.

sinoatrial node (SA node)
Pacemaker of the heart.

sphygmomanometer
Instrument to measure blood pressure.

systemic circulation
Flow of blood from the body cells to the heart and back out from the heart to the cells.

systole
Contraction phase of the heartbeat. From the Greek *systole,* meaning "a contracting."

tricuspid valve
Located between the right atrium and the right ventricle; it has three (tri-) leaflets, or cusps (see Fig. 11–10).

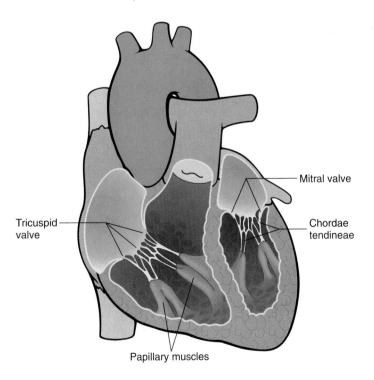

Figure 11-10

Tricuspid and mitral valves. These valves work like parachutes. The chordae tendineae are the connective tissue strings that attach to the papillary muscles projecting from the lining of the ventricles and anchor the valve in place. As the right and left ventricles contract, blood strikes the valves (parachute), which swing up, meet in the midline, and fit tightly together so that blood is prevented from flowing back into the atria.

valve	Structure in veins or in the heart that temporarily closes an opening so that blood flows in only one direction.
vein	Thin-walled vessel that carries blood from body tissues and lungs to the heart. Veins contain valves to prevent backflow of blood.
vena cava (plural: venae cavae)	Largest vein in the body. The superior and inferior venae cavae bring blood into the right atrium of the heart.
ventricle	One of two lower chambers of the heart.
venule	Small vein.

VII. Combining Forms and Terminology

Write the meaning of the medical term in the space provided.

Combining Form	Terminology	Meaning
angi/o	vessel	angiogram _____
		angioplasty _____
aort/o	aorta	aortic stenosis _____
arter/o **arteri/o**	artery	arteriosclerosis _____
		arterial anastomosis _____
		From Greek, anastomoien, meaning "to provide a mouth."
		arteriography _____
		endarterectomy _____
		See Section IX, page 415, under Clinical Procedures.
ather/o	yellowish plaque, fatty substance (the Greek *athere*, means "porridge")	atheroma _____
		The suffix -oma means mass or collection. Atheromas are collections of plaque that protrude into the lumen (opening) of an artery, weakening the muscle lining.
		atherosclerosis _____
		The major form of arteriosclerosis in which deposits of yellow plaque containing cholesterol and lipids are found within the lining of the artery.
		atherectomy _____

atri/o	atrium, upper heart chamber	atrial _____
		atrioventricular _____
brachi/o	arm	brachial artery _____
cardi/o	heart	cardiomegaly _____
		cardiomyopathy _____

Toxic or infectious agents may be the cause, but often the etiology is unknown (idiopathic). **Hypertrophic cardiomyopathy** *is an increase in heart muscle weight, especially along the septum, which causes narrowing (stenosis) of the aortic valve.*

bradycardia _____

Slower than 60 beats per minute. Normal pulse is about 60 to 80 beats per minute.

tachycardia _____

Faster than 100 beats per minute.

cholesterol/o	cholesterol (a lipid substance)	hypercholesterolemia _____
coron/o	heart	coronary arteries _____

These arteries come down over the top of the heart like a crown (corona) (Fig. 11–11).

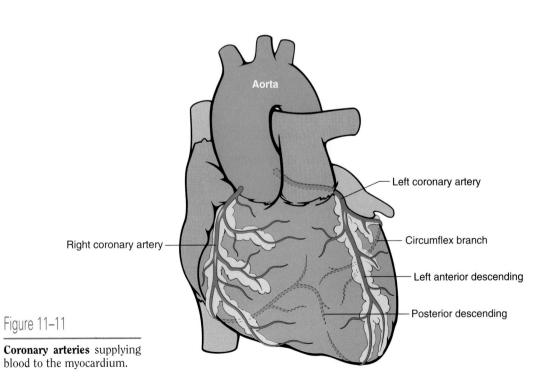

Figure 11–11

Coronary arteries supplying blood to the myocardium.

cyan/o	blue	cyanosis _____

This bluish discoloration of the skin indicates diminished oxygen content of the blood.

myx/o	mucus	myxoma _____

A benign tumor derived from connective tissue, with cells embedded in soft mucoid stromal tissue. These tumors occur most frequently in the left atrium.

ox/o	oxygen	hypoxia _____

Inadequate oxygen at the cellular level.

pericardi/o	pericardium	pericardiocentesis _____

phleb/o	vein	phlebotomy _____

thrombophlebitis _____

Also called phlebitis.

sphygm/o	pulse	sphygmomanometer _____

A manometer measures pressure.

steth/o	chest	stethoscope _____

A misnomer because the examination is by ear, not by eye. Auscultation means listening to sounds within the body using a stethoscope.

thromb/o	clot	thrombolysis _____

valvul/o valv/o	valve	valvuloplasty _____

A balloon-tipped catheter dilates a cardiac valve.

mitral valvulitis _____

Most commonly caused by rheumatic fever.

valvotomy _____

vas/o	vessel	vasoconstriction _____
		Constriction means to tighten or narrow.
		vasodilation _____
vascul/o	vessel	vascular _____
ven/o, ven/i	vein	venous _____
		A venous cutdown is a small surgical incision to permit access to a collapsed vein.
		venipuncture _____
		This procedure is performed for phlebotomy or to start an intravenous infusion.
ventricul/o	ventricle, lower heart chamber	interventricular septum _____

VIII. Pathological Conditions: The Heart and Blood Vessels

Heart

arrhythmias

Abnormal heart rhythms (dysrhythmias).

Arrhythmias are problems with the conduction or electrical system of the heart.
Examples of cardiac arrhythmias are:

1. heart block (atrioventricular block)

Failure of proper conduction of impulses through the AV node to the atrioventricular bundle (bundle of His).

Damage to the SA node may cause its impulses to be too weak to activate the AV node and impulses fail to reach the ventricles. If the failure occurs only occasionally, the heart misses a beat in a rhythm at regular intervals (partial heart block). If no impulses reach the AV node from the SA node, the ventricles contract slower than the atria and are not coordinated. This is complete heart block.

Implantation of an artificial **cardiac pacemaker** can overcome arrhythmias and establish normal rhythm. The pacemaker is an electronic device used in place of the SA node. The pacemaker power source is implanted subcutaneously in the chest (see Fig. 11–12).

2. flutter

Rapid but regular contractions of atria or ventricles.

This condition can occur in patients with heart disease. The heart rhythm may reach up to 300 beats per minute.

3. fibrillation

Rapid, random, ineffectual, and irregular contractions of the heart (350 beats or more per minute).

In atrial fibrillation, the wave of excitation passes through the atrial myocardium even more quickly than in atrial flutter. In order to restore normal heart rhythm, an electrical device called a **defibrillator** is applied to the chest wall. The electric shock stops the heart and reverses its abnormal rhythm. This is also called **cardioversion. Digoxin** is a drug that slows the heart rate to treat atrial fibrillation. Other drugs can convert fibrillation to normal sinus rhythm.

A device, called an **implantable cardioverter/defibrillator (ICD),** can now be implanted in the chest to sense arrhythmias and correct them. These are pacemaker-sized devices that give shocks to change abnormal rhythms, such as ventricular fibrillation. **Radiofrequency catheter ablation (RFA)** is a nonsurgical

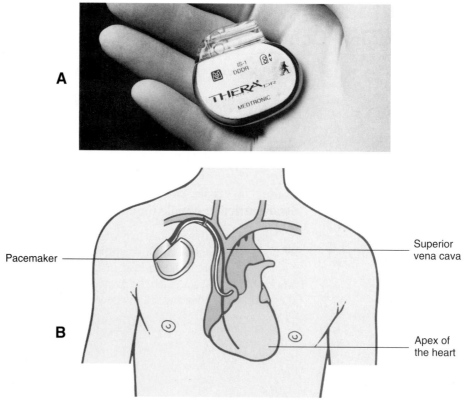

Figure 11–12

(A) A dual-chamber, rate responsive pacemaker (actual size shown) from Medtronic, Inc. is designed to detect body movement and automatically increase or decrease paced heart rates based on levels of physical activity. **(B)** Cardiac leads in both the atrium and ventricle enable a dual-chamber pacemaker to sense and pace in both heart chambers. (From Lewis SM, Heitkemper MM, Dirksen SR: Medical-Surgical Nursing: Assessment and Management of Clinical Problems, 5th ed. St Louis, Mosby, 2000, p. 937.)

treatment used to treat arrhythmias, such as paroxysmal (sharp, sudden spasms) tachycardia. A catheter, placed in blood vessels leading up against heart muscle, delivers a high-frequency current to burn a small portion of the muscle. This injury (ablation) to the muscle destroys the arrhythmia.

Cardiac arrest is the sudden and often unexpected stoppage of heart movement, caused by heart block or ventricular fibrillation (resulting from underlying heart disease).

Palpitations are uncomfortable sensations in the chest associated with different types of arrhythmias. Palpitations do not necessarily indicate serious heart disease (smoking, caffeine, and drugs such as antidepressants can produce palpitations). Two cardiac causes of palpitations are **premature ventricular contractions (PVCs)** and **premature atrial contractions (PACs)**.

congenital heart disease   **Abnormalities in the heart at birth.**

The following conditions are congenital anomalies resulting from some failure in the development of the fetal heart.

1. coarctation of the aorta (CoA)   **Narrowing (coarctation) of the aorta.**

Figure 11–13A shows one form of coarctation of the aorta. Surgical treatment consists of removal of the constricted region and end-to-end anastomosis of the aortic segments.

2. patent ductus arteriosus (PDA)   **A small duct (ductus arteriosus) between the aorta and the pulmonary artery, which normally closes soon after birth, remains open (patent).**

This condition, illustrated in Figure 11–13B, means that oxygenated blood flows from the aorta to the pulmonary artery. The anomaly occurs most often in females

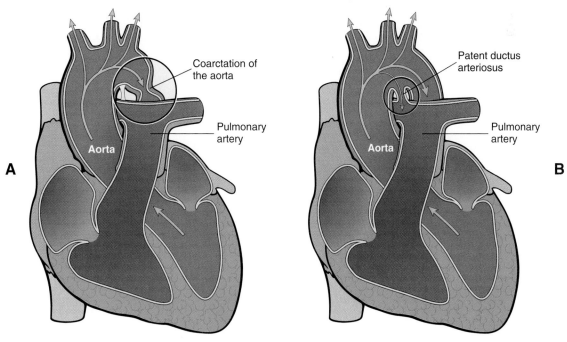

Coarctation of the aorta

Pulmonary artery

Aorta

A

Patent ductus arteriosus

Pulmonary artery

Aorta

B

Figure 11–13

(A) Coarctation of the aorta. Localized narrowing of the aorta reduces the supply of blood to the lower part of the body. **(B) Patent ductus arteriosus.** The ductus arteriosus fails to close after birth, and blood from the aorta flows through it into the pulmonary artery.

and is commonly associated with intrauterine rubella (German measles) infection, prematurity, and infantile respiratory distress syndrome. Treatment is surgery to close the ductus arteriosus. Alternative measures include minimally invasive surgery (a metal clip is used to close the PDA) and use of indomethacin, a drug that blocks the effects of prostaglandin, which naturally keeps the ductus arteriosus open.

3. septal defects

Small holes in the septa between the atria (atrial septal defects) or the ventricles (ventricular septal defects). Figure 11–14A shows a ventricular septal defect.

Although many septal defects close spontaneously, others require surgery. Septal defects can be closed while maintaining a general circulation by means of a **heart-lung machine.** This machine, connected to the patient's circulatory system, relieves the heart and lungs of pumping and oxygenation functions during heart surgery.

Two recent procedures as alternatives to traditional surgery are **trans-catheter closure** (a "clamshell" device is threaded through the blood via a catheter into the heart and into the septal defect, where it is fixed in place to block the hole) and **minimally invasive heart surgery** (through three or four small "puncture" holes in the chest, special instruments are used to repair the defect).

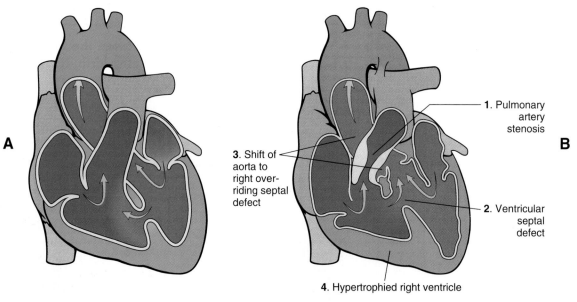

A

B

1. Pulmonary artery stenosis

3. Shift of aorta to right over-riding septal defect

2. Ventricular septal defect

4. Hypertrophied right ventricle

Figure 11–14

(A) Ventricular septal defect. A hole in the ventricular septum causes blood to flow from the left ventricle to the right and into the lungs via the pulmonary artery. **(B) Tetralogy of Fallot** showing the four defects. The flow of blood is indicated by the *arrows.* (Part **B** modified from Kumar V, Cotran RS, Robbins SL: Basic Pathology, 7th ed. Philadelphia, WB Saunders, 2003, p. 367.)

4. tetralogy of Fallot (fă-LŌ)   **A congenital malformation of the heart involving four (tetra-) distinct defects.**

The condition, named for Etienne Fallot, the French physician who described it in 1888, is illustrated in Figure 11–14B. The four defects are:

1. **Pulmonary artery stenosis.** This means that blood is not adequately passed to the lungs for oxygenation.
2. **Ventricular septal defect.** The gap in the septum allows deoxygenated blood to pass into the left ventricle, and from there to the aorta.
3. **Shift of the aorta to the right,** so that the aorta overrides the interventricular septum. Oxygen-poor blood passes even more easily from the right ventricle to the aorta.
4. **Hypertrophy of the right ventricle.** The myocardium has to work harder to pump blood through a narrowed pulmonary artery.

An infant with this condition is described as a "blue baby" because of the extreme degree of **cyanosis** present at birth. Other congenital conditions such as **transposition of the great vessels** (pulmonary artery arises from the left ventricle and the aorta from the right ventricle) cause cyanosis and hypoxia as well. Surgery is necessary to repair these congenital defects.

congestive heart failure (CHF)   **The heart is unable to pump its required amount of blood (more blood enters the heart from the veins than leaves through the arteries).**

Blood accumulates in the lungs (left-sided heart failure) causing **pulmonary edema** (fluid seeps out of capillaries into the tiny air sacs of the lungs). Damming back of blood resulting from right-sided heart failure results in accumulation of fluid in the abdominal organs (liver and spleen) and subcutaneous tissue of the legs. The most common cause of CHF in the United States is high blood pressure and coronary artery disease. Therapy includes lowering dietary intake of sodium and diuretics to promote loss of fluids.

Drugs (**angiotensin-converting enzyme [ACE] inhibitors** and **beta-blockers**) improve the performance of the heart and its pumping activity. These drugs decrease pressure inside blood vessels to treat hypertension (high blood pressure). If drug therapy and lifestyle changes fail to control congestive heart failure, heart transplantation may be the only treatment option. While waiting for a transplant, patients may need a device to assist the heart's pumping. A **left ventricular assist device (LVAD)** is a booster pump implanted in the abdomen, with a cannula (tube) inserted into the left ventricle. It pumps blood out of the heart to all parts of the body. The LVAD is sometimes called a "bridge to transplant."

coronary artery disease (CAD) **Disease of the arteries surrounding the heart.**

The coronary arteries are a pair of blood vessels that arise from the aorta and supply oxygenated blood to the heart. After blood leaves the heart via the aorta, a portion is at once led back over the surface of the heart through the coronary arteries. Figure 11–11 shows the right and left coronary arteries as they branch from the aorta.

Coronary artery disease is usually the result of **atherosclerosis.** This is the deposition of fatty compounds on the inner lining of the coronary arteries (any other artery can be similarly affected). The ordinarily smooth lining of the artery becomes roughened as the atherosclerotic plaque collects in the artery.

The plaque first causes plugging of the coronary artery. Next, the roughened lining of the artery may rupture or cause abnormal clotting of blood, leading to a **thrombotic occlusion** (blocking of the coronary artery by a clot). Blood flow is decreased **(ischemia)** or stopped entirely, leading to death **(necrosis)** of a part of the myocardium. The area of dead myocardial tissue is known as an **infarction.** The infarcted area is eventually replaced by scar tissue. Figure 11–15 illustrates coronary artery occlusion leading to ischemia and infarction of heart muscle. Figure 11–16 is a photograph of myocardium after an acute myocardial infarction.

A new term, **acute coronary syndromes (ACS),** describes the consequences after plaque rupture in coronary arteries. These consequences are **unstable angina** (chest pain at rest or chest pain of increasing frequency) and **myocardial infarction** (see Fig. 11–17).

Patients with ACS benefit from early angiography (x-ray imaging of coronary arteries) and surgery to improve blood flow to the heart muscle (revascularization). Drugs used to treat patients with ACS are anticoagulants (low–molecular-weight heparin) and antiplatelets, such as aspirin and clopidogrel (Plavix).

For acute attacks of angina, **nitroglycerin** is given sublingually. This drug, one of several called **nitrates,** is a powerful vasodilator that increases coronary blood flow and lowers blood pressure to decrease the work of the heart.

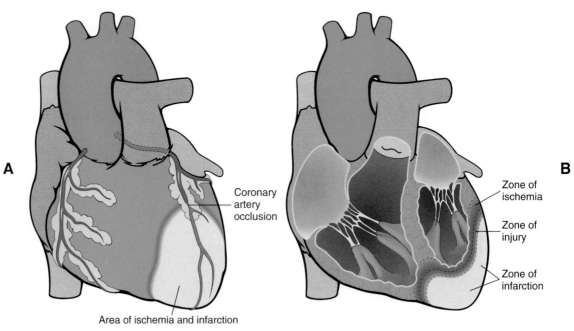

A

Coronary artery occlusion

Area of ischemia and infarction

B

Zone of ischemia

Zone of injury

Zone of infarction

Figure 11–15

(A) Ischemia and **infarction** produced by coronary artery occlusion. **(B)** Internal view of the heart showing an area damaged by myocardial infarction.

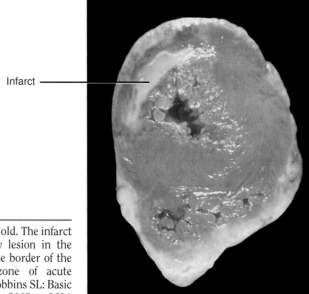

Infarct ⎯⎯⎯⎯

Figure 11-16

Acute myocardial infarction (MI), 5 to 7 days old. The infarct is visible as a well-demarcated, pale yellow lesion in the posterolateral region of the left ventricle. The border of the infarct is surrounded by a dark red zone of acute inflammation. (From Kumar V, Cotran RS, Robbins SL: Basic Pathology, 7th ed. Philadelphia, WB Saunders, 2003, p. 369.)

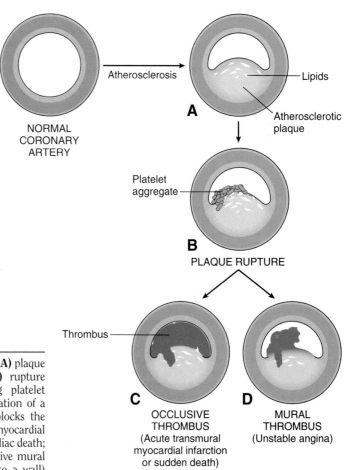

Figure 11-17

Acute coronary syndromes caused by **(A)** plaque formation from lipid collection; **(B)** rupture or erosion of the plaque, causing platelet aggregation on the plaque; **(C)** formation of a thrombus that is occlusive, totally blocks the artery, and produces an acute myocardial infarction (heart attack) or sudden cardiac death; or **(D)** formation of a partially occlusive mural thrombus (mural means pertaining to a wall) which causes unstable angina (chest pain at rest or with increasing frequency).

Physicians advise patients to avoid risk factors such as smoking, obesity, and lack of exercise, and they prescribe effective drugs to prevent CAD and ACS. These drugs include **aspirin** (to prevent aggregation of platelets), **beta-blockers** (to reduce the force and speed of the heartbeat and to lower blood pressure), **ACE inhibitors** (to reduce high blood pressure and the risk of future heart attack even if the patient is not hypertensive), **calcium channel blockers** (to relax muscles in blood vessels), and **statins** (to lower cholesterol levels).

Cardiac surgeons perform an open heart operation called **coronary artery bypass grafting (CABG)** to treat coronary artery disease by replacing clogged vessels. Cardiologists perform **percutaneous transluminal coronary angioplasty (PTCA),** in which catheterization with balloons and stents opens clogged coronary arteries.

An innovative method of treatment is **transmyocardial laser revascularization (TMLR).** A laser makes holes in the heart muscle to induce **angiogenesis** (growth of new blood vessels). Gene therapy (giving DNA or viruses containing DNA to promote expression of factors that lead to angiogenesis) is another new technique to restore damaged heart muscle.

endocarditis

Inflammation of the inner lining of the heart caused by bacteria (bacterial endocarditis).

Damage to the heart valves from infection or trauma produces lesions called **vegetations** (resembling cauliflower) that break off into the bloodstream as **emboli** (material that travels through the blood). The emboli lodge in other vessels (leading to a TIA or stroke) or in small vessels of the skin, where multiple pinpoint hemorrhages known as **petechiae** (from the Italian *petechio,* meaning a fleabite) form. Antibiotics can cure bacterial endocarditis.

hypertensive heart disease

High blood pressure affecting the heart.

This condition results from narrowing of arterioles, which leads to increased pressure in arteries. The heart is affected (left ventricular hypertrophy) because it pumps more vigorously to overcome the increased resistance in the arteries.

mitral valve prolapse (MVP)

Improper closure of the mitral valve (Fig. 11–18).

This condition occurs because the mitral valve enlarges and prolapses into the left atrium during systole. The physician hears a midsystolic click on auscultation (listening with a stethoscope). Most people with MVP live normal lives, but because prolapsed valves can on rare occasions become infected, persons with MVP are advised to have preventive antibiotics at the time of dental procedures if the murmur is present.

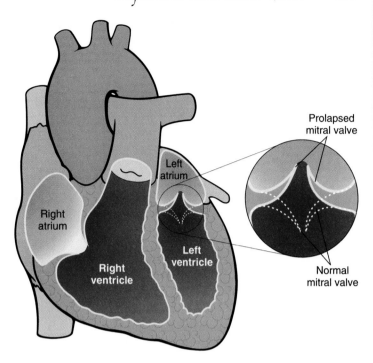

Figure 11–18

**Position of a normal mitral valve
and prolapsed mitral valve.**

murmur	**An extra heart sound, heard between normal beats.**

Murmurs are heard with the aid of a stethoscope and are usually caused by a valvular defect or disease that disrupts the smooth flow of blood in the heart. They are also heard in cases of interseptal defects when blood flows abnormally between chambers through holes in the septa. Functional murmurs are not caused by valve or septal defects and do not seriously endanger a person's health.

A **bruit** (brū-Ē) is an abnormal sound or murmur heard on auscultation. A **thrill,** which is a vibration felt on palpation of the chest, often accompanies a murmur.

pericarditis	**Inflammation of the membrane (pericardium) surrounding the heart.**

In most instances, pericarditis results from disease elsewhere in the body (such as pulmonary infection). Bacteria and viruses cause the condition, or the etiology may be idiopathic. Malaise, fever, and chest pain occur, as well as accumulation of fluid within the pericardial cavity. Compression of the heart caused by collection of fluid is called **cardiac tamponade** (tăm-pō-NŎD). If a considerable amount of fluid is present, pressure on the pulmonary veins may slow the return of blood from the lungs. Excess fluid is drained by pericardiocentesis.

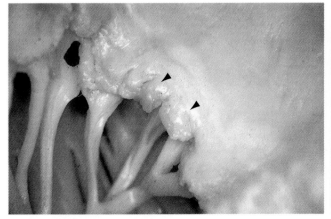

A

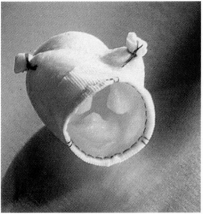

B

Figure 11-19

(A) Acute rheumatic mitral valvulitis with chronic rheumatic heart disease. Small vegetations are visible along the line of closure of the mitral valve leaflet (*arrows*). Previous episodes of rheumatic valvulitis have caused fibrous thickening and fusion of the chordae tendineae of the valves. **(B) Porcine xenograft valve.** A xenograft valve (xen/o means stranger) is tissue that is transferred from an animal of one species (pig) to one of another species (human). (**A** from Kumar V, Cotran RS, Robbins SL: Basic Pathology, 7th ed. Philadelphia, WB Saunders, 2003, p. 377; **B** from Lewis SM, Heitkemper MM, Dirksen SR: Medical-Surgical Nursing: Assessment and Management of Clinical Problems, 5th ed. St Louis, Mosby, 2000, p. 972.)

rheumatic heart disease	**Heart disease caused by rheumatic fever.**

Rheumatic fever is a childhood disease that follows after a streptococcal infection. The heart valves can be damaged by inflammation and scarred (with **vegetations**), so that they do not open and close normally (see Fig. 11–19A). **Mitral stenosis,** atrial fibrillation, and congestive heart failure, caused by weakening of the myocardium, also can result from rheumatic heart disease. Treatment consists of reduced activity, drugs to control arrhythmia, surgery to repair a damaged valve, and anticoagulant therapy to prevent emboli from forming. Mechanical or porcine (pig) valve implants can replace deteriorated heart valves. Figure 11–19B shows a porcine (pig) valve implant.

Blood Vessels

aneurysm	**Local widening (dilation) of an arterial wall.**

An aneurysm (Greek, *aneurysma,* widening) is usually caused by atherosclerosis and hypertension or a congenital weakness in the vessel wall. Aneurysms are common in the aorta, but may occur in peripheral vessels as well. The danger of an aneurysm is rupture and hemorrhage. Treatment depends on the vessel involved, the site, and the health of the patient. In aneurysms of small vessels in the brain **(berry aneurysms),** treatment is occlusion of the vessel with small clips. For larger arteries, such as the aorta, the aneurysm is resected and a synthetic graft is sewn within the aneurysm. Figure 11–20A shows an abdominal aortic aneurysm, and Figure 11–20B illustrates a synthetic graft in place. Stent grafts may also be placed less invasively as an alternative to surgery in some patients.

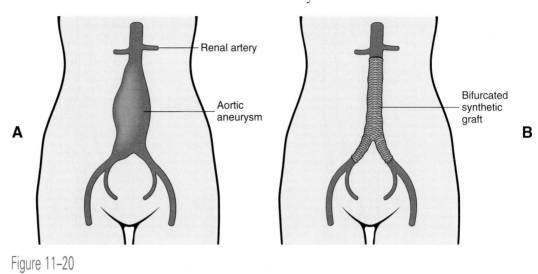

Figure 11–20

(A) Abdominal aortic aneurysm. A dissecting aortic aneurysm is splitting or dissection of the wall of the aorta by blood entering a tear or hemorrhage within the walls of the vessel. **(B) Bifurcated synthetic graft** in place.

hypertension (HTN)	**High blood pressure.**

Most high blood pressure is **essential hypertension,** with no identifiable cause. In adults, a blood pressure equal to or greater than 140/90 mmHg is considered high. Diuretics, beta-blockers, ACE inhibitors, and calcium channel blockers are used as treatment for essential hypertension. Losing weight, limiting sodium (salt) intake, stopping smoking, and reducing fat in the diet can reduce hypertension.

In **secondary hypertension,** the HTN is caused by another associated lesion, such as glomerulonephritis, pyelonephritis, or disease of the adrenal glands.

peripheral vascular disease (PVD)	**Blockage of blood vessels outside the heart.**

Any artery can be affected, such as the **carotid** (neck), **femoral** (thigh), and **popliteal** (back of the knee). A sign of PVD in the lower extremities is **intermittent claudication** (absence of pain or discomfort in a leg at rest, but pain, tension, and weakness after walking has begun). Treatment is exercise, avoidance of nicotine, which causes vessel constriction, and control of risk factors such as hypertension, hyperlipidemia, and diabetes. Surgical treatment includes endarterectomy, angioplasty, and bypass grafting (from the normal proximal vessel around the diseased area to a normal vessel distally).

Raynaud disease	**Short episodes of pallor and cyanosis in the fingers and toes.**

Of uncertain cause, it is marked by intense constriction and vasospasm of arterioles and may be secondary to some other, more serious disorder. Episodes can be triggered by cold temperatures, emotional stress, or cigarette smoking. Protecting the body from cold and use of vasodilators are effective treatments.

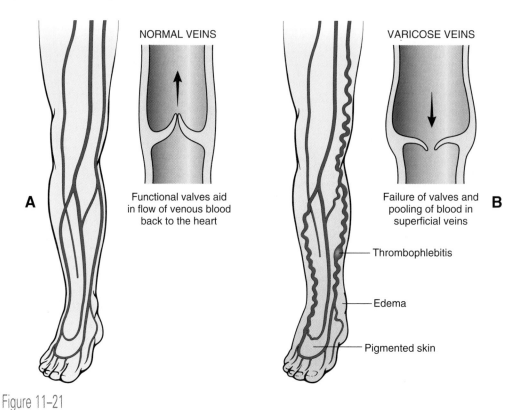

NORMAL VEINS

Functional valves aid
in flow of venous blood
back to the heart

A

VARICOSE VEINS

Failure of valves and
pooling of blood in
superficial veins

B

— Thrombophlebitis

— Edema

— Pigmented skin

Figure 11–21

Normal and varicose veins. The slow flow in veins makes an individual susceptible to clot formation. Thrombotic occlusion of varicose veins is known as thrombophlebitis. If a thrombus becomes loosened from its place in the vein, it can travel to the lungs **(pulmonary embolism)** and block a blood vessel there. When blood pools in the lower parts of the leg, fluid leaks from distended small capillaries, causing **edema.**

varicose veins	**Abnormally swollen and twisted veins, usually occurring in the legs.**

This condition is caused by damaged valves that fail to prevent the backflow of blood (Fig. 11–21). The blood then collects in the veins, which distend to many times their normal size. Because of the slow flow of blood in the varicose veins and frequent injury to the vein, thrombosis may occur as well. **Hemorrhoids** (piles) are varicose veins near the anus.

Physicians now treat varicose veins with sclerosing injections or laser treatment. Surgical intervention is rare.

Study Section

Practice spelling each term and know its meaning.

acute coronary syndromes	The consequences of plaque rupture in coronary arteries: unstable angina and myocardial infarction.

angina (pectoris)	Chest pain resulting from a temporary difference between the supply and the demand of oxygen to the heart muscle.
angiotensin-converting enzyme (ACE) inhibitors	Antihypertensive drugs that block the conversion of angiotensin I to angiotensin II and reduce blood vessel constriction. They prevent heart attacks, CHF, stroke, and death. See page 859 for names of ACE inhibitors and other cardiovascular drugs.
auscultation	Listening with a stethoscope.
beta-blockers	Drugs used to treat angina, hypertension, and arrhythmias. They block the action of epinephrine (Adrenalin) at receptor sites on cells, slowing the heartbeat and reducing the workload on the heart.
bruit	An abnormal sound heard on auscultation.
calcium channel blockers	Drugs used to treat angina and hypertension. They dilate blood vessels by blocking the influx of calcium into muscle cells lining vessels.
cardiac tamponade	Pressure on the heart caused by fluid in the pericardial space.
claudication	Pain, tension, and weakness in a leg after walking has begun, but absence of pain at rest.
digoxin	A drug that treats arrhythmias and strengthens the heartbeat.
emboli (singular: **embolus**)	Collections of material (clots or other substances) that travel to and suddenly block a blood vessel.
infarction	Area of dead tissue.
nitrates	Drugs used in the treatment of angina. They dilate blood vessels, increasing blood flow and oxygen to myocardial tissue.
nitroglycerin	A nitrate drug used in the treatment of angina.
occlusion	Closure of a blood vessel.
palpitations	Uncomfortable sensations in the chest related to cardiac arrhythmias.
patent	Open.
petechiae	Small, pinpoint hemorrhages.
statins	Drugs used to lower cholesterol in the bloodstream.
thrill	Vibration felt on palpation of the chest.
vegetations	Clumps of platelets, clotting proteins, microorganisms, and red blood cells on the endocardium in conditions such as bacterial endocarditis and rheumatic heart disease.

IX. Laboratory Tests, Clinical Procedures, and Abbreviations

Laboratory Tests

lipid tests

Measurement of cholesterol and triglycerides in a blood sample.

High levels of lipids are associated with atherosclerosis. The National Guideline for total cholesterol in the blood is less than 200 mg/dL. **Saturated fats** (animal origin, such as milk, butter, and meats) increase cholesterol in the blood, while **polyunsaturated fats** (vegetable origin, corn and safflower oil) decrease blood cholesterol.

Treatment of hyperlipidemia includes proper diet (low fat, high fiber intake) and exercise. Niacin (a vitamin) also helps reduce lipids. Drug therapy includes **statins,** which reduce the risk of heart attack, stroke, and cardiovascular death. Statins lower cholesterol by reducing its production in the liver. Examples are simvastatin (Zocor), atorvastatin (Lipitor), and pravastatin (Pravachol).

lipoprotein electrophoresis

Lipoproteins (combinations of fat and protein) are physically separated in a blood sample.

Examples of lipoproteins are **low-density lipoprotein (LDL),** and **high-density lipoprotein (HDL).** High levels of LDL are associated with atherosclerosis. The National Guideline for LDL is less than 130 mg/dL in normal individuals and less than 100 mg/dL in patients with CAD, PVD, and diabetes mellitus. High levels of HDL protect adults from atherosclerosis. Factors that increase HDL are estrogen, exercise, and alcohol in moderation.

serum enzyme tests

Chemicals measured in the blood as evidence of a heart attack.

Damaged heart muscle releases enzymes into the bloodstream. The substances tested for are **creatine kinase (CK), troponin-I (cTnI),** and **troponin-T (cTnT).** Troponin is a protein released into circulation after myocardial injury.

Clinical Procedures

Diagnostic

X-Ray

angiography

X-ray imaging of blood vessels after injection of contrast material.

Arteriography is x-ray imaging of arteries after injection of contrast into the aorta or an artery.

digital subtraction angiography (DSA)	**Video equipment and a computer produce x-ray images of blood vessels.**

After taking an initial x-ray and storing it in a computer, physicians inject contrast material and take a second image of that area. The computer compares the two images and subtracts the first from the second, leaving an image of vessels with contrast.

Ultrasound Tests

Doppler ultrasound

Sound waves measure movement of blood flow.

An instrument focuses sound waves on blood vessels and echoes bounce off red blood cells. The examiner can hear various alterations in blood flow caused by vessel obstruction.

echocardiography (ECHO)

High-frequency sound waves and echoes produce images of the heart.

ECHOs show the structure and movement of the heart. In **transesophageal echocardiography (TEE)**, a transducer placed in the esophagus provides ultrasound and Doppler information. This technique detects cardiac masses, prosthetic valve function, aneurysms, and pericardial fluid.

Nuclear Cardiology

positron emission tomography (PET) scan

Images showing blood flow and function of the myocardium following uptake of radioactive substances.

PET scanning can detect coronary artery disease (CAD), myocardial function, and differences between ischemic heart disease and cardiomyopathy.

technetium (Tc) 99m Sestamibi scan

Technetium 99m sestamibi is injected IV and taken up in the area of an MI.

This scan is also used with an exercise tolerance test **(ETT-MIBI).** Sestamibi is a radioactive tracer compound used to define areas of poor blood flow in heart muscle.

thallium 201 scan

Concentration of a radioactive substance is measured in the myocardium.

Thallium studies show the viability of heart muscle. Infarcted or scarred myocardium shows up as "cold spots."

Magnetic Resonance Imaging (MRI)

cardiac MRI

Images of cardiac tissue are produced with magnetic waves.

These images in multiple planes give information about aneurysms, cardiac output, and patency of coronary arteries.

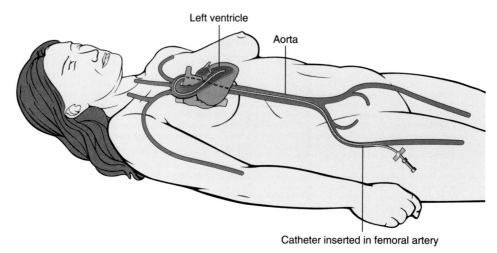

Left ventricle

Aorta

Catheter inserted in femoral artery

Figure 11–22

Left-sided cardiac catheterization. The catheter is passed retrograde (backward) from the femoral artery into the aorta and then into the left ventricle. For right-sided cardiac catheterization, the cardiologist inserts a catheter through the femoral vein and advances it to the right atrium and right ventricle and into the pulmonary artery.

Other Diagnostic Procedures

cardiac catheterization

A thin, flexible tube is guided into the heart via a vein or an artery.

This procedure detects pressures and patterns of blood flow in the heart. Contrast may be injected and x-ray images taken of the heart and blood vessels (see Fig. 11–22).

electrocardiography (ECG, EKG)

Recording of electricity flowing through the heart.

Normal sinus rhythm begins in the SA node and is between 60 to 100 beats per minute. Figure 11–23 shows normal sinus rhythm and ventricular fibrillation on ECG strips.

Holter monitoring

An ECG device is worn during a 24-hour period to detect cardiac arrhythmias.

Rhythm changes are correlated with symptoms recorded in a diary.

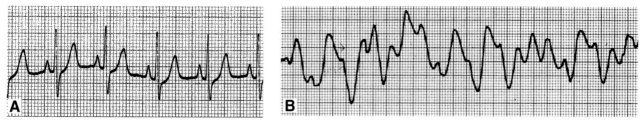

Figure 11–23

(A) Normal sinus rhythm as seen on ECG (EKG) strip. **(B) Ventricular fibrillation** as seen on an ECG strip. (A modified from Wiederhold R: Electrocardiography: The Monitoring and Diagnostic Leads, 2nd ed. Philadelphia, WB Saunders, 1999, p. 37; **B** from Lewis SM, Heitkemper MM, Dirksen SR: Medical-Surgical Nursing: Assessment and Management of Clinical Problems, 5th ed. St Louis, Mosby, 2000, p. 934.)

stress test	**Exercise tolerance test (ETT) determines the heart's response to physical exertion (stress).**

A common protocol uses three minute stages at set speeds and elevation of a treadmill. Continual monitoring of vital signs and ECG rhythms are important in the diagnosis of CAD and left ventricular function.

Treatment Procedures

cardioversion (defibrillation)	**Very brief discharges of electricity, applied across the chest to stop arrhythmias.**
coronary artery bypass graft (CABG)	**Arteries and veins are anastomosed to coronary arteries to detour around blockages.**

Internal mammary (breast) and radial (arm) arteries and saphenous (leg) grafts are used to keep the myocardium supplied with oxygenated blood (see Fig. 11–24). Cardiac surgeons perform minimally invasive CABG surgery with smaller incisions instead of the traditional sternotomy to open the chest. Vein and artery grafts are removed endoscopically with small incisions as well.

endarterectomy	**Surgical removal of the diseased inner layers of an artery.**

Fatty deposits (atheromas) and thromboses are removed to open clogged arteries.

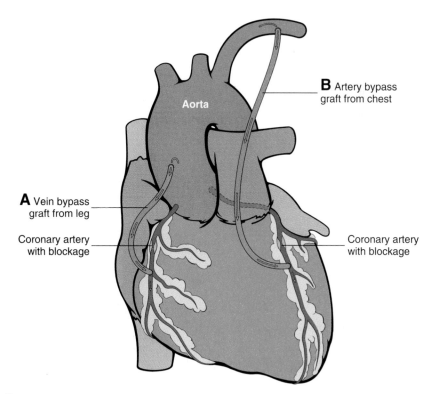

Figure 11-24

Coronary artery bypass graft (CABG) surgery with anastomosis of vein and arterial grafts. **(A)** Section of a vein is removed from the leg and anastomosed (upside down because of its directional valves) to a coronary artery to bypass an area of arteriosclerotic blockage. **(B)** An internal mammary artery is grafted to a coronary artery to bypass a blockage.

extracorporeal circulation

A heart-lung machine diverts blood from the heart and lungs while the heart is being repaired.

Blood leaves the body, enters the heart-lung machine, where it is oxygenated, and then returns to a blood vessel (artery) to circulate through the bloodstream. The machine is an **extracorporeal membrane oxygenator (ECMO).**

heart transplantation

A donor heart is transferred to a recipient.

While waiting for a transplant, a patient may need a **left ventricular assist device (LVAD),** which is a booster pump implanted in the abdomen with a cannula (flexible tube) to the left ventricle.

percutaneous coronary intervention (PCI)

A balloon-tipped catheter is inserted into a coronary artery to open the artery; stents are put in place.

The cardiologist places the catheter in the femoral or radial artery and then threads it up the aorta into the coronary artery. **Stents** (expandable slotted tubes that serve as permanent scaffolding devices) create wide lumens and make restenosis less likely. Now stents are coated with antiproliferative drugs to prevent scar tissue formation that could lead to restenosis. Stents also are placed in carotid, renal, and other peripheral arteries (see Fig. 11–25).

PCI includes percutaneous transluminal coronary angioplasty (PTCA), stent placement, laser angioplasty (a small laser on the tip of a catheter vaporizes plaque), and atherectomy.

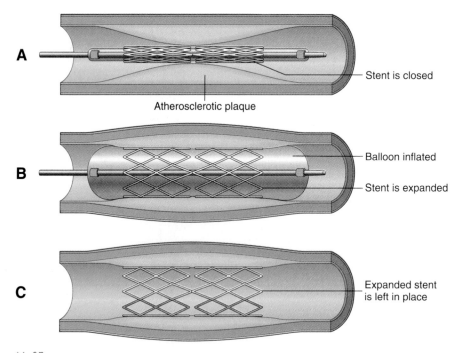

A — Stent is closed

Atherosclerotic plaque

B — Balloon inflated
— Stent is expanded

C — Expanded stent is left in place

Figure 11–25

Placement of an intracoronary artery stent. (A) The stent is positioned at the site of the lesion. **(B)** The balloon is inflated, expanding the stent. **(C)** The balloon is then deflated and removed, and the implanted stent is left in place. Coronary stents are stainless-steel scaffolding devices that help hold open arteries, such as the coronary, renal, and carotid arteries.

thrombolytic therapy	**Drugs to dissolve clots are injected into the bloodstream of patients with coronary thrombosis.**

Tissue plasminogen activator **(tPA)** and **streptokinase** restore blood flow to the heart and limit irreversible damage to heart muscle. The drugs are given within 12 hours after the onset of a heart attack. Thrombolytic agents reduce mortality in patients with myocardial infarction by 25 percent.

Abbreviations

ACE inhibitors	Angiotensin-converting enzyme inhibitors	**ECG, EKG**	Electrocardiogram
ACS	Acute coronary syndromes	**ECHO**	Echocardiography
AF	Atrial fibrillation	**ETT**	Exercise tolerance test
AMI	Acute myocardial infarction	**ETT-MIBI**	Exercise tolerance test combined with a radioactive tracer (sestamibi) scan
AS	Aortic stenosis	**HDL**	High-density lipoproteins; high blood levels are associated with lower incidence of coronary artery disease
ASD	Atrial septal defect		
AV, A-V	Atrioventricular	**HMG**	Hydroxymethyl glutaryl CoA reductase, an enzyme that blocks the synthesis of cholesterol
BBB	Bundle branch block		
BP	Blood pressure	**HTN**	Hypertension
CABG	Coronary artery bypass graft	**ICD**	Implantable cardioverter/defibrillator
CAD	Coronary artery disease	**LDL**	Low-density lipoproteins
CCU	Coronary care unit	**LMWH**	Low-molecular-weight heparin
Cath	Catheterization	**LV**	Left ventricle
CHF	Congestive heart failure	**LVAD**	Left ventricular assist device
CK	Creatine kinase; released into the bloodstream following injury to heart or skeletal muscles	**LVH**	Left ventricular hypertrophy
		MI	Myocardial infarction
CoA	Coarctation of the aorta	**MR**	Mitral regurgitation
CTNI (cTnI)	Cardiac troponin I; troponin is a protein released into the bloodstream after myocardial injury	**MUGA**	Multiple-gated acquisition scan; a radioactive test of heart function
		MVP	Mitral valve prolapse
CTNT (cTnT)	Cardiac troponin T	**NSR**	Normal sinus rhythm
CVP	Central venous pressure (measured with a catheter in the superior vena cava)	**NSTEMI**	Non ST-elevation myocardial infarction
		PAC	Premature atrial contraction
DSA	Digital subtraction angiography	**PCI**	Percutaneous coronary intervention
DVT	Deep venous thrombosis		
ECC	Extracorporeal circulation		

Continued on following page

PDA	Patent ductus arteriosus	**Tc**	Technetium
PTCA	Percutaneous transluminal coronary angioplasty; balloon angioplasty	**TEE**	Transesophageal echocardiography
PVC	Premature ventricular contraction	**TMLR**	Transmyocardial laser revascularization
RFA	Radiofrequency catheter ablation	**tPA**	Tissue-type plasminogen activator; a drug used to prevent thrombosis
SA, S-A	Sinoatrial	**UA**	Unstable angina
SOB	Shortness of breath	**VFib**	Ventricular fibrillation
SPECT	Single photon emission computerized tomography (used for myocardial imaging with sestamibi scans)	**VSD**	Ventricular septal defect
		VT	Ventricular tachycardia
SSCP	Substernal chest pain	**WPW**	Wolff-Parkinson-White syndrome; an abnormal ECG pattern often associated with paroxysmal tachycardia
STEMI	ST-elevation myocardial infarction		

X. Practical Applications

Operating Schedule: General Hospital

Match the treatment in column I with a diagnosis in column II. Answers are found at the end of Answers to Exercises, page 431.

Column I—Operation

1. Coronary artery bypass graft _____

2. Left carotid endarterectomy _____

3. Sclerosing injections and laser treatment _____

4. LV aneurysmectomy _____

5. Atrial septal defect repair _____

6. Left ventricular assist device _____

7. Pericardiocentesis _____

8. Aortic valve replacement _____

9. Pacemaker implantation _____

10. Femoral-popliteal bypass graft _____

Column II—Diagnosis

A. congestive heart failure
B. cardiac tamponade (fluid in the space surrounding the heart)
C. atherosclerotic occlusion of a main artery leading to the head
D. congenital hole in the wall of the upper chamber of the heart
E. disabling angina and extensive coronary atherosclerosis despite medical therapy
F. peripheral vascular disease
G. heart block
H. varicose veins
I. protrusion of the wall of a lower heart chamber
J. aortic stenosis

Medical Language As Written

1. The main determinants of death after acute myocardial infarction are the extent of left ventricular damage and occurrence of arrhythmias.

2. Evaluation of risk factors for sudden cardiac death is important in patients with coronary artery disease. Risk factors include a family history of sudden cardiac death and early myocardial infarction (before age 50 years), hypertension and left ventricular hypertrophy, smoking, diabetes mellitus, and markedly elevated serum cholesterol levels.

3. A 24-year-old woman with a history of palpitations [heartbeat is unusually strong, rapid, or irregular, so that patient is aware of it] and vague chest pains enters the hospital. With the patient supine, you hear a midsystolic click that is followed by a grade 3/6 [moderately loud—6/6 is loud and 1/6 is quiet] honking murmur. Your diagnosis: mitral valve prolapse (click-murmur syndrome).

4. A 47-year-old man had a myocardial infarction in November 1984. On March 3, 1985, he was readmitted to the hospital with an acute inferior myocardial infarction, documented by electrocardiograms and blood enzyme elevations. On April 8, the patient developed a loud systolic murmur and his blood pressure fell sharply. A diagnosis of rupture of the ventricular septum was made, and he was transferred to the surgical service. Right cardiac catheterization confirmed the presence of a left-to-right shunt [of blood] at the ventricular level. Emergency surgery was attempted, but the patient died suddenly. Autopsy diagnosis: ruptured ventricular septum secondary to myocardial infarction.

XI. Exercises

Remember to check your answers carefully with those given in Section XII, Answers to Exercises.

A. Match the following terms with their meanings below.

aorta   inferior vena cava   superior vena cava
arteriole   mitral valve   tricuspid valve
atrium   pulmonary artery   ventricle
capillary   pulmonary vein   venule

1. valve that lies between the right atrium and the right ventricle _____

2. smallest blood vessel _____

3. carries oxygenated blood from the lungs to the heart _____

4. largest artery in the body _____

5. brings oxygen-poor blood into the heart from the upper parts of the body _____

6. upper chamber of the heart _____

7. carries oxygen-poor blood to the lungs from the heart _____

8. small artery _____

9. valve that lies between the left atrium and the left ventricle _____

10. brings blood from the lower half of the body to the heart _____

11. a small vein _____

12. lower chamber of the heart _____

B. Trace the path of blood through the heart. Begin as the blood enters the right atrium from the venae cavae (and include the valves within the heart).

1. _____   7. _____

2. _____   8. _____

3. _____   9. _____

4. _____   10. _____

5. _____   11. _____

6. capillaries of the lung   12. aorta

C. Complete the following sentences.

1. The pacemaker of the heart is the _____.

2. The sac-like membrane surrounding the heart is the _____.

3. The wall of the heart between the right and the left atria is the _____.

4. The relaxation phase of the heartbeat is called _____.

5. Specialized conductive tissue in the wall between the ventricles is the _____.

6. The inner lining of the heart is the _____.

7. The contractive phase of the heartbeat is called _____.

8. A gas released as a metabolic product of catabolism is _____.

9. Specialized conductive tissue at the base of the wall between the two upper heart chambers is the

_____.

10. The inner lining of the pericardium, adhering to the outside of the heart, is the

_____.

11. An abnormal heart sound caused by improper closure of heart valves is a

_____.

12. The beat of the heart as felt through the walls of arteries is called the _____.

D. Complete the following terms from their definitions.

1. hardening of arteries: arterio _____

2. disease condition of heart muscle: cardio _____

3. enlargement of the heart: cardio _____

4. inflammation of a vein: phleb _____

5. condition of rapid heartbeat: _____ cardia

6. condition of slow heartbeat: _____ cardia

7. high levels of cholesterol in the blood: hyper _____

8. surgical repair of a valve: valvulo _____

9. condition of deficient oxygen: hyp _____

10. pertaining to an upper heart chamber: _____ al

11. narrowing of the mitral valve: mitral _____

12. breakdown of a clot: thrombo _____

E. Give the meanings for the following terms.

1. cyanosis _____

2. phlebotomy _____

3. arterial anastomosis _____

4. aneurysmorrhaphy _____

5. atheroma _____

6. arrhythmia _____

7. sphygmomanometer _____

8. stethoscope _____

9. mitral valvulitis _____

10. atherosclerosis _____

11. vasoconstriction _____

12. vasodilation _____

F. Match the following pathological conditions of the heart with their meanings below.

atrial septal defect	endocarditis	mitral valve prolapse
coarctation of the aorta	fibrillation	patent ductus arteriosus
congestive heart failure	flutter	pericarditis
coronary artery disease	hypertensive heart disease	tetralogy of Fallot

1. inflammation of the inner lining of the heart _____

2. rapid but regular atrial or ventricular contractions _____

3. small hole between the upper heart chambers; congenital anomaly _____

4. improper closure of the valve between the left atrium and ventricle during systole

_____

5. blockage of the arteries surrounding the heart leading to ischemia _____

6. high blood pressure affecting the heart _____

7. rapid, random, ineffectual, and irregular contractions of the heart _____

8. inflammation of the sac surrounding the heart _____

9. inability of the heart to pump its required amount of blood _____

10. congenital malformation involving four separate heart defects _____

11. congenital narrowing of the large artery leading from the heart _____

12. a small duct between the aorta and the pulmonary artery, which normally closes soon after birth, remains open _____

G. Give the meanings for the following terms.

1. heart block _____

2. cardiac arrest _____

3. palpitations _____

4. artificial cardiac pacemaker _____

5. thrombotic occlusion _____

6. angina _____

7. myocardial infarction _____

8. necrosis _____

9. infarction _____

10. ischemia _____

11. nitroglycerin _____

12. digoxin _____

13. bruit _____

14. thrill _____

15. acute coronary syndromes _____

H. Match the following terms with their descriptions.

aneurysm	essential hypertension	Raynaud disease
auscultation	murmur	rheumatic heart disease
claudication	peripheral vascular disease	secondary hypertension
emboli	petechiae	vegetations

1. lesions that form on heart valves after damage by infection _____

2. clots that travel to and suddenly block a blood vessel _____

3. small, pinpoint hemorrhages _____

4. an extra heart sound, heard between normal beats and caused by a valvular defect or condition that disrupts the smooth flow of blood through the heart _____

5. listening with a stethoscope _____

6. heart disease caused by rheumatic fever _____

7. high blood pressure in arteries when the etiology is idiopathic _____

8. high blood pressure related to kidney disease _____

9. short episodes of pallor and numbness in fingers and toes caused by a temporary constriction of arterioles in the skin _____

10. local widening of an artery _____

11. pain, tension, and weakness in a limb after walking has begun _____

12. blockage of arteries in the lower extremities; etiology is atherosclerosis _____

I. Give short answers for the following.

1. Name types of drugs used to treat acute coronary syndromes _____ _____.

2. When damaged valves in veins fail to prevent the backflow of blood, the condition that results is called _____.

3. If veins are swollen and twisted in the rectal region, the condition is known as _____.

4. Name the four defects in tetralogy of Fallot from their descriptions:

   A. Narrowing of the artery leading to the lungs from the heart _____.

   B. Gap in the wall between the ventricles _____.

C. The large vessel leading from the left ventricle moves over the interventricular septum

_____ .

D. Excessive development of the wall of the right lower heart chamber

_____ .

J. Select from the following terms to complete the definitions below.

angiography   echocardiography   lipoprotein electrophoresis
cardiac MRI   electrocardiography   serum enzyme test
cardioversion   endarterectomy   stress test
coronary artery bypass graft   lipid test   thallium 201 scan

1. surgical removal of the innermost linings of an artery thickened with fatty deposits

   _____

2. application of brief electrical discharges across the chest to stop a cardiac arrhythmia; defibrillation

   _____

3. measurement of levels of fatty substances (cholesterol and triglycerides) in the bloodstream

   _____

4. measurement of the heart's response to physical exertion (patient monitored while jogging on a

   treadmill) _____

5. measurement of blood creatine kinase (CK) and troponin-T after myocardial infarction

   _____

6. injection of contrast into vessels and x-ray imaging _____

7. recording of the electricity in the heart _____

8. IV injection of a radioactive substance and measurement of its accumulation in heart muscle

   _____

9. high-frequency sound waves and echoes produce images of the heart _____

10. separation of HDL and LDL from a blood sample _____

11. anastomosis of vessel grafts to existing coronary arteries to maintain blood supply to the

    myocardium _____

12. beaming of magnetic waves at the heart, imaging the heart's structure _____

K. Give the meanings for the following terms.

1. digital subtraction angiography _____

2. heart transplantation _____

3. ETT-MIBI _____

4. Doppler ultrasound _____

5. Holter monitoring _____

6. thrombolytic therapy _____

7. extracorporeal circulation _____

8. cardiac catheterization _____

9. percutaneous coronary intervention _____

10. stent _____

L. Identify the following cardiac dysrhythmias from their abbreviations.

1. AF _____

2. VT _____

3. VFib _____

4. PVC _____

5. PAC _____

M. Identify the following abnormal cardiac conditions from their abbreviations.

1. CHF _____

2. VSD _____

3. MI _____

4. PDA _____

5. MVP _____

6. AS _____

7. CAD _____

8. ASD _____

N. Match the following abbreviations for cardiac procedures with their explanations below.

ECHO   ICD   TEE
ETT   LVAD   TMLR
ETT-MIBI   RFA

1. A laser makes a hole in heart muscle to induce growth of new blood vessels (angiogenesis).

   _____

2. A booster pump implanted in the abdomen with a cannula leading to the heart is a "bridge to

   transplant." _____

3. Ultrasound images of the heart are taken through the esophagus. _____

4. A device implanted in the chest that senses and corrects arrhythmias via shock waves.

   _____

5. A catheter delivers a high-frequency current to damage a small portion of the heart muscle and

   reverse an abnormal heart rhythm. _____

6. Procedure determines the heart's response to physical exertion (stress). _____

7. High-frequency sound waves are pulsed through the chest wall and bounce off heart structures,

   creating an image of heart structure. _____

8. Radioactive test of heart function with stress test. _____

O. Spell the term correctly from its definition.

1. pertaining to the heart: _____ ary

2. not a normal heart rhythm: arr _____

3. abnormal condition of blueness: _____ osis

4. relaxation phase of the heartbeat: _____ tole

5. chest pain: _____ pectoris

6. inflammation of a vein: _____ itis

7. widening of a vessel: vaso _____

8. enlargement of the heart: cardio _____

9. hardening of arteries with fatty plaque: _____ sclerosis

10. swollen veins in the rectal region: _____ oids

P. Match the following surgical terms with their meanings below.

aneurysmorrhaphy	embolectomy	pericardiocentesis
atherectomy	endarterectomy	valvotomy
CABG	PCI	

1. incision of a heart valve _____

2. removal of a clot that has traveled into a blood vessel and suddenly caused occlusion

   _____

3. coronary artery bypass graft (to relieve ischemia) _____

4. surgical puncture to remove fluid from the pericardial space _____

5. balloon-tipped catheter and stents placed into a coronary artery _____

6. removal of the inner linings of an artery to make it wider _____

7. suture (repair) of a ballooned-out portion of an artery _____

8. removal of plaque from an artery _____

Q. Select the term that best completes each sentence.

1. Bill was having pain in his chest that radiated up his neck and down his arm. He called Dr. Dan, who thought Bill should report to the emergency department immediately. The first test they performed was a(an) **(stress test, ECG, CABG)**.

2. Dr. Kelly explained to the family that their observation about the bluish color of baby Charles's skin helped him make the diagnosis of a(an) **(thrombotic, aneurysmal, septal)** defect in the baby's heart, which needed immediate attention.

3. Mr. Duggan had a fever of unknown origin. When the doctors completed an echocardiogram and saw vegetations on his mitral valve, they suspected **(bacterial endocarditis, hypertensive heart disease, angina)**.

4. Claudia's hands turned red, almost purple, whenever she went out into the cold or became stressed. Her physician thought it might be wise to evaluate her for **(varicose veins, Raynaud disease, intermittent claudication)**.

5. Daisy's heart felt like it was skipping beats every time she drank coffee. Her physician suggested that she wear a **(Holter monitor, LVAD, CABG)** for 24 hours to assess the nature of the arrhythmia.

6. Paola's father and grandfather died of heart attacks. Her physician tells her that she has inherited a tendency to accumulate fats in her bloodstream. Blood tests reveal high levels of **(enzymes, lipids, nitroglycerin)**. Discussing her family history with her **(gynecologist, hematologist, cardiologist)**, she understands that she has familial **(hypocholesterolemia, hypercholesterolemia, cardiomyopathy)**.

7. While exercising, Bernard complained of a pain (cramp) in his calf muscle. The pain disappeared when he was resting. After performing **(Holter monitoring, Doppler ultrasound, echocardiography)** on his leg to assess blood flow, Dr. Shaw found **(stenosis, fibrillation, endocarditis)** indicating poor circulation. She recommended a daily exercise program, low-fat diet, careful foot care, and antiplatelet drug therapy to treat Bernard's intermittent **(palpitations, hypertension, claudication)**.

8. Fernanda noticed that 6-week-old Luis had a slightly bluish or **(jaundiced, cyanotic, diastolic)** coloration to his skin. She consulted a pediatric **(dermatologist, hematologist, cardiologist)**, who performed **(echocardiography, PET scan, endarterectomy)** and diagnosed Luis' condition as **(endocarditis, congestive heart disease, tetralogy of Fallot)**.

9. Seventy-eight-year-old John Smith had coronary artery disease and high blood pressure for the past 10 years. His history included an acute heart attack or **(MI, PDA, CABG)**. He was often tired and complained of **(dyspnea, nausea, migraine headaches)** and swelling in his ankles. His physician diagnosed his condition as **(aortic aneurysm, congestive heart failure, congenital heart disease)** and recommended restricted salt intake, diuretics, and an **(ACE inhibitor, antibiotic, analgesic)**.

10. Arlette had a routine checkup that included **(auscultation, vasoconstriction, vasodilation)** of her chest with a **(catheter, stent, stethoscope)** to listen to her heart. Her physician noticed a midsystolic murmur characteristic of **(DVT, MVP, LDL)**. An echocardiogram confirmed the diagnosis.

XII. Answers to Exercises

A

1. tricuspid valve
2. capillary
3. pulmonary vein
4. aorta
5. superior vena cava
6. atrium
7. pulmonary artery
8. arteriole
9. mitral valve
10. inferior vena cava
11. venule
12. ventricle

B

1. right atrium
2. tricuspid valve
3. right ventricle
4. pulmonary valve
5. pulmonary artery
6. capillaries of the lung
7. pulmonary veins
8. left atrium
9. mitral valve
10. left ventricle
11. aortic valve
12. aorta

C

1. sinoatrial (SA) node
2. pericardium
3. interatrial septum
4. diastole
5. atrioventricular bundle or bundle of His
6. endocardium
7. systole
8. carbon dioxide (CO_2)
9. atrioventricular (AV) node
10. visceral pericardium (the outer lining is the parietal pericardium)
11. murmur
12. pulse

XIII. Pronunciation of Terms

Pronunciation Guide

ā as in āpe   ă as in ăpple
ē as in ēven   ĕ as in ĕvery
ī as in īce   ĭ as in ĭnterest
ō as in ōpen   ŏ as in pŏt
ū as in ūnit   ŭ as in ŭnder

To test your understanding of the terminology in this chapter, write the meaning of each term in the space provided. In addition, you may wish to cover the terms and write them by looking at your definitions. Make sure your spelling is correct. The page number after each term indicates where it is defined or used in the text so you can easily check your responses.

Vocabulary and Terminology

Term	Pronunciation	Meaning
angiogram (396)	ĂN-jē-ō-grăm	
angioplasty (396)	ĂN-jē-ō-plăs-tē	
aorta (394)	ā-ŎR-tă	
aortic stenosis (396)	ā-ŎR-tĭk stĕ-NŌ-sĭs	
arrhythmia (399)	ā-RĬTH-mē-ă	
arterial anastomosis (396)	ăr-TĒ-rē-ăl ă-năs-tō-MŌ-sĭs	
arteriography (396)	ăr-tē-rē-ŎG-ră-fē	
arteriole (394)	ăr-TĒ-rē-ōl	
arteriosclerosis (396)	ăr-tē-rē-ō-sklĕ-RŌ-sĭs	
artery (394)	ĂR-tĕ-rē	
atherectomy (396)	ă-thĕ-RĔK-tō-mē	
atheroma (396)	ăth-ĕr-Ō-mă	
atherosclerosis (396)	ăth-ĕr-ō-sklĕ-RŌ-sĭs	
atrial (397)	Ā-trē-ăl	
atrioventricular bundle (394)	ā-trē-ō-vĕn-TRĬK-ū-lăr BŬN-dl	
atrioventricular node (394)	ā-trē-ō-vĕn-TRĬK-ū-lăr nōd	
atrium (plural: atria) (394)	Ā-trē-ŭm (Ā-trē-ă)	
brachial artery (397)	BRĀ-kē-ăl ĀR-tĕ-rē	
bradycardia (397)	brād-ē-KĂR-dē-ă	

bundle of His (394)	BŬN-dl of Hĭss	_____
capillary (394)	KĂP-ĭ-lăr-ē	_____
carbon dioxide (394)	kăr-bŏn dī-ŎK-sīd	_____
cardiomegaly (397)	kăr-dē-ō-MĔG-ă-lē	_____
cardiomyopathy (397)	kăr-dē-ō-mī-ŎP-ă-thē	_____
coronary arteries (397)	KŎR-ō-năr-ē ĂR-tĕ-rēz	_____
cyanosis (398)	sī-ă-NŌ-sĭs	_____
deoxygenated blood (394)	dē-ŎK-sĭ-jĕ-NĀ-tĕd blŭd	_____
diastole (394)	dī-ĂS-tō-lē	_____
endocardium (394)	ĕn-dō-KĂR-dē-ŭm	_____
endothelium (394)	ĕn-dō-THĒ-lē-um	_____
hypercholesterolemia (397)	hī-pĕr-kō-lĕs-tĕr-ŏl-Ē-mē-ă	_____
hypoxia (398)	hī-PŎK-sē-ă	_____
interventricular septum (399)	ĭn-tĕr-vĕn-TRĬK-ū-lăr SĔP-tŭm	_____
mitral valve (394)	MĪ-trăl vălv	_____
mitral valvulitis (398)	MĪ-trăl văl-vū-LĪ-tĭs	_____
myocardium (394)	mī-ō-KĂR-dē-ŭm	_____
myxoma (398)	mĭk-SŌ-mă	_____
oxygen (394)	ŎK-sĭ-jĕn	_____
pacemaker (394)	PĀS-mā-kĕr	_____
pericardiocentesis (398)	pĕr-ĭ-kăr-dē-ō-sĕn-TĒ-sĭs	_____
pericardium (395)	pĕr-ĭ-KĂR-dē-ŭm	_____
phlebotomy (398)	flĕ-BŎT-ō-mē	_____
pulmonary artery (395)	PŬL-mō-nĕr-ē ĂR-tĕr-ē	_____
pulmonary circulation (395)	PŬL-mō-nĕr-ē sĕr-kŭ-LĀ-shŭn	_____
pulmonary valve (395)	PŬL-mō-nĕr-ē vălv	_____
pulmonary vein (395)	PŬL-mō-nĕr-ē vān	_____

septum (plural: septa) (395)   SĔP-tŭm (SĔP-tă)   _____

sinoatrial node (395)   sī-nō-Ā-trē-ăl nōd   _____

sphygmomanometer (395)   sfĭg-mō-mă-NŎM-ĕ-tĕr   _____

stethoscope (398)   STĔTH-ō-skōp   _____

systemic circulation (395)   sĭs-TĔM-ĭk sĕr-kū-LĀ-shŭn   _____

systole (395)   SĬS-tō-lē   _____

tachycardia (397)   tăk-ē-KĂR-dē-ă   _____

thrombolysis (398)   thrŏm-BŎL-ĭ-sĭs   _____

thrombophlebitis (398)   thrŏm-bō-flĕ-BĪ-tis   _____

tricuspid valve (395)   trī-KŬS-pĭd vălv   _____

valvotomy (398)   văl-VŎT-ō-mē   _____

valvuloplasty (398)   văl-vū-lō-PLĂS-tē   _____

vascular (399)   VĂS-kū-lăr   _____

vasoconstriction (399)   văz-ō-kŏn-STRĬK-shŭn   _____

vasodilation (399)   văz-ō-dī-LĀ-shŭn   _____

vein (396)   vān   _____

vena cava (plural: venae cavae) (396)   VĒ-nă KĀ-vă (VĒ-nē KĀ-vē)   _____

venipuncture (399)   vĕ-nĭ-PŬNK-chŭr   _____

venous (399)   VĒ-nŭs   _____

ventricle (396)   VĔN-trĭ-k'l   _____

venule (396)   VĔN-ū'l   _____

Pathology, Laboratory Tests, and Clinical Procedures

Term	Pronunciation	Meaning
ACE inhibitors (411)	ĀCE ĭn-HĬB-ĭ-tŏrz	_____
acute coronary syndromes (410)	ă-KŪT kŏr-ō-NĂR-ē SĬN-drōmz	_____
aneurysm (408)	ĂN-ū-rĭzm	

angina (411)	ăn-JĪ-nă or ĂN-jĭ-nă	_____
angiography (412)	ăn-jē-ŎG-ră-fē	_____
atrioventricular block (399)	ā-trē-ō-vĕn-TRĬK-ū-lăr blŏk	_____
auscultation (411)	ăw-skŭl-TĀ-shŭn	_____
beta-blocker (411)	BĀ-tă-BLŎK-ĕr	_____
bruit (411)	BRŪ-ē	_____
calcium channel blocker (411)	KĂL-sē-ŭm CHĂ-nĕl BLŎK-ĕr	_____
cardiac arrest (401)	KĂR-dē-ăk ā-RĔST	_____
cardiac catheterization (414)	KĂR-dē-ăk kăth-ĕ-tĕr-ĭ-ZĀ-shŭn	_____
cardiac MRI (413)	KĂR-dē-ăk MRI	_____
cardiac tamponade (411)	KĂR-dē-ăk tăm-pō-NŎD	_____
cardioversion (415)	kăr-dē-ō-VĔR-zhŭn	_____
claudication (411)	klăw-dĕ-KĀ-shŭn	_____
coarctation of the aorta (401)	kō-ărk-TĀ-shŭn of the ā-ŎR-tă	_____
congenital heart disease (401)	kŏn-GĔN-ĭ-tăl hărt dĭ-ZĒZ	_____
congestive heart failure (403)	kŏn-GĔS-tĭv hărt FĀL-ŭr	_____
coronary artery disease (404)	kŏr-ō-NĂR-ē ĂR-tĕ-rē dĭ-ZĒZ	_____
coronary artery bypass graft (415)	kŏr-ō-NĂR-ē ĂR-tĕ-rē BĪ-păs grăft	_____
digoxin (411)	dĭj-ŎK-sĭn	_____
digital subtraction angiography (413)	DĬJ-ĭ-tăl sŭb-TRĂK-shŭn ăn-jē-ŎG-ră-fē	_____
Doppler ultrasound (413)	DŎP-lĕr ŬL-tră-sŏnd	_____
echocardiography (413)	ĕk-ō-kăr-dē-ŌG-ră-fē	_____
electrocardiography (414)	ē-lĕk-trō-kăr-dē-ŌG-ră-fē	_____

XIV. Review Sheet

Write the meanings of each word part in the space provided. Check your answers with the information in the chapter or in the Glossary (Medical Terms—English) at the end of the book.

COMBINING FORMS

Combining Form	Meaning	Combining Form	Meaning
aneurysm/o		myx/o	
angi/o		ox/o	
aort/o		pericardi/o	
arter/o, arteri/o		phleb/o	
ather/o		pulmon/o	
atri/o		sphygm/o	
axill/o		steth/o	
brachi/o		thromb/o	
cardi/o		valv/o	
cholesterol/o		valvul/o	
coron/o		vas/o	
cyan/o		vascul/o	
isch/o		ven/o, ven/i	
my/o		ventricul/o	

SUFFIXES

Suffix	Meaning	Suffix	Meaning
-constriction	_____	-oma	_____
-dilation	_____	-osis	_____
-emia	_____	-plasty	_____
-graphy	_____	-sclerosis	_____
-lysis	_____	-stenosis	_____
-megaly	_____	-tomy	_____
-meter	_____		

PREFIXES

Prefix	Meaning	Prefix	Meaning
a-, an-	_____	hypo-	_____
brady-	_____	inter-	_____
de-	_____	peri-	_____
dys-	_____	tachy-	_____
endo-	_____	tetra-	_____
hyper-	_____	tri-	_____

chapter

Respiratory System

This chapter is divided into the following sections

In this chapter you will

■ Name the organs of the respiratory system and describe their location and function.

■ Identify various pathological conditions that affect the system.

■ Recognize medical terms that pertain to respiration.

■ Identify clinical procedures and abbreviations related to the system.

■ Apply your new knowledge to understanding medical terms in their proper contexts, such as medical reports and records.

I. Introduction

We usually think of **respiration** as the mechanical process of breathing, the exchange of air between the lungs and the external environment. This exchange of air at the lungs is called **external respiration.** In external respiration, oxygen is inhaled (inhaled air contains about 21 percent oxygen) into the air spaces (sacs) of the lungs and immediately passes into tiny capillary blood vessels surrounding the air spaces. Simultaneously, carbon dioxide, a gas produced when oxygen and food combine in cells, passes from the capillary blood vessels into the air spaces of the lungs to be exhaled (exhaled air contains about 16 percent oxygen).

While external respiration occurs between the outside environment and the capillary bloodstream of the lungs, another form of respiration occurs simultaneously between the individual body cells and the tiny capillary blood vessels that surround them. This is **internal (cellular) respiration,** which involves an exchange of gases at the cells within all organs of the body. Here, oxygen passes out of the bloodstream into tissue cells. At the same time, carbon dioxide passes from tissue cells into the bloodstream to travel to the lungs for exhalation.

II. Anatomy and Physiology of Respiration

Label Figure 12–1 as you read the following paragraphs.

Air enters the body via the **nose** [1] and passes through the **nasal cavity** [2], lined with a mucous membrane and fine hairs **(cilia)** to help filter out foreign bodies, as well as to warm and moisten the air. **Paranasal sinuses** [3] are hollow, air-containing spaces within the skull that communicate with the nasal cavity. They, too, have a mucous membrane lining. Besides producing mucus, a lubricating fluid, the sinuses lighten the bones of the skull and help produce sound.

After passing through the nasal cavity, the air next reaches the **pharynx (throat).** There are three divisions of the pharynx. The first is the **nasopharynx** [4]. It contains the **pharyngeal tonsils,** or **adenoids** [5], which are collections of lymphatic tissue. They are more prominent in children, and if enlarged, can obstruct air passageways. Below the nasopharynx and closer to the mouth is the second division of the pharynx, the **oropharynx** [6]. The **palatine tonsils** [7], two rounded masses of lymphatic tissue, are in the oropharynx. The third division of the pharynx, the **laryngopharynx** [8], serves as a common passageway for food from the mouth and air from the nose. It divides into two branches: the **larynx (voice box)** [9] and the **esophagus** [10].

The esophagus leads into the stomach and carries food to be digested. The larynx contains the vocal cords and is surrounded by pieces of cartilage for support. The thyroid cartilage is the largest and is commonly referred to as the Adam's apple. As expelled air passes the vocal cords, they vibrate to produce sounds. The tension of the vocal cords determines the high or low pitch of the voice.

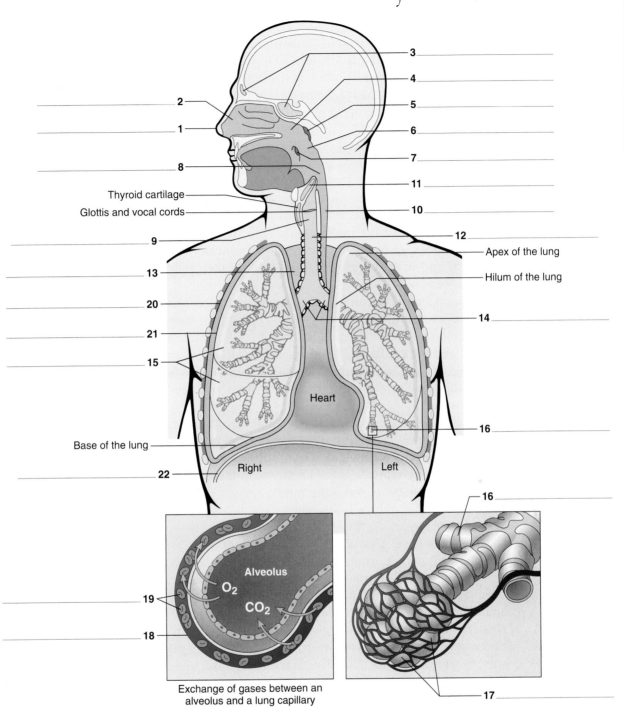

Thyroid cartilage

Glottis and vocal cords

Apex of the lung

Hilum of the lung

Heart

Base of the lung

Right

Left

Alveolus

O_2

CO_2

Exchange of gases between an
alveolus and a lung capillary

Figure 12–1

Organs of the respiratory system.

Because food entering from the mouth and air entering from the nose mix in the pharynx, what prevents food or drink into the larynx and respiratory system during swallowing? Even if a small quantity of solid or liquid matter finds its way into the air passages, aspirated food can cause irritation in the lungs and breathing can stop. The **epiglottis** [11], a flap of cartilage attached to the root of the tongue, prevents choking or aspiration of food. It acts as a lid over the opening of the larynx. During swallowing, when food and liquid move through the throat, the epiglottis closes over the larynx. Figure 12–2 shows the larynx from a superior view.

On its way to the lungs, air passes from the larynx to the **trachea (windpipe)** [12], a vertical tube about $4\frac{1}{2}$ inches long and 1 inch in diameter. The trachea is kept open by 16 to 20 C-shaped rings of cartilage separated by fibrous connective tissue that stiffen the front and sides of the tube.

In the region of the **mediastinum** [13], the trachea divides into two branches called **bronchial tubes,** or **bronchi** [14] (singular: **bronchus**). Each bronchus leads to a separate **lung** [15] and divides and subdivides into smaller and finer tubes, somewhat like the branches of a tree.

The smallest of the bronchial branches are the **bronchioles** [16]. At the end of bronchioles are clusters of air sacs called **alveoli** [17] (singular: **alveolus**). Each alveolus is lined with a one-cell layer of epithelium. This very thin wall permits an exchange of gases between the alveolus and the **capillary** [18] surrounding it. Blood flowing through the capillary accepts oxygen from the alveolus while depositing carbon dioxide into the alveolus. **Erythrocytes** [19] in the blood carry oxygen to all parts of the body and carbon dioxide to the lungs for exhalation.

Each lung is covered by a double-folded membrane called the **pleura.** The outer layer of the pleura, nearest the ribs, is the **parietal pleura** [20], and the inner layer, closest to the lung, is the **visceral pleura** [21]. A serous (thin, watery fluid) secretion moistens the pleura and facilitates movements of the lungs within the chest (thorax).

The two lungs are not quite mirror images of each other. The slightly larger right lung, is divided into three **lobes,** while the smaller left lung has two lobes. One lobe of the lung may be removed without damage to the rest. The uppermost part of the lung is the **apex,** and the lower area is the **base.** The **hilum** of the lung is the midline region where blood vessels, nerves, lymphatic tissue, and bronchial tubes enter and exit.

The lungs extend from the collarbone to the **diaphragm** [22] in the thoracic cavity. The diaphragm is a muscular partition separating the thoracic from the abdominal cavity and aiding in the process of breathing. It contracts and descends with each **inhalation (inspiration).** The downward movement of the diaphragm enlarges the area in the thoracic cavity, decreasing internal air pressure, so that air flows into the lungs to equalize the pressure. When the lungs are full, the diaphragm relaxes and elevates, making the area in the thoracic cavity smaller, thus increasing air pressure in the chest. Air then is expelled out of the lungs to equalize the pressure; this is **exhalation (expiration).** Figure 12–3 shows the position of the diaphragm in inspiration and expiration.

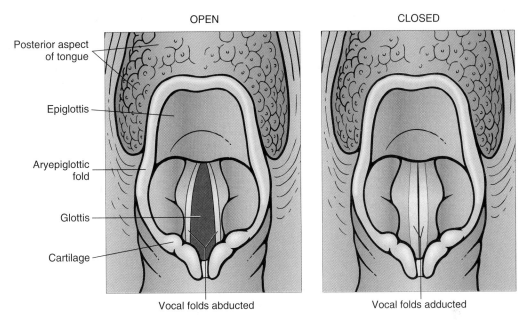

OPEN

CLOSED

Posterior aspect
of tongue

Epiglottis

Aryepiglottic
fold

Glottis

Cartilage

Vocal folds abducted

Vocal folds adducted

Figure 12–2

The larynx from a superior view.

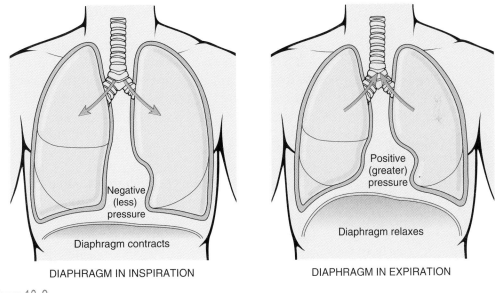

Negative
(less)
pressure

Diaphragm contracts

DIAPHRAGM IN INSPIRATION

Positive
(greater)
pressure

Diaphragm relaxes

DIAPHRAGM IN EXPIRATION

Figure 12–3

Position of the diaphragm during inspiration (inhalation) and expiration (exhalation).

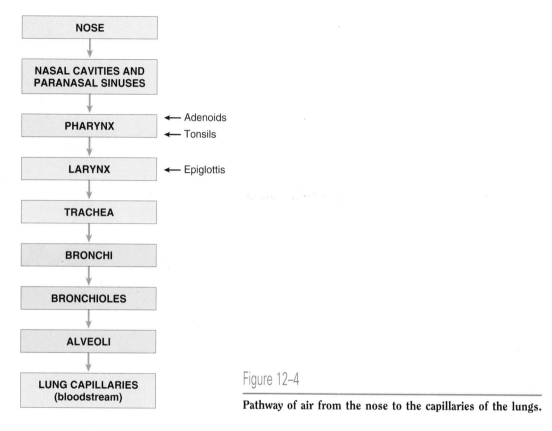

Figure 12–4

Pathway of air from the nose to the capillaries of the lungs.

Figure 12–4 is a flow diagram reviewing the pathway of air from the nose, where air enters the body, to the capillaries of the lungs, where oxygen enters the bloodstream.

III. Vocabulary

This list reviews terminology introduced in the previous section. Short definitions and additional information will reinforce your understanding. See Section X, pages 477-480, of this chapter for pronunciation of terms.

adenoids	Collections of lymph tissue in the nasopharynx; also called pharyngeal tonsils.
alveolus (plural: **alveoli**)	Air sac in the lung.
apex of the lung	Uppermost portion of the lung. The apex is the top, end, or tip of a structure. **Apical** means pertaining to the apex.
base of the lung	Lower portion of the lung; from the Greek, *basis,* foundation.
bronchioles	Smallest branches of the bronchi.
bronchus (plural: **bronchi**)	Branch of the trachea (windpipe) that is a passageway into the air spaces of the lung; bronchial tube.
carbon dioxide (CO$_2$)	A gas produced by body cells when oxygen and food combine; exhaled through the lungs.

cilia	Thin hairs attached to the mucous membrane epithelium lining the respiratory tract. They clear bacteria and foreign substances from the lung. Smoking cigarettes impairs the function of cilia.
diaphragm	Muscle separating the chest and abdomen. It is the most important muscle for breathing.
epiglottis	Lid-like piece of cartilage that covers the larynx, preventing food from entering the larynx and trachea during swallowing.
expiration	Breathing out (exhalation).
glottis	Opening to the larynx.
hilum (of lung)	Midline region where the bronchi, blood vessels, and nerves enter and exit the lungs. **Hilar** means pertaining to the hilum.
inspiration	Breathing in (inhalation).
larynx	Voice box.
lobe	Division of a lung.
mediastinum	Region between the lungs in the chest cavity. It contains the trachea, heart, aorta, esophagus, and bronchial tubes.
oxygen (O$_2$)	Gas that passes into the bloodstream at the lungs and travels to all body cells.
palatine tonsil	One of a pair of almond-shaped masses of lymphoid tissue in the oropharynx (palatine means pertaining to the roof of the mouth).
paranasal sinus	One of the air cavities in the bones near the nose.
parietal pleura	The outer fold of pleura lying closest to the ribs and wall of the thoracic cavity.
pharynx	Throat; composed of the nasopharynx, oropharynx, and laryngopharynx.
pleura	Double-folded membrane surrounding each lung.
pleural cavity	Space between the folds of the pleura.
pulmonary parenchyma	The essential cells of the lung, those performing its main function; the air sacs (alveoli) and small bronchioles.
trachea	Windpipe.
visceral pleura	The inner fold of pleura lying closest to the lung tissue.

IV. Combining Forms, Suffixes, and Terminology

Write the meanings of the medical terms in the spaces provided.

Combining Forms

Combining Form	Meaning	Terminology	Meaning
adenoid/o	adenoids	adenoidectomy	*adenords, cutting, inscision*
		adenoid hypertrophy	
alveol/o	alveolus, air sac	alveolar	
bronch/o **bronchi/o**	bronchial tube, bronchus	bronchospasm	

This is a chief characteristic of asthma and bronchitis.

bronchiectasis _____

Caused by weakening of the bronchial wall by infection.

bronchodilator _____

This drug causes dilation, or enlargement, of the opening of a bronchus to improve ventilation to the lungs. An example is albuterol, delivered via an inhaler.

Combining Form	Meaning	Terminology
bronchiol/o	bronchiole, small bronchus	bronchiolitis

Figure 12–5 shows the relationship among bronchioles, alveoli, and the blood vessels surrounding them. Bronchiolitis is an acute viral infection occurring in infants less than 18 months of age.

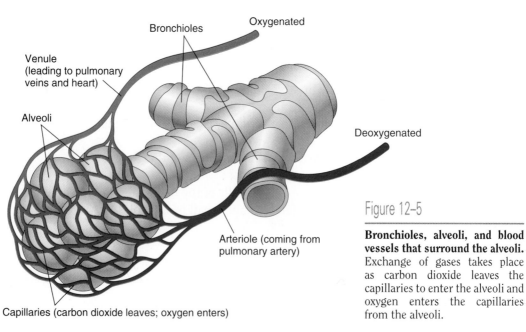

Figure 12–5

Bronchioles, alveoli, and blood vessels that surround the alveoli. Exchange of gases takes place as carbon dioxide leaves the capillaries to enter the alveoli and oxygen enters the capillaries from the alveoli.

capn/o	carbon dioxide	hypercapnia _____
coni/o	dust	pneumoconiosis _____

See page 457, Section V, under Pathological Terms.

cyan/o	blue	cyanosis _____

Caused by deficient oxygen in the blood.

epiglott/o	epiglottis	epiglottitis _____

Characterized by fever, sore throat, and an erythematous, swollen epiglottis.

laryng/o	larynx, voice box	laryngeal _____
		laryngospasm _____

Spasmodic closure of the larynx.

laryngitis _____

lob/o	lobe of the lung	lobectomy _____

Figure 12–6 shows four different types of pulmonary resections.

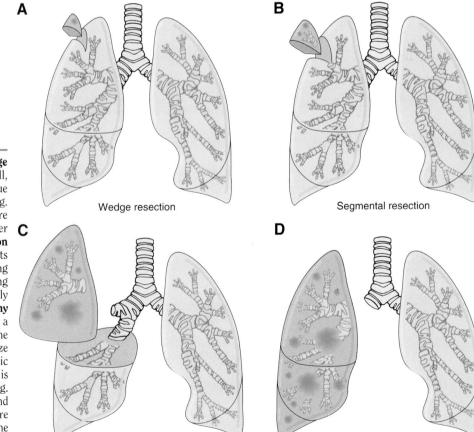

A Wedge resection

B Segmental resection

C Lobectomy

D Pneumonectomy

Figure 12–6

Pulmonary resections. (A) Wedge resection is removal of a small, localized area of diseased tissue near the surface of the lung. Pulmonary function and structure are relatively unchanged after healing. **(B) Segmental resection** is removal of a bronchiole and its alveoli (one or more lung segments). The remaining lung tissue expands to fill previously occupied space. **(C) Lobectomy** is removal of an entire lobe of a lung. Following lobectomy, the remaining lung increases in size to fill the space in the thoracic cavity. **(D) Pneumonectomy** is removal of an entire lung. Techniques (removal of ribs and elevation of the diaphragm) are used to reduce the size of the empty thoracic space.

mediastin/o   mediastinum   mediastinoscopy _____

An endoscope is inserted through an incision in the chest.

nas/o   nose   paranasal sinuses _____

Para- means near in this term.

nasogastric intubation _____

orth/o   straight, upright   orthopnea _____

An abnormal condition in which breathing (-pnea) is easier in the upright position. A major cause of orthopnea is congestive heart failure (the lungs fill with fluid when the patient is lying flat). Physicians assess the degree of orthopnea by the number of pillows a patient requires to sleep comfortably (e.g., two-pillow orthopnea).

ox/o   oxygen   hypoxia _____

Tissues have a decreased amount of oxygen, and cyanosis can result.

pector/o   chest   expectoration _____

Expectorated sputum can contain mucus, blood, cellular debris, pus, and microorganisms.

pharyng/o   pharynx, throat   pharyngeal _____

phon/o   voice   dysphonia _____

Hoarseness or other voice impairment.

phren/o   diaphragm   phrenic nerve _____

The motor nerve to the diaphragm.

pleur/o   pleura   pleurodynia _____

-dynia means pain. The intercostals muscles are inflamed.

pleural effusion _____

An effusion is the escape of fluid from blood vessels or lymphatics into a cavity or into tissue spaces.

pneum/o   air, lung   pneumothorax _____
pneumon/o

-thorax means chest. Air accumulates in the pleural cavity, between the pleura (Fig. 12–7).

pneumonectomy _____

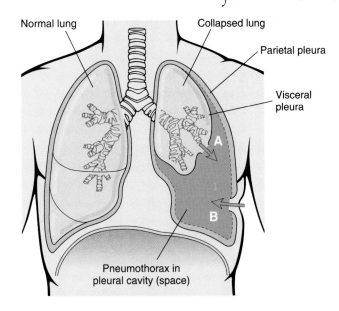

Normal lung

Collapsed lung

Parietal pleura

Visceral pleura

A

B

Pneumothorax in pleural cavity (space)

Figure 12–7

Pneumothorax. Air gathers in the pleural cavity. This condition can **(A)** occur with lung disease or **(B)** follow trauma to and perforation of (a hole through) the chest wall.

pulmon/o	lung	pulmonary	_____
rhin/o	nose	rhinorrhea	_____
		rhinoplasty	_____
sinus/o	sinus, cavity	sinusitis	_____
spir/o	breathing	spirometer	_____
		expiration	_____

Note that the s is omitted.

respiration _____

Cheyne-Stokes respiration *is marked by rhythmic changes in the depth of breathing. The pattern occurs every 45 seconds to 3 minutes. The cause is heart failure or brain damage, both of which affect the respiratory center in the brain.*

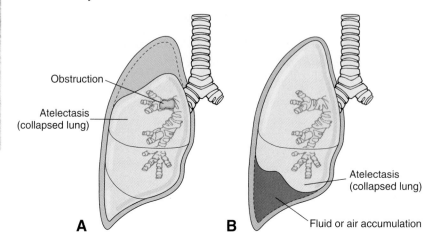

Figure 12–8

Two forms of atelectasis. (A) An obstruction prevents air from reaching distal airways, and alveoli collapse. The most frequent cause is blockage of a bronchus by a mucous or mucopurulent (pus-filled) plug, as might occur postoperatively. **(B)** Accumulations of fluid, blood, or air within the pleural cavity collapse the lung. This can occur with congestive heart failure (poor circulation leads to fluid build up in the pleural cavity) or because of leakage of air caused by a pneumothorax.

tel/o	complete	atelectasis _____

Incomplete expansion (-ectasis) of a lung; collapsed lung. Atelectasis may occur after surgery when a patient experiences pain and does not take deep breaths (Fig. 12–8).

thorac/o	chest	thoracotomy _____
		thoracic _____
tonsill/o	tonsils	tonsillectomy _____

The oropharyngeal (palatine) tonsils are removed.

trache/o	trachea, windpipe	tracheotomy _____
		tracheal stenosis _____

Having an endotracheal tube in place for a prolonged period may lead to tracheal trauma or the formation of scar tissue.

Suffixes			
Suffix	**Meaning**	**Terminology**	**Meaning**
-ema	condition	empyema _____	

Em- means in. Empyema (pyothorax) a collection of pus in the pleural cavity.

-osmia	smell	anosmia _____	

Figure 12–9

This man is sleeping with a **nasal CPAP** (continuous positive airway pressure) mask in place. The pressure supplied by air coming from the compressor opens the oropharynx and nasopharynx. (From Lewis SM, Heitkemper MM, Dirksen SR: Medical-Surgical Nursing: Assessment and Management of Clinical Problems, 5th ed. St. Louis, Mosby, 2000, p. 590.)

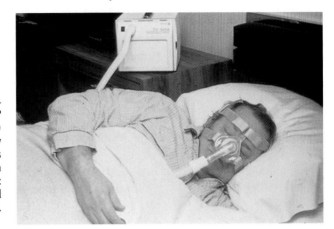

-pnea	breathing	apnea _____

Sleep apnea is sudden cessation of breathing during sleep. It can result in hypoxia, leading to cognitive impairment, hypertension, and arrhythmias. Obstructive sleep apnea (OSA) involves narrowing or occlusion in the upper airway. Continuous positive airway pressure (CPAP) is a device that delivers air into the airway. See Figure 12–9.

dyspnea _____

Paroxysmal (sudden) nocturnal (at night) dyspnea may occur in patients with congestive heart failure when they recline in bed. Patients often describe the sensation as "air hunger."

hyperpnea _____

An increase in the depth of breathing, occurring normally with exercise and abnormally with any condition in which the supply of oxygen is inadequate.

tachypnea _____

Excessively rapid and shallow breathing; hyperventilation.

-ptysis	spitting	hemoptysis _____
-sphyxia	pulse	asphyxia _____

Blockage of breathing and severe hypoxia leads to hypoxemia, hypercapnia, loss of consciousness, and death (lack of pulse).

-thorax	pleural cavity, chest	hemothorax _____
		pyothorax _____

Empyema of the chest.

V. Diagnostic and Pathological Terms

Diagnostic Terms

auscultation

Listening to sounds within the body.

This procedure, performed with a stethoscope, is used chiefly for diagnosing conditions of the lungs, pleura, heart, and abdomen, as well as to determine the condition of the fetus during pregnancy.

percussion

Tapping on a surface to determine the difference in the density of the underlying structure.

Tapping over a solid organ produces a dull sound without resonance. Percussion over an air-filled structure, such as the lung, produces a resonant, hollow note. When the lungs or the pleural space are filled with fluid and become more dense, as in pneumonia, resonance is replaced by dullness.

pleural rub

Scratchy sound produced by the motion of inflamed or irritated pleural surfaces rubbing against each other; also called a friction rub.

Pleural rub occurs when the pleura are thickened by inflammation, scarring, or neoplastic cells. It is heard by auscultation and can be felt by placing the fingers on the chest wall.

rales (crackles)

Abnormal crackling sounds heard during inspiration when there is fluid, blood, or pus in the alveoli.

Rhonchi are coarse, loud rales usually caused by secretions in the bronchial tubes.

sputum

Material expelled from the chest by coughing or clearing the throat.

Purulent (containing pus) sputum is often green or brown. It results from infection and may also be seen with asthma. Blood-tinged sputum makes physicians suspicious of tuberculosis or malignancy.

stridor

Strained, high-pitched, noisy sound made on inspiration; associated with obstruction of the larynx or trachea.

wheezes

Continuous high-pitched whistling sounds heard when air is forced through a narrow space during inspiration or expiration.

Usually caused by tightening of the larger airways in patients with asthma.

Pathological Terms

Upper Respiratory Disorders

croup

Acute viral infection in infants and children; characterized by obstruction of the larynx, barking cough, and stridor.

The most common causative agents are influenza viruses or respiratory syncytial viruses (RSVs).

diphtheria

Acute infection of the throat and upper respiratory tract caused by the diphtheria bacterium *(Corynebacterium).*

Inflammation occurs, and a leathery, opaque membrane (Greek, *diphthera,* "leather membrane") forms in the pharynx and respiratory tract.

Immunity to diphtheria (by production of antibodies) is induced by the administration of weakened toxins (antigens) beginning between the sixth and the eighth weeks of life. These injections are usually given in combination with pertussis and tetanus toxins and are called **DPT** injections.

epistaxis

Nosebleed.

Epistaxis is from the Greek meaning "a dropping." It commonly results from irritation of nasal mucous membranes, trauma, vitamin K deficiency, clotting abnormalities, or hypertension.

pertussis

Bacterial infection of the pharynx, larynx, and trachea caused by *Bordetella pertussis,* a highly contagious bacterium. Also known as whooping cough.

Pertussis is characterized by **paroxysmal** (sudden) coughing that ends in a loud whooping inspiration.

Bronchial Tube Disorders

asthma

Chronic inflammatory disorder characterized by airway obstruction caused by edema, bronchoconstriction, and increased mucus production.

Associated symptoms of asthma are dyspnea, wheezing, and cough. Etiology can involve allergy or infection. Triggers to asthmatic attacks include exercise, strong odors, cold air, stress, allergens (e.g., dust, molds, pollens, or foods) and medications (aspirin, beta-blockers). Asthma treatments are inhaled anti-inflammatory agents (long-term control with glucocorticoids), bronchodilators (quick-relief control with albuterol and theophylline), and trigger avoidance by patient education. Other conditions, such as gastroesophageal reflux (GERD), sinusitis, allergic rhinitis, or medications can impede asthma control.

bronchiectasis

Chronic dilation of a bronchus secondary to infection in the lower lobes of the lung.

This condition is caused by chronic infection with loss of elasticity of the bronchi. Secretions puddle and do not drain normally. Symptoms are cough, fever, and expectoration of foul-smelling, **purulent** (pus-containing) sputum. Treatment is **palliative** (noncurative) and includes antibiotics, mucolytics, bronchodilators, respiratory therapy, and surgical resection if other treatment is not effective.

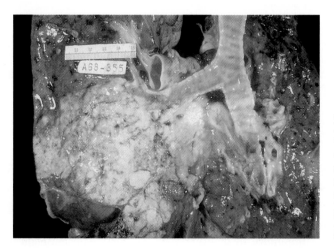

Figure 12–10

Bronchogenic carcinoma. The gray-white tumor tissue is infiltrating the substance of the lung. This tumor was identified as a squamous cell carcinoma. Squamous cell carcinomas arise in major bronchi and spread to local hilar lymph nodes. (From Kumar V, Cotran RS, Robbins SL: Basic Pathology, 7th ed. Philadelphia, WB Saunders, 2003, p. 501.)

bronchogenic carcinoma (lung cancer)

Cancerous tumors arising from a bronchus (see Fig. 12–10).

This group of malignant tumors, often associated with cigarette smoking, is the most frequent fatal malignancy. Lung cancers are divided into two general categories: **non–small cell lung cancer (NSCLC)** and **small cell lung cancer (SCLC).**

NSCLC comprises 90 percent of lung cancers, and there are two main types: adenocarcinoma (derived from mucus-secreting cells) and squamous cell carcinoma (derived from the lining of a bronchus). For localized tumors, surgery may be curative. When disease is locally advanced (lymph nodes or mediastinum), chemotherapy and radiation therapy are options. Doctors treat metastatic disease (to liver, brain, and bones) with chemotherapy and radiation therapy (irradiation).

SCLC derives from small, round to oval secretory cells in pulmonary epithelium. It grows rapidly early in its course and quickly spreads outside the lung. Palliative treatment includes surgery, radiation therapy, and chemotherapy.

chronic bronchitis

Inflammation of the bronchi persisting over a long time.

Infection and cigarette smoking are etiological factors. Symptoms include excessive secretion of mucus, a productive cough, and obstruction of respiratory passages. Chronic bronchitis, asthma, and emphysema (a lung disease) are all components of **chronic obstructive pulmonary disease (COPD).**

cystic fibrosis

Inherited disorder of exocrine glands resulting in thick, mucous secretions that do not drain normally.

The exocrine glands affected are the pancreas (insufficient secretion of enzymes), sweat glands (abnormal salt production), and epithelium (lining cells) of the respiratory tract. Chronic airway obstruction, infection, bronchiectasis, and respiratory failure are the end result. Therapy includes replacement of pancreatic enzymes and treatment of pulmonary obstruction and infection.

The gene responsible for cystic fibrosis is known, and persons carrying the gene may be identified. There is no known cure, although lung transplantation can extend life and restore lung function.

Lung Disorders

atelectasis

Incomplete (atel/o) expansion (-ectasis) of alveoli; collapsed, functionless, airless lung or portion of a lung. Caused by tumor or other obstruction of the bronchus, or poor respiratory effort.

In atelectasis, the bronchioles and alveoli (pulmonary parenchyma) resemble a collapsed balloon. Common causes of atelectasis include poor inspiration effort in the postoperative period, blockage of a bronchus or smaller bronchial tube by secretions, tumor, or a chest wound that permits air, fluid, or blood to accumulate in the pleural cavity. Acute atelectasis requires removal of the underlying cause (tumor, foreign body, mucous plug) and therapy to open airways. Respiration can also be limited by pain.

emphysema

Hyperinflation of air sacs with destruction of alveolar walls.

Loss of elasticity and the breakdown of alveolar walls result in expiratory flow limitation. There is a strong association between cigarette smoking and emphysema. As a result of the destruction of lung parenchyma, including blood vessels, pulmonary artery pressure rises and the right side of the heart must work harder to pump blood. This leads to right ventricular hypertrophy and heart failure **(cor pulmonale).**

pneumoconiosis

Abnormal condition caused by dust in the lungs, with chronic inflammation, infection, and bronchitis.

Various forms are named according to the type of dust particle inhaled: **anthracosis**—coal (anthrac/o) dust (black lung disease); **asbestosis**—asbestos (asbest/o) particles (in shipbuilding and construction trades); **silicosis**—silica (silic/o = rocks) or glass (grinder's disease).

pneumonia

Acute inflammation and infection of alveoli, which fill with pus or products of the inflammatory reaction.

Etiological agents are pneumococci, staphylococci, and other bacteria, fungi, or viruses. Infection damages alveolar membranes so that an **exudate** (fluid, blood cells, and debris) consolidates in alveoli. **Lobar pneumonia** involves an entire lobe of a lung. **Bronchopneumonia,** common in infants and the elderly, involves patchy consolidation in the lung parenchyma. Treatment includes appropriate antibiotics and, if necessary, oxygen and mechanical ventilation.

Community-acquired pneumonia results from a contagious respiratory infection, caused by a variety of viruses, bacteria, or mycoplasma (a type of bacteria). It is usually treated at home with oral antibiotics.

Hospital-acquired pneumonia or **nosocomial pneumonia** results from being hospitalized (Greek, *nosokomeion* means "hospital"). For example, patients may contract pneumonia while on mechanical ventilation or from a hospital-acquired infection.

pulmonary abscess

A large collection of pus (bacterial infection) in the lungs.

pulmonary edema	**Swelling and fluid in the air sacs and bronchioles.**

This condition is most commonly caused by the inability of the heart to pump blood (congestive heart failure). Blood backs up in the pulmonary blood vessels, and fluid seeps out into the alveoli and bronchioles. Acute pulmonary edema requires immediate medical attention, including drugs (diuretics, vasodilators), oxygen in high concentrations, and keeping the patient in a sitting position (to decrease venous return to the heart).

pulmonary embolism (PE) **Clot (thrombus) or other material lodges in vessels of the lung.**

The clot travels from distant veins, usually in the legs. Occlusion can produce an area of dead (necrotic) tissue called a **pulmonary infarction.** PE often causes acute pleuritic chest pain (pain on inspiration) and may be associated with blood in the sputum, fever, and respiratory insufficiency. It is diagnosed by ventilation/perfusion scans that reveal areas of lung that lack perfusion. Other useful tests include computerized tomography (CT) scans that reveal obstruction of pulmonary vessels.

pulmonary fibrosis **Formation of scar tissue in the connective tissue of the lungs.**

This condition may be the result of any inflammation or irritation caused by tuberculosis, pneumonia, or pneumoconiosis.

sarcoidosis **Chronic inflammatory disease of unknown cause in which small nodules or tubercles develop in lungs, lymph nodes, and other organs.**

Bilateral hilar lymphadenopathy or lung involvement is visible on chest x-ray in 90 percent of cases. Many patients are asymptomatic and retain adequate pulmonary function. Others have more active disease and impaired pulmonary function. Corticosteroid drugs are used to prevent progression in these patients.

tuberculosis (TB) **Infectious disease caused by *Mycobacterium tuberculosis;* lungs are usually involved, but any organ in the body may be affected.**

Rod-shaped bacteria called **bacilli** invade the lungs, producing small tubercles (from the Latin word *tuber* meaning a swelling) of infection. Early tuberculosis is usually asymptomatic and detected on routine chest x-ray. Symptoms of advanced disease are cough, weight loss, night sweats, hemoptysis, and pleuritic pain. Antituberculous chemotherapy (isoniazid, rifampin) is effective in most cases. Immunocompromised patients are particularly susceptible to antibiotic-resistant tuberculosis. It is important and often necessary to treat TB with several drugs at the same time to prevent drug resistance.

The PPD skin test (see page 464, Section VI, under Clinical Procedures) is given to most hospital and medical employees because TB is highly contagious.

Pleural Disorders

mesothelioma **Rare malignant tumor arising in the pleura and associated with exposure to asbestos.**

Mesotheliomas are composed of mesothelium, which forms the lining of the pleural surface.

pleural effusion	**Abnormal accumulation of fluid in the pleural space (cavity).**

Two types of pleural effusions are exudates (fluid from tumors, infections, trauma, and other diseases) and transudates (fluid from congestive heart failure, pulmonary embolism, or cirrhosis).

pleurisy (pleuritis)	**Inflammation of the pleura.**

This condition causes pleurodynia and dyspnea and, in chronic cases, pleural effusion.

pneumothorax	**Collection of air in the pleural space.**

Pneumothorax may occur in the course of a pulmonary disease (emphysema, carcinoma, tuberculosis, or lung abscess) when rupture of any pulmonary lesions near the pleural surface allows communication between an alveolus or bronchus and the pleural cavity. It may also follow trauma and perforation of the chest wall or prolonged high-flow oxygen delivered by a respirator in an intensive care unit (ICU).

Study Section

Practice spelling each term and know its meaning.

anthracosis	Coal dust accumulation in the lungs.
asbestosis	Asbestos particles accumulate in the lungs.
bacilli (singular: **bacillus**)	Rod-shaped bacteria (cause of tuberculosis).
chronic obstructive pulmonary disease (COPD)	Chronic condition of persistent obstruction of air flow through bronchial tubes and lungs. COPD is caused by smoking, chronic infection, and, in a minority of cases, asthma. Patients with predominant chronic bronchitis COPD are referred to as *blue bloaters* (cyanotic, stocky build) while those with predominant emphysema are called *pink puffers* (short of breath, but with near normal blood oxygen levels, and no change in skin color).
cor pulmonale	Failure of the right side of the heart to pump a sufficient amount of blood to the lungs because of underlying lung disease.
exudate	Fluid, cells, or other substances (pus) that slowly leave cells or capillaries through pores or small breaks in cell membranes.
hydrothorax	Collection of fluid in the pleural cavity.

Continued on following page

palliative	Relieving symptoms, but not curing the disease.
paroxysmal	Pertaining to a sudden occurrence, such as a spasm or seizure; oxysm/o means sudden.
pulmonary infarction	An area of dead (necrotic) tissue in the lung.
purulent	Containing pus.
rhonchi	Coarse, loud rales caused by secretions in bronchial tubes.
silicosis	Silica or glass dust in the lungs; occurs in mining occupations.

VI. Clinical Procedures and Abbreviations

Clinical Procedures

X-Rays

chest x-ray

Radiographic imaging of the thoracic cavity.

Chest x-ray views are taken in the frontal (coronal) plane (see Fig. 12–11) as posteroanterior (PA) or anteroposterior (AP) views and in the sagittal plane as lateral views. **Chest tomograms** are a series of x-ray images each showing a "slice" of the chest at different depths. Tomograms detect small masses not seen on regular films.

computed tomography (CT scan of the chest)

Computer-generated x-ray images show thoracic structures in cross-section.

This test is for diagnosis of lesions difficult to assess by conventional x-ray studies, such as those in the hilum, mediastinum, and pleura.

pulmonary angiography

X-ray images taken after injecting radiopaque contrast into the pulmonary artery or right side of the heart.

This study visualizes the pulmonary circulation to locate obstructions or pathological conditions, such as a pulmonary embolus.

Magnetic Imaging

magnetic resonance imaging (MRI)

Magnetic waves create detailed images of the chest in frontal, lateral, and cross-sectional (axial) planes.

This test is helpful in locating lesions difficult to assess by CT scan (see Fig. 12–12).

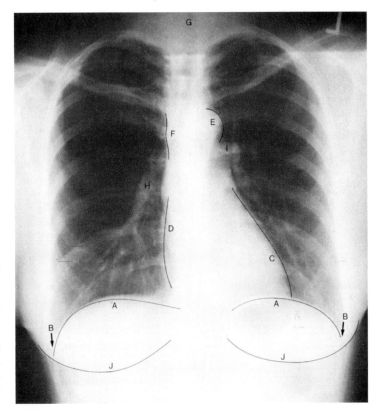

Figure 12-11

A **normal chest x-ray** taken from the posteroanterior (PA) view. The backwards L in the upper corner is placed on the film to indicate the left side of the patient's chest. **(A)** diaphragm; **(B)** costophrenic angle; **(C)** left ventricle; **(D)** right atrium; **(E)** aortic arch; **(F)** superior vena cava; **(G)** trachea; **(H)** right bronchus; **(I)** left bronchus; **(J)** breast shadows. (From Black JM, Hawks JH, Keene AM: Medical-Surgical Nursing: Clinical Management for Positive Outcomes, 6th ed. Philadelphia, WB Saunders, 2001, p. 1644.)

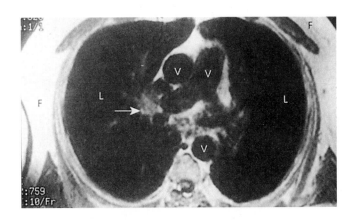

Figure 12-12

MRI of the upper chest, transverse (axial) view. Notice the lungs (L) fat (F) and vessels (V). A hilar tumor (*arrow*) is easily identified. (From Ballinger PW, Frank ED: Merrill's Atlas of Radiographic Positions and Radiologic Procedures, 10th ed. vol 3. St. Louis, Mosby, 2003, p. 388.)

Radioactive Test

ventilation-perfusion (V/Q) scan

Detection device records radioactivity after injection of a radioisotope or inhalation of small amount of radioactive gas (xenon).

This test can identify areas of the lung not receiving air flow (ventilation) or blood flow (perfusion).

Other Procedures

bronchoscopy

Fiber-optic or rigid endoscope inserted into the bronchial tubes for diagnosis, biopsy, or collection of specimens.

A physician places the bronchoscope through the throat, larynx, and trachea into the bronchi. In **bronchial alveolar lavage (bronchial washing),** fluid is injected and withdrawn. In transbronchial biopsies, a forceps is used to grasp tissue or a brush **(bronchial brushing)** is inserted through the bronchoscope (see Fig. 12–13).

endotracheal intubation

Placement of a tube through the mouth into the pharynx, larynx, and trachea to establish an airway (see Fig. 12–14).

This procedure also allows a person to be placed on a **ventilator** (an apparatus that moves air in and out of the lungs).

laryngoscopy

Visual examination of the voice box.

A lighted, flexible endoscope is passed through the mouth or nose into the larynx.

lung biopsy

Removal of lung tissue followed by microscopic examination.

Specimens may be obtained by bronchoscopy or thoracotomy (open-lung biopsy).

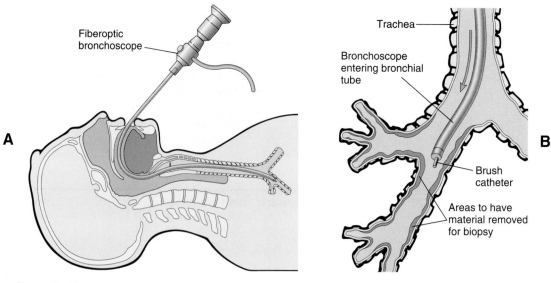

Figure 12–13

(A) Fiberoptic bronchoscopy. A bronchoscope is passed through the nose, throat, larynx, and trachea into a bronchus. **(B)** A **bronchoscope,** with brush catheter, in place in a bronchial tube.

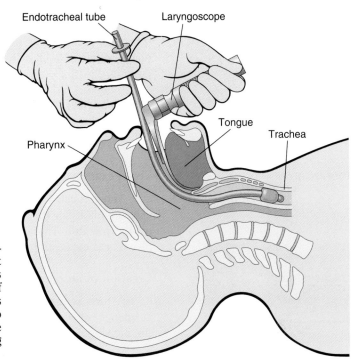

Endotracheal tube   Laryngoscope

Tongue

Trachea

Pharynx

Figure 12–14

Endotracheal intubation. The patient is in a supine position; the head is hyperextended, the lower portion of the neck is flexed, and the mouth is opened. A **laryngoscope** is used to hold the airway open, to expose the vocal cords, and as a guide for placing the ET tube into the trachea.

mediastinoscopy

Endoscopic visual examination of the mediastinum.

An incision is made above the breastbone (suprasternal) for inspection and biopsy of lymph nodes.

pulmonary function tests (PFTs)

Tests that measure the ventilation mechanics of the lung (airway function, lung volume, and capacity of the lungs to exchange oxygen and carbon dioxide efficiently).

PFTs are used for many reasons: (1) to evaluate patients with shortness of breath (SOB); (2) to follow patients with known respiratory diagnoses; (3) to evaluate disability; and (4) to assess lung function before surgery or therapy (chemotherapy). A **spirometer** measures the volume and rate of air passing in and out of the lung.

PFTs determine if lung disease is obstructive, restrictive, or both. In **obstructive lung disease** airways are narrowed, which results in resistance to airflow during breathing. A hallmark PFT value in obstructive disease is decreased expiratory flow rate or **FEV$_1$** (forced expiratory volume in the first second). Examples of obstructive lung diseases are asthma, COPD, bronchiectasis, cystic fibrosis, and bronchiolitis.

In **restrictive lung disease** expansion of the lung is limited by disease that affects the chest wall, pleura, or lung tissue itself. A hallmark PFT value in restrictive disease is decreased total lung capacity (TLC). Examples of lung conditions that stiffen and scar the lung are pulmonary fibrosis, radiation damage, and pneumoconiosis. Other causes of restrictive lung disease are neuromuscular conditions that affect the lung, such as myasthenia gravis, muscular dystrophy, and diaphragmatic weakness and paralysis.

The ability of gas to diffuse across the alveolar-capillary membrane is assessed by the diffusion capacity of the lung for carbon monoxide **(DLco).** A patient breathes in a small amount of carbon monoxide (CO), and the length of time it takes the gas to enter the bloodstream is measured.

thoracentesis

Surgical puncture to remove fluid from the pleural space.

This procedure is used to obtain pleural fluid for diagnosis or to drain a pleural effusion. A chest tube may be inserted to allow further drainage of fluid (see Fig. 12–15).

thoracotomy

Major surgical incision of the chest.

The incision is large, cutting into bone, muscle, and cartilage. It is necessary for lung biopsies and resections (lobectomy and pneumonectomy).

thorascopy

Visual examination of the chest via small incisions and use of an endoscope.

Video-assisted thorascopy (VATS) allows a surgeon to view the chest from a video monitor. The thorascope is equipped with a camera that magnifies the image on the monitor. Thoracoscopy can diagnose and treat conditions of the lung, pleura, and mediastinum.

tracheostomy

Creation of an opening into the trachea through the neck.

A tube is inserted to create an airway. The tracheostomy tube may be permanent as well as an emergency device (see Fig. 12–16). A tracheotomy is the incision necessary to create a tracheostomy.

tuberculin test

Determines past or present tuberculosis infection based on a positive skin reaction.

Examples are **Heaf and tine tests,** using purified protein derivative **(PPD)** applied with multiple punctures of the skin and **Mantoux test,** by intradermal injection.

tube thoracostomy

Chest tube is passed through an opening in the skin of the chest to continuously drain a pleural effusion.

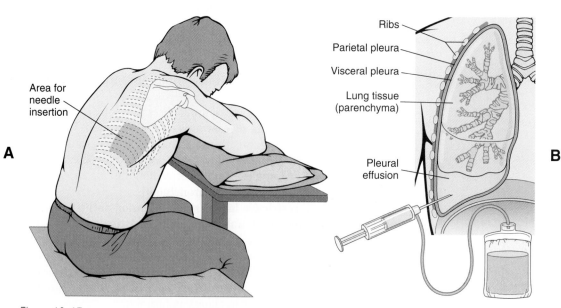

Area for needle insertion

Ribs
Parietal pleura
Visceral pleura
Lung tissue (parenchyma)
Pleural effusion

A

B

Figure 12–15

Thoracentesis. (A) The patient is sitting in the correct position for the procedure; it allows the chest wall to be pulled outward in an expanded position. **(B)** The needle is inserted close to the base of the effusion so the gravity can help with drainage, but it is kept as far away from the diaphragm as possible.

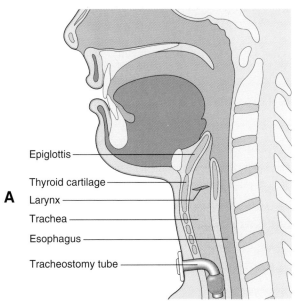

Epiglottis

Thyroid cartilage

A

Larynx

Trachea

Esophagus

Tracheostomy tube

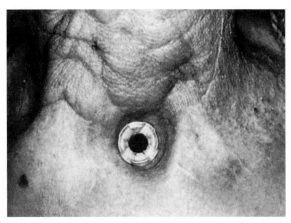

B

Figure 12–16

(A) Tracheostomy with tube in place. **(B) Healed tracheostomy incision** after laryngectomy. (**B** from Black JM, Hawks JH, Keene AM: Medical-Surgical Nursing: Clinical Management for Positive Outcomes, 6th ed. Philadelphia, WB Saunders, 2001, p. 1672.)

Abbreviations

ABGs	arterial blood gases
AFB	acid-fast bacillus (organism causing tuberculosis)
ARDS	adult (or acute) respiratory distress syndrome (a group of symptoms—tachypnea, dyspnea, tachycardia, hypoxemia, cyanosis—resulting in acute respiratory failure)
BAL	bronchial aveolar lavage
Bronch	bronchoscopy
COPD	chronic obstructive pulmonary disease (airway obstruction associated with emphysema and chronic bronchitis)
CPAP	continuous positive airway pressure
CPR	cardiopulmonary resuscitation (three basic steps: *a*irway opened by tilting the head, *b*reathing restored by mouth-to-mouth breathing, *c*irculation restored by external cardiac compression)
CTA	clear to auscultation
CXR	chest x-ray

DLco	diffusion in capacity of the lung for carbon monoxide
DOE	dyspnea on exertion
DPI	dry powder inhaler
DPT	diphtheria, pertussis, tetanus (injection in an infant to provide immunity to these diseases)
FEV$_1$	Forced expirations volume in first second
FVC	forced vital capacity
ICU	intensive care unit
LLL	left lower lobe (of lung)
LUL	left upper lobe (of lung)
MDI	metered-dose inhaler; used to deliver aerosolized medications to patients with respiratory disease
NIV	noninvasive ventilation
NSCLC	non–small cell lung cancer

OSA	obstructive sleep apnea
Paco2	carbon dioxide partial pressure; amount of carbon dioxide in arterial blood
Pao2	oxygen partial pressure; amount of oxygen in arterial blood
PCP	*Pneumocystis carinii* pneumonia (a type of pneumonia seen in patients with AIDS)
PE	pulmonary embolism
PEEP	positive end expiratory pressure (a common mechanical ventilator setting in which airway pressure is maintained above atmospheric pressure)
PFTs	pulmonary function tests
PND	paroxysmal nocturnal dyspnea
PPD	purified protein derivative (substance used in a tuberculosis test)
RDS	respiratory distress syndrome (condition of the newborn marked by dyspnea and cyanosis and related to absence of surfactant, a substance that permits normal expansion of lungs); also called hyaline membrane disease

RLL	right lower lobe (of lung)
RSV	respiratory syncytial virus; in tissue culture forms syncytia or giant cells (cytoplasm flows together). It is a common cause of bronchiolitis, bronchopneumonia, and the common cold
RUL	right upper lobe (of lung)
SCLC	small cell lung cancer
SIMV	synchronized intermittent mandatory ventilation
SOB	shortness of breath
TB	tuberculosis
TLC	total lung capacity
URI	upper respiratory infection
VAP	ventilation-associated pneumonia
VATS	video-assisted thorascopy
V/Q scan	ventilation-perfusion scan. Radioactive test of lung ventilation and blood perfusion throughout the lung capillaries (lung scan)

VII. Practical Applications

This section contains actual medical reports using terms that you have studied in this and previous chapters. Explanations of more difficult terms are added in brackets. Answers to the questions are on page 477 after Answers to Exercises.

Case Report

A 22-year-old known heroin abuser was admitted to an emergency room comatose with shallow respirations. Routine laboratory studies and chest x-rays were done after the patient was aroused. He was then transferred to the ICU. He complained of left-sided chest pain. Examination of the chest x-ray showed three fractured ribs on the right and a large right pleural effusion. Further questioning of a friend revealed that he had fallen and struck the corner of a table after injecting heroin.

The diagnosis was traumatic hemothorax secondary to fractured ribs, and a thoracotomy tube was inserted into the right pleural space. No blood could be obtained despite maneuvering of the tube. Another chest x-ray showed that the tube was correctly placed in the right pleural space, but the fractured ribs and pleural effusion were on the left. The radiologist then realized that he had reversed the first film. A second tube was inserted into the left pleural space, and 1500 mL (6-7 cups) of blood were evacuated.

Necropsy Report and Questions

Adenocarcinoma, bronchogenic, left lung, with extensive mediastinal, pleural, and pericardial involvement. Metastasis to tracheobronchial lymph nodes, liver, lumbar vertebrae. Pulmonary emboli, multiple, recent, with recent infarct of left lower lobe. The tumor apparently originated at the left main bronchus and extends peripherally. Parenchyma (alveoli) is particularly atelectatic with a centrally located area of hemorrhage in the lower lobe.

Questions on the Case Report

1. **What was the patient's primary disease?**
   (A) blood clots in the lung
   (B) mediastinal, pleural, and pericardial inflammation
   (C) lung cancer
2. **Which was *not* an area of metastasis?**
   (A) backbones
   (B) bone marrow
   (C) hepatocytes
3. **What event was probably the cause of death?**
   (A) infarction of lung tissue caused by pulmonary emboli
   (B) COPD
   (C) myocardial infarction
4. **What best describes the pulmonary parenchyma in the lower left lobe?**
   (A) Alveoli are filled with tumor.
   (B) Alveoli are collapsed, with central area of bleeding.
   (C) Alveoli are filled with pus and blood.

X-Ray Reports and Bronchoscopy

1. CXR: Complete opacification of left hemithorax with deviation of mediastinal structures of right side. Massive pleural effusion.
2. Chest tomograms: Mass most compatible with LUL bronchogenic carcinoma. Possible left paratracheal adenopathy or direct involvement of mediastinum.
3. Bronchoscopy: Larynx, trachea, carina (area of bifurcation or forking of the trachea), and left lung all within normal limits. On the right side there was irregularity and roughening of the bronchial mucosa on the lateral aspect of the bronchial wall. This irregularity extended into the RUL, and the apical and posterior segments (divisions of lobes of the lung) each contained inflamed irregular mucosa. Conclusion: Suspicious for infiltrating tumor, but may be nonspecific inflammation. Bronchial washings, brushings, and bxs [biopsies] taken. Bronchial biopsy diagnosis: squamous cell carcinoma. Washings and brushings showed no malignant cells.

VIII. Exercises

Remember to check your answers carefully with those given in Section IX, Answers to Exercises.

A. Match the following anatomical structures with their descriptions below.

adenoids	epiglottis	paranasal sinuses
alveoli	hilum	parietal pleura
bronchi	larynx	pharynx
bronchioles	mediastinum	trachea
cilia	palatine tonsils	visceral pleura

1. Outer fold of pleura lying closest to the ribs _____.

2. Collections of lymph tissue in the nasopharynx _____.

3. Windpipe _____.

4. Lid-like piece of cartilage that covers the voice box _____.

5. Branches of the windpipe that lead into the lungs _____.

6. Region between the lungs in the chest cavity _____.

7. Air-containing cavities in the bones around the nose _____.

8. Thin hairs attached to the mucous membrane lining the respiratory tract _____.

9. Inner fold of pleura closest to lung tissue _____.

10. Throat _____.

11. Air sacs of the lung _____.

12. Voice box _____.

13. Smallest branches of bronchi _____.

14. Collections of lymph tissue in the oropharynx _____.

15. Midline region of the lungs where bronchi, blood vessels, and nerves enter and exit the lungs

_____.

B. Complete the following sentences.

1. The apical part of the lung is the _____.

2. The gas that passes into the bloodstream at the lungs is _____.

3. Breathing in air is called _____.

4. Divisions of the lungs are known as _____.

5. The gas produced by cells and exhaled through the lungs is _____.

6. The space between the visceral and the parietal pleura is the _____.

7. Breathing out air is called _____.

8. The essential cells of the lung that perform its main function are pulmonary _____.

9. The exchange of gases in the lung is _____ respiration.

10. The exchange of gases at the tissue cells is _____ respiration.

C. Give meanings for the following medical terms.

1. bronchiectasis _____

2. pleuritis _____

3. pneumothorax _____

4. anosmia _____

5. laryngectomy _____

6. nasopharyngitis _____

7. phrenic _____

8. alveolar _____

9. glottis _____

10. tracheal stenosis _____

D. Complete the medical terms for the following respiratory symptoms.

1. excessive carbon dioxide in the blood: hyper _____

2. breathing is possible only in an upright position: _____ pnea

3. difficult breathing: _____ pnea

4. condition of blueness of skin: _____ osis

5. spitting up blood: hemo _____

6. deficiency of oxygen: hyp _____

7. condition of pus in the pleural cavity: pyo _____ or em _____

8. hoarseness; voice impairment: dys _____

9. blood in the pleural cavity: hemo _____

10. nosebleed: epi _____

E. Give the meanings of the following medical terms.

1. rales (crackles) _____

2. auscultation _____

3. sputum _____

4. percussion _____

5. rhonchi _____

6. pleural rub _____

7. purulent _____

8. paroxysmal nocturnal dyspnea _____

9. hydrothorax _____

10. pulmonary infarction _____

11. stridor _____

12. wheeze _____

F. Match the following terms with their descriptions below.

asbestosis	chronic bronchitis	emphysema
asthma	croup	pertussis
atelectasis	cystic fibrosis	sarcoidosis
bronchogenic carcinoma	diphtheria	

1. acute infectious disease of the throat caused by *Corynebacterium* _____

2. acute respiratory syndrome in children and infants that is marked by obstruction of the larynx and

   stridor _____

3. hyperinflation of air sacs with destruction of alveolar walls _____

4. inflammation of tubes that lead from the trachea; over a long period of time _____

5. chronic inflammation disorder characterized by airway obstruction _____

6. lung or a portion of a lung is collapsed _____

7. malignant neoplasm originating in a bronchus _____

8. whooping cough _____

9. inherited disease of exocrine glands; mucous secretions lead to airway obstruction _____

10. type of pneumoconiosis; dust particles are inhaled _____

11. inflammatory disease in which small nodules form in lungs and lymph nodes _____

G. Use the following terms or abbreviations to complete the sentences below:

CPAP	fibrosis	PaO_2
DLco	obstructive lung disease	palliative
exudate	OSA	restrictive lung disease
FEV_1	$PaCO_2$	rhonchi

1. Sarah had a pulmonary function test in which she inhaled as much air as she could and the air that

   she expelled in the first second was measured. This PFT is a _____.

2. Dr. Smith heard loud _____ when he auscultated Kate's chest. Her bronchial tubes were obstructed with thick mucous secretions.

3. Karl was asked to breathe in a small amount of carbon monoxide and then blood samples were taken to detect the gas in his bloodstream. This is a PFT to assess how well gases can diffuse across

   the alveolar membrane and it is called _____.

4. Formation of scar tissue in the connective tissue of the lungs is pulmonary _____.

5. A purulent _____ consists of white blood cells, microorganisms (dead and alive), and other debris.

6. Myasthenia gravis and muscular dystrophy are examples of neuromuscular conditions that produce

   _____.

7. Chronic bronchitis and asthma are examples of _____.

8. Patients with a small pharyngeal airway that closes during sleep may experience

   _____.

9. With nasal _____, positive pressure (air coming from a compressor) opens the oropharynx and nasopharynx, preventing obstructive sleep apnea.

10. Doctors realized that they could not cure Jean's adenocarcinoma of the lung. They used

    _____ measures to relieve her uncomfortable symptoms.

11. During an apneic period, a patient experiences severe hypoxemia (decreased

    _____) and hypercapnia (increased _____).

H. Give the meanings of the following medical terms.

1. pulmonary abscess _____

2. pulmonary edema _____

3. pneumoconiosis _____

4. pneumonia _____

5. pulmonary embolism _____

6. tuberculosis _____

7. pleural effusion _____

8. pleurisy _____

9. anthracosis _____

10. mesothelioma _____

11. adenoid hypertrophy _____

12. pleurodynia _____

13. expectoration _____

14. tachypnea _____

I. Match the clinical procedure or abbreviation with its description.

bronchial alveolar lavage   mediastinoscopy   tracheostomy
bronchoscopy   pulmonary angiography   tube thoracostomy
endotracheal intubation   pulmonary function tests   tuberculin tests
laryngoscopy   thoracentesis   V/Q scan

1. Placement of a tube through the mouth into the trachea to establish an airway _____

2. Injection or inhalation of radioactive material and recording images of its distribution in the lungs

_____

3. PPD, tine, and Mantoux tests _____

4. Puncture of the chest wall to obtain fluid from the pleural cavity _____

5. Tests that measure the ventilation mechanics of the lung _____

6. An opening is made into the trachea through the neck to establish an airway _____

7. Visual examination of the bronchi _____

8. Fluid is injected into the bronchi and withdrawn for examination _____

9. Insertion of an endoscope into the larynx to view the voice box _____

10. X-ray images taken after injecting contrast into the pulmonary artery _____

11. Visual examination of the area between the lungs _____

12. Chest tube is passed through a small skin incision to continuously drain the pleural spaces

_____

J. Give the meanings of the following abbreviations and then select the letter of the sentences that follow that is the best association for each.

Column I

1. DOE _____ ____

2. PND _____ ____

3. VATS _____ ____

4. CPR _____ ____

5. NSCLC _____ ____

6. ARDS _____ ____

7. COPD _____ ____

8. PFTs _____ ____

9. PPD _____ ____

10. DPT _____ ____

Column II

A. Patients with congestive heart failure and pulmonary edema experience this symptom when they recline in bed.

B. Chronic bronchitis and emphysema are examples.

C. Substance used in the test for tuberculosis.

D. Adenocarcinoma and squamous cell carcinoma are types.

E. Visual examination of the chest via endoscope and a video monitor.

F. Injection in an infant to provide immunity.

G. A spirometer is used for these respiratory tests.

H. This symptom means that a patient has difficulty breathing and becomes short of breath when exercising.

I. Three basic steps: (A) airway opened by tilting the head; (B) breathing restored by mouth-to-mouth breathing; (C) circulation restored by external cardiac compression.

J. A group of symptoms resulting in acute respiratory failure.

K. Match the respiratory system procedures with their meanings.

laryngectomy   rhinoplasty   thoracotomy
lobectomy   thoracentesis   tonsillectomy
pneumonectomy   thorascopy

1. removal of lymph tissue in the oropharynx _____

2. surgical puncture of the chest to remove fluid from the pleural space _____

3. surgical repair of the nose _____

4. incision of the chest for lung biopsy _____

5. removal of the voice box _____

6. removal of a region of a lung _____

7. endoscopic examination of the chest _____

8. pulmonary resection _____

L. Circle the terms that best complete the meanings of the sentences.

1. Ruth was having difficulty taking a deep breath, and her chest x-ray showed accumulation of fluid in her pleural spaces. Dr. Smith ordered **(PPD, tracheotomy, thoracentesis)** to relieve the pressure on her lungs.

2. Dr. Wong used her stethoscope to perform **(percussion, auscultation, thoracentesis)** on the patient's chest.

3. Before surgery on Mrs. Hope, an 80-year-old woman with lung cancer, her physicians ordered **(COPD, bronchoscopy, PFTs)** to determine the functioning of her lungs.

4. Sylvia produced yellow-colored sputum and had a high fever. Her physician told her that she probably had **(pneumonia, pulmonary embolism, pneumothorax)** and needed antibiotics.

5. The night before her thoracotomy for lung biopsy, Mrs. White was told by her anesthesiologist that he would place a/an **(thoracostomy tube, mediastinoscope, endotracheal tube)** down her throat to keep her airways open during surgery.

6. Early in her pregnancy, Sonya had a routine **(PET scan, CXR, MRI)**, which revealed a/an **(epiglottic, alveolar, mediastinal)** mass in the area between her chest. After delivery of her child, the mass was removed, and biopsy revealed a malignant thymoma (tumor of the thymus gland).

7. Five-year-old Seth was allergic to cats and experienced wheezing, coughing, and difficult breathing at night when he was trying to sleep. After careful evaluation by a **(cardiologist, pulmonologist, neurologist)**, his parents were told that Seth had **(pleurisy, sarcoidosis, asthma)** involving inflammation of his **(nasal passages, pharynx, bronchial tubes)**.

8. Daisy had a habit of picking her nose. During the winter months, heat in her house caused drying of her nasal **(mucus, mucous, pleural)** membranes. She had frequent bouts of **(epistaxis, croup, stridor)**.

9. Seventy-five-year-old Beatrice had been a pack-a-day smoker all her life. Over the previous 3 months she noticed a persistent cough, weight loss, blood in her sputum **(hemoptysis, hematemesis, asbestosis)**, and dyspnea. A chest CT revealed a mass. Biopsy confirmed the diagnosis of **(tuberculosis, pneumoconiosis, adenocarcinoma)**, which is a type of **(small cell, non–small cell, lymph node)** lung cancer.

10. Carrie's lungs were normal at birth, but thick bronchial secretions soon blocked her **(arterioles, venules, bronchioles)**, which became inflamed. She was losing weight, and tests revealed inadequate amounts of pancreatic enzymes necessary for digestion of fats and proteins. Her pediatrician diagnosed her hereditary condition as **(chronic bronchitis, asthma, cystic fibrosis)**.

IX. Answers to Exercises

A

1. parietal pleura
2. adenoids
3. trachea
4. epiglottis
5. bronchi
6. mediastinum
7. paranasal sinuses
8. cilia
9. visceral pleura
10. pharynx
11. alveoli
12. larynx
13. bronchioles
14. palatine tonsils
15. hilum

B

1. uppermost part
2. oxygen
3. inspiration; inhalation
4. lobes
5. carbon dioxide
6. pleural cavity
7. expiration; exhalation
8. parenchyma
9. external
10. internal

C

1. chronic dilation of a bronchus
2. inflammation of pleura
3. air in the chest (pleural cavity)
4. lack of sense of smell
5. removal of the voice box
6. inflammation of the nose and throat
7. pertaining to the diaphragm
8. pertaining to an air sac
9. opening to the larynx
10. narrowing of the windpipe

D

1. hypercapnia
2. orthopnea
3. dyspnea
4. cyanosis
5. hemoptysis
6. hypoxia
7. pyothorax; empyema
8. dysphonia
9. hemothorax
10. epistaxis

E

1. abnormal crackling sounds heard on inspiration when there is fluid, blood, or pus in the alveoli
2. listening to sounds within the body
3. material expelled from the chest by coughing or clearing the throat
4. tapping on the surface to determine the underlying structure
5. coarse, loud rales caused by bronchial secretions
6. abnormal grating sound produced by the motion of pleural surfaces rubbing against each other (caused by inflammation or tumor cells)
7. pus-filled
8. sudden attack of difficult breathing associated with lying down at night (caused by congestive heart failure and pulmonary edema as the lungs fill with fluid)
9. fluid in the pleural cavity
10. area of dead tissue in the lung
11. strained, high-pitched inspirational sound
12. continuous high-pitched whistling sound heard when air is forced through a narrow space

F

1. diphtheria
2. croup
3. emphysema
4. chronic bronchitis
5. asthma
6. atelectasis
7. bronchogenic carcinoma
8. pertussis
9. cystic fibrosis
10. asbestosis
11. sarcoidosis

G

1. FEV_1 (forced expiratory volume in first second)
2. rhonchi
3. DLCO (diffusion capacity of the lung for carbon monoxide)
4. fibrosis
5. exudate
6. restrictive lung disease
7. obstructive lung disease
8. OSA (obstructive sleep apnea)
9. CPAP (continuous positive airway pressure)
10. palliative
11. PaO_2, $PaCO_2$

H

1. collection of pus in the lungs
2. swelling, fluid collection in the air sacs and bronchioles
3. abnormal condition of dust in the lungs
4. acute inflammation and infection of alveoli; they become filled with fluid and blood cells
5. floating clot or other material blocking the blood vessels of the lung
6. an infectious disease caused by rod-shaped bacilli and producing tubercles (nodes) of infection
7. collection of fluid in the pleural cavity
8. inflammation of pleura

9. abnormal condition of coal dust in the lungs (black-lung disease)
10. malignant tumor arising in the pleura; composed of mesothelium (epithelium

that covers the surfaces of membranes such as pleura and peritoneum)
11. excessive growth of cells in the adenoids (lymph tissue in the nasopharynx)

12. pain of the pleura (irritation of pleural surfaces leads to intercostal pain)
13. coughing up of material from the chest
14. rapid breathing; hyperventilation

I

1. endotracheal intubation
2. lung scan
3. tuberculin tests
4. thoracentesis
5. pulmonary function tests
6. tracheostomy
7. bronchoscopy
8. bronchial alveolar lavage
9. laryngoscopy
10. pulmonary angiography
11. mediastinoscopy
12. tube thoracostomy

J

1. dyspnea on exertion. H
2. paroxysmal nocturnal dyspnea. A
3. video-assisted thorascopy. E
4. cardiopulmonary resuscitation. I
5. non-small cell lung cancer. D
6. acute (adult) respiratory distress syndrome. J
7. chronic obstructive pulmonary disease. B
8. pulmonary function tests. G
9. purified protein derivative. C
10. diphtheria, pertussis, and tetanus. F

K

1. tonsillectomy
2. thoracentesis
3. rhinoplasty
4. thoracotomy
5. laryngectomy
6. lobectomy
7. thorascopy
8. pneumonectomy

L

1. thoracentesis
2. auscultation
3. PFTs
4. pneumonia
5. endotracheal tube
6. CXR; mediastinal
7. pulmonologist; asthma; bronchial tubes
8. mucous; epistaxis
9. hemoptysis; adenocarcinoma; non–small cell
10. bronchioles; cystic fibrosis

Answers to Practical Applications

1. C
2. B
3. A
4. B

X. Pronunciation of Terms

Pronunciation Guide

ā as in āpe　ă as in ăpple
ē as in ēven　ĕ as in ĕvery
ī as in īce　ĭ as in ĭnterest
ō as in ōpen　ŏ as in pŏt
ū as in ūnit　ŭ as in ŭnder

To test your understanding of the terminology in this chapter, write the meaning of each term in the space provided. In addition, you may wish to cover the terms and write them by looking at your definitions. Make sure your spelling is correct. The page number after each term indicates where it is defined or used in the text so you can easily check your responses.

Vocabulary and Terminology

Term	Pronunciation	Meaning
adenoidectomy (448)	ăd-ĕ-noyd-ĔK-tō-mē	
adenoid hypertrophy (448)	ĂD-ĕ-noyd hī-PĔR-trō-fē	
adenoids (446)	ĂD-ĕ-noydz	
alveolar (448)	ăl-VĒ-ō-lăr	
alveolus (alveoli) (446)	ăl-VĒ-ō-lŭs (ăl-VĒ-ō-lī)	
anosmia (452)	ăn-ŎS-mē-ă	
apex of the lung (446)	Ā-pĕkz of the lŭng	
apical (446)	Ā-pĭ-kăl	
apnea (453)	ăp-NĒ-ă	
asphyxia (453)	ăs-FĬK-sē-ă	
atelectasis (452)	ă-tĕ-LĔK-tă-sĭs	
base of the lung (446)	bās of the lung	
bronchiectasis (448)	brŏng-kē-ĔK-tă-sĭs	
bronchiole (446)	BRŎNG-kē-ŏl	
bronchiolitis (448)	brŏng-kē-ō-LĪ-tĭs	
bronchodilator (448)	brŏng-kō-DĪ-lā-tĕr	
bronchospasm (448)	BRŎNG-kō-spăzm	
bronchus (bronchi) (446)	BRŎNG-kŭs (BRŎNG-kī)	
carbon dioxide (446)	KĂR-bŏn dī-ŎK-sīd	
cilia (447)	SĬL-ē-ă	
cyanosis (449)	sī-ă-NŌ-sĭs	
diaphragm (447)	DĪ-ă-frăm	
dysphonia (450)	dĭs-FŌ-nē-ă	
dyspnea (453)	DĬSP-nē-ă	
empyema (452)	ĕm-pī-Ē-mă	

epiglottis (447)	ĕp-ĭ-GLŎT-ĭs	
epiglottitis (449)	ĕp-ĭ-glŏ-TĪ-tĭs	
expectoration (450)	ĕk-spĕk-tō-RĀ-shŭn	
expiration (447)	ĕks-pir-RĀ-shun	
glottis (447)	GLŎ-tĭs	
hemoptysis (453)	hē-MŎP-tĭ-sĭs	
hemothorax (453)	hē-mō-THŌ-răks	
hilum of the lung (447)	HĪ-lŭm of the lŭng	
hilar (447)	HĪ-lăr	
hypercapnia (449)	hī-pĕr-KĂP-nē-ă	
hyperpnea (453)	hī-PĔRP-nē-ă	
hypoxia (450)	hī-PŎK-sē-ă	
inspiration (447)	ĭn-spĭ-RĀ-shun	
laryngeal (449)	lă-RĬN-jē-ăl or lăr-ĭn-JĒ-ăl	
laryngospasm (449)	lă-RĬNG-gō-spăzm	
laryngitis (449)	lă-rĭn-JĪ-tĭs	
larynx (447)	LĂR-ĭnks	
lobectomy (449)	lō-BĔK-tō-mē	
mediastinoscopy (450)	mē-dē-ă-stī-NŎS-kō-pē	
mediastinum (447)	mē-dē-ă-STĪ-nŭm	
nasogastric intubation (450)	nā-zō-GĂS-trĭk ĭn-too-BĀ-shun	
orthopnea (450)	ŏr-thŏp-NĒ-ă	
oxygen (447)	ŎKS-ĭ-jĕn	
palatine tonsil (447)	PĂL-ĭ-tīn TŎN-sĭl	
paranasal sinus (447)	pă-ră-NĀ-zăl SĪ-nĭs	
parietal pleura (447)	pă-RĪ-ĕ-tăl PLOO-răh	

pharyngeal (450)	fă-RĬN-jē-ăl or făr-ĭn-JĒ-ăl	
pharynx (447)	FĂR-ĭnkz	
phrenic nerve (450)	FRĔN-ĭk nĕrv	
pleura (447)	PLOOR-ă	
pleural cavity (447)	PLOOR-ăl KĂ-vĭ-tē	
pleurodynia (450)	ploor-ō-DĬN-ē-ă	
pneumoconiosis (457)	nū-mō-kō-nē-Ō-sĭs	
pneumonectomy (450)	nū-mō-NĔK-tō-mē	
pneumothorax (450)	nū-mō-THŌ-răks	
pulmonary (451)	PŬL-mō-năr-ē	
pulmonary parenchyma (447)	pŭl-mō-NĂR-ē pă-RĔN-kă-mă	
pyothorax (453)	pī-ō-THŌ-răks	
respiration (451)	rĕs-pĕ-RĀ-shĕn	
rhinoplasty (451)	RĪ-nō-plăs-tē	
rhinorrhea (451)	rī-nō-RĒ-ăh	
sinusitis (451)	sī-nū-SĪ-tĭs	
spirometer (451)	spī-RŎM-ĕ-tĕr	
tachypnea (453)	tăk-ĭp-NĒ-ă	
thoracic (452)	thōr-RĂ-sĭk	
thoracoscopy (464)	thōr-ră-KŎS-kō-pē	
thoracotomy (452)	thōr-ră-KŎT-ō-mē	
tonsillectomy (452)	tŏn-sĭ-LĔK-tō-mē	
trachea (447)	TRĀ-kē-ă	
tracheal stenosis (452)	TRĀ-kē-ăl stĕ-NŌ-sĭs	
tracheotomy (452)	trā-kē-ŎT-ō-mē	
visceral pleura (447)	VĬ-sĕr-ăl PLOO-ră	

Pathological Conditions, Laboratory Tests, and Clinical Procedures

Term	Pronunciation	Meaning
anthracosis (459)	ăn-thră-KŌ-sĭs	
asbestosis (459)	ăs-bĕs-TŌ-sĭs	
asthma (455)	ĂZ-mă	
atelectasis (457)	ă-tĕ-LĔK-tă-sĭs	
auscultation (454)	ăw-skŭl-TĀ-shŭn	
bacilli (459)	bă-SĬL-ī	
bronchial alveolar lavage (462)	BRŎNG-kē-ăl ăl-vē-Ō-lar lă-VĂJ	
bronchiectasis (455)	brŏng-kē-ĔK-tă-sĭs	
bronchogenic carcinoma (456)	brŏng-kō-JĔN-ĭk kăr-sĭ-NŌ-mă	
bronchoscopy (462)	brŏng-KŎS-kō-pē	
chest tomograms (460)	chĕst TŌ-mō-grămz	
chronic bronchitis (456)	KRŎ-nĭk brŏng-KĪ-tĭs	
chronic obstructive pulmonary disease (459)	KRŎ-nĭk ŏb-STRŬK-tĭv PŬL-mō-nă-rē dĭ-ZĒZ	
computed tomography (460)	kom-PŪ-tid tō-MŎG-ră-fē	
cor pulmonale (459)	kŏr pŭl-mō-NĂ-lē	
croup (455)	kroop	
cystic fibrosis (456)	SĬS-tĭk fī-BRŌ-sĭs	
diphtheria (455)	dĭf-THĔR-ē-ă	
emphysema (457)	ĕm-fĭ-ZĒ-mă	
endotracheal intubation (462)	ĕn-dō-TRĀ-kē-ăl ĭn-tū-BĀ-shŭn	
epistaxis (455)	ĕp-ĭ-STĂK-sĭs	
exudate (459)	ĔK-sū-dāt	
hydrothorax (459)	hī-drō-THŎR-ăks	

laryngoscopy (462)	lăr-ĭng-GŎS-kō-pē	
lung biopsy (462)	lŭng BĪ-ŏp-sē	
magnetic resonance imaging (460)	măg-NĔ-tik RĔ-zō-năns Ĭm-ă-gĭng	
mediastinoscopy (463)	mē-dē-ă-stī-NŎS-kō-pē	
mesothelioma (458)	mĕz-ō-thē-lē-Ō-mă	
obstructive lung disease (463)	ŏb-STRŬK-tĭv lŭng dĭ-ZĒZ	
palliative (460)	PĂL-ē-ă-tĭv	
paroxysmal (460)	păr-ŏk-SĬZ-măl	
percussion (454)	pĕr-KŬSH-ŭn	
pertussis (455)	pĕr-TŬS-ĭs	
pleural effusion (459)	PLOOR-ăl ĕ-FŪ-zhŭn	
pleural rub (454)	PLOOR-ăl rŭb	
pleurisy (459)	PLOOR-ă-sē	
pneumonia (457)	nū-MŌ-nē-ă	
pneumothorax (459)	nū-mō-THŎR-ăks	
pulmonary abscess (457)	PŬL-mō-nă-rē ĂB-sĕs	
pulmonary angiography (460)	PŬL-mō-nă-rē ăn-jē-ŎG-ră-fē	
pulmonary edema (458)	PŬL-mō-nă-rē ĕ-DĒ-mă	
pulmonary embolism (458)	PŬL-mō-nă-rē ĔM-bō-lĭzm	
pulmonary fibrosis (458)	PŬL-mō-nă-rē fĭ-BRŌ-sĭs	
pulmonary function test (463)	PŬL-mō-nă-rē FŬNK-shŭn tĕst	
pulmonary infarction (460)	PŬL-mō-nă-rē ĭn-FĂRK-shŭn	
purulent (460)	PŪ-roo-lĕnt	
rales (454)	răhlz	
restrictive lung disease (463)	rē-STRĬK-tĭv lŭng dĭ-ZĒZ	

rhonchi (460)   RŎNG-kī   _____

sarcoidosis (458)   săr-koy-DŌ-sĭs   _____

silicosis (460)   sĭ-lĭ-KŌ-sĭs   _____

sputum (454)   SPŬ-tŭm   _____

stridor (454)   STRĪ-dŏr   _____

thoracentesis (464)   thō-ră-sĕn-TĒ-sĭs   _____

thorascopy (464)   thō-RĂS-kō-pē   _____

thoracotomy (464)   thō-ră-KŎ-tō-mē   _____

tracheostomy (464)   trā-kē-ŎS-tō-mē   _____

tuberculin test (464)   too-BĔR-kū-lĭn tĕst   _____

tuberculosis (458)   too-bĕr-kū-LŌ-sĭs   _____

tube thoracostomy (464)   tūb thŏr-ă-KŎS-tō-mē   _____

ventilation-
perfusion scan (462)   vĕn-tĭ-LĀ-shŭn-
pĕr-FŪ-shŭn scăn   _____

wheezes (454)   wēz-ĕz   _____

XI. Review Sheet

Write the meanings of the word parts in the spaces provided. Check your answers with the information in the chapter or in the glossary (Medical Terms—English) at the end of the book.

COMBINING FORMS

Combining Form	Meaning	Combining Form	Meaning
adenoid/o	_____	pector/o	_____
alveol/o	_____	pharyng/o	_____
bronch/o	_____	phon/o	_____
bronchi/o	_____	phren/o	_____
bronchiol/o	_____	pleur/o	_____
capn/o	_____	pneum/o	_____
coni/o	_____	pneumon/o	_____
cyan/o	_____	pulmon/o	_____
epiglott/o	_____	py/o	_____
hydr/o	_____	rhin/o	_____
laryng/o	_____	sinus/o	_____
lob/o	_____	spir/o	_____
mediastin/o	_____	tel/o	_____
nas/o	_____	thorac/o	_____
or/o	_____	tonsill/o	_____
orth/o	_____	trache/o	_____
ox/o	_____		

SUFFIXES

Suffix	Meaning	Suffix	Meaning
-algia	_____	-plasty	_____
-capnia	_____	-pnea	_____
-centesis	_____	-ptysis	_____
-dynia	_____	-rrhea	_____
-ectasis	_____	-scopy	_____
-ectomy	_____	-sphyxia	_____
-ema	_____	-stenosis	_____
-lysis	_____	-stomy	_____
-osmia	_____	-thorax	_____
-oxia	_____	-tomy	_____
-phonia	_____	-trophy	_____

PREFIXES

Prefix	Meaning	Prefix	Meaning
a-, an-	_____	hyper-	_____
brady-	_____	hypo-	_____
dys-	_____	para-	_____
em-	_____	per-	_____
eu-	_____	re-	_____
ex-	_____	tachy-	_____

chapter

Blood System

This chapter is divided into the following sections

In this chapter you will

- Identify terms relating to the composition, formation, and function of blood.
- Differentiate among the different types of blood groups.
- Identify terms related to blood clotting.
- Build words and recognize combining forms used in the blood system.
- Describe various pathological conditions affecting blood.
- Differentiate among various laboratory tests, clinical procedures, and abbreviations used in connection with the blood system.
- Apply your new knowledge to understanding medical terms in their proper contexts, such as medical reports and records.

I. Introduction

The primary function of blood is to maintain a constant environment for the other living tissues of the body. Blood transports foods, gases, and wastes to and from the cells of the body. Food, digested in the stomach and small intestine, passes into the bloodstream through the lining cells of the small intestine. Blood then carries these nutrients to all body cells. Oxygen enters the body through the air sacs of the lungs. Blood cells then transport the oxygen to cells throughout the body. Blood also helps remove the waste products released by cells. It carries gaseous waste (such as carbon dioxide) to the lungs to be exhaled. It carries solid waste, such as urea, to the kidneys to be expelled in the urine.

Blood transports chemical messengers called hormones from their sites of secretion in glands, such as the thyroid or pituitary, to distant sites where they regulate growth, reproduction, and energy production. These hormones will be discussed later in the endocrine chapter.

Finally, blood contains proteins and white blood cells that fight infection, and platelets (thrombocytes) that help the blood to clot.

II. Composition and Formation of Blood

Blood is composed of **cells,** or formed elements, suspended in a clear, straw-colored liquid called **plasma.** The cells constitute 45 percent of the blood volume and include **erythrocytes** (red blood cells), **leukocytes** (white blood cells), and **platelets** or **thrombocytes** (clotting cells). The remaining 55 percent of blood is plasma, a solution of water, proteins, sugar, salts, hormones, and vitamins.

Cells

Beginning at birth all blood cells originate in the marrow cavity of bones. Both the red blood cells that carry oxygen and the white blood cells that fight infection arise from the same blood-forming or hematopoietic **stem cells.** Under the influence of proteins in the bloodstream and bone marrow, stem cells change their size and shape to become specialized, or **differentiated.** In this process, the cells change in size from large (immature cells) to small (mature forms) and the cell nucleus shrinks (in red cells, the nucleus actually disappears). Figure 13–1 illustrates these changes in the formation of blood cells. Use Figure 13–1 as a reference as you learn the names of mature blood cells and their earlier forms.

Erythrocytes

As a red blood cell matures (from erythroblast to erythrocyte), it loses its nucleus and assumes the shape of a biconcave disk. This shape (a depressed or hollow surface on each side of the cell, resembling a cough drop with a thin central portion) allows for a large surface area so that absorption and release of gases (oxygen and carbon dioxide) can take place. Red cells contain the unique protein **hemoglobin,** composed of **heme** (iron-containing pigment) and **globin** (protein). Hemoglobin enables the erythrocyte to carry oxygen. The combination of oxygen and hemoglobin (oxyhemoglobin) produces the bright red color of blood.

Erythrocytes originate in the bone marrow. A hormone called **erythropoietin** (secreted by the kidney) stimulates their production (-*poiesis* means formation). Erythrocytes live

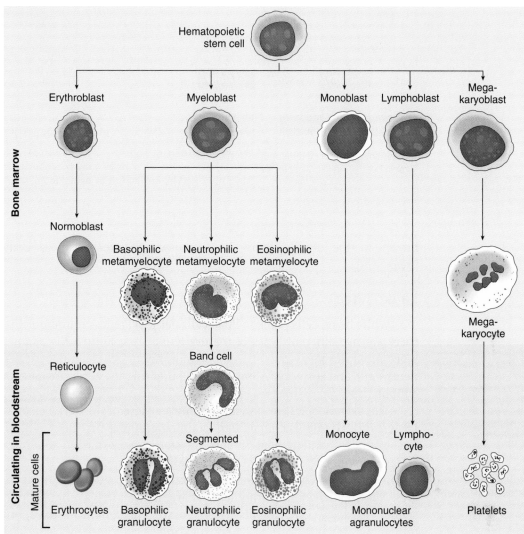

Figure 13–1

Stages in blood cell development (hematopoiesis). Notice that the suffix -blast is used to indicate immature forms of all cells. Band cells are identical to segmented granulocytes except that the nucleus is U-shaped and its lobes are connected by a band rather than by a thin thread, as in segmented forms.

and fulfill their role of transporting gases for about 120 days in the bloodstream. After this time, cells (called **macrophages**) in the spleen, liver, and bone marrow destroy the worn-out erythrocytes. Two to ten million red cells are destroyed each second, but because they are constantly replaced, the number of circulating cells remains constant (4 to 6 million per μL).

Macrophages break down erythrocytes and the hemoglobin within them into their heme and globin (protein) portions. The heme releases iron and decomposes into a yellow/orange pigment called **bilirubin.** The iron in hemoglobin is reutilized to form new red cells or is stored in the spleen, liver, or bone marrow. Bilirubin is excreted into bile by the liver, and from bile it enters the small intestine, where it is excreted in the stool. Its color then turns

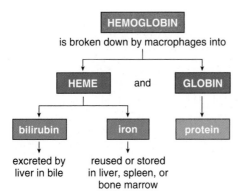

Figure 13–2

The breakdown of hemoglobin.

brown in the stool. Figure 13–2 reviews the sequence of events in hemoglobin breakdown.

Leukocytes

White blood cells (7000 to 9000 cells per μL) are less numerous than erythrocytes, but there are five different types of mature leukocytes. Figure 13–1 shows these five mature types of white blood cells: three polymorphonuclear granulocytic leukocytes (basophil, neutrophil, and eosinophil) and two mononuclear agranulocytic leukocytes (monocyte and lymphocyte).

The **granulocytes,** or **polymorphonuclear leukocytes,** are the most numerous (about 60 percent). **Basophils** contain dark-staining granules that stain with a basic (alkaline) dye. The granules contain heparin (an anticlotting substance) and histamine (a chemical released in allergic responses). **Eosinophils** contain granules that stain with eosin, a red acidic dye. They increase in allergic responses and engulf substances that trigger the allergies. **Neutrophils** contain granules that are neutral; they do not stain intensely with either acidic or basic dye. Neutrophils are **phagocytes** (**phag/o** means to eat or swallow) that accumulate at sites of infection, where they ingest and destroy bacteria. Figure 13–3 shows phagocytosis by a neutrophil.

Specific proteins, called **colony-stimulating factors** (CSFs) promote the growth of granulocytes in bone marrow. **G-CSF** (granulocyte CSF) and **GM-CSF** (granulocyte macrophage CSF), are given to restore granulocyte production in cancer patients. Erythropoietin, like CSFs, is produced by recombinant DNA techniques. It stimulates red blood cell production.

Although all granulocytes are **polymorphonuclear** (they have multilobed nuclei), the term **polymorphonuclear leukocyte (poly)** is used most often to describe the **neutrophil,** which is the most numerous of the granulocytes.

Mononuclear (containing one large nucleus) leukocytes do not have large numbers of granules in their cytoplasm, but they may have a few granules. These are **lymphocytes** and **monocytes** (see Fig. 13–1). Lymphocytes are made in lymph nodes and circulate both in the bloodstream and in the parallel circulating system, the lymphatic system.

Lymphocytes play an important role in the **immune** response that protects the body against infection. They can directly attack foreign matter and, in addition, make **antibodies,** which neutralize and can lead to the destruction of foreign **antigens** (bacteria and viruses). Monocytes are phagocytic cells that also fight disease. They move

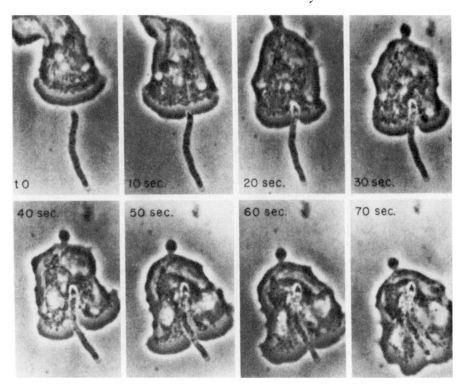

Figure 13-3

Phagocytosis (ingestion) of a bacterium by a neutrophil. (From Hirsch JG: Cinemicrophotographic observations of granule lysis in polymorphonuclear leukocytes during phagocytosis, J Exp Med 1962; 116:827, by copyright permission of Rockefeller University Press.)

from the bloodstream into tissues (as **macrophages**) and dispose of dead and dying cells and other tissue debris by phagocytosis.

Table 13–1 reviews the different types of leukocytes, their numbers in the blood, and their function.

 Table 13–1. **LEUKOCYTES**

Leukocyte	Percentage of Leukocytes in Blood	Function
GRANULOCYTES		
Basophil	0–1	Contains heparin (prevents clotting) and histamine (involved in allergic responses)
Eosinophil	1–4	Phagocytic cell involved in allergic reactions
Neutrophil	50–70	Phagocytic cell that accumulates at sites of infection
MONONUCLEARS		
Lymphocyte	20–40	Controls the immune response; makes antibodies to antigens
Monocyte	3–8	Phagocytic cell that becomes a macrophage and digests bacteria and tissue debris

Platelets

Platelets, or thrombocytes, are formed in red bone marrow from giant cells with multi-lobed nuclei called **megakaryocytes** (see Fig. 13–1). Tiny fragments of a megakaryocyte break off to form platelets. The main function of platelets is to help blood to clot. Specific terms related to blood clotting are discussed later in this chapter.

Plasma

Plasma, the liquid part of the blood, consists of water, dissolved proteins, sugar, wastes, salts, hormones, and other substances. The four major plasma proteins are **albumin, globulins, fibrinogen,** and **prothrombin** (the last two are clotting proteins).

Albumin maintains the proper proportion (and concentration) of water in the blood. Because albumin cannot pass easily through capillary walls, it remains in the blood and carries smaller molecules bound to its surface. It attracts water from the tissues back into the bloodstream and thus opposes the water's tendency to leave the blood and leak out into tissue spaces. **Edema** (swelling) results when too much fluid from blood "leaks" out into tissues. This happens in a mild form when a person ingests too much salt (water is retained in the blood and seeps out into tissues) and in a severe form when a person is burned in a fire. In this situation albumin escapes from capillaries as a result of the burn injury. Then water cannot be held in the blood; it escapes through the skin and blood volume drops.

Globulins are another part of blood containing plasma proteins. These are alpha, beta, and gamma globulins. The gamma globulins are **immunoglobulins,** which are antibodies that bind to and sometimes destroy antigens (foreign substances). Examples of immunoglobulin antibodies are **IgG** (found in high concentration in plasma) and **IgA** (found in breast milk, saliva, tears, and respiratory mucus). Other immunoglobulins are **IgM, IgD,** and **IgE.** Immunoglobulins are separated from other plasma proteins by **electrophoresis.** In this process, an electric current passes through a solution of plasma.

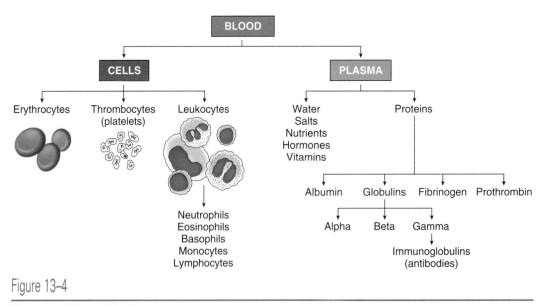

Figure 13-4

The composition of blood.

The different proteins in plasma separate as they migrate at different speeds to the source of the electricity.

Plasmapheresis (-apheresis means to remove) is the process of separating plasma from cells and then removing the plasma from the patient. In plasmapheresis, the entire blood sample is spun in a centrifuge machine, and the plasma, being lighter in weight than the cells, moves to the top of the sample.

Figure 13–4 reviews the composition of blood.

III. Blood Groups

Transfusions of "whole blood" (cells and plasma) are used to replace blood lost after injury, during surgery, or in severe shock. A patient who is severely anemic and needs only red blood cells will receive a transfusion of packed red cells (whole blood with most of the plasma removed). Human blood falls into four main groups: A, B, AB, and O. There are harmful effects of transfusing blood from a donor of one blood group into a recipient who has blood of another blood group. Therefore, before blood is transfused, both the blood donor and the blood recipient are tested to be certain that the transfused blood will be compatible with the recipient.

Each of the blood groups has a specific combination of factors called **antigens** and **antibodies.** Blood group antigens are inherited, and antibodies are acquired by 6 months of age after exposure to antigens. The antigen and antibody factors of blood groups are:

Type A, containing **A antigen** and **anti-B antibody**

Type B, containing **B antigen** and **anti-A antibody**

Type AB, containing **A and B antigens** and **no anti-A or anti-B antibodies**

Type O, containing **no A or B antigens** and **both anti-A and anti-B antibodies**

The problem in transfusing blood from a type A donor into a type B recipient is that A antigens (from the A donor) will react adversely with the anti-A antibodies in the recipient's type B bloodstream. The accidental adverse reaction is **hemolysis,** or breakdown of blood cells. Intravascular hemolysis may lead to **disseminated intravascular coagulation (DIC),** a serious coagulopathy. Similar problems can occur in other transfusions if the donor's antigens are incompatible with the recipient's antibodies.

People with type O blood are known as universal donors because their blood contains neither A nor B antigens. The anti-A and anti-B antibodies in O blood do not have an effect in the recipient because the antibodies are diluted in the recipient's bloodstream. Those with type AB blood are known as universal recipients because their blood contains neither anti-A nor anti-B antibodies, so that neither the A nor the B group antigens will cause hemolysis in their blood.

Besides A and B antigens, many other antigens are located on the surface of red blood cells. One of these is called the **Rh factor** (named because it was first found in the blood of a rhesus monkey). The term Rh-positive refers to a person who is born with the Rh antigen on her or his red blood cells. An Rh-negative person does not have the Rh antigen. There are no anti-Rh antibodies normally present in the blood of an Rh-positive or an Rh-negative person. However, if Rh-positive blood is transfused into an Rh-negative person, the recipient may, but not always, begin to develop antibodies that would cause hemolysis of Rh-positive blood if another transfusion were to occur subsequently.

The same reactions occur during pregnancy if the fetus of an Rh-negative woman happens to be Rh-positive. This situation is described in Chapter 4 as an example of an antigen–antibody reaction.

Table 13–2. BLOOD GROUPS

Type	Percentage in Population	Red Cell Antigens	Plasma Antibodies
A	41	A	Anti-B
B	10	B	Anti-A
AB	4	A and B	Neither anti-A nor anti-B
O	45	Neither A nor B	Anti-A and anti-B
Rh positive	85	Rh factor	No anti-Rh
Rh negative	15	No Rh factor	Anti-Rh (occurs if an Rh-negative person is given Rh-positive blood)

Table 13–2 shows the blood group types, their frequency of occurrence in the population, and their antigens and antibodies.

IV. Blood Clotting

Blood clotting, or **coagulation,** is a complicated process involving many different substances and chemical reactions. The final result (usually taking less than 15 minutes) is the formation of a **fibrin clot** from the plasma protein **fibrinogen.** Platelets are important in beginning the process following injury to tissues or blood vessels. The platelets clump, or aggregate, at the site of injury. Then in combination with a protein tissue factor, other clotting factors and calcium promote the formation of a fibrin clot. One of the clotting factors is clotting factor VIII. It is missing in some people who are born with hemophilia. Other hemophiliacs are missing factor IX. Figure 13–5 reviews the basic sequence of events in the clotting process.

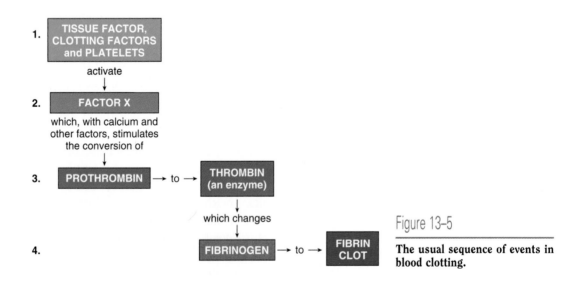

Figure 13–5

The usual sequence of events in blood clotting.

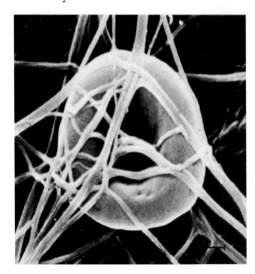

Figure 13–6

A red blood cell enmeshed in threads of fibrin. (From Page J, et al: Blood: The River of Life. Washington DC, U.S. News Books, 1981, p. 79.)

The fibrin threads form the clot by trapping red blood cells and platelets and plasma (Fig. 13–6 shows a red blood cell trapped by fibrin threads). Then the clot retracts into a tight ball, leaving behind a clear fluid called **serum.** Normally, clots (thrombi) do not form in blood vessels unless the vessel is damaged or the flow of blood is impeded. Anticoagulant substances in the bloodstream inhibit blood clotting, so thrombi and emboli (floating clots) do not form. **Heparin,** produced by tissue cells (especially in the liver), is an example of an anticoagulant. Other drugs such as **warfarin (Coumadin),** are given to patients with thromboembolic diseases to prevent the formation of clots and emboli.

V. Vocabulary

This list will help you review many of the new terms introduced in the text. Short definitions will reinforce your understanding of the terms. See Section XII of this chapter for help in pronouncing the more difficult terms.

albumin   Protein in blood; maintains the proper amount of water in the blood.

antibody   Protein (immunoglobulin) produced by lymphocytes in response to bacteria, viruses, or other antigens. An antibody is specific to an antigen and inactivates it.

antigen   A substance (usually foreign) that stimulates the production of an antibody.

basophil   Granulocytic white blood cell with granules that stain blue when exposed to a basic dye.

bilirubin	Orange-yellow pigment in bile. It is formed by the breakdown of hemoglobin when red blood cells die.
coagulation	Blood clotting.
colony-stimulating factor (CSF)	Protein that stimulates the growth and proliferation of white blood cells (granulocytes).
differentiation	Change in structure and function of a cell as it matures; specialization.
electrophoresis	Method of separating serum proteins by electrical charge.
eosinophil	Granulocytic white blood cell with granules that stain red with the acidic dye eosin; associated with allergic reactions.
erythrocyte	Red blood cell. There are about 5 million per microliter (μL) or cubic millimeter (mm^3) of blood.
erythropoietin (EPO)	Hormone secreted by the kidneys that stimulates formation of red blood cells.
fibrin	Protein threads that form the basis of a blood clot.
fibrinogen	Plasma protein that is converted to fibrin in the clotting process.
globulins	Part of blood containing different plasma proteins. Immunoglobulins and alpha and beta globulins are examples.
granulocyte	White blood cell with numerous dark-staining granules: eosinophil, neutrophil, and basophil.
heme	Iron-containing nonprotein portion of the hemoglobin molecule.
hemoglobin	Blood protein containing iron; carries oxygen in red blood cells.
hemolysis	Destruction or breakdown of blood (red blood cells).
heparin	Anticoagulant found in blood and tissue cells.
immune reaction	Response of the immune system to foreign invasion.
immunoglobulin	Protein (globulin) with antibody activity; examples are IgG, IgM, IgA, IgE, IgD. Immun/o means protection.
leukocyte	White blood cell.

lymphocyte	Mononuclear leukocyte that produces antibodies.
macrophage	Monocyte that migrates from the blood to tissue spaces. It is a large phagocyte.
megakaryocyte	Large platelet precursor cell formed in the bone marrow.
monocyte	Large mononuclear phagocytic leukocyte formed in bone marrow. Monocytes become macrophages as they leave the blood and enter body tissues.
mononuclear	Pertaining to a cell (leukocyte) with a single round nucleus; lymphocytes and monocytes are mononuclear leukocytes.
neutrophil	Granulocytic leukocyte formed in bone marrow; a phagocyte with neutral-staining granules; also called a **polymorphonuclear leukocyte,** or **poly.**
plasma	Liquid portion of blood; contains water, proteins, salts, nutrients, hormones, and vitamins.
plasmapheresis	Removal of plasma from withdrawn blood by centrifuge. Cells are retransfused into the donor. Fresh-frozen plasma or salt solution is used to replace withdrawn plasma.
platelet	Smallest blood cell (thrombocyte); clumps at sites of injury to prevent bleeding and facilitate clotting.
prothrombin	Plasma protein; converted to thrombin in the clotting process.
reticulocyte	Immature erythrocyte with a network of strands (reticulin) that can be seen after staining the cells with special dyes.
Rh factor	Antigen on red blood cells of Rh-positive individuals. The factor was first identified in the blood of a rhesus monkey.
serum	Plasma minus clotting proteins and cells. Clear, yellowish fluid that separates from blood when it is allowed to clot. It is formed from plasma, but does not contain protein-coagulation factors.
stem cell	Bone marrow cell that gives rise to different types of blood cells; hematopoietic stem cell.
thrombin	Enzyme that converts fibrinogen to fibrin during coagulation.
thrombocyte	Platelet.

VI. Combining Forms, Suffixes, and Terminology

Write the meanings of the medical terms in the spaces provided.

Combining Forms

Combining Form	Meaning	Terminology	Meaning
bas/o	base (*alkaline,* the opposite of acid)	basophil _____ *-phil means attraction to.*	
chrom/o	color	hypochromic _____ *Pertaining to a type of anemia with decreased hemoglobin in erythrocytes.*	
coagul/o	clotting	anticoagulant _____ coagulopathy _____ *Disseminated intravascular coagulopathy (DIC) results from clotting and anticlotting processes in response to injury or disease.*	
cyt/o	cell	cytology _____	
eosin/o	red, dawn, rosy	eosinophil _____	
erythr/o	red	erythrocytopenia _____ *-penia means deficiency.*	
granul/o	granules	granulocyte _____	
hem/o	blood	hemolysis _____ *Destruction of red blood cells. See hemolytic anemia, page 502, Section VII, Pathological Conditions.*	
hemat/o	blood	hematocrit _____ *-crit means to separate. The hematocrit gives the percentage of red blood cells in a volume of blood. See page 507, Section VIII, under Laboratory Tests.*	
hemoglobin/o	hemoglobin	hemoglobinopathy _____	

is/o	same, equal	anisocytosis _____

An abnormality of red blood cells; they are of unequal (anis/o) size; -cytosis means an increase in the number of cells.

kary/o	nucleus	megakaryocyte _____

leuk/o	white	leukocytopenia _____

Usually is shortened to leukopenia.

mon/o	one, single	monocyte _____

The cell has a single, rather than a multilobed, nucleus.

morph/o	shape, form	morphology _____

myel/o	bone marrow	myeloblast _____

-blast indicates an immature cell.

myelogenous _____

-genous means pertaining to produced in.

neutr/o	neutral (neither base nor acid)	neutropenia _____

This term refers to neutrophils.

nucle/o	nucleus	mononuclear _____

polymorphonuclear _____

phag/o	eat, swallow	phagocyte _____

poikil/o	varied, irregular	poikilocytosis _____

Irregularity in the shape of red blood cells. Poikilocytosis occurs in certain types of anemia.

sider/o	iron	sideropenia _____

spher/o	globe, round	spherocytosis _____

In this condition, the erythrocyte has a round shape, making the cell fragile and easily able to be destroyed.

thromb/o	clot	thrombocytopenia _____

Suffixes			
Suffix	Meaning	Terminology	Meaning

-apheresis	removal, carry away	plasmapheresis	_____
		A centrifuge spins blood to remove plasma from the other parts of blood.	
		leukapheresis	_____
		plateletpheresis	_____
		Note that the "a" of apheresis is dropped in this term. Platelets are removed from the donor's blood (and used in a patient), and the remainder of the blood is reinfused into the donor.	
-blast	immature, embryonic	monoblast	_____
		erythroblast	_____
-cytosis	abnormal condition of cells (increase in cells)	macrocytosis	_____
		Macrocytes are erythrocytes that are larger (macro-) than normal size.	
		microcytosis	_____
		These are erythrocytes that are smaller (micro-) than normal size. Table 13–3 reviews terms related to abnormalities of red blood cell morphology.	

Table 13–3. **ABNORMALITIES OF RED BLOOD CELL MORPHOLOGY**

ABNORMALITY	DESCRIPTION
Anisocytosis	Cells are **unequal** in size
Hypo**chromia**	Cells have reduced **color** (less hemoglobin)
Macrocytosis	Cells are **large**
Microcytosis	Cells are **small**
Poikilocytosis	Cells are **irregularly shaped**
Spherocytosis	Cells are **rounded**

-emia	blood condition	leukemia _____

See page 504, Section VII, Pathological Conditions.

-globin	protein	hemoglobin _____

-globulin	protein	immunoglobulin _____

-lytic	pertaining to destruction	thrombolytic therapy _____

Used to dissolve clots.

-oid	derived from	myeloid _____

-osis	abnormal condition	thrombosis _____

-penia	deficiency	granulocytopenia _____
		pancytopenia _____

-phage	eat, swallow	macrophage _____

A large phagocyte that destroys worn-out red blood cells and foreign material.

-philia	attraction for (an increase in cell numbers)	eosinophilia _____
		neutrophilia _____

-phoresis	carrying, transmission	electrophoresis _____

-poiesis	formation	hematopoiesis _____
		erythropoiesis _____

Erythropoietin is produced by the kidneys to stimulate erythrocyte formation.

		myelopoiesis _____

-stasis	stop, control	hemostasis _____

VII. Pathological Conditions

Any abnormal or pathological condition of the blood is generally referred to as a blood **dyscrasia** (disease). The blood dyscrasias discussed in this section are organized in the following manner: diseases of red blood cells, disorders of blood clotting, diseases of white blood cells, and disease of the bone marrow.

Diseases of Red Blood Cells

anemia	**Deficiency in erythrocytes or hemoglobin.**

The most common type of anemia is **iron-deficiency anemia;** it is caused by a lack of iron, which is required for hemoglobin production (see Fig. 13–7). Other types of anemia include:

1. aplastic anemia

Failure of blood cell production due to aplasia (absence of development, formation) of bone marrow cells.

The cause of most cases of aplastic anemia is unknown (idiopathic), but some cases have been linked to benzene exposure and to antibiotics such as chloramphenicol. **Pancytopenia** occurs as stem cells fail to produce leukocytes, platelets, and erythrocytes. Blood transfusions prolong life, allowing the marrow time to resume its normal functioning, and antibiotics control infections. Bone marrow transplants and drugs that inhibit the immune system have been successful as therapy in cases where spontaneous recovery is unlikely.

2. hemolytic anemia

Reduction in red cells due to excessive destruction.

One example of hemolytic anemia is **congenital spherocytic anemia** (also called **hereditary spherocytosis**). Instead of their normal biconcave shape, erythrocytes are spheroidal. This shape makes them fragile and easily destroyed (hemolysis). Shortened red cell survival results in increased reticulocytes in blood as the bone marrow compensates for hemolysis of mature erythrocytes. Because the spleen destroys red cells, removing the spleen usually improves this anemia. Figure 13–8 shows the altered shape of erythrocytes in hereditary spherocytosis.

A 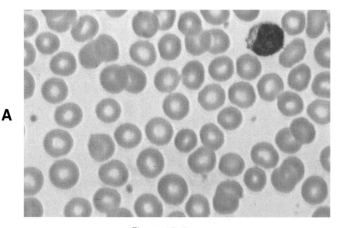 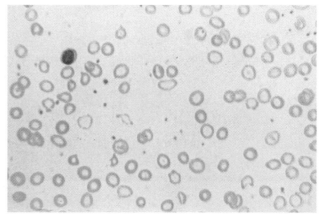 **B**

Figure 13-7

Normal red blood cells and iron-deficiency anemia. (A) Normal red cells. Erythrocytes are fairly uniform in size and shape. The red cells are normal in hemoglobin content (normochromic) and size (normocytic). **(B) Iron-deficiency anemia.** Many erythrocytes are smaller (microcytic) than the nucleus of the small lymphocyte and have increased central pallor (hypochromic). Red cells in this slide demonstrate variation in size (anisocytosis) and shape (poikilocytosis). (From Tkachuk DC, Hirschmann JV, McArthur JR: Atlas of Clinical Hematology. Philadelphia, WB Saunders, 2002, p. 4.)

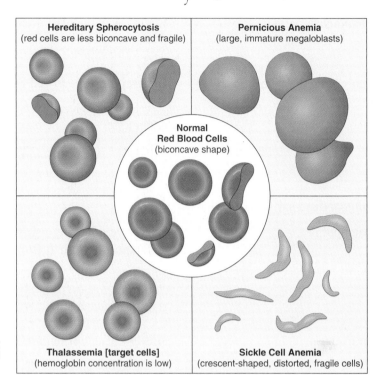

Figure 13–8

Normal red blood cells and several types of anemia.

Inside figure:

Hereditary Spherocytosis
(red cells are less biconcave and fragile)

Pernicious Anemia
(large, immature megaloblasts)

Normal Red Blood Cells
(biconcave shape)

Thalassemia [target cells]
(hemoglobin concentration is low)

Sickle Cell Anemia
(crescent-shaped, distorted, fragile cells)

3. pernicious anemia

Lack of mature erythrocytes caused by inability to absorb vitamin B$_{12}$ into the body. (Pernicious means "ruinous" or "hurtful.")

Vitamin B$_{12}$ is necessary for the proper development and maturation of erythrocytes. Although vitamin B$_{12}$ is a common constituent of food matter (liver, kidney, sardines, egg yolks, oysters), it cannot be absorbed into the bloodstream without the aid of a special substance called **intrinsic factor** that is normally found in gastric juice. Individuals with pernicious anemia lack this factor in their gastric juice, and the result is unsuccessful maturation of red blood cells, with an excess of large, immature, and poorly functioning cells in the bone marrow and large, often oral red cells (macrocytes) in the circulation. Treatment is administration of vitamin B$_{12}$ for life. Figure 13–8 illustrates pernicious anemia.

4. sickle cell anemia

A hereditary condition characterized by abnormal shape of erythrocytes and by hemolysis.

The crescent, or sickle, shape of the erythrocyte is caused by an abnormal type of hemoglobin (hemoglobin S) in the red cell (see Fig. 13–8). The distorted, fragile erythrocytes cannot pass through small blood vessels normally, leading to thrombosis and infarction (dead tissue). Symptoms include arthralgias, acute attacks of abdominal pain, and ulcerations of the extremities. The genetic defect (presence of the hemoglobin S gene) is particularly prevalent in black persons of African or African-American ancestry and appears with different degrees of severity. Individuals who inherit just one gene for the trait usually do not have symptoms.

5. thalassemia

An inherited defect in the ability to produce hemoglobin, usually seen in persons of Mediterranean background.

This condition presents in varying forms and degrees of severity and usually leads to hypochromic anemia with diminished hemoglobin content in red cells (see Fig. 13–8). *Thalassa* is a Greek word meaning "sea."

hemochromatosis | **Excess iron deposits throughout the body.**

Hepatomegaly, skin pigmentation, diabetes, and cardiac failure may occur.

polycythemia vera | **General increase in red blood cells (erythremia).**

Blood consistency is viscous (thick) because of greatly increased numbers of erythrocytes. The bone marrow is hyperplastic, and leukocytosis and thrombocytosis commonly accompany the increase in red blood cells. Treatment consists of reduction of red cell volume to normal levels by phlebotomy (removal of blood from a vein) and by suppressing blood cell production with myelotoxic drugs.

Disorders of Blood Clotting

hemophilia | **Excessive bleeding caused by hereditary lack of one of the protein substances (either factor VIII or factor IX) necessary for blood clotting.**

Although the platelet count of a hemophiliac patient is normal, deficiency in clotting factors (VIII or IX), result in a prolonged coagulation time. Treatment consists of administration of the deficient factor.

purpura | **Multiple pinpoint hemorrhages and accumulation of blood under the skin.**

Hemorrhages into the skin and mucous membranes produce red-purple discoloration of the skin. Purpura can be caused by having too few platelets (thrombocytopenia). The cause may be immunologic, meaning the body produces an antiplatelet factor that harms its own platelets. **Autoimmune thrombocytopenic purpura** (previously idiopathic thrombocytopenia purpura) is a condition in which a patient makes an antibody that destroys platelets. Bleeding time is prolonged; splenectomy (the spleen is the site of platelet destruction) and drug therapy with corticosteroids are common treatments.

Diseases of White Blood Cells

leukemia | **An increase in cancerous white blood cells.**

Malignant leukocytes fill the marrow and bloodstream. The terms **acute** and **chronic** discriminate between leukemias of primarily immature (acute) or mature (chronic) leukocytes.

Acute leukemias have common clinical characteristics: abrupt, stormy onset of symptoms, fatigue, fever, bleeding, bone pain and tenderness, lymphadenopathy, splenomegaly, hepatomegaly, and CNS symptoms, such as headache, vomiting, and paralysis. Four types of leukemia are:

1. **Acute myelogenous (myelocytic) leukemia (AML).** Immature granulocytes (myeloblasts) predominate. Platelets and erythrocytes are diminished because of infiltration and replacement of the bone marrow by large numbers of myeloblasts (see Fig. 13–9A).
2. **Acute lymphocytic leukemia (ALL).** Immature lymphocytes (lymphoblasts) predominate. This form is seen most often in children and adolescents; onset is sudden (Fig. 13–9B).
3. **Chronic myelogenous (myelocytic) leukemia (CML).** Both mature and immature granulocytes are present in the marrow and bloodstream. This is a slowly progressive illness with which patients (often adults over

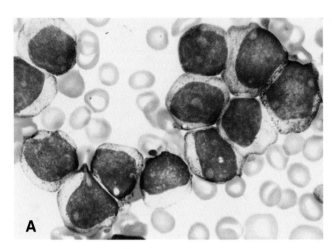 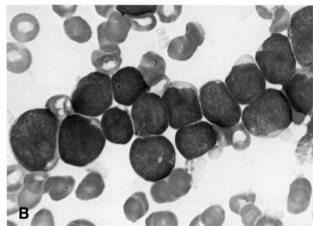

Figure 13–9

Acute leukemia. (A) Acute myeloblastic leukemia. Myeloblasts (immature granulocytes) predominate. AML affects primarily adults. The majority of patients achieve remission with intensive chemotherapy, but relapse is common. Hematopoietic stem cell transplantation may be a curative therapy. **(B) Acute lymphoblastic leukemia.** Lymphoblasts (immature lymphocytes) predominate. ALL is a disease of children and young adults. Most children are cured with chemotherapy. (Courtesy Dr. Robert W. McKenna, Department of Pathology, University of Texas Southwestern Medical School, Dallas, TX; from Kumar V, Cotran RS, Robbins SL: Basic Pathology, 7th ed. Philadelphia, WB Saunders, 2003, p. 424.)

55 years old) may live for many years without encountering life-threatening problems. New therapies (such as the drug Gleevec) target abnormal proteins responsible for malignancy.

4. **Chronic lymphocytic leukemia (CLL).** Abnormal numbers of relatively mature lymphocytes predominate in the marrow, lymph nodes, and spleen. This most common form of leukemia usually occurs in the elderly and follows a slowly progressive course.

All forms of leukemia are treated with chemotherapy, using drugs that prevent cell division and selectively injure rapidly dividing cells. Effective treatment can lead to a **remission** (disappearance of signs of disease). **Relapse** occurs when leukemia cells reappear in the blood and bone marrow, necessitating further treatment.

Transplantation of normal bone marrow from donors of similar tissue type is successful in restoring normal bone marrow function in some patients with acute leukemia. This procedure is performed following high-dose chemotherapy, which is administered to eliminate the leukemic cells.

granulocytosis **Abnormal increase in granulocytes in the blood.**

An increase in neutrophils in the blood may occur in response to infection or inflammation of any type. **Eosinophilia** is an increase in eosinophilic granulocytes, seen in certain allergic conditions, such as asthma, or in parasitic infections (tapeworm, pinworm). **Basophilia** is an increase in basophilic granulocytes seen in certain types of leukemia.

mononucleosis	**An infectious disease marked by increased numbers of leukocytes and enlarged cervical lymph nodes.**

This disease is caused by the Epstein-Barr virus (EBV). Lymphadenitis is present, with fever, fatigue, asthenia (weakness), and pharyngitis. Atypical lymphocytes are present in the blood, liver (hepatomegaly), and spleen (splenomegaly).

Mononucleosis is usually transmitted by direct oral contact (salivary exchange during kissing) and affects primarily young adults. No treatment is necessary for EBV infections. Antibiotics are not effective for self-limited viral illnesses. Rest during the period of acute symptoms and slow return to normal activities is advised.

Diseases of Bone Marrow Cells

multiple myeloma	**Malignant neoplasm of bone marrow.**

The malignant cells destroy bone tissue and cause overproduction of immunoglobulins, including **Bence Jones protein,** an immunoglobulin fragment found in urine. The condition leads to osteolytic lesions, hypercalcemia, anemia, renal damage, and increased susceptibility to infection. Treatment is with analgesics, radiotherapy, **palliative** (relieving, not curing) doses of chemotherapy, and special orthopedic supports.

VIII. Laboratory Tests, Clinical Procedures, and Abbreviations

Laboratory Tests

antiglobulin test (Coombs test)	**Test for the presence of antibodies that coat and damage erythrocytes**

This test determines the presence of antibodies in infants of Rh-negative women or in patients with autoimmune hemolytic anemia.

bleeding time	**Time required for blood to stop flowing from a tiny puncture wound.**

Normal time is 8 minutes or less. The Simplate or Ivy method is used. Platelet disorders and the use of aspirin prolong bleeding time.

coagulation time	**Time required for venous blood to clot in a test tube.**

Normal time is less than 15 minutes.

complete blood count (CBC)	**Determination of the number of red and white blood cells, platelets, hemoglobin, hematocrit, and red cell indices—MCH, MCV, MCHC** (see Abbreviations).

erythrocyte sedimentation rate (ESR or sed rate)	**Speed at which erythrocytes settle out of plasma.**

Venous blood is collected into an anticoagulant, and the blood is placed in a tube in a vertical position. The distance that the erythrocytes fall in a given period of time is the sedimentation rate. The rate increases with infections, joint inflammation, and tumor, which increase the fibrinogen content of the blood.

hematocrit (Hct)	**Percentage of erythrocytes in a volume of blood.**

A sample of blood is spun in a centrifuge so that the erythrocytes fall to the bottom of the sample.

hemoglobin test (H, Hg, HGB)	**Total amount of hemoglobin in a sample of peripheral blood.**

partial thromboplastin time (PTT)	**Measures the presence of plasma factors that act in a portion of the coagulation pathway.**

This test is used to follow patients taking anticoagulants, such as heparin.

platelet count	**Number of platelets per cubic millimeter (mm^3) or microliter (μL) of blood.**

Platelets normally average between 150,000 and 350,000 per mm^3 (cu mm) or μL.

prothrombin time (PT)	**Test of the ability of blood to clot.**

The test measures the time elapsed between the addition of calcium and tissue factor (thromboplastin) to a plasma sample and the appearance of a visible clot.

red blood cell count (RBC)	**Number of erythrocytes per cubic millimeter (mm^3) or microliter (μL) of blood.**

The normal number is 4 to 6 million per mm^3 or μL.

red blood cell morphology	**Microscopic examination of a stained blood smear to determine the shape of individual red cells.**

Abnormal morphology includes anisocytosis, poikilocytosis, and sickle cells.

white blood cell count (WBC)	**Number of leukocytes per cubic millimeter (mm^3) or microliter (μL).**

Automated counting devices record numbers with seconds. Normal number of leukocytes average between 5000 and 10,000 per mm^3 or μL.

white blood cell differential	**Determines the percentage of the total WBC made up by different types of leukocytes.**

Some instruments can produce automated differentials, but otherwise the cells are stained and counted under a microscope by a technician. Percentages of neutrophils, eosinophils, basophils, monocytes, lymphocytes, and immature cells are determined.

The term "shift to the left" describes an increase in immature neutrophils in the blood.

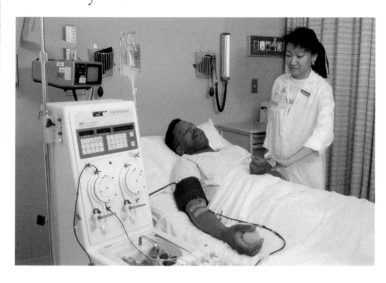

Figure 13-10

Leukapheresis. This machine is an automated blood cell separator that removes large numbers of white blood cells and returns red cells, platelets, and plasma to the individual. (From Black JM, Hawks JH, Keene AM: Medical-Surgical Nursing: Clinical Management for Positive Outcomes, 6th ed. Philadelphia, WB Saunders, 2001, p. 2170.)

Clinical Procedures

apheresis

Separation of blood into component parts and removal of a select part from the blood.

This procedure can remove toxic substances or autoantibodies from the blood and can collect blood cells. Leukapheresis, plateletpheresis, and plasmapheresis are examples (see Fig. 13–10). If plasma is removed from the patient and fresh plasma is given, the procedure is termed **plasma exchange.**

blood transfusion

Whole blood or cells are taken from a donor and infused into a patient.

Appropriate testing to ensure a match of red blood cell type (A, B, AB, or O) is essential. Tests are also performed to detect the presence of hepatitis and the acquired immunodeficiency syndrome (AIDS) virus. **Autologous transfusion** is the collection and later reinfusion of a patient's own blood or blood components.

bone marrow biopsy

Microscopic examination of a core of bone marrow removed with a needle.

This procedure is helpful in the diagnosis of blood disorders such as anemia, cell deficiencies, and leukemia. Bone marrow may also be removed by brief suction produced by a syringe, which is termed a **bone marrow aspirate.**

hematopoietic stem cell transplant

Peripheral stem cells from a compatible donor are administered into a recipient's vein.

Patients with malignant hematologic disease, such as AML, ALL, CLL, CML, and multiple myeloma, are candidates for this treatment. First the donor is treated with a drug that mobilizes stem cells into the blood. Then stem cells are removed from the donor, a process like leukapheresis in Figure 13–10. Meanwhile, the patient undergoes a conditioning process in which radiation and chemotherapy are administered to kill malignant marrow cells and inactivate the patient's immune system so that subsequent stem cells will not be rejected. A cell suspension containing the donor's stem cells, which will repopulate the bone marrow, is then given through a vein to the recipient. A **bone marrow transplant** follows the same procedure, except bone marrow cells are removed and used rather than peripheral stem cells (see Fig. 13–11). Problems encountered subsequently may be serious infection, **graft versus host disease** (immune reaction of the donor's cells to the recipient's), and relapse of the original disease despite the treatment.

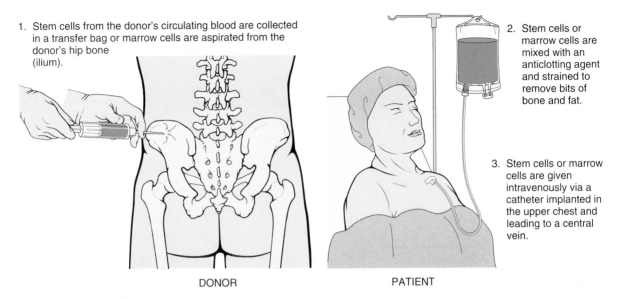

1. Stem cells from the donor's circulating blood are collected in a transfer bag or marrow cells are aspirated from the donor's hip bone (ilium).

2. Stem cells or marrow cells are mixed with an anticlotting agent and strained to remove bits of bone and fat.

3. Stem cells or marrow cells are given intravenously via a catheter implanted in the upper chest and leading to a central vein.

DONOR   PATIENT

Figure 13–11

Hematopoietic stem cell and bone marrow transplant. This is an **allogeneic** (all/o means other, different) **transplant** in which a relative or unrelated person having a close HLA (human leukocyte antigen) type is the donor. It has a high rate of morbidity (causing disease) and mortality (causing death) because of complications of incompatibility such as GVHD (graft versus host disease). In an **autologous transplant,** stem cells or bone marrow cells are removed from the patient during a remission phase and given back to the patient after intensive chemotherapy (drug treatment).

Abbreviations

ABO	three main blood types	**ESR**	erythrocyte sedimentation rate
ALL	acute lymphocytic leukemia	**G-CSF**	granulocyte colony-stimulating factor
AML	acute myelogenous leukemia	**GM-CSF**	granulocyte macrophage colony-stimulating factor
ASCT	autologous stem cell transplant	**g/dL**	gram per deciliter (deciliter = one tenth of a liter)
baso	basophils		
BMT	bone marrow transplant	**GVHD**	graft versus host disease
CBC	complete blood count	**Hct**	hematocrit
CLL	chronic lymphocytic leukemia	**H, Hg, HGB**	hemoglobin
CML	chronic myelogenous leukemia	**H and H**	hemoglobin and hematocrit
DIC	disseminated intravascular coagulation	**HLA**	human leukocyte antigen
diff.	differential count (white blood cells)	**IgA, IgD, IgE, IgG, IgM**	immunoglobulins
EBV	Epstein-Barr virus, the cause of mononucleosis	**lymphs**	lymphocytes
eos	eosinophils	**MCH**	mean corpuscular hemoglobin, average amount of hemoglobin per cell
EPO	erythropoietin		

Continued on following page

MCHC	mean corpuscular hemoglobin concentration, average concentration of hemoglobin in a single red cell. When MCHC is low, the cell is hypochromic.	**PT**	prothrombin time
		PTT	partial thromboplastin time
		RBC	red blood cell (red blood cell count)
MCV	mean corpuscular volume, average volume or size of a single red blood cell. When MCV is high, the cells are macrocytic, and when low, the cells are microcytic.	**sed rate**	erythrocyte sedimentation rate
		segs	segmented, mature white blood cells
mm³	cubic millimeter (one millionth of a liter)	**SMAC**	Sequential Multiple Analyzer Computer, an automated chemistry system that determines substances in serum
		µL	microliter (one millionth of a liter; a liter equals 1.057 quarts)
mono	monocyte		
poly, PMN, PMNL	polymorphonuclear leukocyte, neutrophil	**WBC**	white blood cell (white blood cell count)

IX. Practical Applications

Answers to the questions are on page 521 after Answers to Exercises.

Normal Laboratory Values

WBC 5000–10,000/mm³ or µL
Differential:

Segs (polys)	54%–62%
Lymphs	20%–40%
Eos	1%–3%
Baso	0%–1%
Mono	3%–7%

RBC	(M)	4.5–6.0 million per mm³ or µL
	(F)	4.0–5.5 million per mm³ or µL
Hct	(M)	40–50%
	(F)	37–47%
HGB	(M)	14–16 g/dL
	(F)	12–14 g/dL

Platelets 150,000–350,000/mm³ or µL

Three Short Cases

1. **A 65-year-old Swedish woman visits her physician complaining of shortness of breath and swollen ankles. Lab tests reveal that her hematocrit is 18.0 and her hemoglobin 5.8. Her blood smear shows macrocytes and her blood level of vitamin B$_{12}$ is very low. What is a likely diagnosis?**
   (A) aplastic anemia
   (B) hemochromatosis
   (C) pernicious anemia

2. A 22-year-old college student visits the clinic with a fever and complaining of a sore throat. Blood tests show a WBC of 28,000 per mm^3 or μL with 95% myeloblasts (polys are 5%). Platelet count is 15,000 per mm^3 or μL, hemoglobin is 10 g/dL, hematocrit is 22.5. What is your diagnosis?

   (A) chronic lymphocytic leukemia

   (B) acute myelogenous leukemia

   (C) thalassemia

3. A 35-year-old female goes to her physician complaining of spots on her legs and bleeding gums. On examination, she has minute purple spots covering her legs and evidence of dried blood in her mouth. Her CBC shows hemoglobin 14 g/dL, hematocrit 42%, WBC 5000 per mm^3 or μL with normal differential, platelet count 4000/mm^3 or μL (with megakaryocytes in bone marrow). What is your diagnosis?

   (A) sickle cell anemia

   (B) hemolytic anemia

   (C) autoimmune thrombocytopenic purpura

Multiple Myeloma

Multiple myeloma is a neoplastic proliferation of plasma cells. The clinical manifestations of the disease result from the effects of the myeloma tumor cell mass in the bone marrow as well as from the myeloma proteins produced by the malignant cells. The effects of the tumor cell mass include lytic skeletal lesions, hypercalcemia, anemia, leukopenia, and thrombocytopenia. Clinical features related to the myeloma proteins include hyperviscosity (excessive thickness), coagulopathy, and renal insufficiency (tubules get plugged with protein material). There is no curative therapy for multiple myeloma, but chemotherapy is used and aimed at improving quality of life and delaying disease progression. Autologous or allogeneic stem cell transplantation may be beneficial as well.

X. Exercises

Remember to check your answers carefully with those given in Section XI, Answers to Exercises.

A. Match the following cells with their meanings as given below.

basophil   hematopoietic stem cell   neutrophil
eosinophil   lymphocyte   platelet
erythrocyte   monocyte

1. mononuclear white blood cell (agranulocyte) formed in lymph tissue; it is a phagocyte and the

   precursor of a macrophage _____

2. thrombocyte or cell that helps blood clot _____

3. cell in the bone marrow that gives rise to different types of blood cells _____

4. mononuclear leukocyte formed in lymph tissue; produces antibodies _____

5. leukocyte with dense, reddish granules having an affinity for red acidic dye; associated with allergic

   reactions _____

6. red blood cell _____

7. leukocyte (polymorphonuclear granulocyte) formed in the bone marrow and having neutral-

   straining granules _____

8. leukocyte (granulocyte) whose granules have an affinity for basic dye; releases histamine and

   heparin _____

B. Give the meanings of the following terms.

1. coagulation _____

2. granulocyte _____

3. mononuclear _____

4. polymorphonuclear _____

5. globulins _____

6. erythroblast _____

7. megakaryocyte _____

8. macrophage _____

9. hemoglobin _____

10. plasma _____

11. reticulocyte _____

12. myeloblast _____

C. Give the medical terms for the following descriptions.

1. liquid portion of blood _____

2. orange-yellow pigment produced from hemoglobin when red blood cells are destroyed

    _____

3. iron-containing nonprotein part of hemoglobin _____

4. proteins in plasma; separated into alpha, beta, and gamma types

    _____

5. hormone secreted by the kidneys to stimulate bone marrow to produce red blood cells

    _____

6. foreign material that stimulates the production of an antibody _____

7. plasma protein that maintains the proper amount of water in the blood _____

8. proteins made by lymphocytes in response to antigens in the blood _____

D. Give short answers for the following.

1. Name four types of plasma proteins. _____

2. What is the Rh factor? _____

3. What is hemolysis? _____

4. A person with type A blood has _____ antigens and _____ antibodies in his or her blood.

5. A person with type B blood has _____ antigens and _____ antibodies in her or his blood.

6. A person with type O blood has _____ antigens and _____ antibodies in her or his blood.

7. A person with type AB blood has _____ antigens and _____ antibodies in her or his blood.

8. Can you transfuse blood from a type A donor into a type B recipient? _____

   Why? _____

9. Can you transfuse blood from a type AB donor into a type O recipient? _____

   Why? _____

10. What is electrophoresis? _____

11. What is immunoglobulin? _____

12. What is differentiation? _____

13. What is plasmapheresis? _____

E. Match the following terms related to clotting with their meanings as given below.

coagulation   heparin   thrombin
fibrin   prothrombin   warfarin (Coumadin)
fibrinogen   serum

1. anticoagulant substance found in liver cells, bloodstream, and tissues _____

2. protein threads that form the basis of a blood clot _____

3. plasma protein that is converted to thrombin in the clotting process _____

4. plasma minus clotting proteins and cells _____

5. drug given to patients to prevent formation of clots _____

6. plasma protein that is converted to fibrin in the clotting process _____

7. process of clotting _____

8. enzyme that helps convert fibrinogen to fibrin _____

F. Divide the following terms into component parts and give meanings of the complete terms.

1. anticoagulant _____

2. hemoglobinopathy _____

3. cytology _____

4. leukocytopenia _____

5. morphology _____

6. megakaryocyte _____

7. sideropenia _____

8. phagocyte _____

9. myeloblast _____

10. plateletpheresis _____

11. monoblast _____

12. myelopoiesis _____

13. hemostasis _____

14. thrombolytic _____

15. hematopoiesis _____

G. Match the following terms concerning red blood cells with their meanings as given below.

anisocytosis	hemoglobin	microcytosis
erythrocytopenia	hemolysis	poikilocytosis
erythropoiesis	hypochromic	polycythemia vera
hematocrit	macrocytosis	spherocytosis

1. any irregularity in the shape of red blood cells _____

2. oxygen-containing protein in red blood cells _____

3. formation of red blood cells _____

4. deficiency in numbers of red blood cells _____

5. destruction of red blood cells _____

6. pertaining to reduction of hemoglobin in red blood cells _____

7. variation in size of red blood cells _____

8. abnormal numbers of round, rather than normally biconcave-shaped, red blood cells

_____

9. increase in number of small red blood cells _____

10. general increase in numbers of red blood cells; erythremia _____

11. increase in numbers of large red blood cells _____

12. separation of blood so that the percentage of red blood cells in relation to the volume of a blood

sample is measured _____

L. Give the meanings of the following abbreviations and then select from the sentences that follow the best association for each.

Column I

1. HGB _____ ____

2. GVHD _____ ____

3. ALL _____ ____

4. PTT _____ ____

5. CML _____ ____

6. G-CSFs _____ ____

7. IgA, IgE, IgD _____ ____

8. CLL _____ ____

9. Hct _____ ____

10. AML _____ ____

Column II

A. Blood protein that helps transport oxygen to body tissues.

B. Malignant condition of white blood cells in which immature granulocytes predominate; normal bone marrow is replaced by myeloblasts.

C. Malignant condition of white blood cells in which immature lymphocytes predominate; children are affected and onset is sudden.

D. Test used to follow patients who are taking certain anticoagulants.

E. Percentage of erythrocytes in a volume of blood.

F. Malignant condition of white blood cells in which both mature and immature granulocytes are present; a slowly progressive illness.

G. Immune reaction by a recipient's cells to a donor's cells; a possible outcome of hematopoietic stem cell or bone marrow transplant.

H. Proteins containing antibodies.

I. Malignant condition of white blood cells in which relatively mature lymphocytes predominate in lymph nodes, spleen, and bone marrow; usually seen in elderly patients.

J. Proteins that stimulate the formation and proliferation of white blood cells.

M. Circle the terms that best complete the meanings of the sentences.

1. Gary, a 1-year-old African-American baby, was failing to gain weight normally. He seemed pale and without energy. His blood tests showed a decreased hemoglobin (5.0 g/dL) and decreased hematocrit (16.5%). After a blood smear revealed abnormally shaped red cells, the physician told Gary's mother that her son had (**iron-deficiency anemia, hemophilia, sickle cell anemia**).

2. While in the hospital, Mr. Klein was told he had an elevated (**red blood cell, white blood cell, platelet**) count with a "left shift." This was information that confirmed his diagnosis of a systemic infection.

3. While taking Coumadin, a blood thinner, Mr. Ratzan's physician made sure to check his (**prothrombin time, hematocrit, sed rate**).

4. When they checked Babette's blood type during her prenatal examination, she was AB⁻. Her physician told her that she and her baby might have the condition of (**Rh incompatibility, multiple myeloma, pernicious anemia**).

5. Bobby was diagnosed at a very early age with a bleeding disorder called **(hemophilia, thalassemia, eosinophilia)**. He needed factor VIII regularly, especially after even the slightest traumatic injury.

6. Bill was a 9-year-old boy who suddenly noticed many black and blue marks all over his legs. He had a fever and was tired all the time. The physician did a blood test that revealed pancytopenia. A bone marrow biopsy confirmed the diagnosis of **(acute lymphocytic leukemia, polycythemia vera, aplastic anemia)**.

7. Suzy and her friends had been staying up late for weeks, cramming for exams. She developed a sore throat, fatigue, and swollen lymph nodes in her neck. Dr. Smith did a blood test, and the results showed lymphocytosis and antibodies to EBV in the bloodstream. His diagnosis was **(leukapheresis, lymphocytopenia, mononucleosis)**.

8. Suzy was experiencing heavy menstrual periods **(menorrhea, menorrhagia, hemoptysis)**. Because of the bleeding, she frequently felt tired and weak and was probably sideropenic. Her physician performed blood tests that revealed her problem as **(thrombocytopenia, pernicious anemia, iron-deficiency anemia)**.

9. Dr. Harris examined a highly allergic patient and sent a blood sample to a **(pulmonary, cardiovascular, hematologic)** pathologist. The physician stained the blood smear and found an abundance of leukocytes with dense, reddish granules. She made the diagnosis of **(basophilia, eosinophilia, neutrophilia)**.

10. George's blood cell counts had been falling in recent weeks. His scheduled laparotomy was canceled because blood tests revealed **(pancytopenia, plasmapheresis, myelopoiesis)**. Bone marrow biopsy determined that the cause was **(hyperplasia, hypoplasia, differentiation)** of all cellular elements.

XI. Answers to Exercises

A

1. monocyte
2. platelet
3. hematopoietic stem cell
4. lymphocyte
5. eosinophil
6. erythrocyte
7. neutrophil
8. basophil

B

1. blood clotting
2. white blood cell with dense, dark-staining granules (neutrophil, basophil, and eosinophil)
3. pertaining to (having) one (prominent) nucleus (monocytes and lymphocytes are mononuclear leukocytes)
4. pertaining to (having) a many-shaped nucleus (neutrophils are polymorphonuclear leukocytes)
5. plasma proteins in blood; immunoglobulins are examples
6. immature red blood cell
7. forerunner (precursor) of platelets (formed in the bone marrow)
8. large phagocytes formed from monocytes and found in tissues; they destroy worn-out red blood cells and engulf foreign material
9. blood protein found in red blood cells; enables the erythrocyte to carry oxygen
10. liquid portion of blood
11. immature, developing red blood cell with a network of granules in its cytoplasm
12. immature bone marrow cell that is the forerunner of granulocytes

C

1. plasma
2. bilirubin
3. heme
4. globulins
5. erythropoietin
6. antigen
7. albumin
8. antibodies

Continued on following page

D

1. albumin, globulins, fibrinogen, and prothrombin
2. an antigen normally found on red blood cells of Rh-positive individuals
3. destruction of red blood cells when incompatible bloods are mixed
4. A; anti-B
5. B; anti-A
6. no A or B; anti-A and anti-B
7. A and B; no anti-A and no anti-B
8. no; the A antigens will agglutinate with the anti-A antibodies in the B person's bloodstream
9. no; the A and B antigens will agglutinate with the anti-A and anti-B antibodies in the O person's bloodstream
10. a method of separating substances (such as proteins) by electrical charge
11. a type of gamma globulin (blood protein) that contains antibodies
12. change in the structure and function (specialization) of a cell as it matures
13. the process of using a centrifuge to separate or remove blood cells from plasma.

E

1. heparin
2. fibrin
3. prothrombin
4. serum
5. warfarin (Coumadin)
6. fibrinogen
7. coagulation
8. thrombin

F

1. anti/coagul/ant—a substance that prevents clotting
2. hemoglobin/o/pathy—disease (abnormality) of hemoglobin
3. cyt/o/logy—study of cells
4. leuk/o/cyt/o/penia—deficiency of white (blood) cells
5. morph/o/logy—study of the shape or form (of cells)
6. mega/kary/o/cyte—cell with a large (mega-) nucleus (kary); platelet precursor
7. sider/o/penia—deficiency of iron
8. phag/o/cyte—cell that eats or swallows other cells
9. myel/o/blast—immature bone marrow cell (gives rise to granulocytes)
10. platelet/pheresis—separation of platelets from the rest of the blood
11. mon/o/blast—immature monocyte
12. myel/o/poiesis—formation of bone marrow cells
13. hem/o/stasis—controlling or stopping the flow of blood
14. thromb/o/lytic—pertaining to destruction of clots
15. hemat/o/poiesis—formation of blood

G

1. poikilocytosis
2. hemoglobin
3. erythropoiesis
4. erythrocytopenia
5. hemolysis
6. hypochromic
7. anisocytosis
8. spherocytosis
9. microcytosis
10. polycythemia vera
11. macrocytosis
12. hematocrit

H

1. lack of iron leading to insufficient hemoglobin production
2. lack of mature erythrocytes due to inability to absorb vitamin B_{12} into the bloodstream (gastric juice lacks a factor that helps absorb B_{12})
3. abnormal shape (crescent-shape) of erythrocytes caused by an abnormal type of hemoglobin (hereditary disorder)
4. lack of all types of blood cells due to lack of development of bone marrow cells
5. defect in the ability to produce hemoglobin, leading to hypochromia

I

1. multiple pinpoint hemorrhages due to a deficiency of platelets (patient makes an antibody that destroys her or his own platelets)
2. abnormal condition of excess numbers of granulocytes (eosinophilia and basophilia)
3. excessive bleeding caused by a hereditary lack of factor VIII or factor IX necessary for clotting
4. excessive deposits of iron in tissues of the body
5. malignant neoplasm of bone marrow
6. infectious disease marked by increased numbers of mononuclear leukocytes

J

1. E
2. G
3. D
4. B
5. F
6. A
7. H
8. C

K

1. red blood cell morphology
2. hematocrit
3. platelet count
4. coagulation time
5. erythrocyte sedimentation rate
6. white blood cell differential
7. antiglobulin (Coombs) test
8. bone marrow transplant
9. bleeding time
10. bone marrow biopsy
11. red blood cell count
12. autologous transfusion

L

1. hemoglobin. A
2. graft versus host disease. G
3. acute lymphocytic leukemia. C
4. partial thromboplastin time. D

5. chronic myelogenous (myelocytic) leukemia. F
6. granulocyte colony-stimulating factors. J
7. immunoglobulins. H

8. chronic lymphocytic leukemia. I
9. hematocrit. E
10. acute myelogenous (myelocytic) leukemia. B

M

1. sickle cell anemia
2. white blood cell
3. prothrombin time
4. Rh incompatibility

5. hemophilia
6. aplastic anemia
7. mononucleosis

8. menorrhagia; iron-deficiency anemia
9. hematologic; eosinophilia
10. pancytopenia; hypoplasia

Answers to Practical Applications

1. C
2. B
3. C

XII. Pronunciation of Terms

Pronunciation Guide	
ā as in āpe	ă as in ăpple
ē as in ēven	ĕ as in ĕvery
ī as in īce	ĭ as in ĭnterest
ō as in ōpen	ŏ as in pŏt
ū as in ūnit	ŭ as in ŭnder

To test your understanding of the terminology in this chapter, write the meaning of each term in the space provided. In addition, you may wish to cover the terms and write them by looking at your definitions. Make sure your spelling is correct. The page number after each term indicates where it is defined or used in the text so you can easily check your responses.

Vocabulary and Terminology

Term	Pronunciation	Meaning
albumin (495)	ăl-BŪ-mĭn	
anisocytosis (499)	ăn-ī-sō-sī-TŌ-sĭs	
antibody (495)	ĂN-tĭ-bŏd-ē	
anticoagulant (498)	ăn-tĭ-cō-ĂG-ū-lănt	
antigen (495)	ĂN-tĭ-jĕn	
basophil (495)	BĀ-sō-fĭl	
bilirubin (496)	bĭl-ĭ-ROO-bĭn	

coagulation (496)	kō-ăg-ū-LĀ-shŭn	_____
coagulopathy (498)	kō-ăg-ū-LŎP-ă-thē	_____
colony-stimulating factor (496)	KŎL-ō-nē STĬM-ū-lā-tĭng FĂK-tŏr	_____
cytology (498)	sī-TŎL-ō-jē	_____
differentiation (496)	dĭf-ĕr-ĕn-shē-Ā-shŭn	_____
electrophoresis (496)	ē-lĕk-trō-fō-RĒ-sis	_____
eosinophil (496)	ē-ō-SĬN-ō-fĭl	_____
eosinophilia (501)	ē-ō-sĭn-ō-FĬL-ē-ă	_____
erythroblast (500)	ě-RĬTH-rō-blăst	_____
erythrocytopenia (498)	ě-rĭth-rō-sī-tō-PĒ-nē-ă	_____
erythropoiesis (501)	ě-rĭth-rō-poy-Ē-sĭs	_____
erythropoietin (496)	ě-rĭth-rō-PŌ-ě-tĭn	_____
fibrin (496)	FĪ-brĭn	_____
fibrinogen (496)	fī-BRĬN-ō-jěn	_____
globulins (496)	GLŎB-ū-lĭnz	_____
granulocyte (496)	GRĂN-ū-lō-sīt	_____
granulocytopenia (501)	grăn-ū-lō-sī-tō-PĒ-nē-ă	_____
hematopoiesis (501)	hē-mă-tō-poy-Ē-sĭs	_____
hemoglobin (496)	HĒ-mō-glō-bĭn	_____
hemoglobinopathy (498)	hē-mō-glō-bĭn-ŎP-ă-thē	_____
hemolysis (496)	hē-MŎL-ĭ-sĭs	_____
hemostasis (501)	hē-mŏ-STĀ-sĭs	_____
heparin (496)	HĔP-ă-rĭn	_____
hypochromic (498)	hī-pō-KRŌ-mĭk	_____
immunoglobulin (496)	ĭm-ū-nō-GLŎB-ū-lĭn	_____
leukapheresis (500)	loo-kă-fě-RĒ-sĭs	_____
leukocytopenia (499)	loo-kō-sī-tō-PĒ-nē-ă	_____

lymphocyte (497)	LĬM-fō-sīt	_____
macrocytosis (500)	măk-rō-sī-TŌ-sĭs	_____
macrophage (497)	MĂK-rō-făj	_____
megakaryocyte (497)	mĕg-ă-KĀR-ē-ō-sīt	_____
microcytosis (500)	mī-krō-sī-TŌ-sĭs	_____
monoblast (500)	MŎN-ō-blăst	_____
monocyte (497)	MŎN-ō-sīt	_____
mononuclear (497)	mŏn-ō-NŪ-klē-ăr	_____
morphology (499)	mŏr-FŎL-ō-jē	_____
myeloblast (499)	MĪ-ĕ-lō-blăst	_____
myeloid (501)	MĪ-ĕ-loyd	_____
myelogenous (499)	mī-ĕ-LŎJ-ĕn-ŭs	_____
myelopoiesis (501)	mī-ĕ-lō-poy-Ē-sĭs	_____
neutropenia (499)	nū-trō-PĔ-nē-ă	_____
neutrophil (497)	NŪ-trō-fĭl	_____
neutrophilia (501)	nū-trō-FĬL-ē-ă	_____
pancytopenia (501)	păn-sī-tō-PĒ-nē-ă	_____
phagocyte (499)	FĂG-ō-sīt	_____
plasma (497)	PLĂZ-mă	_____
plasmapheresis (497)	plăz-mă-fĕ-RĒ-sĭs	_____
plateletpheresis (500)	plăt-lĕt-fĕ-RĒ-sĭs	_____
poikilocytosis (499)	poy-kĭ-lō-sī-TŌ-sĭs	_____
polymorphonuclear (499)	pŏl-ē-mŏr-fō-NŪ-klē-ăr	_____
prothrombin (497)	prō-THRŎM-bĭn	_____
reticulocyte (497)	rĕ-TĬK-ū-lō-sīt	_____
serum (497)	SĔ-rŭm	_____
sideropenia (499)	sĭd-ĕr-ō-PĒ-nē-ă	_____

spherocytosis (499)	sphĕr-ō-sī-TŌ-sĭs	_____
stem cell (497)	stĕm sĕl	_____
thrombin (497)	THRŎM-bĭn	_____
thrombocyte (497)	THRŎM-bō-sīt	_____
thrombocytopenia (499)	thrŏm-bō-sī-tō-PĒ-nē-ă	_____
thrombolytic therapy (501)	thrŏm-bō-LĬ-tĭk THĔR-ă-pē	_____
thrombosis (501)	thrŏm-BŌ-sĭs	_____

Pathological Conditions, Laboratory Tests, and Clinical Procedures

Term	Pronunciation	Meaning
acute lymphocytic leukemia (504)	ă-KŪT lĭm-fō-SĬ-tĭk loo-KĒ-mē-ă	_____
acute myelogenous leukemia (504)	ă-KŪT mī-ĕ-LŎJ-ĕ-nŭs loo-KĒ-mē-ă	_____
antiglobulin test (506)	ăn-tē-GLŎB-ū-lĭn tĕst	_____
apheresis (508)	ă-fĕ-RĒ-sĭs	_____
aplastic anemia (502)	ā-PLĂS-tĭk ă-NĒ-mē-ă	_____
autologous transfusion (508)	ăw-TŎL-ō-gŭs trăns-FŪ-zhŭn	_____
bleeding time (506)	BLĒ-dĭng tīm	_____
blood transfusion (508)	blŭd trăns-FŪ-zhŭn	_____
bone marrow biopsy (508)	bōn MĂ-rō BĪ-ŏp-sē	_____
chronic lymphocytic leukemia (505)	KRŎ-nĭk lĭm-fō-SĬ-tĭk loo-KĒ-mē-ă	_____
chronic myelogenous leukemia (504)	KRŎ-nĭk mī-ĕ-LŎJ-ĕ-nŭs loo-KĒ-mē-ă	_____
coagulation time (506)	kō-ăg-ū-LĀ-shŭn tīm	_____
complete blood count (506)	kŏm-PLĒT blŭd kount	_____
dyscrasia (502)	dĭs-KRĀ-zē-ă	_____
erythrocyte sedimentation rate (507)	ĕ-RĬTH-rō-sīt sĕd-ĕ-mĕn-TĀ-shŭn rāt	_____

granulocytosis (505)	grăn-ū-lō-sī-TŌ-sis	_____
hematocrit (507)	hē-MĂT-ō-krĭt	_____
hematopoietic stem cell transplant (508)	hē-mă-tō-pō-Ĕ-tĭk stĕm sel TRĂNS-plant	_____
hemochromatosis (504)	hē-mō-krō-mă-TŌ-sĭs	_____
hemoglobin test (507)	HĒ-mō-glō-bĭn tĕst	_____
hemolytic anemia (502)	hē-mō-LĬ-tĭk ă-NĒ-mē-ă	_____
hemophilia (504)	hē-mō-FĬL-ē-ă	_____
intrinsic factor (503)	ĭn-TRĬN-sĭk FĂK-tŏr	_____
mononucleosis (506)	mŏ-nō-nū-klē-Ō-sĭs	_____
multiple myeloma (506)	MŬL-tĭ-p'l mī-ĕ-LŌ-mă	_____
palliative (506)	PĂL-ē-ă-tĭv	_____
partial thromboplastin time (507)	PĂR-shŭl thrŏm-bō-PLĂS-tĭn tīm	_____
pernicious anemia (503)	pĕr-NĬSH-ŭs ă-NĒ-mē-ă	_____
platelet count (507)	PLĀT-lĕt kount	_____
polycythemia vera (504)	pŏl-ē-sī-THĒ-mē-ă VĔR-ă	_____
prothrombin time (507)	prō-THRŎM-bĭn tīm	_____
purpura (504)	PŬR-pū-ră	_____
red blood cell count (507)	rĕd blŭd sĕl kount	_____
red blood cell morphology (507)	rĕd blŭd sĕl mŏr-FŎL-ō-jē	_____
relapse (505)	RĒ-lăps	_____
remission (505)	rē-MĬSH-ŭn	_____
sickle cell anemia (503)	SĬK'l sĕl ă-NĒ-mē-ă	_____
thalassemia (503)	thāl-ă-SĒ-mē-ă	_____
white blood cell count (507)	whĭte blŭd sĕl kount	_____
white blood cell differential (507)	whĭte blŭd sĕl dĭ-fĕr-ĔN-shŭl	_____

XIII. Review Sheet

Write the meanings of the word parts in the spaces provided. Check your answers with the information in the chapter or in the glossary (Medical Terms—English) at the end of the book.

COMBINING FORMS

Combining Form	Meaning	Combining Form	Meaning
bas/o		leuk/o	
chrom/o		mon/o	
coagul/o		morph/o	
cyt/o		myel/o	
eosin/o		neutr/o	
erythr/o		nucle/o	
granul/o		phag/o	
hem/o		poikil/o	
hemat/o		sider/o	
hemoglobin/o		spher/o	
is/o		thromb/o	
kary/o			

SUFFIXES

Suffix	Meaning	Suffix	Meaning
-apheresis	_____	-osis	_____
-blast	_____	-penia	_____
-cytosis	_____	-phage	_____
-emia	_____	-philia	_____
-globin	_____	-phoresis	_____
-globulin	_____	-plasia	_____
-lytic	_____	-poiesis	_____
-oid	_____	-stasis	_____

PREFIXES

Prefix	Meaning	Prefix	Meaning
a-, an-	_____	micro-	_____
anti-	_____	mono-	_____
hypo-	_____	pan-	_____
macro-	_____	poly-	_____
mega-	_____		

chapter

Lymphatic and Immune Systems

This chapter is divided into the following sections

In this chapter you will

■ Identify the structures and analyze terms related to the lymphatic system.
■ Learn terms that describe basic elements of the immune system.
■ Recognize terms that describe various pathological conditions affecting the lymphatic and immune systems.
■ Identify laboratory tests, clinical procedures, and abbreviations that are pertinent to the lymphatic and immune systems.
■ Apply your new knowledge to understanding medical terms in their proper contexts, such as medical reports and records.

I. Introduction

Lymph is a clear, watery fluid (the term *lymph* comes from the Latin, meaning "clear spring water") that surrounds body cells and flows in a system of lymph vessels that extends throughout the body.

Lymph differs from blood, but it has a close relationship with the blood systems. Lymph fluid does not contain erythrocytes or platelets, but it is rich in two types of white blood cells (leukocytes): **lymphocytes** and **monocytes.** The liquid part of lymph is similar to blood plasma in that it contains water, salts, sugar, and wastes of metabolism such as urea and creatinine, but it differs in that it contains less protein. Lymph actually originates from the blood. It is the fluid that filters out of tiny blood vessels into the spaces between cells. This fluid that surrounds body cells is called **interstitial fluid.** Interstitial fluid passes continuously into specialized thin-walled vessels called **lymph capillaries,** which are found coursing through tissue spaces (Fig. 14–1). The fluid in the lymph capillaries, now called **lymph** instead of interstitial fluid, passes through larger lymphatic vessels and through deposits of lymph tissues (called **lymph nodes**), finally to reach large lymph vessels in the upper chest. Lymph enters these large lymphatic vessels, which then empty into the bloodstream. Figure 14–2 illustrates the relationship between the blood and the lymphatic systems.

The lymphatic system has several functions. First, it is a drainage system to transport needed proteins and fluid that have leaked out of the blood capillaries (and into the interstitial fluid) back to the bloodstream via the veins. Second, the lymphatic vessels in the intestines absorb lipids (fats) from the small intestine and transport them to the bloodstream.

A third function of the lymphatic system relates to the **immune system:** the defense of the body against foreign organisms such as bacteria and viruses. Lymphocytes and monocytes, originating in lymph nodes and organs such as the spleen and thymus gland, protect the body by producing antibodies, by mounting a cellular attack on foreign cells, or by phagocytosis (engulfing and destroying foreign matter).

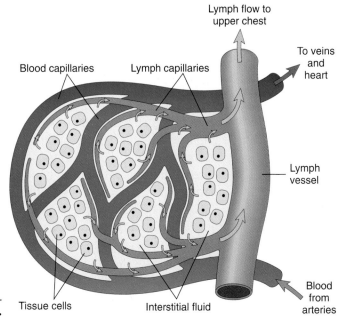

Figure 14–1

Interstitial fluid and lymph capillaries.

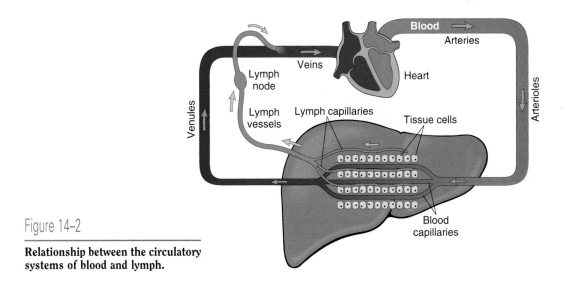

Figure 14–2

Relationship between the circulatory systems of blood and lymph.

II. Lymphatic System

Anatomy

Label Figure 14–3A as you read the following paragraphs.

Lymph capillaries [1] begin at the spaces around cells throughout the body. Like blood capillaries, they are thin-walled tubes. Lymph capillaries carry lymph from the tissue spaces to larger **lymph vessels** [2]. Lymph vessels have thicker walls than those of lymph capillaries and, like veins, contain valves so that lymph flows in only one direction, toward the thoracic cavity. Collections of stationary lymph tissue, called **lymph nodes** [3], are located along the path of the lymph vessels. These masses of lymph cells and vessels are surrounded by a fibrous, connective tissue capsule (Fig. 14–4).

Lymph nodes not only produce lymphocytes but also filter lymph and trap substances from inflammatory and cancerous lesions. Special cells, called **macrophages,** located in lymph nodes (as well as in the spleen, liver, lungs, brain, and spinal cord), phagocytose foreign substances. When bacteria are present in lymph nodes that drain a particular area of the body, the nodes become swollen with collections of cells and their engulfed debris and become tender. Lymph nodes also fight disease when specialized lymphocytes **(B-cell lymphocytes),** present in the nodes, produce antibodies. Other lymphocytes **(T-cell lymphocytes)** attack bacteria and foreign cells by accurately recognizing a cell surface protein as foreign, attaching to the foreign or cancerous cells, poking holes in them, and injecting toxic chemicals into the cells.

Label the major sites of lymph node concentration on Figure 14–3. These are the **cervical** [4], **axillary** (armpit) [5], **mediastinal** [6], and **inguinal** (groin) [7] regions of the body. Remember that **tonsils** are masses of lymph tissue in the throat near the back of the mouth (oropharynx), and **adenoids** are enlarged lymph tissue in the part of the throat near the nasal passages (nasopharynx).

Lymph vessels all lead toward the thoracic cavity and empty into two large ducts in the upper chest. These are the **right lymphatic duct** [8] and the **thoracic duct** [9]. The thoracic duct drains the lower body and the left side of the head, whereas the right lymphatic duct drains the right side of the head and chest (a much smaller area) (Fig. 14–3B). Both ducts carry the lymph into **large veins** [10] in the neck where lymph then merges with the blood system.

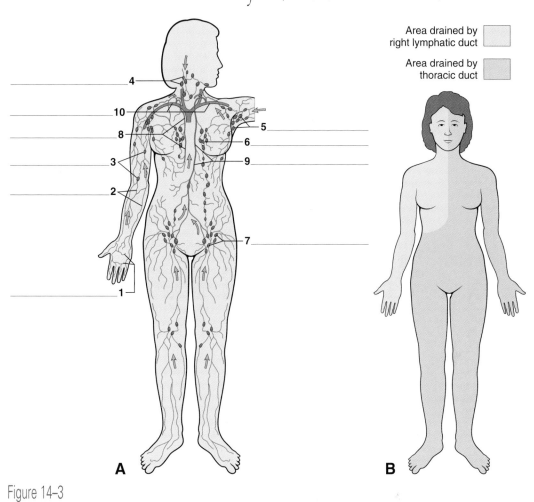

Area drained by right lymphatic duct

Area drained by thoracic duct

Figure 14-3

Lymphatic system. (A) Label the figure according to the descriptions in the text. **(B)** Note the different regions of the body drained by the right lymphatic duct and the thoracic duct.

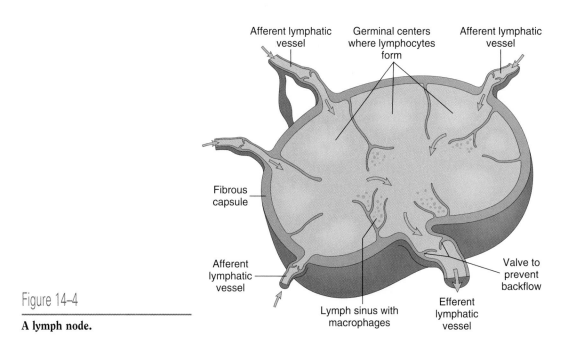

Afferent lymphatic vessel

Germinal centers where lymphocytes form

Afferent lymphatic vessel

Fibrous capsule

Afferent lymphatic vessel

Lymph sinus with macrophages

Efferent lymphatic vessel

Valve to prevent backflow

Figure 14-4

A lymph node.

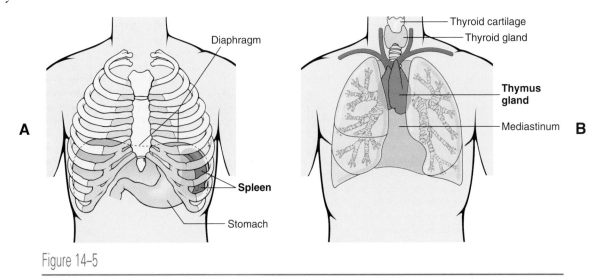

A

B

Figure 14–5

(A) Spleen and adjacent structures. **(B) Thymus gland** in its location in the mediastinum between the lungs.

Spleen and Thymus Gland

The spleen and the thymus gland are organs composed of lymph tissue.

The **spleen** (Fig. 14–5A) is located in the left upper quadrant of the abdomen, adjacent to the stomach. Although the spleen is not essential to life, it has several important functions:

1. Destruction of old erythrocytes by macrophages. Because of hemolytic activity in the spleen, red cell breakdown liberates hemoglobin, which is converted to bilirubin in the liver and then is added to the bloodstream.
2. Filtration of microorganisms and other foreign material from the blood.
3. Activation of lymphocytes as it filters out antigens from the blood. Activated B-cell lymphocytes produce antibodies.
4. Storage of blood, especially erythrocytes and platelets. A large number of platelets collect in the splenic blood pool.

The spleen is easily and frequently injured. A sharp blow or injury to the upper abdomen (as from the impact of a car's steering wheel) may cause rupture of the spleen. Massive hemorrhage can occur when the spleen is ruptured, and immediate surgical removal (splenectomy) may be necessary. After splenectomy, the liver, bone marrow, and lymph nodes take over the functions of the spleen.

The **thymus gland** (Fig. 14–5B) is a lymphatic organ located in the upper mediastinum between the lungs. During fetal life and childhood it is quite large, but it becomes smaller with age. The thymus gland is composed of nests of lymphoid cells resting on a connective tissue stroma. It plays an important role in the body's ability to protect itself from disease (immunity), especially in fetal life and the early years of growth. It is known that a thymectomy (removal of the thymus gland) performed in an animal during the first weeks of life impairs the ability of the animal to make antibodies and to produce immune cells that fight against foreign antigens such as bacteria and viruses.

III. Immune System

The immune system is the body's special defense response against foreign organisms. This system includes the **lymphoid organs** (lymph nodes, spleen, and thymus gland) and their products (**lymphocytes** and **antibodies**) and **macrophages** (phagocytes that are found in the blood, brain, liver, lymph nodes, and spleen).

Immunity is the body's ability to resist foreign organisms and toxins (poisons) that damage tissues and organs. **Natural immunity** is a **genetic predisposition** present in the body at birth. It is not dependent on a specific immune response or a previous contact with an infectious agent. When bacteria enter the body, natural immunity protects the body as **phagocytes** such as neutrophils (white blood cells) migrate to the site of infection and ingest the bacteria. They release proteins that attract other immune cells and cause localized inflammation. **Macrophages** move in to clear away the dead cells and debris as the infection subsides. Other cells, known as **natural killer (NK) cells** are primitive lymphocytes that destroy tumor cells and virally infected cells.

Besides possessing natural immunity, a person may **acquire immunity.** In this way, the body develops powerful, specific immunity (such as antibodies and cells) against invading antigens. **Acquired active immunity** occurs in several ways. First, **having a disease** causes the production of antibodies that fight against foreign organisms and then remain in the body to protect against further infection by the same organism. Next, receiving a **vaccination** containing a modified pathogen or toxin stimulates lymphocytes to produce antibodies without having undergone an attack of the disease. An example is vaccination against smallpox, using the cowpox virus, which produces immunity but no infection. Finally, immunity can also be acquired through the transfer of immune cells (lymphocytes or hematopoietic stem cell) from a donor, as in a stem cell transplant, which stimulates the growth of immune cells in the bone marrow of the recipient.

When immediate protection is needed, **acquired passive immunity** is administered. In this case, the patient receives immune serum (antiserum) containing antibodies produced in another animal. Examples are **antitoxins** given in cases of poisonous snake bites and rabies infections. Injections of immunoglobulins (antibodies) also provide protection against disease or lessen its severity. Newborns receive passive acquired immunity as **maternal antibodies** pass through the placenta or in breast milk after birth. Figure 14–6 reviews the various types of immunity.

The immune response involves two major disease fighters: **B-cell lymphocytes** and **T-cell lymphocytes.** B cells are involved in **humoral immunity.** They produce antibodies in response to specific antigens. B cells originate from bone marrow stem cells. When a B cell is confronted with a specific type of antigen, it transforms into an antibody-producing cell called a **plasma cell.** Plasma cells produce antibodies called **immunoglobulins,** such as **IgA, IgD, IgE, IgG,** and **IgM.** Immunoglobulins travel to the site of an infection to react with and neutralize antigens. IgG, the most abundant immunoglobulin, crosses the placenta to provide immunity for newborns. IgE is important in causing allergic reactions and fighting parasitic infections.

T-cell lymphocytes are involved in **cell-mediated immunity.** They originate from stem cells in the bone marrow and are processed in the thymus gland, where they are acted on

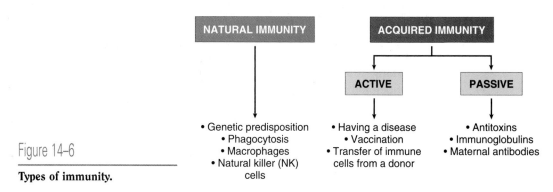

Figure 14–6

Types of immunity.

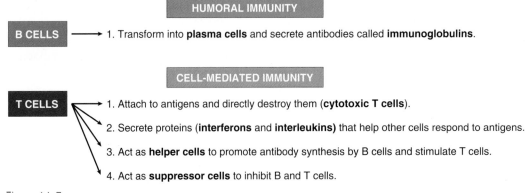

Figure 14-7

Functions of B-cell (humoral immunity) and T-cell lymphocytes (cell-mediated immunity).

by thymic hormones. When a T cell encounters an antigen, the T cell multiplies rapidly to produce cells that destroy the antigen (bacteria, viruses, and cancer cells). T cells also react to transplanted tissues and skin grafts.

Some T cells are **cytotoxic cells (T8 cells)** that act directly on antigens to destroy them. Others produce proteins called **cytokines (interferons** and **interleukins)** that aid other cells in antigen destruction. One special class of T cells, **helper cells (T4 cells),** promotes antibody production by B cells and stimulates cytotoxic T cells. **Suppressor T cells** inhibit the activity of B and T cells. Disease may occur when the normal ratio of helper to suppressor cells (normally 2:1) is altered. For example, in AIDS (acquired immunodeficiency syndrome) the number of helper (T4) cells is diminished. Figure 14–7 summarizes the functions of T- and B-cell lymphocytes.

Another important cell of the immune system is a **dendritic cell.** This cell, derived from monocytes, specializes in recognizing and digesting foreign antigens. The antigens are then presented on the surface of the dendritic cell, which stimulates a B- and T-cell response that destroys the antigen. Immunity can be transferred by exposing dendritic cells in culture to an antigen (tumor protein) and then infusing the cells into a patient. The antigen-sensitive dendritic cells are then able to stimulate the patient's B and T cells to attack the antigen-presenting dendritic cells. Clinical experiments that use sensitized dendritic cells to treat cancer and AIDS are under way.

Immunotherapy is the use of immunologic techniques to treat disease, especially cancer. Examples are:

- **Vaccines** that use killed tumor cells, purified protein antigens, or tumor cells genetically modified to produce **cytokines** that enhance the immune response.
- **Dendritic cells** incubated outside the body with antigens and then reinfused into the patient to stimulate T-cell response.
- **Monoclonal antibodies (MOAB)** produced in a laboratory by special cloning techniques (making multiple copies of cells or genes). Rituxan (anti-CD20) is an example of a monoclonal antibody that kills tumors of B-cell lymphocytes (non-Hodgkin lymphoma). The antibody can be linked to various toxins or radioactive particles and then delivered to tumor cells.
- **Donor lymphocyte infusions** in which T-cell lymphocytes, infused after an allogeneic (from an unrelated donor) stem cell or bone marrow transplant, attack tumor cells of the recipient and cure leukemia.

IV. Vocabulary

This list will help you review many of the new terms introduced in the text. Short definitions will reinforce your understanding of the terms. See Section XI of this chapter for help in pronouncing the more difficult terms.

acquired immunity	Formation of antibodies and lymphocytes after exposure to an antigen.
adenoids	Masses of lymph tissue in the nasopharynx.
antibody	Protein produced by lymphocytes that destroys antigens.
axillary node	One of 20 to 30 lymph nodes in the armpit (underarm).
B cell	Lymphocyte that originates in the bone marrow and transforms into a plasma cell to secrete antibodies. The B refers to the bursa of Fabricius, an organ in birds in which B-cell differentiation and growth were first noted to occur.
cell-mediated immunity	An immune response involving T-cell lymphocytes; antigens are destroyed by direct action of cells, as opposed to antibodies.
cervical node	One of many lymph nodes in the neck region.
cytokine	Protein that aids cells to destroy antigens. Examples are interferons, interleukins, and colony-stimulating factors (G-CSF and GM-CSF).
cytotoxic cell	T-cell lymphocyte that directly kills foreign cells; also called **T8 cell**.
dendritic cell	Cell that captures antigens and presents them to T cells.
helper T cell	Lymphocyte that aids B cell in recognizing antigens and stimulating antibody production; also called **T4 cell**.
humoral immunity	Immune response in which B cells transform into plasma cells and secrete antibodies.
immune response	The body's capacity to resist all types of organisms and toxins that can damage tissue and organs; immunity.
immunoglobulins	Antibodies (gamma globulins) such as IgA, IgE, IgG, IgM, and IgD that are secreted by plasma cells in humoral immunity.
immunotherapy	Use of immunologic knowledge and techniques to treat disease. Examples are vaccines, dendritic cells, monoclonal antibodies, and donor lymphocyte infusions.
inguinal node	One of several lymph nodes in the groin region (area where the legs join the trunk of the body).
interferons	Antiviral proteins (cytokines) secreted by T cells; they also stimulate macrophages to ingest bacteria.

interleukins	Proteins (cytokines) that stimulate the growth of B- or T-cell lymphocytes and activate specific components of the immune response.
interstitial fluid	Fluid in the spaces between cells. This fluid becomes lymph when it enters lymph capillaries.
lymph	Thin, watery fluid found within lymphatic vessels and collected from tissues throughout the body. Latin, *lympha* means "water."
lymph capillaries	Tiniest lymphatic vessels.
lymphoid organs	Lymph nodes, spleen, and thymus gland.
lymph node	Stationary lymph tissue along lymph vessels.
lymph vessel	Carrier of lymph throughout the body; lymph vessels empty lymph into veins in the upper part of the chest.
macrophage	Large phagocyte found in lymph nodes and other tissues of the body.
mediastinal node	One of many lymph nodes in the area between the lungs in the thoracic (chest) cavity.
monoclonal antibody	An antibody produced in a laboratory to attack antigens. It is useful in immunotherapy and cancer treatment.
natural immunity	A person's own genetic ability to fight off disease.
natural killer (NK) cell	Lymphocyte that recognizes and destroys foreign cells (viruses and tumor cells) by releasing cytotoxins.
plasma cell	Lymphoid cell that secretes an antibody and originates from B-cell lymphocytes.
right lymphatic duct	Large lymph vessel in the chest that receives lymph from the upper right part of the body.
spleen	Organ near the stomach that produces, stores, and eliminates blood cells.
suppressor T cell	Lymphocyte that inhibits the activity of B- and T-cell lymphocytes.
T cell	Lymphocyte formed in the thymus gland; it acts directly on antigens to destroy them or produce chemicals such as interferons and interleukins that are toxic to antigens.
thoracic duct	Large lymph vessel in the chest that receives lymph from below the diaphragm and from the left side of the body above the diaphragm; it empties the lymph into veins in the upper chest.
thymus gland	Organ in the mediastinum that produces T-cell lymphocytes and aids in the immune response.

tonsils	Masses of lymph tissue in the back of the oropharynx.
toxin	Poison; a protein produced by certain bacteria, animals, or plants.
vaccination	Introduction of altered antigens (viruses or bacteria) to produce an immune response and protection against disease. The term comes from the Latin "*vacca*," meaning "cow," and was used when the first inoculations were given with organisms that caused the disease cow pox to produce immunity to smallpox.
vaccine	Weakened or killed microorganisms administered to induce immunity to infection or disease.

V. Combining Forms, Prefixes, and Terminology

Write the meanings of the medical terms in the spaces provided.

Combining Forms

Combining Form	Meaning	Terminology	Meaning
immun/o	protection	auto<u>immun</u>e disease	_____

Examples are rheumatoid arthritis and lupus erythematosus. These are chronic, disabling diseases caused by the abnormal production of antibodies to normal body tissues. Symptoms are inflammation of joints, skin rash, and fever. Glucocorticoid drugs (prednisone) and other immunosuppressants (imuran, methotrexate) are effective as treatment, but make patients susceptible to infection.

immunoglobulin _____

immunosuppression _____

This may occur because of exposure to drugs (corticosteroids) or as the result of disease (AIDS and cancer). Immunosuppressed patients are susceptible to infection with fungi, PCP, and other parasites.

lymph/o	lymph	<u>lymph</u>opoiesis	_____

<u>lymph</u>edema _____

Interstitial fluid collects within the spaces between cells secondary to obstruction of lymph vessels and nodes. Radiation therapy may destroy lymphatics and produce lymphedema, as in breast cancer treatment.

<u>lymph</u>ocytopenia _____

<u>lymph</u>ocytosis _____

<u>lymphoid</u> _____

-oid means resembling or derived from. Lymphoid organs include lymph nodes, spleen, and thymus gland.

lymphaden/o	lymph node (gland)	<u>lymphadenopathy</u> _____	
		<u>lymphadenitis</u> _____	
splen/o	spleen	<u>splenomegaly</u> _____	
		<u>splenectomy</u> _____	
		<u>hypersplenism</u> _____	

A syndrome marked by splenomegaly and often associated with blood cell destruction, anemia, leukopenia, and thrombocytopenia.

thym/o	thymus gland	<u>thymoma</u> _____	
		<u>thymectomy</u> _____	
tox/o	poison	<u>toxic</u> _____	

Prefix			
Prefix	**Meaning**	**Terminology**	**Meaning**
ana-	again, anew	<u>anaphylaxis</u> _____	

-phylaxis means protection. This is an exaggerated or unusual hypersensitivity to previously encountered foreign proteins or other antigens. Vasodilation and a decrease in blood pressure can be life threatening.

inter-	between	<u>interstitial fluid</u> _____	

-stitial means pertaining to standing or positioned.

VI. Disorders of the Lymphatic and Immune Systems

Immunodeficiency

acquired immunodeficiency syndrome (AIDS)

Syndrome associated with suppression of the immune system and marked by opportunistic infections, secondary neoplasms, and neurological problems.

This syndrome is caused by the **human immunodeficiency virus (HIV).** HIV destroys T-cell helper lymphocytes (also called **CD4+ cells**) and thus disrupts the cell-mediated immune response. Infectious diseases associated with AIDS are opportunistic infections because HIV lowers resistance and allows infection by

Table 14–1. OPPORTUNISTIC INFECTIONS WITH AIDS

Infection	Description
Candidiasis	Yeast-like fungus *(Candida)* normally present in the mouth, skin, intestinal tract, and vagina overgrows, causing infections of the mouth (thrush), respiratory tract, and skin.
Cryptococcus (Crypto)	Yeast-like fungus *(Cryptococcus)* causes lung, brain, and blood infections. Pathogen is found in pigeon droppings, nesting places, air, water, and soil.
Cryptosporidiosis	One-celled parasitic *(Cryptosporidium)* infection of the gastrointestinal tract and brain and spinal cord. Organism is commonly found in farm animals.
Cytomegalovirus (CMV)	Virus causes enteritis and retinitis (inflammation of the retina at the back of the eye). Found in saliva, semen, cervical secretions, urine, feces, blood, and breast milk, but usually causes disease only when the immune system is compromised.
Herpes simplex	Viral infection causes small blisters on the skin of the lips or nose or on the genitals. Herpes also can cause encephalitis.
Histoplasmosis (Histo)	Fungal infection caused by inhalation of dust contaminated with *Histoplasma capsulatum;* causes fever, chills, and lung infection. Pathogen is found in bird and bat droppings.
Mycobacterium avium-intracellulare (MAI)	Bacterial disease with fever, malaise, night sweats, anorexia, diarrhea, weight loss, and lung and blood infections.
Pneumocystis carinii pneumonia (PCP)	One-celled organism causes lung infection, with fever, cough, and chest pain. Pathogen is found in air, water, and soil and is carried by animals. It is treated with trimethoprim and sulfamethoxazole (Bactrim), a combination of antibiotics, or with pentamidine. Aerosolized pentamidine, which is inhaled, can prevent occurrence of PCP.
Toxoplasmosis (Toxo)	Parasitic infection involving the central nervous system (CNS) and causing fever, chills, visual disturbances, confusion, hemiparesis (slight paralysis in one-half of the body), and seizures. Pathogen is acquired by eating uncooked lamb or pork, unpasteurized dairy products, raw eggs, or vegetables.
Tuberculosis (TB)	Bacterial disease *(Mycobacterium tuberculosis)* involving the lungs. Symptoms are fever, loss of weight, anorexia, and low energy.

bacteria and parasites that are easily otherwise contained by normal defenses. Table 14–1 lists many of these opportunistic infections.

Malignancies associated with AIDS are **Kaposi sarcoma** (a cancer arising from the lining cells of capillaries, which produce bluish-red skin nodules) and **lymphoma** (cancer of lymph nodes).

Persons exposed to HIV and who have antibodies in their blood against HIV are **HIV-positive.** HIV is found in blood, semen, vaginal and cervical secretions, saliva, and other body fluids. Transmission of HIV may occur by three routes: sexual contact, blood inoculation (sharing of contaminated needles, accidental needle sticks, contact with contaminated blood or blood products), and passage of the virus from infected mothers to their newborns. Table 14–2 summarizes the common routes of transmission of HIV.

Table 14–2. COMMON ROUTES OF TRANSMISSION

Route	People Affected
Receptive anal intercourse	Men and women
Receptive vaginal intercourse	Women
Sharing of needles and equipment (users of IV drugs)	Men and women
Contaminated blood (transfusion) or blood products (hemophiliacs)	Men and women
From mother *in utero*	Neonates

HIV-infected patients may remain asymptomatic for as many as 10 years. Symptoms associated with HIV are lymphadenopathy, neurologic disease, oral thrush (fungal infection), night sweats, fatigue, and evidence of opportunistic infections.

Drugs that are used to treat AIDS are inhibitors of the viral enzyme called **reverse transcriptase (RT).** After invading the CD4+ lymphocyte, HIV releases RT to help it grow and multiply inside the cell. Examples of **RT inhibitors (RTIs)** are zidovudine and lamivudine (Epivir). A second class of anti-HIV drugs are inhibitors of the viral protease (proteolytic) enzyme. HIV needs protease at a later stage than it needs RT to make viral parts that will spread throughout the body. Combinations of **protease inhibitors** (nelfinavir, amprenavir) and RT inhibitors have greatly increased the effectiveness of anti-HIV therapy, and in many cases have abolished evidence of the presence of the viral infection in affected people.

Hypersensitivity

allergy

Abnormal hypersensitivity acquired by exposure to an antigen.

Allergic (all/o = other) reactions occur when a person is exposed to a sensitizing agent **(allergen),** and the immune response that follows on reexposure to the allergen is damaging to the body. These reactions can vary from allergic rhinitis or hay fever (caused by pollen or animal dander) to systemic **anaphylaxis,** in which an extraordinary hypersensitivity reaction occurs throughout the body, leading to hypotension, shock, respiratory distress, and edema of the larynx. Anaphylaxis can be life threatening, but the patient usually survives if the airways are kept open and treatment is given immediately with epinephrine and antihistamines.

Other allergies include asthma (pollens, dust, molds), urticaria, or hives (foods, drugs), and **atopic dermatitis** (soaps, cosmetics, chemicals). **Atopic** means related to atopy, a hypersensitivity or allergic state arising from an inherited predisposition. A person who is atopic is prone to allergies.

Malignancies

lymphoma

Malignant tumor of lymph nodes and lymph tissue.

There are many types of lymphoma, varying according to the particular cell type and degree of differentiation. Some examples are:

Hodgkin disease—Malignant tumor of lymph tissue in the spleen and lymph nodes. This disease is characterized by lymphadenopathy (lymph nodes enlarge), splenomegaly, fever, weakness, and loss of weight and appetite. The diagnosis is often made by identifying a malignant cell (Reed-Sternberg cell) in the lymph nodes (Fig. 14–8). If disease is localized, the treatment of choice is radiotherapy

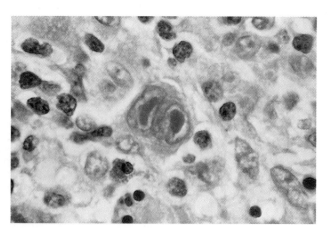

Figure 14–8

Hodgkin disease. Notice the binucleate **Reed-Sternberg cell** in the center of the slide. It is found in lymph nodes and is surrounded by lymphocytes. (Courtesy Dr. Robert W. McKenna, Department of Pathology, University of Texas Southwestern Medical School, Dallas, TX; From Kumar V, Cotran RS, Robbins SL: Basic Pathology, 7th ed. Philadelphia, WB Saunders, 2003, p. 432.)

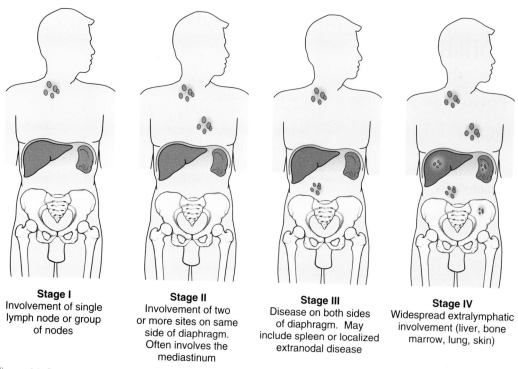

| **Stage I**
Involvement of single lymph node or group of nodes | **Stage II**
Involvement of two or more sites on same side of diaphragm. Often involves the mediastinum | **Stage III**
Disease on both sides of diaphragm. May include spleen or localized extranodal disease | **Stage IV**
Widespread extralymphatic involvement (liver, bone marrow, lung, skin) |

Figure 14-9

Staging of Hodgkin disease involves assessing the extent of spread of the disease. Lymph node biopsies, laparotomy with liver and lymph node biopsies, and splenectomy may be necessary for staging.

(using high-dose radiation). If the disease is more widespread, chemotherapy is given alone or in combination with radiotherapy. There is a very high probability of cure with available treatments. Figure 14-9 illustrates staging of Hodgkin disease.

Non-Hodgkin lymphoma—Types of this disease include **follicular lymphoma** (composed of collections of small lymphocytes in a follicle or nodule arrangement) and **large cell lymphoma** (composed of large lymphocytes that infiltrate nodes and tissues diffusely). Chemotherapy and radiation may cure or stop the progress of this disease.

multiple myeloma

Malignant tumor of bone marrow cells.

This is a tumor composed of plasma cells (antibody-producing B-cell lymphocytes) associated with high levels of one of the specific immunoglobulins, usually IgG. **Waldenstrom macroglobulinemia** is another tumor of malignant B-cell lymphocytes. This disease involves B cells that produce large quantities of IgM (a globulin of high molecular weight). Increased IgM concentration impairs the passage of blood through capillaries in the brain and eyes, causing a hyperviscosity syndrome (thickening of the blood).

thymoma

Malignant tumor of the thymus gland.

Some symptoms of thymoma are cough, dyspnea, dysphagia, fever, chest pain, weight loss, and anorexia. Often, the tumor is associated with other disorders, such as myasthenia gravis and cytopenias.

Surgery is the principal method of treating thymoma; postoperative radiation therapy is used for patients with evidence of spread of the tumor.

G. Match the following terms with their meanings below.

AIDS   Hodgkin disease   lymphoid organs
allergen   hypersplenism   thymectomy
anaphylaxis   lymphedema

1. syndrome marked by enlargement of the spleen and associated with anemia, leukopenia, and

   thrombocytopenia _____

2. an extraordinary hypersensitivity to a foreign protein; marked by hypotension, shock, and respiratory

   distress _____

3. an antigen capable of causing allergy (hypersensitivity) _____

4. disorder in which the immune system is suppressed by exposure to HIV _____

5. removal of a mediastinal organ _____

6. malignant tumor of lymph nodes and spleen marked by the presence of Reed-Sternberg cells in

   lymph nodes _____

7. tissue that produces lymphocytes—spleen, thymus, tonsils, and adenoids _____

8. swelling of tissues due to interstitial fluid accumulation _____

H. Match the following terms or abbreviations related to AIDS with their meanings below.

CD4+ lymphocytes   HIV   PCP
ELISA   Kaposi sarcoma   protease inhibitor
HAART   opportunistic infections   RT inhibitor

1. a cancerous condition associated with AIDS (bluish-red skin nodules appear)

   _____

2. human immunodeficiency virus; the retrovirus that causes AIDS _____

3. white blood cells that are destroyed by the AIDS virus _____

4. pneumonia (*Pneumocystis carinii* pneumonia) that occurs in AIDS patients

   _____

5. group of infectious diseases associated with AIDS _____

6. combination of drugs to treat AIDS _____

7. test to detect anti-HIV antibodies _____

8. drug used to treat AIDS by blocking the growth of the AIDS virus _____

9. drug used to treat AIDS by blocking the production of a proteolytic enzyme

_____

I. Complete the following terms according to their definitions. Pay close attention to the proper spelling of each term.

1. chronic, disabling diseases caused by abnormal production of antibodies to normal tissue:

   auto _____ diseases

2. a hypersensitivity or allergic state with an inherited predisposition: a _____

3. a malignant tumor of lymph nodes; histiocytic and lymphocytic are types of this disease:

   non-_____

4. fluid that lies between cells throughout the body: inter _____ fluid

5. formation of lymphocytes or lymphoid tissue: lympho _____

6. chronic swelling of a part of the body due to collection of fluid between tissues secondary to

   obstruction of lymph vessels and nodes: lymph _____

7. an unusual or exaggerated allergic reaction to a foreign protein: ana _____

8. introduction of altered antigens to produce an immune response and protection from disease:

   vac _____

9. test that separates immunoglobulins: immuno _____

J. Circle the correct term to complete each sentence.

1. Mr. Blake had been HIV-positive for 5 years before he developed **(PCP, thymoma, multiple myeloma)** and was diagnosed with **(Hodgkin disease, non-Hodgkin lymphoma, AIDS)**.

2. Mary developed rhinitis, rhinorrhea, and red eyes every spring when pollen was prevalent. She consulted her doctor about her bad **(hypersplenism, allergies, lymphadenitis)**.

3. Paul felt some marble-sized lumps in his left groin. His doctor told him that he had an infection in his foot and had developed secondary **(axillary, cervical, inguinal)** lymphadenopathy.

4. Mr. Jones was referred to a dermatologist and an oncologist when his primary physician noticed purple spots on his arms and legs. Because he had AIDS, his physician was worried about **(Kaposi sarcoma, splenomegaly, thrombocytopenic purpura)**.

5. Fifteen-year-old Peter was allergic to nuts. His allergy was so severe that he carried epinephrine with him at all times to prevent **(acquired immunity, anaphylaxis, immunosuppression)** in case he came in contact with peanut butter at school.

6. When she was in her mid-twenties, Rona was diagnosed with lymph node malignancy known as **(sarcoidosis, Kaposi sarcoma, Hodgkin disease)**. Because the disease was primarily in her chest, her **(inguinal, mediastinal, axillary)** lymph nodes were irradiated (radiation therapy) and she was cured. When she developed lung cancer in her mid-forties, her oncologist told her she had an **(iatrogenic, hereditary, metastatic)** radiation-induced secondary tumor.

7. Mary has suffered from hay fever, asthma, and chronic dermatitis ever since she was a young child. She has been particularly bothered by the severely pruritic (itching), erythematous (reddish) patches on her hands. Her dermatologist gave her topical steroids for her **(toxic, atopic, opportunistic)** dermatitis and told her to avoid soaps, cosmetics, and irritating chemicals.

8. Bernie noticed pain in his pelvis, spine, and ribs and was evaluated by his physician. Blood tests showed high levels of plasma cells and abnormal globulins. Increased numbers of plasma cells were revealed on **(chest x-ray, stem cell transplant, bone marrow biopsy)**. Radiologic studies showed bone loss. The physician's diagnosis was multiple **(sclerosis, thymoma, myeloma)**.

9. AIDS is caused by **(herpes simplex virus, monoclonal antibodies, human immunodeficiency virus)**. Lymphocytes called **(CD4+ helper cells, suppressor cells, B cells)** are destroyed, which disrupts **(humoral immunity, cell-mediated immunity, natural immunity)**, leading to **(anaphylaxis, atopy, opportunistic infections)**.

10. Drugs used to treat AIDS are **(immunosuppressants, protease inhibitors, interferons)**. Other anti-AIDS drugs are **(reverse transcriptase inhibitors, monoclonal antibodies, immunoglobulins)**.

X. Answers to Exercises

A

1. lymph nodes
2. thoracic duct
3. spleen
4. adenoids
5. thymus gland
6. lymph capillaries
7. right lymphatic duct
8. interstitial fluid

B

1. groin region
2. armpit region
3. neck (of the body) region
4. space between the lungs in the chest

C

1. humoral immunity
2. T cells
3. cell-mediated immunity
4. B cells

D

1. plasma cell
2. macrophage
3. helper cell
4. natural killer (NK) cell
5. suppressor cell
6. dendritic cell

E

1. A
2. C
3. B
4. D
5. G
6. F
7. E

F

1. splenectomy
2. splenomegaly
3. lymphopoiesis
4. thymoma
5. lymphadenitis
6. lymphocytopenia
7. toxic
8. lymphadenopathy

G

1. hypersplenism
2. anaphylaxis
3. allergen
4. AIDS
5. thymectomy
6. Hodgkin disease
7. lymphoid organs
8. lymphedema

H

1. Kaposi sarcoma
2. HIV
3. T4 helper lymphocytes
4. PCP
5. opportunistic infections
6. ELISA (enzyme-linked immunosorbent assay)
7. HAART
8. RT inhibitor
9. protease inhibitor

I

1. autoimmune
2. atopy
3. non-Hodgkin lymphoma
4. interstitial
5. lymphopoiesis
6. lymphedema
7. anaphylaxis
8. vaccination
9. immunoelectrophoresis

J

1. PCP; AIDS
2. allergies
3. inguinal
4. Kaposi sarcoma
5. anaphylaxis
6. Hodgkin disease; mediastinal; iatrogenic
7. atopic
8. bone marrow biopsy; myeloma
9. human immunodeficiency virus; CD4+ helper cells; cell-mediated immunity; opportunistic infections
10. protease inhibitors; reverse transcriptase inhibitors

Answers to Practical Applications

1. B
2. A
3. A
4. B
5. B
6. A
7. B
8. C

XI. Pronunciation of Terms

Pronunciation Guide

ā as in āpe   ă as in ăpple
ē as in ēven   ĕ as in ĕvery
ī as in īce   ĭ as in ĭnterest
ō as in ōpen   ŏ as in pŏt
ū as in ūnit   ŭ as in ŭnder

To test your understanding of the terminology in this chapter, write the meaning of each term in the space provided. In addition, you may wish to cover the terms and write them by looking at your definitions. Make sure your spelling is correct. The page number after each term indicates where it is defined or used in the text so you can easily check your responses.

Vocabulary and Terminology

Term	Pronunciation	Meaning
acquired immunity (537)	ă-KWĪ-erd ĭ-MŪ-nĭ-tē	_____
acquired immunodeficiency syndrome (540)	ă-KWĪ-ĕrd ĭm-ū-nō-dĕ-FĬSH-ĕn-sē SĬN-drōm	_____
adenoids (537)	ĂD-ĕ-noydz	_____
allergen (544)	ĂL-ĕr-jĕn	_____
allergy (542)	ĂL-ĕr-jē	_____
anaphylaxis (544)	ăn-ă-fă-LĂK-sĭs	_____
antibody (537)	ĂN-tĭ-bŏ-dē	_____
atopy (544)	ĂT-ō-pē	_____
autoimmune disease (539)	āw-tō-ĭ-MŪN dĭ-ZĒZ	_____
axillary node (537)	ĂKS-ĭ-lăr-ē nōd	_____
B cell (537)	B sĕl	_____
cell-mediated immunity (537)	sĕl-MĒ-dē-ā-tĕd ĭ-MŪ-nĭ-tē	_____
cervical node (537)	SĔR-vĭ-k'l nōd	_____
cytokine (537)	SĪ-tō-kĭne	_____
cytotoxic cell (537)	sī-tō-TŎK-sĭk sĕl	_____
dendritic cell (537)	dĕn-DRĬ-tik sĕl	_____
ELISA test (545)	ĕ-LĪ-ză tĕst	_____
helper T cell (537)	HĔL-pĕr T sĕl	_____
Hodgkin disease (544)	HŎJ-kĭn dĭ-ZĒZ	_____

human immunodeficiency virus (544)	HŪ-măn ĭm-ū-nō-dĕ-FĬSH-ĕn-sē VĪ-rŭs	_____
humoral immunity (537)	HŪ-mŏr-ăl ĭ-MŪ-nĭ-tē	_____
hypersensitivity (542)	hī-pĕr-sĕn-sĭ-TĬV-ĭ-tē	_____
hypersplenism (540)	hī-pĕr-SPLĔN-ĭzm	_____
immune response (537)	ĭ-MŪN rĕ-SPŎNS	_____
immunoelectrophoresis (545)	ĭm-ū-nō-ē-lĕk-trō-phŏr-Ē-sĭs	_____
immunoglobulins (537)	ĭm-ū-nō-GLŎB-ū-lĭnz	_____
immunosuppression (539)	ĭm-ū-nō-sū-PRĔ-shun	_____
immunotherapy (537)	ĭ-mū-nō-THĔR-ă-pē	_____
inguinal node (537)	ĬNG-gwĭ-năl nōd	_____
interferons (537)	ĭn-tĕr-FĔR-ŏnz	_____
interleukins (538)	ĭn-tĕr-LOO-kĭnz	_____
interstitial fluid (538)	ĭn-tĕr-STĬSH-ăl FLOO-ĭd	_____
Kaposi sarcoma (544)	KĂ-pō-sē (kă-PŌs-sē) săr-KŌ-mă	_____
lymph (538)	lĭmf	_____
lymphadenitis (540)	lĭm-FĂH-dĕ-nī-tĭs	_____
lymphadenopathy (540)	lĭm-făd-ĕ-NŎP-ăh-thē	_____
lymph capillaries (538)	lĭmf KĂP-ĭ-lă-rēz	_____
lymphedema (539)	lĭmf-ĕ-DĒ-mă	_____
lymph node (538)	lĭmf nōd	_____
lymphocytes (530)	LĬM-fō-sītz	_____
lymphocytosis (539)	lĭm-fō-sī-TŌ-sĭs	_____
lymphocytopenia (539)	lĭm-fō-sī-tō-PĒ-nē-ă	_____
lymphoid organs (538)	LĬM-foid ŎR-gănz	_____
lymphoma (542)	lĭm-FŌ-mă	_____
lymphopoiesis (539)	lĭm-fō-poy-Ē-sĭs	_____
lymph vessel (538)	lĭmf VĔS-ĕl	_____

D. Facial Bones

All the facial bones, except one, are joined together by sutures, so they are immovable. The mandible (lower jaw bone) is the only facial bone capable of movement. This ability is necessary for activities such as mastication (chewing) and speaking.

Figure 15–5 shows the facial bones; label it as you read the following descriptions of the facial bones:

Nasal bones [1]—Two slender nasal (**nas/o** means nose) bones support the bridge of the nose. They join with the frontal bone superiorly and form part of the nasal septum.

Lacrimal bones [2]—Two paired lacrimal (**lacrim/o** means tear) bones are located at the corner of each eye. These thin, small bones contain fossae for the lacrimal gland (tear gland) and canals for the passage of the lacrimal duct.

Maxillary bones [3]—Two large bones compose the massive upper jawbones **(maxillae).** They are joined by a suture in the median plane. If the two bones do not come together normally before birth, the condition known as **cleft palate** results.

Mandibular bone [4]—This is the lower jawbone **(mandible).** Both the maxilla and the mandible contain the sockets called **alveoli** in which the teeth are embedded. The mandible joins the skull at the region of the temporal bone, forming the temporomandibular joint (TMJ) on either side of the skull.

Zygomatic bones [5]—Two bones, one on each side of the face, form the high portion of the cheek.

Vomer [6]—This thin, single, flat bone forms the lower portion of the nasal septum.

Sinuses, or air cavities, are located in specific places within the cranial and facial bones to lighten the skull and warm and moisten air as it passes through. Figure 15–6 shows the sinuses of the skull.

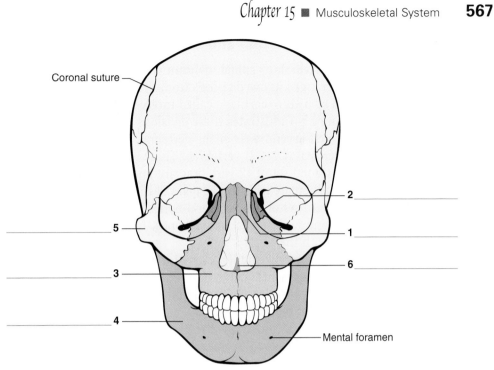

Coronal suture

2

5

1

3

6

4

Mental foramen

Figure 15–5

Facial bones.

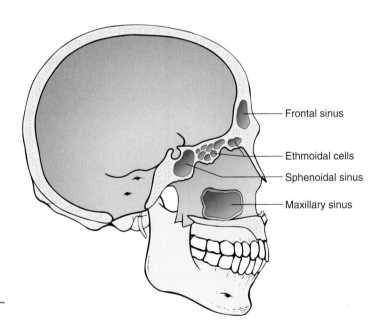

Frontal sinus

Ethmoidal cells

Sphenoidal sinus

Maxillary sinus

Figure 15–6

Sinuses of the skull.

E. Vertebral Column and Structure of Vertebrae

The **vertebral,** or **spinal, column** is composed of 26 bone segments, called vertebrae, that are arranged in five divisions from the base of the skull to the tailbone. The bones are separated by pads of cartilage called **intervertebral disks (discs).**

Figure 15–7 illustrates these divisions of the vertebral column.

The first seven bones of the vertebral column, forming the bony aspect of the neck, are the **cervical (C1–C7) vertebrae.** These vertebrae do not articulate (join) with the ribs.

The second set of 12 vertebrae are known as the **thoracic (T1–T12) vertebrae.** These vertebrae articulate with the 12 pairs of ribs.

The third set of five vertebral bones are the **lumbar (L1–L5) vertebrae.** They are the strongest and largest of the backbones. Like the cervical vertebrae, these bones do not articulate with the ribs.

The **sacrum** is a slightly curved, triangularly shaped bone. At birth it is composed of five separate segments (sacral bones); these gradually become fused in the young child.

The **coccyx** is the tailbone, and it, too, is a fused bone, having been formed from four small coccygeal bones.

Figure 15–8A illustrates the general structure of a vertebra. Although the individual vertebrae in the separate regions of the spinal column are all slightly different in structure, they do have several parts in common.

A vertebra is composed of an inner, thick, round portion called the **vertebral body** [1]. Between the body of one vertebra and the bodies of the vertebrae lying beneath and above are intervertebral cartilaginous disks, which help provide flexibility and cushion most shocks to the vertebral column.

The **vertebral arch** [2] is the posterior part of the vertebra, and it consists of a single **spinous process** [3], two **transverse processes** [4], and two **laminae** [5]. The **neural canal** [6] is the space between the vertebral body and the vertebral arch through which the spinal cord passes. Figure 15–8B shows a lateral view of several vertebrae. Note the location of the spinal cord running through the neural canal.

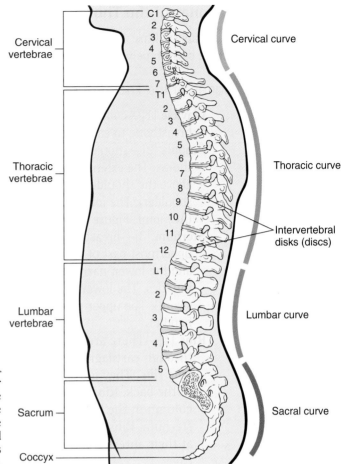

Figure 15-7

Vertebral column. Notice the four curves of the vertebral column. The sacral and thoracic curvatures are present at birth. The cervical curvature develops when an infant holds its head erect. The lumbar curvature develops as an infant begins to stand and walk.

Cervical vertebrae
Thoracic vertebrae
Lumbar vertebrae
Sacrum
Coccyx

C1
2
3
4
5
6
7
T1
2
3
4
5
6
7
8
9
10
11
12
L1
2
3
4
5

Cervical curve
Thoracic curve
Intervertebral disks (discs)
Lumbar curve
Sacral curve

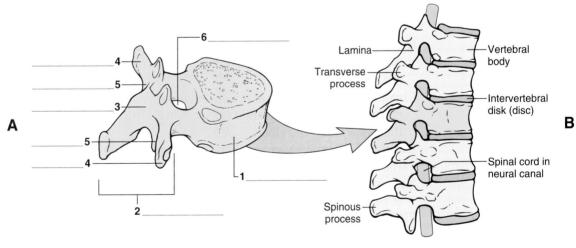

A

6
4
5
3
5
4
1
2

Lamina
Transverse process
Spinous process

Vertebral body
Intervertebral disk (disc)
Spinal cord in neural canal

B

Figure 15-8

(A) General structure of a vertebra, viewed from above. **(B) Series of vertebrae,** lateral view, to show the position of the spinal cord behind the vertebral bodies and intervertebral discs.

The **ilium** is the uppermost and largest portion. Dorsally, the two parts of the ilium do not meet. Rather, they join the sacrum on either side to form the sacroiliac joints. The connection between the iliac bones and the sacrum is very firm, and very little motion occurs at these joints. The superior part of the ilium is known as the **iliac crest.** It is filled with red bone marrow and serves as an attachment for abdominal wall muscles.

The **ischium** (**isch/o** means back) is the posterior part of the pelvis. The ischium and the muscles attached to it are what you sit on.

The **pubis** is the anterior part, and the two pubic bones join by way of a cartilaginous disk. This area is called the **pubic symphysis.** Like the sacroiliac joints, this area is quite rigid.

The region within the ring of bone formed by the pelvic girdle is called the **pelvic cavity.** The rectum, sigmoid colon, bladder, and female reproductive organs lie within the pelvic cavity and are protected by the rigid architecture of the pelvic girdle.

Bones of the Leg and Foot

Femur [12]—thigh bone; this is the longest bone in the body. At its proximal end it has a rounded head that fits into a depression, or socket, in the pelvis. This socket is called the **acetabulum.** The acetabulum was named because of its resemblance to a rounded cup the Romans used for vinegar (acetum). The head of the femur and the acetabulum form the "ball and socket" joint otherwise known as the hip joint.

Patella [13]—kneecap; this is a small, flat bone that lies in front of the articulation between the femur and one of the lower leg bones called the tibia. It is a sesamoid bone surrounded by protective tendons and held in place by muscle attachments. Together with the femur and tibia, it forms the knee joint.

Tibia [14]—largest of two bones of the lower leg; the tibia runs under the skin in the front part of the leg. It joins with the femur and patella proximally, and at its distal end (ankle) forms a flare that is the bony prominence (medial **malleolus**) at the inside of the ankle. The tibia is commonly called the **shin bone.**

Fibula [15]—smaller of two lower leg bones; this thin bone, well hidden under the leg muscles, runs parallel to the tibia. At its distal part, it forms a flare, which is the bony prominence (lateral **malleolus**) on the outside of the ankle. The tibia, fibula, and **talus** (the first of the tarsal bones) come together to form the **ankle joint.**

Tarsals [16]—bones of the hind part of the foot; these seven short bones resemble the carpal bones of the wrist but are larger. The **calcaneus** is the largest of these bones and is also called the **heel bone** (Fig. 15–11). The **talus** is one of three bones that form the ankle joint.

Metatarsals [17]—bones of the midfoot; there are five metatarsal bones, which are similar to the metacarpals of the hand. Each leads to the phalanges of the toes.

Phalanges of the toes [18]—bones of the forefoot; similar to the hand, there are two phalanges in the big toe and three in each of the other toes.

Figure 15–11 illustrates the bones of the foot.

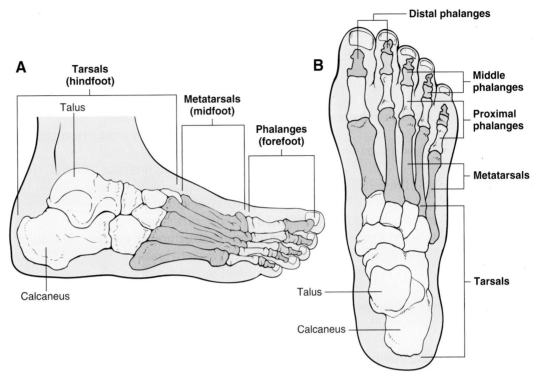

Figure 15-11

(A) Bones of the foot, lateral view. **(B) Bones of the foot,** as viewed from above.

G. Vocabulary

This list will help you review many of the new terms introduced in the text. Short definitions will reinforce your understanding of the terms. See Section IX of this chapter for help in pronouncing the more difficult terms.

acetabulum	Rounded depression, or socket, in the pelvis, which joins the femur (thigh bone), forming the hip joint.
acromion	Outward extension of the shoulder bone forming the point of the shoulder. It overlies the shoulder joint and articulates with the clavicle.
articular cartilage	Thin layer of cartilage occurring at the ends of long bones and covering any part of any bone that comes together with another bone to form a joint.
bone	Dense, hard connective tissue composing the skeleton. Examples are long bones (femur), short bones (carpals), flat bones (scapula), and sesamoid bones (patella).
calcium	One of the mineral constituents of bone. **Calcium phosphate** is the major calcium salt in bones.
cancellous bone	Spongy, porous, trabecular bone.

H. Combining Forms and Suffixes

These are divided into two groups: general terms and terms related to specific bones. Write the meanings of the medical terms in the spaces provided.

GENERAL TERMS			
Combining Forms			
Combining Forms	Meaning	Terminology	Meaning
calc/o **calci/o**	calcium	hypercalcemia _____	
		decalcification _____	
		de- means less or lack of; -fication is the process of making.	
kyph/o	humpback (posterior curvature in the thoracic region)	kyphosis _____	
		The term (from Greek meaning hill or mountain) indicates a hump on the back. A person's height is reduced, and kyphosis may lead to pressure on the spinal cord or peripheral nerves.	
lamin/o	lamina (part of the vertebral arch)	laminectomy _____	
		An operation often performed to relieve the symptoms of compression of the spinal cord or spinal nerve roots. It involves removal of the lamina and spinous process.	
lord/o	curve, swayback (anterior curvature in the lumbar region)	lordosis _____	
		This term is used to describe the normal anterior curvature of the spinal column in the lumbar region. An excessive, abnormal anterior curvature, or swayback condition, is known as hyperlordosis. The word lordosis is derived from Greek, describing a person leaning backward in a lordly fashion.	
lumb/o	loins, lower back	lumbar _____	
		lumbosacral _____	
myel/o	bone marrow	myelopoiesis _____	
orth/o	straight	orthopedics _____	
		Ped/o means child.	
oste/o	bone	osteitis _____	
		osteodystrophy _____	
		osteogenesis _____	
		Osteogenesis imperfecta *is a genetic disorder involving defective development of bones, which are brittle and fragile; fractures occur with the slightest trauma.*	

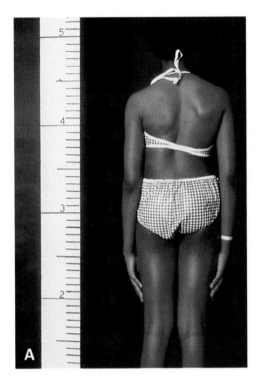
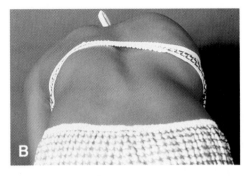

Figure 15–12

Moderate thoracic idiopathic adolescent scoliosis.
(A) Notice the scapular asymmetry in the upright
position. This results from rotation of the spine
and attached rib cage. **(B)** Bending forward reveals
mild rib hump deformity. (From Zitelli BJ, Davis
HW: Atlas of Pediatric Physical Diagnosis, 4th ed.
St. Louis, Mosby, 2002, p. 756.)

scoli/o	crooked, bent (lateral curvature)	<u>scoli</u>osis _____
		The spinal column is bent abnormally to the side. Scoliosis is the most common spinal deformity in adolescent girls (Fig. 15–12).
spondyl/o (used to make words about conditions of the structure)	vertebra	<u>spondyl</u>osis _____
		Degeneration of the intervertebral disks in the cervical, thoracic, and lumbar regions. Symptoms include pain and restriction of movement.
vertebr/o (used to describe the structure)	vertebra	<u>vertebr</u>al _____

| **Suffixes** | | | |
Suffix	Meaning	Terminology	Meaning
-blast	embryonic or immature cell	osteo<u>blast</u> _____	
		This cell synthesizes collagen and protein to form bone tissue.	
-clast	to break	osteo<u>clast</u> _____	
		This cell breaks down bone to remove bone tissue.	
-listhesis	slipping	spondylo<u>listhesis</u> _____	
		(spŏn-dĭ-lō-lĭs-THĒ-sĭs), the forward slipping (subluxation) of a vertebra over a lower vertebra.	

-malacia	softening	osteomalacia _____	

A condition in which vitamin D deficiency leads to decalcification of bones; known as rickets in children.

-physis	to grow	epiphysis _____	
		pubic symphysis _____	
-porosis	pore, passage	osteoporosis _____	

Loss of bony tissue and decreased mass of bone. See page 582, Section II (I), Pathological Conditions and Fractures.

-tome	instrument to cut	osteotome _____	

This surgical chisel is designed to cut bone.

TERMS RELATED TO SPECIFIC BONES
Combining Forms

Combining Forms	Meaning	Terminology	Meaning
acetabul/o	acetabulum (hip socket)	acetabular	*hip socket*
calcane/o	calcaneus (heel bone)	calcaneal	*heel of the foot*

The calcaneus is one of the tarsal (hindfoot) bones.

Combining Forms	Meaning	Terminology	Meaning
carp/o	carpals (wrist bones)	carpal	*wrist*
clavicul/o	clavicle (collar bone)	supraclavicular	*collar*

supra- means above.

Combining Forms	Meaning	Terminology	Meaning
cost/o	ribs (true ribs, false ribs, and floating ribs)	subcostal	
		chondrocostal	

Cartilage that is attached to the ribs.

Combining Forms	Meaning	Terminology	Meaning
crani/o	cranium (skull bones)	craniotomy	
		craniotome	
femor/o	femur (thigh bone)	femoral	
fibul/o	fibula (smaller lower leg bone)	fibular	

See perone/o.

Combining Forms	Meaning	Terminology	Meaning
humer/o	humerus (upper arm bone)	humeral	

ili/o	ilium (upper part of pelvic bone)	iliac _____
isch/o	ischium (posterior part of pelvic bone)	ischial _____
malleol/o	malleolus (process on each side of the ankle)	malleolar _____
		The medial malleolus is at the lower end of the tibia, and the lateral malleolus is at the lower end of the fibula.
mandibul/o	mandible (lower jaw bone)	mandibular _____
maxill/o	maxilla (upper jaw bone)	maxillary _____
metacarp/o	metacarpals (hand bones)	metacarpectomy _____
metatars/o	metatarsals (foot bones)	metatarsalgia _____
olecran/o	olecranon (elbow)	olecranal _____
patell/o	patella (kneecap)	subpatellar _____
pelv/i	pelvis (hipbone)	pelvimetry _____
perone/o	fibula	peroneal _____
phalang/o	phalanges (finger and/or toe bones)	phalangeal _____
pub/o	pubis (anterior part of the pelvic bone)	pubic _____
radi/o	radius (lower arm bone—thumb side)	radial _____
scapul/o	scapula (shoulder bone)	scapular _____
stern/o	sternum (breastbone)	sternal _____
tars/o	tarsals (bones of the hindfoot)	tarsectomy _____
tibi/o	tibia (shin bone)	tibial _____
uln/o	ulna (lower arm bone—little finger side)	ulnar _____

I. Pathological Conditions and Fractures

Ewing sarcoma

Malignant bone tumor.

Pain and swelling are common, especially if the tumor involves the shaft (medullary cavity) of a long bone. This tumor usually occurs at an early age (5-15 years old), and combined treatment with surgery, radiotherapy and chemotherapy represents the best chance for cure (60-70 percent of patients are cured if metastasis has not occurred).

exostosis

Bony growth arising from the surface of bone (ex- means out, -ostosis means condition of bone).

Osteochondromas (composed of cartilage and bone) are **exostoses** and are usually found on the metaphyses of long bones near the epiphyseal plates.

A **bunion** is a swelling of the metatarsophalangeal joint near the base of the big toe and is accompanied by the buildup of soft tissue and underlying bone at the distal/medial aspect of the first metatarsal.

fracture

Traumatic breaking of a bone.

A **closed fracture** means that a bone is broken but there is no open wound in the skin, whereas an **open** (compound) **fracture** means a bone is broken and a fragment of bone protrudes through an open wound in the skin. A **pathological fracture** is caused by disease of the bone such as tumor or infection, making it weak. **Crepitus** is the crackling sound produced when ends of bones rub each other or rub against roughened cartilage.

Some examples of fractures (Fig. 15–13) are the following:

Colles fracture—Occurs near the wrist joint at the lower end of the radius.
comminuted fracture—Bone is splintered or crushed into several pieces. A simple fracture means that a bone breaks in only one place and is therefore not comminuted.
compression fracture—Bone is compressed; often occurs in vertebrae.
greenstick fracture—Bone is partially broken; it breaks on one surface and only bends on the other, as when a green stick breaks; occurs in children.
impacted fracture—Fracture in which one fragment is driven firmly into the other.

Treatment of fractures involves **reduction,** which is restoration of the bone to its normal position. A **closed reduction** is manipulative reduction without a surgical incision; in an **open reduction,** an incision is made into the fracture site. A **cast** (solid mold of the body part) is applied to fractures to immobilize the injured bone. In some cases, metal plates, screws, rods, or pins (internal fixation) are utilized to stabilize and maintain an open reduction.

osteogenic sarcoma

Malignant tumor arising from bone (osteosarcoma).

This is the most common type of malignant bone tumor. Osteoblasts multiply, forming large, bony tumors, especially at the ends of long bones (half the lesions are located just below or just above the knee) (Fig. 15–14). Metastasis takes place through the bloodstream and often occurs to the lungs. Surgical resection followed by chemotherapy improves the survival rate.

Malignant tumors from other parts of the body (breast, prostate, lung, thyroid gland, and kidney) may metastasize to bones; and are called **metastatic bone lesions.**

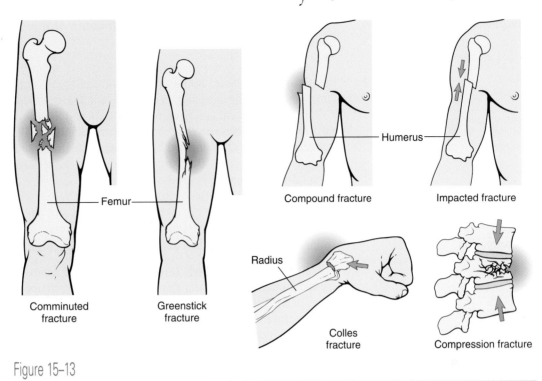

Femur

Humerus

Radius

Comminuted
fracture

Greenstick
fracture

Compound fracture

Impacted fracture

Colles
fracture

Compression fracture

Figure 15–13

Types of fractures.

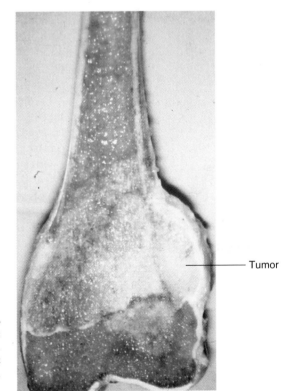

Tumor

Figure 15–14

Osteosarcoma. The tumor has grown through the cortex of the bone and elevated the periosteum. (From Kumar V, Cotran RS, Robbins SL: Basic Pathology, 7th ed. Philadelphia, WB Saunders, 2003, p. 767.)

osteomalacia

Softening of bone, with inadequate amounts of mineral (calcium) in the bone.

Osteomalacia occurs primarily as a disease of infancy and childhood and is then known as **rickets.** Bones fail to receive adequate amounts of calcium and phosphorus; they become soft, bend easily, and become deformed.

In these individuals, vitamin D is deficient in the diet, which prevents calcium and phosphorus from being absorbed into the bloodstream from the intestines. Vitamin D is formed by the action of sunlight on certain compounds (such as cholesterol) in the skin; thus rickets is more common in large, smoky cities during the winter months.

Treatment most often consists of administration of large daily doses of vitamin D and an increase in dietary intake of calcium and phosphorus.

osteomyelitis

Inflammation of the bone and bone marrow secondary to infection.

Bacteria enter the body through a wound and spread to the bone. Children are most often affected, and the infection usually occurs near the ends of long bones of the legs and arms. Adults can be affected too, usually as the result of an open fracture.

The lesion begins as an inflammation with pus collection. Pus tends to spread down the medullary cavity and outward to the periosteum. Antibiotic therapy corrects the condition if the infection is treated quickly. If treatment is delayed, an **abscess** can form. An abscess is a walled-off area of infection that can be difficult or impossible to penetrate with antibiotics. Surgical drainage of an abscess is usually necessary.

osteoporosis

Decrease in bone density (mass); thinning and weakening of bone.

This condition is also called **osteopenia** because the interior of bones is diminished in structure, as if the steel skeleton of a building had rusted and been worn down (Fig. 15–15). Osteoporosis commonly occurs in older women as a consequence of estrogen deficiency with menopause. Lack of estrogen promotes excessive bone resorption (osteoclast activity) and less bone deposition. Weakened bones are subject to fractures (as in the hip); loss of height and kyphosis occur as vertebrae collapse (Fig. 15–16).

Estrogen replacement therapy and increased intake of calcium may be helpful for some patients. A weight-bearing daily exercise program is also important as is the avoidance of smoking. Bisphosphonates (Fosamax) may be taken to decrease osteoclast activity and increase bone mineral content.

Osteoporosis can occur with atrophy caused by disuse, as in a limb that is in a cast, in the legs of a paraplegic, or in a bedridden patient. It may also occur in men as part of the aging process and in patients who have been given corticosteroid (hormones made by the adrenal gland and used to treat inflammatory conditions) therapy.

talipes

Congenital abnormality of the hindfoot (involving the talus).

Several varieties of talipes are known. They are thought to result from congenital anomalies, abnormal positioning of the fetus, or both while in the womb. The most common form is **talipes equinovarus (equin/o** means horse), or **clubfoot.** In this congenital deformity, the patient cannot stand with the sole of the foot flat on the ground. The defect can be corrected by orthopedic splinting in the early months of infancy or, if that fails, by surgery.

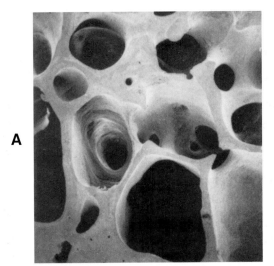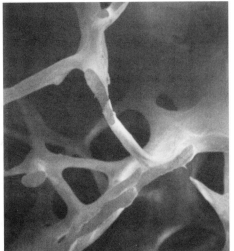

Figure 15–15

Scanning electromicrograph of (A) normal bone and **(B) bone with osteoporosis.** Notice the thinning and wide separation of the trabeculae in the osteoporotic bone. (Reproduced from Dempster DW, Shane E, Horbert W, et al: A simple method for correlative light and scanning electron microscopy of human iliac crest bone biopsies: qualitative observations in normal and osteoporotic subjects. J Bone Miner Res 1986; 1:15-21, with permission of the American Society for Bone and Mineral Research.)

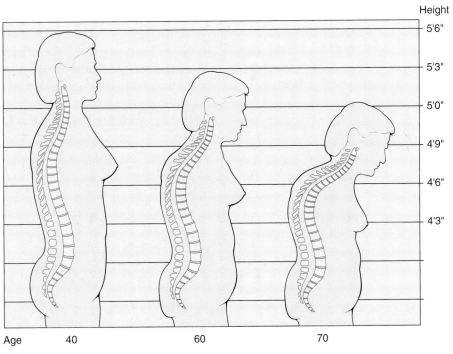

Figure 15–16

Kyphosis. Loss of bone mass due to osteoporosis produces posterior curvature of the spine in the thoracic region. A normal spine is shown at 40 years of age, and osteoporotic changes are illustrated at 60 and at 70 years of age. The changes in the spine can cause a loss of as much as 6 to 9 inches in height.

III. Joints

A. Types of Joints

A joint (articulation) is a coming together of two or more bones. Some joints are immovable, such as the **suture joints** between the skull bones. Other joints, such as those between the vertebrae, are partially movable. Most joints, however, allow considerable movement. These freely movable joints are called **synovial joints.** Examples of synovial joints are the ball-and-socket type (the hip and shoulder joints) and the hinge type (elbow, knee, and ankle joints). Label the structures in Figure 15–17 as you read the following description of a synovial joint:

The bones in a synovial joint are surrounded by a **joint capsule** [1] composed of fibrous tissue. **Ligaments** (thickened fibrous bands of connective tissue) anchor one bone to another and thereby add considerable strength to the joint capsule in critical areas. Bones at the joint are covered with a smooth surface called the **articular cartilage** [2]. The **synovial membrane** [3] lies under the joint capsule and lines the **synovial cavity** [4] between the bones. The synovial cavity is filled with a special lubricating fluid produced by the synovial membrane. This **synovial fluid** contains water and nutrients that nourish as well as lubricate the joints so that friction on the articular cartilage is minimal.

B. Bursae

Bursae (singular: **bursa**) are closed sacs of synovial fluid lined with a synovial membrane and are located near but not within a joint. Bursae are present wherever two types of tissue are closely opposed and need to slide past one another with as little friction as possible. Bursae serve as layers of lubrication between the tissues. Common sites of bursae are between **tendons** (connective tissue that connects a muscle to bone) and bones, between **ligaments** (connective tissue binding bone to bone) and bones, and between skin and bones in areas where bony anatomy is prominent.

Some common locations of bursae are at the elbow joint (olecranon bursa), knee joint (prepatellar bursa), and shoulder joint (subacromial bursa). Figure 15–18A shows a lateral view of the knee joint with bursae. Figure 15–18B is a frontal view of the knee showing ligaments that provide stability for the joint.

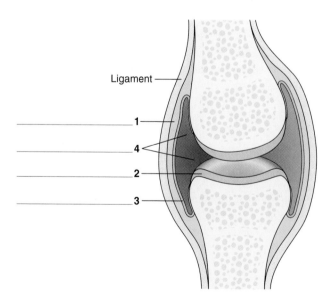

Figure 15–17

Structure of a synovial joint.

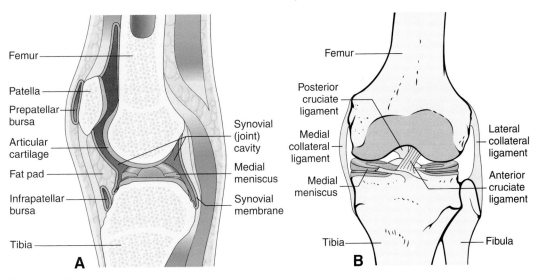

Femur

Patella

Prepatellar bursa

Articular cartilage

Fat pad

Infrapatellar bursa

Tibia

Synovial (joint) cavity

Medial meniscus

Synovial membrane

A

Femur

Posterior cruciate ligament

Medial collateral ligament

Medial meniscus

Lateral collateral ligament

Anterior cruciate ligament

Tibia

Fibula

B

Figure 15–18

(A) Sagittal section of the knee showing bursae and other structures. A **meniscus** (pl., menisci) is a crescent-shaped piece of cartilage that acts as a protective cushion in a synovial joint such as the knee. A "torn cartilage" in the knee is a damaged meniscus and is frequently repaired with arthroscopic surgery. **(B) Frontal section of the knee.** Notice the **anterior cruciate ligament (ACL),** which may be damaged ("torn ligament") with knee injury. Reconstruction of the ACL can require extensive surgery and may involve months of physical therapy for return of normal function.

C. Vocabulary

This list will help you review many of the new terms introduced in this text. Short definitions will reinforce your understanding of the terms. See Section IX of this chapter for help in pronouncing the more difficult terms.

articulation	Joint.
bursa (plural: **bursae**)	Sac of fluid near a joint; promotes smooth sliding of one tissue against another.
ligament	Connective tissue binding bones to other bones; supports, strengthens, and stabilizes the joint.
suture joint	Joint in which apposed surfaces are closely united; motion is minimal.
synovial cavity	Space between bones at a synovial joint; contains synovial fluid produced by the synovial membrane.
synovial fluid	Viscous (sticky) fluid within the synovial cavity. Synovial fluid is similar in viscosity to egg white; this accounts for the origin of the term (syn- means like, ov/o means egg).
synovial joint	A freely movable joint.
synovial membrane	Membrane lining the synovial cavity; it produces synovial fluid.
tendon	Connective tissue that binds muscles to bones.

D. Combining Forms and Suffixes

Write the meanings of the medical terms in the spaces provided.

Combining Forms			
Combining Form	Meaning	Terminology	Meaning

ankyl/o   stiff   ankylosis _____

*A fusion of bones across a joint space by either bony tissue **(bony ankylosis)** or growth of fibrous tissue **(fibrous ankylosis).** This immobility and stiffening of the joint most often occurs in rheumatoid arthritis.*

arthr/o   joint   arthroplasty _____

Replacement arthroplasty is the replacement of one or both bone ends by a prosthesis (artificial part) of metal or plastic.

arthrotomy _____

hemarthrosis _____

hydrarthrosis _____

Synovial fluid collects abnormally in the joint.

polyarthritis _____

articul/o   joint   articular cartilage _____

burs/o   bursa   bursitis _____

Causes of this periarticular condition may be related to stress placed on the bursa or to diseases such as gout or rheumatoid arthritis. The bursa becomes inflamed and movement is limited and painful. Intrabursal injection of corticosteroids as well as rest and splinting of the limb are helpful in treatment.

chondr/o   cartilage   achondroplasia _____

This is an inherited condition in which the bones of the arms and legs fail to grow to normal size because of a defect in cartilage and bone formation. Dwarfism occurs, with short limbs and a normal-sized head and trunk.

chondroma _____

chondromalacia _____

***Chondromalacia patellae** is a softening and roughening of the articular cartilaginous surface of the kneecap, resulting in pain, a grating sensation, and mechanical "catching" behind the patella.*

ligament/o	ligament	<u>ligament</u>ous _____
rheumat/o	watery flow	<u>rheumat</u>ologist _____

Various forms of arthritis are marked by collection of fluid in joint spaces.

synov/o	synovial membrane	<u>synov</u>itis _____
ten/o	tendon	<u>ten</u>orrhaphy _____
		<u>ten</u>osynovitis _____

synov/o here refers to the sheath (covering) around the tendon.

tendin/o	tendon	<u>tendin</u>itis _____

Suffixes

Suffix	Meaning	Terminology	Meaning
-desis	to bind, tie together	arthro<u>desis</u> _____	

Bones are fused across the joint space by surgery (artificial ankylosis). This operation is performed when a joint is very painful, unstable, or chronically infected.

-stenosis	narrowing	spinal <u>stenosis</u> _____	

Narrowing of the neural canal or nerve root canals in the lumbar spine. Symptoms (pain, paresthesias, urinary retention, bowel incontinence) come from compression of the cauda equina (nerves that spread out from the lower end of the spinal cord like a horse's tail).

E. Pathological Conditions

arthritis

Inflammation of joints.

Some of the more common forms are:

1. ankylosing spondylitis

Chronic, progressive arthritis with stiffening of joints, primarily of the spine.

Bilateral sclerosis (hardening) of the sacroiliac joints is a diagnostic sign. Joint changes are similar to those seen in rheumatoid arthritis, and the condition can respond to corticosteroids and anti-inflammatory drugs.

2. gouty arthritis

Inflammation of joints caused by excessive uric acid in the body.

A defect in the metabolism of uric acid causes too much of it to accumulate in blood **(hyperuricemia),** joints, and soft tissues near joints. The uric acid crystals (salts) destroy the articular cartilage and damage the synovial membrane.

A joint chiefly affected is the big toe; hence, the condition is often called **podagra** (pod/o means foot, -agra means excessive pain). Treatment consists of drugs to lower uric acid production (allopurinol) and to prevent inflammation (colchicine and indomethacin) and a special diet that avoids foods that are rich in uric acid, such as red meats, red wines, and fermented cheeses.

3. osteoarthritis (OA)

Progressive, degenerative joint disease characterized by loss of articular cartilage and hypertrophy of bone (formation of osteophytes, or bone spurs) at articular surfaces.

This condition, also known as **degenerative joint disease,** occurs mainly in the hips and knees of older individuals and is marked by a narrowing of the joint space (due to loss of cartilage). Treatment consists of aspirin and other analgesics to reduce inflammation and pain and physical therapy to loosen impaired joints. Figure 15–19 compares a normal joint with those that have changes characteristic of osteoarthritis and rheumatoid arthritis.

End-stage osteoarthritis is the most common reason for joint replacement surgery (total joint arthroplasty).

4. rheumatoid arthritis (RA)

Chronic disease in which joints become inflamed and painful. It is believed to be caused by an immune (autoimmune) reaction against joint tissues, particularly against the synovial membrane.

The small joints of the hands and feet are affected first and larger joints later. Women are more commonly afflicted than men. Synovial membranes become inflamed and thickened, damaging the articular cartilage and preventing easy movement (see Fig. 15–19). Sometimes fibrous tissue forms and calcifies, creating a bony **ankylosis** (union) at the joint and preventing any movement at all. Swollen, painful joints accompanied by **pyrexia** (fever) are symptoms.

Diagnosis is by a blood test that shows the presence of the rheumatoid factor (an antibody) and x-rays revealing changes around the affected joints. Treatment consists of heat applications and drugs (aspirin or NSAIDs, and corticosteroids) to reduce inflammation and pain. Disease-modifying antirheumatic drugs (DMARDs), such as methotrexate and gold salts, are also used.

bunion

Abnormal swelling of the medial aspect of the joint between the big toe and the first metatarsal bone.

A bursa often develops over the site, and chronic irritation from ill-fitting shoes can cause a build-up of soft tissue and underlying bone. Bunionectomy (removal of a bony exostosis and associated soft tissue) is indicated if other measures (changing shoes and use of anti-inflammatory agents) fail.

carpal tunnel syndrome (CTS)

Compression (by a wrist ligament) of the median nerve as it passes between the ligament and the bones and tendons of the wrist (the carpal tunnel) (Fig. 15–20).

This condition most often affects middle-aged women, and pain and burning sensations occur in the fingers and hand, sometimes extending to the elbow. Symptoms most often affect the index (2nd) and long fingers, although the thumb and radial half of the ring (4th) finger may also be symptomatic. Excessive wrist movement, arthritis, hypertrophy of bone, and swelling of the wrist can produce CTS.

Treatment is splinting the wrist to immobilize it, use of anti-inflammatory medications, and injection of cortisone into the carpal tunnel. If these measures fail, surgical release of the carpal ligament can be helpful.

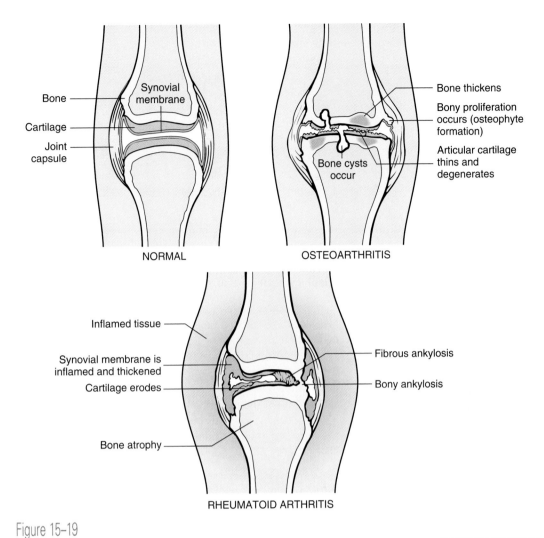

Figure 15-19

Changes in a joint with **osteoarthritis (OA)** and **rheumatoid arthritis (RA).**

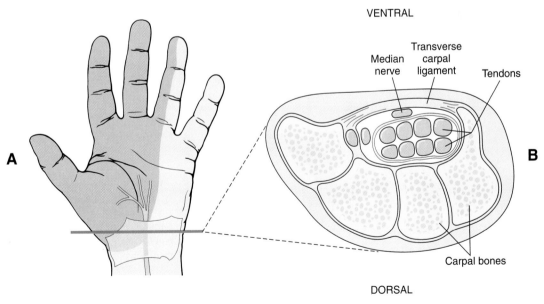

Figure 15-20

Carpal tunnel syndrome (CTS). (A) The median nerve's sensory distribution in the thumb, first three fingers, and palm. **(B)** Cross section of a right hand at the level indicated in (A). Note the position of the median nerve between the carpal ligament and the tendons and carpal bones.

589

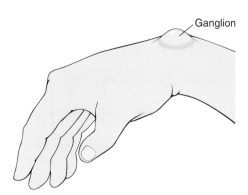

Ganglion

Figure 15–21

Ganglion of the wrist.

dislocation

Displacement of a bone from its joint.

Dislocated bones do not articulate with each other. The most common cause of dislocations is trauma. Some examples of dislocations are **acromioclavicular dislocation** (disruption of the articulation between the acromion and clavicle, also known as a shoulder separation); **shoulder dislocation** (disruption of articulation between the head of the humerus and the glenoid fossa of the scapula); and **hip dislocation** (disruption of articulation between the head of the femur and the acetabulum of the pelvis).

Treatment of dislocations involves **reduction,** which is restoration of the bones to their normal positions. A **subluxation** is a partial or incomplete dislocation.

ganglion

A fluid-filled cyst arising from the joint capsule or a tendon in the wrist.

Most common in the wrist (Fig. 15–21), but can occur in the shoulder, knee, hip, or ankle.

herniation of an intervertebral disk

Abnormal protrusion of a fibrocartilaginous intervertebral disk into the neural canal or spinal nerves.

This condition is commonly referred to as **slipped disk.** Pain is experienced as the protruded disk (Fig. 15–22) presses on spinal nerves or on the spinal cord. Low-back pain and **sciatica** (pain radiating down the leg) are symptoms when the disk protrudes in the lumbar spine. Neck pain and burning pain radiating down an arm are characteristic of a herniated disk in the cervical spine. Bed rest, physical therapy,

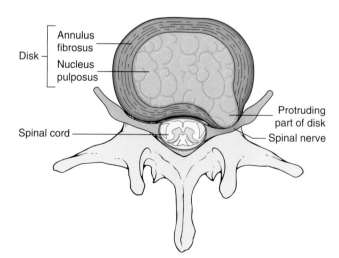

Annulus fibrosus

Disk

Nucleus pulposus

Spinal cord

Protruding part of disk

Spinal nerve

Figure 15–22

Protrusion of an intervertebral disk (looking down on a vertebra). Note how the inner portion (nucleus pulposus) of the disk herniates and presses on the spinal nerve.

and drugs for pain help in initial treatment. In patients with chronic or recurrent disk herniation, **laminectomy** (surgical removal of a portion of the vertebral arch to allow visualization of the protruded disk) and diskectomy (removal of all or part of the protruding disk) may be advised. Spinal fusion of the two vertebrae may be necessary as well. In endoscopic diskectomy the disk is removed by inserting a tube through the skin and aspirating the disk through the tube. Chemonucleolysis is injection of a disk-dissolving enzyme (such as chymopapain) into the center of a herniated disk in an effort to relieve pressure on the compressed nerve or spinal cord.

Lyme disease	**A recurrent disorder marked by severe arthritis, myalgia, malaise, and neurologic and cardiac symptoms.**

Also known as **Lyme arthritis,** the cause of the condition is a spirochete (bacterium) that is carried by a tick. It was first reported in Old Lyme, Connecticut, and is now found throughout the eastern coast of the United States. It is treated with antibiotics.

sprain **Trauma to a joint with pain, swelling, and injury to ligaments.**

Sprains may also involve damage to blood vessels, muscles, tendons, and nerves. A **strain** is a less serious injury involving the overstretching of muscle. Application of ice, elevation of the joint, and application of a gentle compressive wrap are immediate measures to relieve pain and minimize swelling caused by sprains.

systemic lupus erythematosus (SLE) **Chronic inflammatory disease involving joints, skin, kidneys, nervous system, heart, and lungs.**

This condition affects connective tissue (specifically a protein component called **collagen**) in tendons, ligaments, bones, and cartilage all over the body. Typically, there is a red, scaly rash on the face over the nose and cheeks (Fig. 15–23). Patients, usually women, experience joint pain in several joints (polyarthralgia), pyrexia (fever), kidney inflammation, and malaise. SLE is believed to be an autoimmune disease that can be diagnosed by the presence of abnormal antibodies in the bloodstream and characteristic white blood cells called LE cells. Treatment involves giving corticosteroids, hormones made by the adrenal gland that are used to treat inflammatory conditions.

The name lupus (meaning wolf) has been used since the 13th century because physicians thought the shape and color of the skin lesions resembled the bite of a wolf.

Figure 15–23

Butterfly rash that may accompany systemic lupus erythematosus. (From Lewis SM, Heitkemper MM, Dirksen SR: Medical-Surgical Nursing: Assessment and Management of Clinical Problems, 5th ed. St. Louis, Mosby, 2000, p. 1843.)

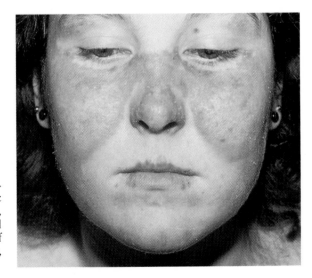

IV. Muscles

A. Types of Muscles

There are three types of muscles in the body. Label Figure 15–24 as you read the following descriptions of the various types of muscles:

Striated muscles [1], also called **voluntary** or **skeletal muscles,** are the muscle fibers that move all bones as well as the face and eyes. Through the central and peripheral nervous system, we have conscious control over these muscles. Striated muscle fibers (cells) have a pattern of dark and light bands, or fibrils, in their cytoplasm. Fibrous tissue that envelops and separates muscles is called **fascia,** which contains the muscle's blood, lymph, and nerve supply.

Smooth muscles [2], also called **involuntary** or **visceral muscles,** are those muscle fibers that move internal organs such as the digestive tract, blood vessels, and secretory ducts leading from glands. These muscles are controlled by the autonomic nervous system. They are called smooth because they have no dark and light fibrils in their cytoplasm. Skeletal muscle fibers are arranged in bundles, whereas smooth muscle forms sheets of fibers as it wraps around tubes and vessels.

Cardiac muscle [3] is striated in appearance but is like smooth muscle in its action. Its movement cannot be consciously controlled. The fibers of cardiac muscle are branching fibers and are found in the heart.

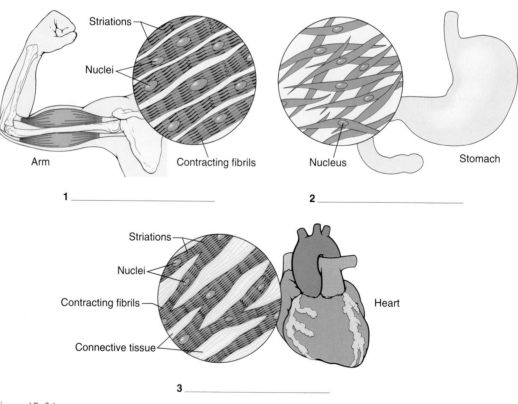

Figure 15–24

Types of muscles.

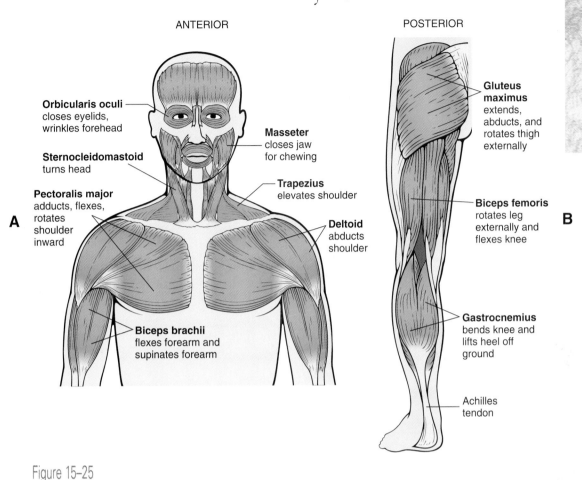

ANTERIOR

POSTERIOR

Orbicularis oculi
closes eyelids,
wrinkles forehead

Sternocleidomastoid
turns head

Pectoralis major
adducts, flexes,
rotates
shoulder
inward

Masseter
closes jaw
for chewing

Trapezius
elevates shoulder

Deltoid
abducts
shoulder

Biceps brachii
flexes forearm and
supinates forearm

A

Gluteus maximus
extends,
abducts, and
rotates thigh
externally

Biceps femoris
rotates leg
externally and
flexes knee

Gastrocnemius
bends knee and
lifts heel off
ground

Achilles tendon

B

Figure 15–25

(A) Selected muscles of the head, neck, torso, and arm and their functions. **(B)** Selected muscles of the posterior aspect of the leg and their functions.

B. Actions of Skeletal Muscles

Skeletal (striated) muscles (more than 600 in the human body) are the muscles that move bones. Figure 15–25 shows some skeletal muscles of the head, neck, and torso and muscles of the posterior aspect of the leg. When a muscle contracts, one of the bones to which it is joined remains virtually stationary as a result of other muscles that hold it in place. The point of attachment of the muscle to the stationary bone is called the **origin (beginning)** of that muscle. When the muscle contracts, however, another bone to which it is attached does move. The point of junction of the muscle to the bone that moves is called the **insertion** of the muscle. Most often, the origin of a muscle lies proximal in the skeleton, whereas its insertion lies distal.

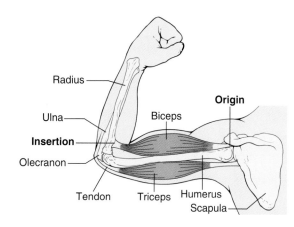

Figure 15–26

Origin and insertion of the biceps in the arm. Note also the origin of the triceps at the scapula and the insertion at the olecranon of the ulna.

Figure 15–26 shows the biceps and triceps muscles in the upper arm. One origin of the biceps is at the scapula, and its insertion is at the radius. Tendons are the connective tissue bands that connect muscles to the bones.

Muscles can perform a variety of actions. Some of the terms used to describe those actions are listed here with a short description of the specific type of movement performed (Fig. 15–27):

Action	Meaning
flexion	Decreasing the angle between two bones; bending a limb.
extension	Increasing the angle between two bones; straightening out a limb.
abduction	Movement away from the midline of the body.
adduction	Movement toward the midline of the body.
rotation	Circular movement around an axis. Internal rotation is toward the midline and external rotation is away from the midline.
dorsiflexion	Decreasing the angle of the ankle joint so that the foot bends backward (upward). This is the opposite movement of stepping on the gas pedal when driving a car.
plantar flexion	The motion that extends the foot downward toward the ground as when pointing the toes or stepping on the gas pedal. Plant/o means sole of the foot.
supination	As applied to the hand and forearm, the act of turning the palm forward, or up.
pronation	As applied to the hand and forearm, the act of turning the palm backward, or down.

Your medical dictionary has a complete list of the muscles of the body, with a description of their origins, insertions, and various actions.

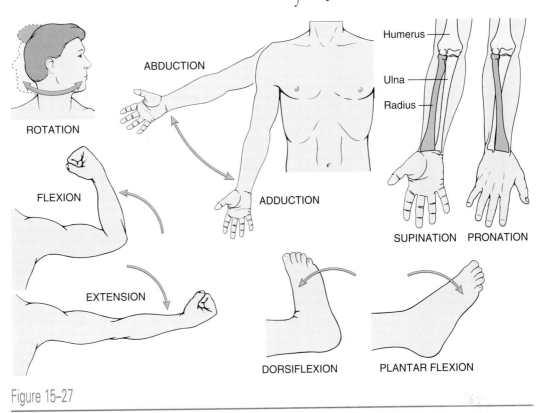

Figure 15–27

Types of muscular actions.

C. Vocabulary

This list will help you review many of the new terms introduced in the text. Short definitions will reinforce your understanding of the terms. See Section IX of this chapter for help in pronouncing the more difficult terms.

abduction	Movement away from the midline of the body.
adduction	Movement toward the midline of the body.
dorsiflexion	Backward (upward) bending of the foot.
extension	Straightening of a flexed limb.
fascia	Fibrous membrane separating and enveloping muscles.
flexion	Bending at a joint.
insertion of a muscle	Connection of the muscle to a bone that moves.
origin of a muscle	Connection of the muscle to a stationary bone.
plantar flexion	Bending the sole of the foot downward toward the ground.

pronation	Turning the palm backward.
rotation	Circular movement around a central point.
skeletal muscle	Muscle connected to bones; voluntary or striated muscle.
smooth muscle	Muscle connected to internal organs; involuntary or visceral muscle.
striated muscle	Skeletal muscle.
supination	Turning the palm forward.
visceral muscle	Smooth muscle.

D. Combining Forms, Suffixes, and Prefixes

Write the meanings of the medical terms in the spaces provided.

Combining Forms

Combining Form	Meaning	Terminology	Meaning
fasci/o	fascia (forms sheaths enveloping muscles)	fasciectomy _____	
fibr/o	fibrous connective tissue	fibromyalgia _____	
		Chronic pain and stiffness in muscles, joints, and fibrous tissue, especially of the back, shoulders, neck, hips, and knees. Fatigue is a common complaint.	
leiomy/o	smooth (visceral) muscle that lines the walls of internal organs	leiomyoma _____	
		leiomyosarcoma _____	
my/o	muscle	myalgia _____	
		electromyography _____	
		myopathy _____	
myocardi/o	heart muscle	myocardial _____	
myos/o	muscle	myositis _____	

plant/o	sole of the foot	<u>plant</u>ar flexion	_____
rhabdomy/o	skeletal (striated) muscle connected to bones	<u>rhabdomy</u>oma	_____
		<u>rhabdomy</u>osarcoma	_____

Suffixes

Suffix	Meaning	Terminology	Meaning
-asthenia	lack of strength	my<u>asthenia</u> gravis	_____

Muscles lose strength because of a failure in transmission of the nervous impulse from the nerve to the muscle cell.

Suffix	Meaning	Terminology	Meaning
-trophy	development, nourishment	a<u>trophy</u>	_____

Decrease in size of an organ or tissue.

		hyper<u>trophy</u>	_____

Increase in size of an organ or tissue.

		amyo<u>trophic</u>	_____

*In **amyotrophic lateral sclerosis** (Lou Gehrig disease), muscles are affected (paralysis occurs) by degeneration of nerves in the spinal cord and lower region of the brain.*

Prefixes

Prefix	Meaning	Terminology	Meaning
ab-	away from	<u>ab</u>duction	_____

duct/o means to lead.

Prefix	Meaning	Terminology	Meaning
ad-	toward	<u>ad</u>duction	_____
dorsi-	back	<u>dorsi</u>flexion	_____
poly-	many, much	<u>poly</u>myalgia	_____

***Polymyalgia rheumatica** is a syndrome marked by aching and morning stiffness in the shoulder, hip, or neck for more than one month.*

E. Pathological Conditions

muscular dystrophy	**A group of inherited diseases characterized by progressive weakness and degeneration of muscle fibers without involvement of the nervous system.**
	Duchenne dystrophy is the most common form. Muscles enlarge (**pseudohypertrophy**) as fat replaces functional muscle cells that have degenerated and atrophied. Onset of muscle weakness occurs soon after birth, and diagnosis can be made by muscle biopsy and electromyography.
polymyositis	**Chronic inflammatory myopathy.**
	This condition is marked by symmetrical muscle weakness and pain, often accompanied by a rash around the eyes, face, and limbs. Evidence that polymyositis is an autoimmune disorder is growing stronger, and some patients recover completely with immunosuppressive therapy.

V. Laboratory Tests, Clinical Procedures, and Abbreviations

Laboratory Tests

antinuclear antibody test (ANA)	**Detects an antibody present in serum of patients with systemic lupus erythematosus (SLE).**
erythrocyte sedimentation rate (ESR)	**Measures the rate at which erythrocytes settle to the bottom of a test tube.**
	Elevated ESR is associated with inflammatory disorders such as rheumatoid arthritis, tumors, and infections, and with chronic infections of bone and soft tissue.
rheumatoid factor test (RF)	**Serum is tested for the presence of an antibody found in patients with rheumatoid arthritis.**
serum calcium (Ca)	**Measurement of calcium level in serum.**
	Hypercalcemia may be caused by disorders of the parathyroid gland and malignancy that affects bone metabolism. Hypocalcemia is seen in critically ill patients with burns, sepsis, and acute renal failure.
serum creatine kinase (CK)	**Measurement of an enzyme (creatine kinase) in serum.**
	This enzyme is normally present in skeletal and cardiac muscle. Increased levels occur in muscular dystrophy, polymyositis, and traumatic injuries.
uric acid test	**Measurement of uric acid in serum.**
	High values are associated with gout.

Clinical Procedures

arthrocentesis	**Surgical puncture to remove fluid from the joint space.**
	Synovial fluid is removed for analysis.

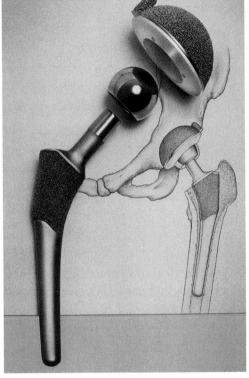

A

B

Figure 15–28

(A) Acetabular and femoral components of a total hip arthroplasty. (B) Radiograph showing a hip after a **Charnley total hip arthroplasty.** (**A** from Jebson LR, Coons DD: Total Hip Arthroplasty, Surg Technol October 1998; **B** from Mercier LR: Practical Orthopedics, 5th ed. St. Louis, Mosby, 2000, p. 237.)

arthrography	**Process of taking x-ray images after injection of contrast material into the joint.**
arthroplasty	**Surgical repair of a joint.**

Total hip arthroplasty is replacement of the femoral head and acetabulum with prostheses that are fastened into the bone (Fig. 15–28).

arthroscopy	**Visual examination of the inside of a joint with an endoscope.**

An orthopedist passes small surgical instruments into a joint (knee, shoulder, ankle) to remove and repair damaged tissue (Fig. 15–29).

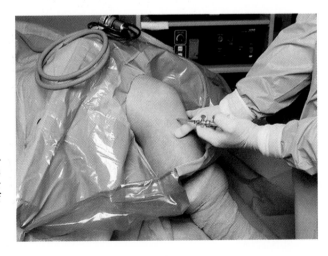

Figure 15–29

Arthroscopy of the knee. An arthroscope is used in the diagnosis of pathological changes. (From Lewis SM, Collier IC, Heitkemper MM: Medical-Surgical Nursing: Assessment and Management of Clinical Problems, 4th ed. St. Louis, Mosby, 1996.)

bone density test

Low-energy x-rays are taken of bones in the spinal column, pelvis, and wrist.

An x-ray detector measures how well x-rays penetrate through bones. Areas of decreased density indicate osteopenia and osteoporosis. Also called **dual-energy x-ray absorptiometry (DEXA).**

bone scan

Uptake of a radioactive substance is measured in bone.

A nuclear medicine physician uses a special scanning device to detect areas of increased uptake (tumors, infection, inflammation, stress fractures). See Figure 15–30.

computed tomography (CT)

X-ray beam is used with a computer to provide cross-sectional images.

CT scans identify soft-tissue abnormalities, bony abnormalities, and musculoskeletal trauma.

diskography

X-ray of cervical or lumbar intervertebral disk after injection of contrast into nucleus pulposus (interior of the disk).

electromyography (EMG)

Process of recording the strength of muscle contraction as a result of electrical stimulation.

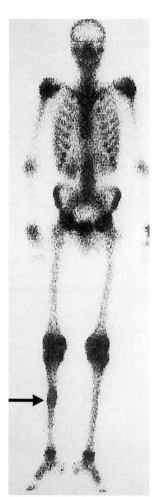

Figure 15–30

A technetium-99m bone scan of a skeleton showing an area of increased radioactive uptake on the right tibia that indicates a bone tumor. (From Walter JB: An Introduction to the Principles of Disease, 3rd ed. Philadelphia, WB Saunders, 1992.)

magnetic resonance imaging (MRI)	**Radio waves and a magnetic field create images of soft tissue.**
muscle biopsy	**Removal of muscle tissue for microscopic examination.**

Abbreviations

AC joint	acromioclavicular joint	**L1–L5**	lumbar vertebrae
ACL	anterior cruciate ligament of the knee	**LE cell**	lupus erythematosus cell
ANA	antinuclear antibody	**NSAID**	nonsteroidal anti-inflammatory drug; often prescribed to treat joint disorders
C1–C7	cervical vertebrae	**Ortho.**	orthopedics, orthopaedics
Ca	calcium	**P**	phosphorus
CK	creatine kinase	**RA**	rheumatoid arthritis
CTS	carpal tunnel syndrome	**RF**	rheumatoid factor
DEXA	dual-energy x-ray absorptiometry; a test of bone density	**ROM**	range of motion
DMARD	disease-modifying antirheumatic drug	**sed rate**	erythrocyte sedimentation rate
DTR	deep tendon reflexes	**SLE**	systemic lupus erythematosus
EMG	electromyography	**T1–T12**	thoracic vertebrae
ESR	erythrocyte sedimentation rate	**TMJ**	temporomandibular joint
IM	intramuscular		

VI. Practical Applications

This section contains an actual medical report using terms that you have studied in this and previous chapters. Explanations of more difficult terms are added in brackets. Answers are on page 617 after Answers to Exercises.

Skeletal Memorial Hospital—Department of Radiology

PA [posteroanterior] and lateral chest: The heart is enlarged in its transverse diameter. The lungs are fully expanded and free of active disease.

Thoracic spine shows a scoliosis of the upper thoracic spine convex to the left. There is 50 percent wedge compression fracture of T6 and slight wedge compression fracture of T5. There is also anterior wedge compression fracture of T12.

Continued on following page

Lumbar spine shows 90 percent compression fractures of L1 and L3 with 30 percent compression fractures L2 and L5. All bones are markedly osteoporotic. There is calcification within the aortic arch. There are gallstones in the right upper quadrant. The findings in the spine are most compatible with osteoporotic compression fractures. During the procedure, the patient had a sickable* episode and fell, striking her head. A skull series, done at no cost to the patient, shows no evidence of bony fracture. The pineal gland is calcified and has a midline location. The sella turcica is normal.

*This word was incorrectly transcribed. The correct term is syncopal.

Operating Schedule—Skeletal Memorial Hospital

Match the operation in column I with an accompanying diagnosis or reason for surgery in column II.

Column I—Operations

1. Excision, osteochondroma, _____
   R calcaneous

2. TMJ arthroscopy with _____
   probable arthrotomy

3. L4–5 laminectomy and _____
   diskectomy

4. Arthroscopy, left knee _____

5. Open reduction, malleolar _____
   fracture

6. R occipital craniotomy _____
   with tumor resection

7. Excision, distal end right _____
   clavicle, with prob.
   acromioplasty

8. Acetabuloplasty with open _____
   reduction hip

Column II—Diagnoses

A. fracture of the ankle
B. ACL rupture
C. neoplastic lesion in brain
D. exostosis on heel bone
E. pelvic fracture
F. pain and malocclusion of jaw bones
G. lower back pain radiating down one leg
H. pain in shoulder joint with bone spur (exostosis) evident on x-ray

VII. Exercises

Remember to check your answers carefully with those given in Section VIII, Answers to Exercises.

A. Complete the following sentences.

1. Bones are composed of bony connective tissue called _____ tissue.

2. Bone cells are called _____.

3. The bones of a fetus are composed mainly of _____.

4. During bone development, immature bone cells called _____ produce bony tissue.

5. Large bone cells called _____ digest bone tissue to shape the bone and smooth it out.

6. Two mineral substances necessary for proper development of bones are _____

   and _____.

7. A round, small bone resembling a sesame seed in shape and covering the knee joint is called a (an)

   _____ bone.

8. The shaft of a long bone is called the _____.

9. The ends of a long bone are called the _____.

10. The cartilaginous area at the end of a long bone where growth takes place is called the

    _____.

11. Red bone marrow is found in spongy or _____ bone.

12. Yellow bone marrow is composed of _____ tissue.

13. The strong membrane surrounding the surface of a bone is the _____.

14. Hard, dense bone tissue lying under the periosteum is _____.

15. A series of canals containing blood vessels lie within the outer dense tissue of bone and are called

    the _____ canals.

16. A thin layer of cartilage covering the ends of bones at the joints is _____.

17. The _____ is a central, hollowed-out area in the shaft of long bones.

18. A physician who treats bones and bone diseases is called a (an) _____.

19. A person who uses his or her hands to manipulate the spinal column (in the belief that diseases are caused by pressure on spinal nerves) is a (an) _____.

20. A doctor who treats patients based on the belief that the body can be healed when bones are in proper position and adequate nutrition is provided is a (an) _____.

B. Give a short description of each term.

1. metaphysis _____

2. sinus _____

3. tubercle _____

4. condyle _____

5. fossa _____

6. tuberosity _____

7. trochanter _____

8. foramen _____

9. fissure _____

10. bone head _____

C. Match the following cranial and facial bones with their meanings as given below.

ethmoid bone	mandible	occipital bone	temporal bone
frontal bone	maxilla	parietal bone	vomer
lacrimal bones	nasal bone	sphenoid bone	zygomatic bone

1. forms the roof and upper side parts of the skull _____

2. delicate bone, composed of spongy, cancellous tissue; supports the nasal cavity and orbits of the eye

_____

3. forms the back and base of the skull _____

4. forms the forehead _____

5. bat-shaped bone extending behind the eyes to form the base of the skull _____

6. bone near the ear and connecting to the lower jaw _____

7. cheekbone _____

8. bone that supports the bridge of the nose _____

9. thin, flat bone forming the lower portion of the nasal septum _____

10. lower jawbone _____

11. upper jawbone _____

12. two paired bones, one located at the corner of each eye _____

D. Name the five divisions of the spinal column.

1. _____   4. _____

2. _____   5. _____

3. _____

E. Identify the following parts associated with a vertebra.

1. space through which the spinal cord passes _____

2. piece of cartilage between each vertebra _____

3. posterior part of a vertebra _____

4. anterior part of a vertebra _____

F. Give the medical names of the following bones.

1. shoulder blade _____   10. wrist bones _____

2. upper arm bone _____   11. backbone _____

3. breastbone _____   12. kneecap _____

4. thigh bone _____   13. shin bone (larger of two lower leg bones)

5. finger bones _____   _____

6. hand bones _____   14. smaller of two lower leg bones _____

7. medial lower arm bone _____   15. three parts of the pelvis are: _____,

8. lateral lower arm bone _____   _____, and _____

9. collar bone _____   16. midfoot bones _____

G. Give the meanings of the following terms associated with bones.

1. foramen magnum _____

2. calcaneus _____

3. acromion _____

4. xiphoid process _____

5. lamina _____

6. malleolus _____

7. acetabulum _____

8. pubic symphysis _____

9. olecranon _____

10. fontanelle _____

11. mastoid process _____

12. styloid process _____

H. Give the meanings of the following terms.

1. osteogenesis _____

2. hypercalcemia _____

3. spondylosis _____

4. epiphyseal _____

5. decalcification _____

6. ossification _____

7. osteitis _____

8. costoclavicular _____

I. Build medical terms.

1. pertaining to the shoulder blade _____

2. instrument to cut the skull _____

3. pertaining to the upper arm bone _____

4. pertaining to below the kneecap _____

5. softening of cartilage _____

6. pertaining to a toe bone _____

7. removal of hand bones _____

8. pertaining to the shin bone _____

9. pertaining to the heel bone _____

10. poor bone development _____

11. removal of the lamina of the vertebral arch _____

12. pertaining to the sacrum and ilium _____

J. Give medical terms for the following.

1. formation of bone marrow _____

2. clubfoot _____

3. humpback _____

4. high levels of calcium in the blood _____

5. benign tumors arising from the bone surface _____

6. brittle bone disease _____

7. lateral curvature of the spine _____

8. anterior curvature of the spine _____

9. forward slipping (subluxation) of a vertebra over a lower vertebra _____

10. instrument to cut bone _____

K. Match the term in column I with its description in column II. Write the letter of the description in the space provided.

Column I

1. greenstick fracture _____

2. closed fracture _____

3. comminuted fracture _____

4. compound (open) fracture _____

5. Colles fracture _____

6. cast _____

7. open reduction _____

8. closed reduction _____

9. impacted fracture _____

10. compression fracture _____

Column II

A. fracture of the lower end of the radius at the wrist

B. break in bone with wound in the skin

C. one side of the bone is fractured; the other side is bent

D. bone is put in proper place without incision of skin

E. mold of the bone applied to fractures to immobilize the injured bone

F. bone is broken by pressure from another bone; often in vertebrae, bone is partially flattened

G. bone is splintered or crushed

H. bone is put in proper place after incision through the skin

I. bone is broken and one side of the fracture is wedged into the other

J. break in the bone without an open skin wound

L. Give the meanings of the following terms.

1. osteoporosis _____

2. osteomyelitis _____

3. osteogenic sarcoma _____

4. crepitus _____

5. osteomalacia _____

6. abscess _____

7. osteopenia _____

8. Ewing sarcoma _____

9. metastatic bone lesion _____

M. Complete the following sentences.

1. A joint in which apposed bones are closely united as in the skull bones is called a (an)

   _____.

2. Connective tissue that binds muscles to bones is a (an) _____.

3. Another term for a joint is a (an) _____.

4. Connective tissue that binds bones to other bones is a (an) _____.

5. Fluid found in a joint is called _____.

6. The membrane that lines the joint cavity is the _____.

7. A sac of fluid near a joint is a (an) _____.

8. Smooth cartilage that covers the surface of bones at joints is _____.

9. Surgical repair of a joint is called _____.

10. Inflammation surrounding a joint is known as _____.

N. Complete the following terms based on the definitions provided.

1. inflammation of a tendon: _____ itis

2. tumor (benign) of cartilage: _____ oma

3. tumor (malignant) of cartilage: _____ oma

4. incision of a joint: arthr _____

5. softening of cartilage: chondro _____

6. abnormal condition of blood in the joint: _____ osis

7. inflammation of a sac of fluid near the joint: _____ itis

8. a doctor who specializes in treatment of joint disorders: _____ logist

9. abnormal condition of a stiffened, immobile joint: _____ osis

10. suture of a tendon: ten _____

O. Select from the following terms to name the abnormal conditions below.

achondroplasia	dislocation	osteoarthritis
ankylosing spondylitis	ganglion	rheumatoid arthritis
bunion	gouty arthritis	systemic lupus erythematosus
carpal tunnel syndrome	Lyme disease	tenosynovitis

1. an inherited condition in which the bones of the arms and the legs fail to grow normally because of

   a defect in cartilage and bone formation; type of dwarfism _____

2. degenerative joint disease; chronic inflammation of bones and joints _____

3. inflammation of joints caused by excessive uric acid in the body (hyperuricemia) _____

4. chronic joint disease; inflamed and painful joints owing to autoimmune reaction against normal

   joint tissue, and synovial membranes become swollen and thickened _____

5. tick-borne bacterium causes this condition marked by arthritis, myalgia, malaise, and neurological

   and cardiac symptoms _____

6. abnormal swelling of a metatarsophalangeal joint _____

7. cystic mass arising from a tendon in the wrist _____

8. chronic, progressive arthritis with stiffening of joints, especially of the spine (vertebrae)

   _____

9. chronic inflammatory disease affecting not only the joints but also the skin (red rash on the face),

   kidneys, heart, and lungs _____

10. inflammation of a tendon sheath _____

11. compression of the median nerve in the wrist as it passes through an area between a ligament and

   tendons, bones, and connective tissue _____

12. displacement of a bone from its joint _____

P. Give the meanings of the following terms.

1. subluxation _____

2. arthrodesis _____

3. pyrexia _____

4. podagra _____

5. sciatica _____

6. herniation of an intervertebral disk _____

7. laminectomy _____

8. sprain _____

9. strain _____

10. hyperuricemia _____

Q. Circle the term that best fits the definition given.

1. fibrous membrane separating and enveloping muscles: **(fascia, flexion)**

2. movement away from the midline of the body: **(abduction, adduction)**

3. connection of the muscle to a stationary bone: **(insertion, origin)** of the muscle

4. connection of the muscle to a bone that moves: **(insertion, origin)** of the muscle

5. muscle that is connected to internal organs; involuntary muscle: **(skeletal, visceral)** muscle

6. muscle that is connected to bones; voluntary muscle: **(skeletal, visceral)** muscle

7. pain of many muscles: **(myositis, polymyalgia)**

8. pertaining to heart muscle: **(myocardial, myasthenia)**

9. process of recording electricity within muscles: **(muscle biopsy, electromyography)**

10. increase in development (size) of an organ or tissue: **(hypertrophy, atrophy)**

R. Match the term for muscle action with its meaning. Write the letter of the meaning in the space provided.

Column I

1. extension _____

2. rotation _____

3. flexion _____

4. adduction _____

5. supination _____

6. abduction _____

7. pronation _____

8. dorsiflexion _____

9. plantar flexion _____

Column II

A. movement away from the midline
B. turning the palm backward
C. turning the palm forward
D. straightening out a limb or joint
E. bending the sole of the foot downward
F. circular movement around an axis
G. bending a limb
H. movement toward the midline
I. backward (upward) bending of the foot

S. Give the meanings of the following abnormal conditions affecting muscles.

1. leiomyosarcoma _____

2. rhabdomyoma _____

3. polymyositis _____

4. fibromyalgia _____

5. muscular dystrophy _____

6. myasthenia gravis _____

7. amyotrophic lateral sclerosis _____

T. Match the term in column I with its meaning in column II. Write the letter of the answer in the space provided.

Column I

1. antinuclear antibody test _____

2. serum creatine kinase _____

3. uric acid test _____

Column II

A. radioactive substance is injected and traced in dense, hard connective tissue
B. chemical found in myoneural space
C. test for presence of an antibody found in the serum of patients with rheumatoid arthritis

4. rheumatoid factor test _____

5. bone scan _____

6. muscle biopsy _____

7. arthroscopy _____

8. acetylcholine _____

9. calcium _____

10. arthrography _____

D. substance necessary for proper bone development
E. visual examination of a joint
F. test tells if patient has gouty arthritis
G. test tells if patient has systemic lupus erythematosus
H. removal of soft connective tissue for microscopic examination
I. process of taking x-ray pictures of a joint
J. elevated blood levels of this enzyme are found in muscular disorders

U. Circle the term that best completes the meaning of the sentence.

1. Selma, a 40-year-old secretary, had been complaining of wrist pain with tingling sensations in her fingers for months. Dr. Ayres diagnosed her condition as **(osteomyelitis, rheumatoid arthritis, carpal tunnel syndrome)**.

2. Daisy tripped while playing tennis and landed on her hand. She had excruciating pain and a **(Ewing, Colles, pathological)** fracture that required casting.

3. In her fifties, Estelle started hunching over more and more. Her doctor realized that she was developing **(gouty arthritis, osteoarthritis, osteoporosis)** and prescribed calcium pills and exercise.

4. Paul had a skiing accident and tore ligaments in his knee. Dr. Miller recommended **(electromyography, hypertrophy, arthroscopic surgery)** to repair the ligaments.

5. For several months after her first pregnancy Elsie noticed a red rash on her face and cheeks. Her joints were giving her pain and she had a slight fever. Her ANA was elevated and her doctor suspected that she had **(SLE, polymyositis, muscular dystrophy)**.

6. David injured his left knee while playing basketball. He was scheduled for arthroscopic repair of his **(ACL, SLE, TMJ)**. However, because his ligament was so long, his **(rheumatologist, orthopedist, chiropractor)** decided to do "open" surgery.

7. James has significant lower back pain radiating down his left leg. MRI shows an intervertebral **(disk, bunion, exostosis)** impinging on spinal nerves at the **(L5–S1, C2–C3, T3–T5)** level. Bed rest produces no improvement. His orthopedist decided to perform a **(tenorrhaphy, laminectomy, bunionectomy)** to relieve pressure on his nerves.

8. Bruce spent two weeks hiking and vacationing on Nantucket Island. A week later he developed a bull's-eye rash on his chest (from a tick bite), fever, muscle pain, and a swollen, tender right ankle. His physician ordered a blood test that revealed **(antigens, antibodies)** to a spirochete bacterium. The physician told Bruce he had contracted **(ankylosing spondylitis, polymositis, Lyme disease)**.

9. Scott likes to eat rich food. Lately he has noticed pain and tenderness in his right toe called **(talipes, podagra, rickets)** and also deposits of hard lumps over his elbows. His doctor orders a serum uric

acid test, which comes back abnormally high revealing (**hemarthrosis, hyperuricemia, hypercalcemia**), consistent with a diagnosis of (**rheumatoid arthritis, gouty arthritis, osteoarthritis**).

10. Selma, a 70-year-old widow, has persistent midback pain, and her (**CXR, ESR, EMG**) shows compression fractures of her (**scapula, femur, vertebrae**) and thinning of her bones. A bone density scan confirms the diagnosis of (**osteomyelitis, osteomalacia, osteoporosis**), and her doctor prescribes calcium, Vitamin D, and Fosamax.

V. Give meanings for the following abbreviations and then select the letter from the sentences that follow that is the best association for each.

Column I

1. ROM _____ ____

2. NSAID _____ ____

3. TMJ _____ ____

4. EMG _____ ____

5. ACL _____ ____

6. SLE _____ ____

7. C1–C5 _____ ____

8. T1–T12 _____ ____

Column II

A. Connection between the lower jawbone and a bone of the skull.

B. Band of fibrous tissue connecting bones in the knee.

C. Bones of the spinal column in the chest region.

D. Test of strength of electrical transmission within muscle.

E. This autoimmune disease affects joints, skin, and other body tissues.

F. Measurement in degrees of a circle assesses the extent a joint can be flexed or extended.

G. Bones of the spinal column in the neck region.

H. Drug used to treat joint diseases.

VIII. Answers to Exercises

A

1. osseous	8. diaphysis	15. haversian
2. osteocytes	9. epiphyses	16. articular cartilage
3. cartilage	10. epiphyseal plate	17. medullary cavity
4. osteoblasts	11. cancellous or trabecular	18. orthopedist
5. osteoclasts	12. fat	19. chiropractor
6. calcium and phosphorus	13. periosteum	20. osteopath
7. sesamoid	14. compact bone	

B

1. flared portion of a long bone that lies between the diaphysis and the epiphyseal plate	4. rounded, knuckle-like process at the joint	8. opening in a bone for blood vessels and nerves
2. hollow cavity within the bone	5. shallow cavity in or on a bone	9. narrow, deep, slit-like opening
3. rounded process for attachment of tendons and muscles	6. rounded process for attachment of muscles and tendons	10. rounded end of a bone separated from the rest of the bone by a neck
	7. large process on the femur for attachment of tendons and muscles	

C

1. parietal bone
2. ethmoid bone
3. occipital bone
4. frontal bone
5. sphenoid bone
6. temporal bone
7. zygomatic bone
8. nasal bone
9. vomer
10. mandible
11. maxilla
12. lacrimal bones

D

1. cervical
2. thoracic
3. lumbar
4. sacral
5. coccygeal

E

1. neural canal
2. intervertebral disk
3. vertebral arch
4. vertebral body

F

1. scapula
2. humerus
3. sternum
4. femur
5. phalanges
6. metacarpals
7. ulna
8. radius
9. clavicle
10. carpals
11. vertebral column
12. patella
13. tibia
14. fibula
15. ilium, ischium, pubis
16. metatarsals

G

1. opening of the occipital bone through which the spinal cord passes
2. heel bone; largest of the tarsal bones
3. lateral extension of the scapula
4. lower portion of the sternum
5. portion of the vertebral arch
6. the bulge on either side of the ankle joint; the lower end of the fibula is the lateral malleolus, and the lower end of the tibia is the medial malleolus
7. depression in the pelvis into which the femur fits
8. area of convergence of the two pubis bones, at the midline
9. bony process at the proximal end of the ulna; elbow joint
10. soft spot between the bones of the skull in an infant
11. round process on the temporal bone behind the ear
12. pole-like process projecting downward from the temporal bone

H

1. formation of bone; osteogenesis imperfecta is known as brittle bone disease
2. excessive calcium in the blood
3. abnormal condition of the vertebrae; degenerative changes in the spine
4. pertaining to the epiphysis
5. removal of calcium from bones
6. formation of bone
7. inflammation of bone; osteitis deformans or Paget disease causes deformed bones such as an enlarged skull
8. pertaining to the ribs and clavicle

I

1. scapular
2. craniotome
3. humeral
4. subpatellar
5. chondromalacia
6. phalangeal
7. metacarpectomy
8. tibial
9. calcaneal
10. osteodystrophy
11. laminectomy
12. sacroiliac

J

1. myelopoiesis
2. talipes
3. kyphosis
4. hypercalcemia
5. exostoses
6. osteogenesis imperfecta
7. scoliosis
8. lordosis
9. spondylolisthesis
10. osteotome

K

1. C
2. J
3. G
4. B
5. A
6. E
7. H
8. D
9. I
10. F

Continued on following page

L

1. increased porosity in bone; decrease in bone density
2. inflammation of bone and bone marrow
3. cancerous tumor of bone; osteoblasts multiply at the ends of long bones
4. crackling sensation as broken bones move against each other

5. softening of bones; rickets in children due to loss of calcium in bones
6. collection of pus
7. deficiency of bone; occurs in osteoporosis

8. malignant tumor of bone, often involving the entire shaft of a long bone
9. malignant tumor that has spread to bone from the breast, lung, kidney, or prostate gland

M

1. suture joint; a synovial joint is a freely movable joint
2. tendon
3. articulation

4. ligament
5. synovial fluid
6. synovial membrane
7. bursa

8. articular cartilage
9. arthroplasty
10. periarthritis

N

1. tendinitis
2. chondroma
3. chondrosarcoma
4. arthrotomy

5. chondromalacia
6. hemarthrosis
7. bursitis

8. rheumatologist
9. ankylosis
10. tenorrhaphy

O

1. achondroplasia
2. osteoarthritis
3. gouty arthritis
4. rheumatoid arthritis

5. Lyme disease
6. bunion
7. ganglion
8. ankylosing spondylitis

9. systemic lupus erythematosus
10. tenosynovitis
11. carpal tunnel syndrome
12. dislocation

P

1. partial or incomplete displacement of a bone from the joint
2. surgical fixation of a joint (binding it together by fusing the joint surfaces)
3. fever; increase in body temperature
4. pain in a big toe from gouty arthritis
5. pain radiating from the back to the leg (along the sciatic nerve); most

commonly caused by a protruding intervertebral disk
6. protrusion of a disk into the neural canal or the spinal nerves
7. removal of a portion of the vertebral arch (lamina) to relieve pressure from a protruding intervertebral disk

8. trauma to a joint with pain, swelling, and injury to ligaments
9. overstretching of a muscle
10. high levels of uric acid in the bloodstream; present in gouty arthritis

Q

1. fascia
2. abduction
3. origin of the muscle
4. insertion of the muscle

5. visceral muscle
6. skeletal muscle
7. polymyalgia

8. myocardial
9. electromyography
10. hypertrophy

R

1. D
2. F
3. G

4. H
5. C
6. A

7. B
8. I
9. E

S

1. malignant tumor of smooth (involuntary, visceral) muscle
2. benign tumor of striated (voluntary, skeletal) muscle
3. inflammation of many muscles; polymyositis rheumatica is a chronic inflammatory condition causing muscle weakness and pain

4. pain of muscle and fibrous tissue (especially of the back); also called fibrositis or rheumatism
5. group of inherited muscular diseases marked by progressive weakness and degeneration of muscles without nerve involvement

6. loss of strength of muscles (often with paralysis) because of a defect at the connection between the nerve and the muscle cell
7. muscles degenerate (paralysis occurs) owing to degeneration of nerves in the spinal cord and lower region of the brain; Lou Gehrig disease

T

1. G	5. A	8. B
2. J	6. H	9. D
3. F	7. E	10. I
4. C		

U

1. carpal tunnel syndrome	5. SLE	8. antibodies; Lyme disease
2. Colles	6. ACL; orthopedist	9. podagra; hyperuricemia; gouty arthritis
3. osteoporosis	7. disk; L5–S1; laminectomy	10. CXR; vertebrae; osteoporosis
4. arthroscopic surgery		

V

1. range of motion. F	5. anterior cruciate ligament. B	8. 1st thoracic vertebra to 12th thoracic vertebra. C
2. nonsteroidal anti-inflammatory drug. H	6. systemic lupus erythematosus. E	
3. temporomandibular joint. A	7. 1st cervical vertebra to 5th cervical vertebra. G	
4. electromyography. D		

Answers to Practical Applications

1. D	4. B	7. H
2. F	5. A	8. E
3. G	6. C	

IX. Pronunciation of Terms

Pronunciation Guide

To test your understanding of the terminology in this chapter, write the meaning of each term in the space provided. In addition, you may wish to cover the terms and write them by looking at your definitions. Make sure your spelling is correct. The page number after each term indicates where it is defined or used in the text so you can easily check your responses.

ā as in āpe   ă as in ăpple
ē as in ēven   ě as in ěvery
ī as in īce   ĭ as in ĭnterest
ō as in ōpen   ŏ as in pŏt
ū as in ūnit   ŭ as in ŭnder

Terms Related to Bones

Term	Pronunciation	Meaning
acetabulum (573)	ăs-ĕ-TĂB-ū-lŭm	_____
acromion (573)	ă-KRŌ-mē-ŏn	_____
articular cartilage (573)	ăr-TĬK-ū-lăr KĂR-tĭ-lăj	_____
calcaneal (578)	kăl-KĀ-nē-ăl	_____
calcaneus (578)	kăl-KĀ-nē-ŭs	_____

calcium (573)	KĂL-sē-ŭm	
cancellous bone (573)	KĂN-sĕ-lŭs bōn	
carpals (578)	KĂR-pălz	
cartilage (574)	KĂR-tĭ-lĭj	
cervical vertebrae (568)	SĔR-vĭ-kăl VĔR-tĕ-brā	
chondrocostal (578)	kŏn-drō-KŎS-tăl	
clavicle (578)	KLĂV-ĭ-k'l	
coccyx (568)	KŎK-sĭks	
collagen (574)	KŎL-ă-jĕn	
Colles fracture (580)	KŎL-ēz FRĂK-shŭr	
comminuted fracture (580)	KŎM-ĭ-nūt-ĕd FRĂK-shŭr	
compact bone (574)	KŎM-păkt bōn	
condyle (574)	KŎN-dīl	
cranial bones (574)	KRĀ-nē-ăl bōnz	
craniotome (578)	KRĀ-nē-ō-tōm	
craniotomy (578)	krā-nē-ŎT-ō-mē	
crepitus (580)	KRĔP-ĭ-tŭs	
decalcification (576)	dē-kăl-sĭ-fĭ-KĀ-shŭn	
diaphysis (574)	dī-ĂF-ĭ-sĭs	
epiphyseal plate (574)	ĕp-ĭ-FĬZ-ē-ăl plāt	
epiphysis (574)	ĕ-PĬF-ĭ-sĭs	
ethmoid bone (564)	ĔTH-moyd bōn	
Ewing sarcoma (580)	Ū-ĭng săr-kō-mă	
exostosis (580)	ĕk-sŏs-TŌ-sĭs	
facial bones (574)	FĀ-shăl bōnz	
femoral (578)	FĔM-ŏr-ăl	
femur (578)	FĒ-mŭr	
fibula (578)	FĬB-ū-lă	

fibular (578)	FĬB-ū-lăr	_____
fissure (574)	FĬSH-ŭr	_____
fontanelle (574)	fŏn-tă-NĔL	_____
foramen (574)	fōr-Ā-mĕn	_____
fossa (574)	FŎS-ă	_____
frontal bone (564)	FRŎN-tăl bōn	_____
haversian canals (574)	hă-VĔR-shăn kă-NĂLZ	_____
humeral (578)	HŪ-mĕr-ăl	_____
humerus (578)	HŪ-mĕr-ŭs	_____
hypercalcemia (576)	hī-pĕr-kăl-SĒ-mē-ă	_____
iliac (579)	ĬL-ē-ăk	_____
ilium (579)	ĬL-ē-ŭm	_____
impacted fracture (580)	ĭm-PĂK-tĕd FRĂK-shŭr	_____
ischial (579)	ĬSH-ē-ăl or Ĭs-kē-ăl	_____
ischium (579)	ĬSH-ē-ŭm or Ĭs-kē-um	_____
kyphosis (576)	kī-FŌ-sĭs	_____
lacrimal bones (566)	LĂ-krĭ-măl bōnz	_____
lamina (576)	LĂM-ĭ-nă	_____
laminectomy (576)	lăm-ĭ-NĔK-tō-mē	_____
lordosis (576)	lŏr-DŌ-sĭs	_____
lumbar vertebrae (568)	LŬM-băr VĔR-tĕ-brā	_____
lumbosacral (576)	lŭm-bō-SĀ-krăl	_____
malleolar (579)	mă-LĒ-ō-lăr	_____
malleolus (574)	măl-LĒ-ō-lŭs	_____
mandible (579)	MĂN-dĭ-b'l	_____
mandibular (579)	măn-DĬB-ū-lăr	_____
manubrium (574)	mă-NŪ-brē-ŭm	_____
mastoid process (574)	MĂs-toyd PRŎS-ĕs	_____

medullary cavity (574)	MĔD-ū-lăr-ē KĂ-vĭ-tē	_____
metacarpals (579)	mĕt-ă-KĂR-pălz	_____
metacarpectomy (579)	mĕt-ă-kăr-PĔK-tō-mē	_____
metaphysis (574)	mĕ-TĂ-fĭ-sĭs	_____
metatarsalgia (579)	mĕt-ă-tăr-SĂL-jă	_____
metatarsals (579)	mĕt-ă-TĂR-sălz	_____
myelopoiesis (576)	mī-ĕ-lō-poy-Ē-sĭs	_____
nasal bone (566)	NĀ-zăl bōn	_____
occipital bone (564)	ŏk-SĬP-ĭ-tăl bōn	_____
olecranal (579)	ō-LĔK-ră-năl	_____
olecranon (574)	ō-LĔK-ră-nŏn	_____
orthopedics (576)	ŏr-thō-PĒ-dĭks	_____
osseous tissue (575)	ŎS-ē-ŭs TĬSH-ū	_____
ossification (575)	ŏs-ĭ-fĭ-KĀ-shŭn	_____
osteitis (576)	ŏs-tē-Ī-tĭs	_____
osteoblast (575)	ŎS-tē-ō-blăst	_____
osteoclast (575)	ŎS-tē-ō-klăst	_____
osteodystrophy (576)	ŏs-tē-ō-DĬS-trō-fē	_____
osteogenesis imperfecta (576)	ŏs-tē-ō-JĔN-ĕ-sĭs ĭm-pĕr-FĔK-tă	_____
osteogenic sarcoma (580)	ŏs-tē-ō-JĔN-ĭk săr-KŌ-mă	_____
osteomalacia (582)	ŏs-tē-ō-mă-LĀ-shă	_____
osteomyelitis (582)	ŏs-tē-ō-mī-ĕ-LĪ-tĭs	_____
osteopenia (582)	ŏs-tē-ō-PĒ-nē-ă	_____
osteoporosis (582)	ŏs-tē-ō-pŏr-Ō-sĭs	_____
osteotome (578)	ŎS-tē-ō-tōm	_____
parietal bones (564)	pă-RĪ-ĭ-tăl bōnz	_____
patella (579)	pă-TĔL-ă	_____

pelvimetry (579)	pĕl-VĬM-ĕ-trē	_____
periosteum (575)	pĕ-rē-ŎS-tē-um	_____
peroneal (579)	pĕr-ō-NĒ-ăl	_____
phalangeal (579)	fă-lăn-JĒ-ăl	_____
phalanges (579)	fă-LĂN-jēz	_____
phosphorus (575)	FŎS-fō-rŭs	_____
pubic symphysis (575)	PŪ-bĭk SĬM-fĭ-sĭs	_____
pubis (579)	PŪ-bĭs	_____
radial (579)	RĀ-dē-ăl	_____
radius (579)	RĀ-dē-ŭs	_____
reduction (580)	rĕ-DŬK-shŭn	_____
ribs (575)	rĭbz	_____
sacral vertebrae (568)	SĀ-krăl VĔR-tĕ-brā	_____
scapula (579)	SKĂP-ū-lă	_____
scapular (579)	SKĂP-ŭ-lăr	_____
scoliosis (577)	skō-lē-Ō-sĭs	_____
sella turcica (575)	SĔ-lă TŬR-sĭ-kă	_____
sinus (575)	SĪ-nŭs	_____
sphenoid bone (564)	SFĔ-noyd bōn	_____
spondylolisthesis (577)	spŏn-dĭ-lō-lĭs-THĒ-sĭs	_____
spondylosis (577)	spŏn-dĭ-LŌ-sĭs	_____
sternum (579)	STĔR-nŭm	_____
styloid process (575)	STĪ-loyd PRŎS-ĕs	_____
subcostal (578)	sŭb-KŎS-tăl	_____
subpatellar (579)	sŭb-pă-TĔL-lăr	_____
supraclavicular (578)	sŭ-pră-klă-VĬK-ū-lăr	_____
suture (575)	SŪ-tŭr	_____

talipes (582)	TĂL-ĭ-pēz	_____
tarsals (579)	TĂR-sălz	_____
tarsectomy (579)	tăr-SĔK-tō-mē	_____
temporal bones (564)	TĔM-pōr-ăl bōnz	_____
temporomandibular joint (575)	tĕm-pŏr-ō-măn-DĬB-ŭ-lăr joynt	_____
thoracic vertebrae (568)	thō-RĂS-ĭk VĔR-tĕ-brā	_____
tibia (579)	TĬB-ē-ă	_____
tibial (579)	TĬB-ē-ăl	_____
trabeculae (575)	tră-BĔK-ū-lē	_____
trochanter (575)	trō-KĂN-tĕr	_____
tubercle (575)	TŪ-bĕr-k'l	_____
tuberosity (575)	tū-bĕ-RŎS-ĭ-tē	_____
ulna (579)	ŬL-nă	_____
ulnar (579)	ŬL-năr	_____
vomer (566)	VŌ-mĕr	_____
xiphoid process (575)	ZĬF-oyd PRŎS-ĕs	_____
zygomatic bones (566)	zī-gō-MĂ-tĭk bōnz	_____

Terms Related to Joints and Muscles

Term	Pronunciation	Meaning
abduction (594)	ăb-DŬK-shŭn	_____
achondroplasia (586)	ā-kŏn-drō-PLĀ-zē-ă	_____
adduction (594)	ă-DŬK-shŭn	_____
amyotrophic lateral sclerosis (597)	ā-mī-ō-TRŌ-fĭk LĂT-ĕr-ăl sklĕ-RŌ-sĭs	_____
ankylosing spondylitis (587)	ăng-kĭ-LŌ-sĭng spŏn-dĭ-LĪ-tĭs	_____
ankylosis (586)	ăng-kĭ-LŌ-sĭs	_____
arthrodesis (587)	ăr-thrō-DĒ-sĭs	_____

arthrotomy (586)	ăr-THRŌT-ō-mē
articular cartilage (586)	ăr-TĬK-ū-lăr KĂR-tĭ-lĭj
articulation (585)	ăr-tĭk-ū-LĀ-shŭn
atrophy (597)	ĂT-rō-fē
bunion (588)	BŬN-yŭn
bursa (plural: bursae) (585)	BĔR-să (BĔR-sē)
bursitis (586)	bŭr-SĪ-tis
carpal tunnel syndrome (588)	KĂR-păl TŬN-nĕl SĬN-drōm
chondroma (586)	kŏn-DRŌ-mă
chondromalacia (586)	kŏn-drō-mă-LĀ-shă
dislocation (590)	dĭs-lō-KĀ-shŭn
dorsiflexion (594)	dŏr-sē-FLĔK-shŭn
extension (594)	ĕk-STĔN-shŭn
fascia (595)	FĂSH-ē-ă
fasciectomy (596)	făsh-ē-ĔK-tō-mē
fibromyalgia (596)	fī-brō-mī-ĂL-jă
flexion (594)	FLĔK-shŭn
ganglion (590)	GĂNG-lē-ŏn
gouty arthritis (587)	GŎW-tē ăr-THRĪ-tĭs
hemarthrosis (586)	hĕm-ăr-THRŌ-sĭs
hydrarthrosis (586)	hī-drăr-THRŌ-sĭs
hypertrophy (597)	hī-PĔR-trō-fē
hyperuricemia (587)	hī-pĕr-ŭr-ĭ-SĒ-mē-ă
leiomyoma (596)	lī-ō-mī-Ō-mă
leiomyosarcoma (596)	lī-ō-mī-ō-săr-KŌ-mă
ligament (585)	LĬG-ă-mĕnt
ligamentous (587)	lĭg-ă-MĔN-tŭs
Lyme disease (591)	līm dĭ-ZĒZ

muscular dystrophy (598)	MŬS-kū-lăr DĬS-tră-fē	_____
myalgia (596)	mī-ĂL-jă	_____
myopathy (596)	mī-ŎP-ă-thē	_____
myositis (596)	mī-ō-SĪ-tĭs	_____
osteoarthritis (588)	ŏs-tē-ō-ăr-THRĪ-tĭs	_____
plantar flexion (594)	PLĂN-tăr FLĔK-shun	_____
podagra (588)	pō-DĂG-ră	_____
polyarthritis (586)	pŏl-ē-ărth-RĪ-tĭs	_____
polymyalgia (597)	pŏl-ē-mĭ-ĂL-jă	_____
polymyositis (598)	pŏl-ē-mī-ō-SĪ-tĭs	_____
pronation (594)	prō-NĀ-shŭn	_____
pyrexia (588)	pī-RĔK-sē-ă	_____
rhabdomyoma (597)	răb-dō-mī-Ō-mă	_____
rhabdomyosarcoma (597)	răb-dō-mī-ō-săr-KŌ-mă	_____
rheumatoid arthritis (588)	ROO-mă-toyd ăr-THRĪ-tĭs	_____
rheumatologist (587)	roo-mă-TŎL-ō-jĭst	_____
rotation (594)	rō-TĀ-shŭn	_____
spinal stenosis (587)	SPĪ-năl stĕ-NŌ-sĭs	_____
sprain (591)	sprān	_____
strain (591)	strān	_____
striated muscle (596)	STRĪ-ā-tĕd MŬS-el	_____
subluxation (590)	sŭb-lŭk-SĀ-shŭn	_____
supination (594)	sū-pĭ-NĀ-shŭn	_____
suture joint (585)	SŪ-chŭr joint	_____
synovial fluid (585)	sĭ-NŌ-vē-ăl FLOO-ĭd	_____
synovial joint (585)	sĭ-NŌ-vē-ăl joint	_____
synovial membrane (585)	sĭ-NŌ-vē-ăl MĔM-brān	_____
synovitis (587)	sĭn-ō-VĪ-tĭs	_____

systemic lupus erythematosus (591)	sĭs-TĔM-ĭk LŪ-pŭs ĕ-rĭ-thē-mă-TŌ-sŭs	_____
tendinitis (587)	tĕn-dĭ-NĪ-tĭs	_____
tendon (585)	TĔN-dŭn	_____
tenorrhaphy (587)	tĕn-ŎR-ă-fē	_____
tenosynovitis (587)	tĕn-ō-sī-nō-VĪ-tĭs	_____
visceral muscle (596)	VĬS-ĕr-ăl MŬS-ĕl	_____

Laboratory Tests and Clinical Procedures

Term	Pronunciation	
antinuclear antibody test (598)	ăn-tē-NŪ-klē-ăr ĂN-tĭ-bŏd-ē tĕst	_____
arthrocentesis (598)	ăr-thrō-sĕn-TĒ-sĭs	_____
arthrography (599)	ăr-THRŎG-ră-fē	_____
arthroplasty (599)	ăr-thrō-PLĂS-tē	_____
arthroscopy (599)	ăr-THRŎS-kō-pē	_____
bone density test (600)	bōn DĔN-sĭ-tē tĕst	_____
bone scan (600)	bōn skăn	_____
computed tomography (600)	kŏm-PŪ-tĕd tō-MŎG-ră-fē	_____
diskography (600)	dĭsk-ŎG-ră-fē	_____
electromyography (600)	ē-lĕk-trō-mī-ŎG-ră-fē	_____
erythrocyte sedimentation rate (598)	ĕ-RĬTH-rō-sīt sĕd-ĭ-mĕn-TĀ-shŭn rāt	_____
magnetic resonance imaging (601)	măg-NĔT-ĭk rĕ-sō-NĂNS ĬM-ĭj-ĭng	_____
muscle biopsy (601)	MŬS'l BĪ-ŏp-sē	_____
rheumatoid factor test (598)	RŌŌ-mă-tŏyd FĂK-tŏr tĕst	_____
serum calcium (598)	SĔR-ŭm KĂL-sē-ŭm tĕst	_____
serum creatine kinase (598)	SĔR-ŭm krĕ-ă-tĭn KĪ-nās	_____
uric acid test (598)	ŬR-ĭk ĂS-ĭd tĕst	_____

X. Review Sheet

Write the meanings of the word parts in the spaces provided. Check your answers with the information in the chapter or in the glossary (Medical Terms—English) at the end of the book.

COMBINING FORMS

Combining Form	Meaning	Combining Form	Meaning
acetabul/o	_____	humer/o	_____
ankyl/o	_____	ili/o	_____
arthr/o	_____	isch/o	_____
articul/o	_____	kyph/o	_____
burs/o	_____	lamin/o	_____
calc/o	_____	leiomy/o	_____
calcane/o	_____	ligament/o	_____
calci/o	_____	lord/o	_____
carp/o	_____	lumb/o	_____
cervic/o	_____	malleol/o	_____
chondr/o	_____	mandibul/o	_____
clavicul/o	_____	maxill/o	_____
coccyg/o	_____	metacarp/o	_____
cost/o	_____	metatars/o	_____
crani/o	_____	my/o	_____
fasci/o	_____	myel/o	_____
femor/o	_____	myocardi/o	_____
fibr/o	_____	myos/o	_____
fibul/o	_____	olecran/o	_____

orth/o _____

oste/o _____

patell/o _____

ped/o _____

pelv/i _____

perone/o _____

phalang/o _____

plant/o _____

pub/o _____

radi/o _____

rhabdomy/o _____

rheumat/o _____

sacr/o _____

sarc/o _____

scapul/o _____

scoli/o _____

spondyl/o _____

stern/o _____

synov/o _____

tars/o _____

ten/o _____

tendin/o _____

thorac/o _____

tibi/o _____

uln/o _____

vertebr/o _____

SUFFIXES

Suffix	Meaning	Suffix	Meaning
-algia	_____	-penia	_____
-asthenia	_____	-physis	_____
-blast	_____	-plasty	_____
-clast	_____	-porosis	_____
-desis	_____	-stenosis	_____
-emia	_____	-tome	_____
-listhesis	_____	-trophy	_____
-malacia	_____		

Continued on following page

PREFIXES

Prefix	Meaning	Prefix	Meaning
a-, an-	_____	hyper-	_____
ab-	_____	meta-	_____
ad-	_____	peri-	_____
dia-	_____	poly-	_____
dorsi-	_____	sub-	_____
epi-	_____	supra-	_____
exo-	_____	sym-	_____

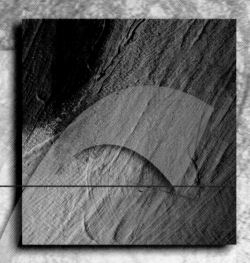

chapter 17

Skin

This chapter is divided into the following sections
   I. Introduction
   II. Structure of the Skin
   III. Accessory Organs of the Skin
   IV. Vocabulary
   V. Combining Forms and Suffixes
   VI. Lesions, Signs and Symptoms, Abnormal Conditions, and Skin Neoplasms
   VII. Laboratory Tests, Clinical Procedures, and Abbreviations
   VIII. Practical Applications
   IX. Exercises
   X. Answers to Exercises
   XI. Pronunciation of Terms
   XII. Review Sheet

In this chapter you will
- Identify the layers of the skin and the accessory structures associated with the skin.
- Build medical words using the combining forms that are related to the specialty of dermatology.
- Describe lesions, symptoms, and pathological conditions that relate to the skin.
- Identify laboratory tests, clinical procedures, and abbreviations that pertain to the skin.
- Apply your new knowledge to understanding medical terms in their proper contexts, such as medical reports and records.

I. Introduction

The skin and its accessory organs (hair, nails, and glands) are the **integumentary system** of the body. Integument means covering, and the skin (weighing 8 to 10 pounds over an area of 22 square feet in an average adult) is the outer covering for the body. It is, however, more than a simple body covering. This complex system of specialized tissues contains glands that secrete several types of fluids, nerves that carry impulses, and blood vessels that aid in the regulation of the body temperature. The following paragraphs review the many important functions of the skin.

First, as a protective membrane over the entire body, the skin guards the deeper tissues of the body against excessive loss of water, salts, and heat and against invasion of pathogens and their toxins. Secretions from the skin are slightly acidic in nature, which contributes to the skin's ability to prevent bacterial invasion. Specialized cells (Langerhans cells) react to the presence of antigens and have an immune function.

Second, the skin contains two types of glands that produce important secretions. These glands under the skin are the **sebaceous** and the **sweat glands.** Sebaceous glands produce **sebum,** an oily secretion, and sweat glands produce **sweat,** a watery secretion. Sebum and sweat pass to the outer edges of the skin through ducts and leave the skin through openings, or pores. Sebum lubricates the surface of the skin, and sweat cools the body as it evaporates from the skin surface.

Third, nerve fibers under the skin are receptors for sensations such as pain, temperature, pressure, and touch. Thus the adjustment of an individual to the environment depends on sensory messages relayed to the brain and spinal cord by sensitive nerve endings in the skin.

Fourth, different tissues in the skin maintain body temperature (thermoregulation). Nerve fibers coordinate thermoregulation by carrying messages to the skin from heat centers in the brain that are sensitive to increases and decreases in body temperature. Impulses from these fibers cause blood vessels to dilate to bring blood to the surface and cause sweat glands to produce the watery secretion that carries heat away.

II. Structure of the Skin

Figure 16–1A shows the three layers of the skin. Label these layers from the outer surface inward.

Epidermis [1]—a thin, cellular membrane layer
Dermis [2]—dense, fibrous, connective tissue layer
Subcutaneous tissue [3]—thick, fat-containing tissue

Epidermis

The epidermis is the outermost, totally cellular layer of the skin. It is composed of **squamous epithelium.** Epithelium is the covering of both the internal and the external surfaces of the body. Squamous epithelial cells are flat and scale-like. In the outer layer of the skin, these cells are arranged in several layers **(strata)** and are therefore called **stratified squamous epithelium.**

The epidermis lacks blood vessels, lymphatic vessels, and connective tissue (elastic fibers, cartilage, fat) and is therefore dependent on the deeper dermis (also called corium) layer and its rich network of capillaries for nourishment. In fact, oxygen and nutrients seep

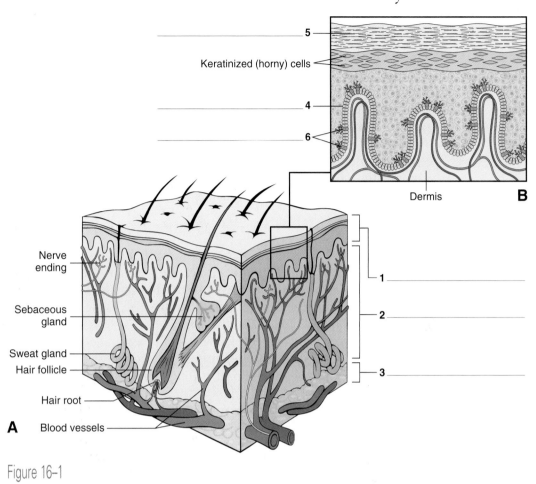

5

Keratinized (horny) cells

4

6

Dermis **B**

Nerve ending

Sebaceous gland

Sweat gland

Hair follicle

Hair root

A   Blood vessels

1

2

3

Figure 16–1

The skin. (A) Three layers of the skin. (B) Epidermis.

out of the capillaries in the dermis, pass through tissue fluid, and supply nourishment to the deeper layers of the epidermis.

Figure 16–1B illustrates the multilayered cells of the epidermis. The deepest layer is called the **basal layer** [4]. The cells in the basal layer are constantly growing and multiplying and give rise to all the other cells in the epidermis. As the basal layer cells divide, they are pushed upward and away from the blood supply of the dermal layer by a steady stream of younger cells. In their movement toward the most superficial layer of the epidermis, called the **stratum corneum** [5], the cells flatten, shrink, lose their nuclei, and die, becoming filled with a hard protein material called **keratin.** The cells are then called horny cells, reflecting their composition of keratin. Finally, within 3 to 4 weeks after beginning as a basal cell in the deepest part of the epidermis, the keratinized cell is sloughed off from the surface of the skin. The epidermis is thus constantly renewing itself, cells dying at the same rate at which they are replaced.

The basal layer of the epidermis contains special cells called **melanocytes** [6]. Melanocytes form and contain a brown-black pigment called **melanin** that is transferred to other epidermal cells and gives color to the skin. The number of melanocytes in all human races is the same, but the amount of melanin within each cell accounts for the color differences among the races. Individuals with darker skin possess more melanin within the melanocytes, not a greater number of melanocytes. The presence of melanin in the epidermis is vital for protection against the harmful effects of ultraviolet radiation, which can manifest themselves as skin cancer. Individuals who are incapable of forming melanin are called **albino.** Skin and hair are white. Their pupils (circular opening in the eye) are red because in the absence of pigment in the retina, the tiny blood vessels are visible in the iris (normally pigmented portion) of the eye.

Melanin production increases with exposure to strong ultraviolet light, and this creates a suntan, which is a protective response. When the melanin cannot absorb all of the ultraviolet rays, the skin becomes sunburned and inflamed (redness, swelling, and pain). Over a period of years, excessive exposure to sun can tend to cause wrinkles, permanent pigmenting changes, and even cancer of the skin. Because dark-skinned people have more melanin, they have fewer wrinkles and they are less likely to develop skin cancer.

Dermis (Corium)

The dermis layer, directly below the epidermis, is composed of blood and lymph vessels and nerve fibers, as well as the accessory organs of the skin, which are the hair follicles, sweat glands, and sebaceous glands. To support the elaborate system of nerves, vessels, and glands, the dermis contains connective tissue cells and fibers that account for the extensibility and elasticity of the skin.

The dermis is composed of interwoven elastic and **collagen** fibers. Collagen (**colla** means glue) is a fibrous protein material found in bone, cartilage, tendons, and ligaments, as well as in the skin. It is tough and resistant but also flexible. In the infant, collagen is loose and delicate, and it becomes harder as the body ages. During pregnancy, overstretching of a woman's skin may break the elastic fibers, resulting in linear markings called striae or stretch marks. Collagen fibers support and protect the blood and nerve networks that pass through the dermis. Collagen diseases affect connective tissues of the body. Examples of these connective tissue collagen disorders are systemic lupus erythematosus and scleroderma (see Section VI, under Abnormal Conditions).

Subcutaneous Layer

The subcutaneous layer of the skin is another connective tissue layer; it specializes in the formation of fat. **Lipocytes** (fat cells) are predominant in the subcutaneous layer, and they manufacture and store large quantities of fat. Obviously, areas of the body and individuals vary as far as fat deposition is concerned. Functionally, this layer of the skin is important in protection of the deeper tissues of the body, as a heat insulator, and for energy storage.

III. Accessory Organs of the Skin

Hair

A hair fiber is composed of a tightly fused meshwork of horny cells filled with the hard protein called **keratin.** Hair growth is similar to the growth of the epidermal layer of the skin. Deep-lying cells in the hair root (see Fig. 16–1) produce horny cells that move upward through the **hair follicles** (shafts that hold the hair fibers). Melanocytes are located at the root of the hair follicle, and they donate the melanin pigment to the horny cells of the hair fiber. Hair turns gray when the melanocytes stop producing melanin.

Of the 5 million hairs on the body, about 100,000 are on the head. They grow about ½ inch (1.3 cm) per month. Cutting the hair has no effect on its rate of growth.

Nails

Nails are hard, keratin plates covering the dorsal surface of the last bone of each toe and finger. They are composed of horny cells that are cemented together tightly and can extend indefinitely unless cut or broken. A nail grows in thickness and length as a result of division of cells in the region of the nail root, which is at the base (proximal portion) of the nail plate.

Fingernails grow about 1 mm per week, which means that they can regrow in 3 to 5 months. Toenails grow more slowly than fingernails; it takes 12 to 18 months for toenails to be replaced completely.

The **lunula** is a semilunar (half-moon), white region at the base of the nail plate, and it is generally found in the thumbnail of most people and in varying degrees in other fingers. Air mixed in with keratin and cells rich in nuclei give the lunula its whitish color. The **cuticle,** a narrow band of epidermis (layer of keratin), is at the base and sides of the nail plate. The **paronychium** is the soft tissue surrounding the nail border. Figure 16–2A illustrates the anatomic structure of a nail.

Nail growth and appearance commonly alter during systemic disease. For example, grooves in nails may occur with high fevers and serious illness, and spoon nails (flattening of the nail plate) occur in iron-deficiency anemia. Onycholysis (**onych/o** = nail) is the loosening of the nail plate with separation from the nail bed. It may occur with infection of the nail (Fig. 16–2B).

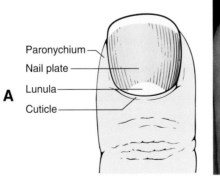
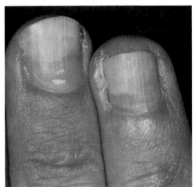

Figure 16-2

(A) Anatomical structure of a nail. (B) Onycholysis. Infection or trauma to the nail may be the cause of the detachment of the nail from its plate. (**B** from Seidel HM: Mosby's Guide to Physical Examination, 5th ed. St. Louis, Mosby, 2003, p. 214.)

Glands

Sebaceous Glands

Sebaceous glands are located in the dermal layer of the skin over the entire body, with the exception of the palms (hands) and soles (feet). They secrete an oily substance called **sebum.** Sebum, containing lipids, lubricates the skin and minimizes water loss. Sebaceous glands are closely associated with hair follicles, and their ducts open into the hair follicle through which the sebum is released. Figure 16–1 shows the relationship of the sebaceous gland to the hair follicle. The sebaceous glands are influenced by sex hormones, which cause them to hypertrophy at puberty and atrophy in old age. Overproduction of sebum during puberty contributes to blackhead (comedo) formation and acne in some individuals.

Sweat Glands

Sweat glands are tiny, coiled glands found on almost all body surfaces (about 2 million in the body). They are most numerous in the palm of the hand (3000 glands per square inch) and on the sole of the foot. Figure 16–1 illustrates how the coiled sweat gland originates deep in the dermis and straightens out to extend up through the epidermis. The tiny opening on the surface is called a **pore.**

Sweat, or perspiration, is almost pure water, with dissolved materials such as salt making up less than 1 percent of the total composition. It is colorless and odorless. The odor produced when sweat accumulates on the skin is caused by the action of bacteria on the sweat.

Sweat cools the body as it evaporates into the air. Perspiration is controlled by the sympathetic nervous system, whose nerve fibers are activated by the heart regulatory center in the hypothalamic region of the brain, which stimulates sweating.

A special variety of sweat gland, active only from puberty onward and larger than the ordinary kind, is concentrated in a few areas of the body near the reproductive organs and in the armpits. These glands (called **apocrine sweat glands**) secrete an odorless sweat, containing substances easily broken down by bacteria on the skin. The bacterial waste products produce a characteristic human body odor. The milk-producing mammary gland is another type of modified sweat gland; it secretes milk after the birth of a child.

IV. Vocabulary

This list will help you review many of the new terms introduced in the text. Short definitions will reinforce your understanding of the terms. See Section XI of this chapter for help in pronouncing the more difficult terms.

albino	Person with skin deficient in pigment (melanin).
apocrine sweat gland	One of the large dermal exocrine glands located in the axilla and genital areas. It secretes sweat that, in action with bacteria, is responsible for human body odor.
basal layer	The deepest region of the epidermis; it gives rise to all the epidermal cells.
collagen	Structural protein found in the skin and connective tissue.
cuticle	Band of epidermis at the base and sides of the nail plate.
dermis	Middle layer of the skin; also called corium.
epidermis	Outermost layer of the skin.
epithelium	Layer of skin cells forming the outer and inner surfaces of the body.
hair follicle	Sac within which each hair grows.
integumentary system	The skin and its accessory structures such as hair and nails.
keratin	Hard protein material found in the epidermis, hair, and nails. Keratin means horn and is commonly found in the horns of animals.
lipocyte	A fat cell.
lunula	The half-moon–shaped, white area at the base of a nail.
melanin	Major pigment that gives the skin color. It is formed by melanocytes in the epidermis.
paronychium	Soft tissue surrounding the nail border.
pore	Tiny opening on the surface of the skin.
sebaceous gland	Oil-secreting gland in the dermis that is associated with hair follicles.
sebum	Oily substance secreted by sebaceous glands.
squamous epithelium	Flat, scale-like cells composing the epidermis.
stratified	Arranged in layers.

stratum (plural: **strata**)   A layer (of cells).

stratum corneum   The outermost layer of the epidermis, which consists of flattened, keratinized (horny) cells.

subcutaneous tissue   The innermost layer of the skin, containing fat tissue.

V. Combining Forms and Suffixes

Write the meanings of the medical terms in the spaces provided.

Combining Forms

Combining Form	Meaning	Terminology	Meaning
adip/o	fat (see **lip/o** and **steat/o**)	adipose _____	
albin/o	white	albinism _____	

Table 16–1 lists combining forms for colors and examples of terms using those combining forms.

caus/o	burn, burning	causalgia _____	

Intensely unpleasant burning sensation in skin and muscles when there is damage to nerves.

Table 16–1. COLORS

Combining Form	Meaning	Terminology
albin/o	white	*albin*ism
anthrac/o	black (as coal)	*anthrac*osis
chlor/o	green	*chlor*ophyll
cirrh/o	tawny yellow	*cirrh*osis
cyan/o	blue	*cyan*osis
eosin/o	rosy	*eosin*ophil
erythr/o	red	*erythr*ocyte
jaund/o	yellow	*jaund*ice
leuk/o	white	*leuk*oderma
lute/o	yellow	corpus *luteum*
melan/o	black	*melan*ocyte
poli/o	gray	*poli*omyelitis
xanth/o	yellow	*xanth*oma

cauter/o	heat, burn	electrocautery _____

A needle or blade used during surgery to burn through tissue. It is very effective in minimizing blood loss.

cutane/o	skin (see **derm/o**)	subcutaneous _____

derm/o **dermat/o**	skin	epidermis _____

dermatitis _____

Atopic dermatitis *is of unknown cause; it is marked by itching and scratching. In 70 percent of cases, there is a family history of the condition. Atopy is an allergic reaction for which there is a genetic predisposition.*

dermatoplasty _____

Skin is transplanted to a body surface damaged by disease or injury.

dermatologist _____

dermabrasion _____

Abrasion means a scraping away. Dermabrasion is a surgical procedure performed to remove acne scars, tattoos, or fine wrinkles.

epidermolysis _____

Loosening of the epidermis with the development of large blisters; occurs after injury.

diaphor/o	profuse sweating (see **hidr/o**)	diaphoresis _____

erythem/o **erythemat/o**	redness	erythema _____

*Flushing; widespread redness of the skin. Erythema infectiosum (fifth disease) is a benign infectious disease, mainly of children. It is marked by fever and **erythematous** rash that begins on the cheeks and later appears on the arms, buttocks, and trunk. It is caused by a parvovirus.*

hidr/o	sweat	anhidrosis _____

Do not confuse hidr/o with hydr/o (water)!

ichthy/o	scaly, dry (fish-like)	ichthyosis _____

A hereditary condition in which the skin is dry, rough, and scaly because of a defect in keratinization. Ichthyosis can also be acquired, appearing with malignancies such as lymphomas and multiple myeloma.

kerat/o	hard, horny tissue	keratosis _____

See page 647, Section VI, under Skin Neoplasms.

leuk/o	white	leukoplakia _____

-plakia means plaques.

lip/o	fat	lipoma _____
		liposuction _____

Removal of subcutaneous fat tissue through a tube that is introduced into the fatty area via a small incision. The fat is aspirated (suctioned) out.

melan/o	black	melanocyte _____
		melanoma _____

This is a malignant skin tumor. See page 648, Section VI, under Skin Neoplasms.

myc/o	fungus (fungi include yeasts, molds, and mushrooms)	dermatomycosis _____

An example is ringworm (athlete's foot).

onych/o	nail (see **ungu/o**)	onycholysis _____

Separation of the nail plate from the nail bed in fungal infections or after trauma.

onychomycosis _____

Fungal infection of the nails, which become white, opaque, thick, and brittle.

paronychia _____

par- means near or beside. Paronychia is the inflammation and swelling of the soft tissue around the nail and is associated with torn cuticles or ingrown nails.

phyt/o	plant	dermatophytosis _____

Examples are fungal infections of the hands and feet; dermatomycosis.

pil/o	hair (see **trich/o**), hair follicle	pilosebaceous _____	

sebace/o means a gland that secretes sebum.

rhytid/o wrinkle rhytidectomy _____

Reconstructive plastic surgery to remove wrinkles and signs of aging skin; also called rhytidoplasty or face lift.

seb/o sebum (oily secretion from sebaceous glands) seborrhea _____

*Excessive secretion from sebaceous glands. **Seborrheic dermatitis** is commonly known as **dandruff.***

squam/o scale-like squamous epithelium _____

Cells are flat and scale-like; pavement epithelium.

steat/o fat steatoma _____

*A cystic collection of sebum (fatty material) that forms in a sebaceous gland and can become infected; **sebaceous cyst.***

trich/o hair trichomycosis _____

ungu/o nail subungual _____

xanth/o yellow xanthoma _____

*Nodules develop under the skin owing to excess lipid deposits. Usually associated with a high cholesterol level. Plaques that appear on the eyelids are **xanthelasmas** (-elasma means a flat plate).*

xer/o dry xeroderma _____

-derma means skin. This is a mild form of ichthyosis.

Suffixes

Suffix	Meaning	Terminology	Meaning
-derma	skin	pyoderma _____	

Impetigo is a purulent skin disease (pyoderma).

leukoderma _____

VI. Lesions, Signs and Symptoms, Abnormal Conditions, and Skin Neoplasms

Cutaneous Lesions

A **lesion** is an area of damaged tissue, caused by disease or trauma. The following terms describe common skin lesions, which are illustrated in Figure 16–3.

crust	**Collection of dried serum and cellular debris.**
	A scab is a crust. It forms from the drying of a body exudate as in eczema, impetigo, and seborrhea.
cyst	**Thick-walled, closed sac or pouch containing fluid or semisolid material.**
	Examples of cysts are the **pilonidal cyst,** which is found over the sacral area of the back in the midline and contains hairs (**pil/o** means hair, **nid/o** means nest); and the **sebaceous cyst,** which is a collection of yellowish, cheesy sebum commonly found on the scalp, vulva, and scrotum.

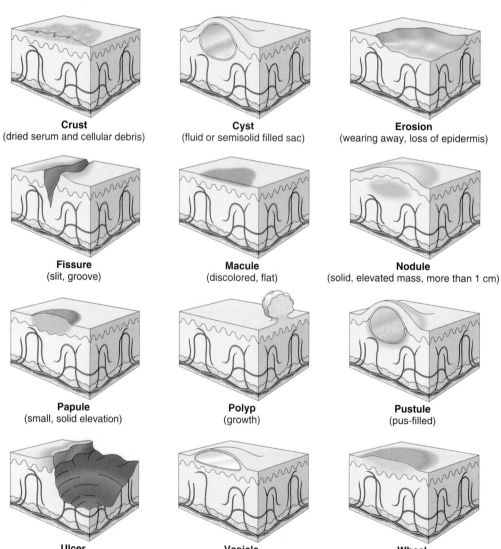

Crust
(dried serum and cellular debris)

Cyst
(fluid or semisolid filled sac)

Erosion
(wearing away, loss of epidermis)

Fissure
(slit, groove)

Macule
(discolored, flat)

Nodule
(solid, elevated mass, more than 1 cm)

Papule
(small, solid elevation)

Polyp
(growth)

Pustule
(pus-filled)

Ulcer
(open sore, erosion)

Vesicle
(clear fluid, blister)

Wheal
(smooth, slightly elevated, edema)

Figure 16–3

Cutaneous lesions.

erosion	**Wearing away or loss of epidermis.**
	Erosions do not penetrate below the dermoepidermal junction. They occur as a result of inflammation or injury and heal without scarring.
fissure	**Groove or crack-like sore.**
	An anal fissure is a break in the skin lining of the anal canal.
macule	**Discolored (often reddened) flat lesion.**
	Freckles, tattoo marks, and flat moles are examples.
nodule	**Solid, elevated lesion more than 1 cm in diameter.**
	An enlarged lymph node is an example. A large nodule is a tumor.
papule	**Small (less than 1 cm in diameter), solid elevation of the skin.**
	Pimples are examples of papules. Papules may become confluent (run together) and form **plaques.**
polyp	**Mushroom-like growth extending on a stalk from the surface of mucous membrane.**
	Polyps are commonly found in the nose and sinuses, urinary bladder, and uterus.
pustule	**Small elevation of the skin containing pus.**
	A pustule is a small **abscess** (collection of pus) on the skin.
ulcer	**Open sore on the skin or mucous membrane.**
	Decubitus ulcers (bedsores) are caused by pressure that results from lying in one position (**decubitus** means "lying down"). Pressure ulcers usually involve loss of tissue substance and pus or exudate formation.
vesicle	**Small collection of clear fluid (serum); blister.**
	Vesicles are found in burns, allergies, and dermatitis. **Bullae** (singular: **bulla**) are large vesicles (Fig. 16–4).

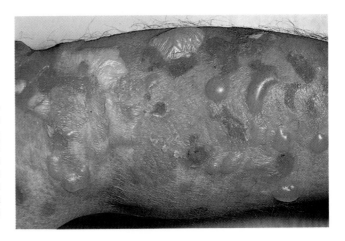

Figure 16–4

Bullae (large blisters) in bullous pemphigoid (a chronic skin disorder in older individuals). The pemphigoid (pemphix means bubble) bullae occur as the entire thickness of the epidermis detaches from its foundation. (From Kumar V, Cotran RS, Robbins SL: Basic Pathology, 7th ed. Philadelphia, WB Saunders, 2003, p. 797.)

wheal   **Smooth, slightly elevated, edematous (swollen) area that is redder or paler than the surrounding skin.**

Wheals may be circumscribed, as in a mosquito bite, or may involve a wide area, as in allergic reactions. Wheals are often accompanied by itching and are seen in hives, anaphylaxis, and insect bites.

Signs and Symptoms

alopecia   **Absence of hair from areas where it normally grows.**

Alopecia, or baldness, may be hereditary (usual progressive loss of scalp hair in men) or it may be caused by disease, injury, or treatment (chemotherapy) or may occur in old age. **Alopecia areata** is an idiopathic condition in which hair falls out in patches. See Figure 16–5A.

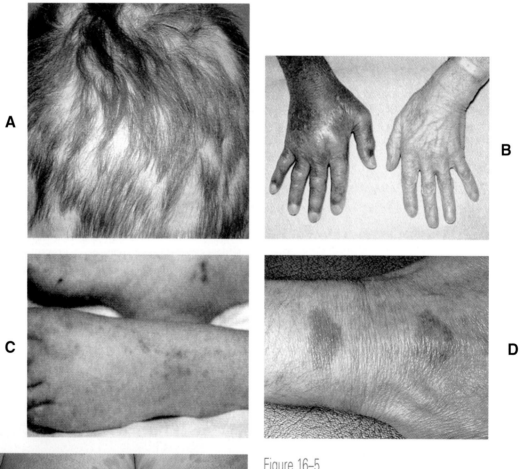

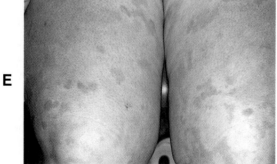

Figure 16–5

Dermatologic signs. (A) Alopecia areata. (B) Ecchymoses, right hand. **(C) Petechiae. (D) Senile purpura.** Fragile blood vessels rupture with minimal trauma. **(E) Urticaria;** erythematous, edematous, often circular plaques. (A-D from Mosby's Medical, Nursing and Allied Health Dictionary, 5th ed. St. Louis, Mosby, 1998; E from Murphy GF, Herzberg AJ: Atlas of Dermatopathology, Philadelphia, WB Saunders, 1996, in Cotran RS, Kumar V, Collins T: Robbins Pathologic Basis of Disease, 6th ed. Philadelphia, WB Saunders, 1999.)

ecchymosis (plural: **ecchymoses**)	**Bluish-black mark (macule) on the skin; black-and-blue mark.**

Ecchymoses (**ec-** means out, **chym/o** means to pour) are caused by hemorrhages into the skin from injury or spontaneous leaking of blood from vessels. See Figure 16–5B.

petechia (plural: **petechiae**)   **A small, pinpoint hemorrhage.**

Petechiae are smaller versions of ecchymoses. See Figure 16–5C.

pruritus   **Itching.**

Pruritus is a symptom associated with most forms of dermatitis and with other conditions as well. It arises as a result of stimulation of nerves in the skin by substances released in allergic reactions or by irritation caused by substances in the blood or by foreign bodies.

purpura   **Merging ecchymoses and petechiae over any part of the body.** See Figure 16–5D.

urticaria (hives)   **Acute allergic reaction in which red, round wheals develop on the skin.** See Figure 16–5E.

Pruritus may be intense, and the cause is commonly allergy to foods (such as shellfish or strawberries). Localized edema (swelling) occurs as well.

Abnormal Conditions

acne   **Papular and pustular eruption of the skin.**

Acne vulgaris (**vulgaris** means "ordinary") is caused by the buildup of sebum and keratin in the pores of the skin. A **blackhead** or **comedo** (plural: **comedones**) is a sebum plug partially blocking the pore (Fig. 16–6). If the pore becomes completely blocked, a **whitehead** forms. Bacteria in the skin break down the sebum, producing inflammation in the surrounding tissue. Papules, pustules, and cysts can thus form. Treatment consists of long-term antibiotic use and medications to dry the skin. Benzoyl peroxide and tretinoin (Retin-A) are medications used to prevent comedo formation; isotretinoin (Accutane) is used in severe cystic acne.

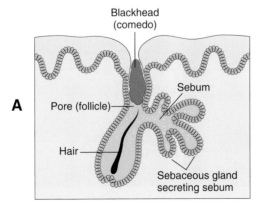 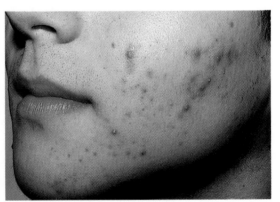

Figure 16–6

(A) Formation of a blackhead (comedo) in a dilated pore filled with sebum, bacteria, and pigment. (B) Acne vulgaris on the face. (B from Callen JP, Paller AS, Greer KE, Swinyer LJ: Color Atlas of Dermatology, 2nd ed. Philadelphia, WB Saunders, 2000, p. 151.)

burns	**Injury to tissues caused by heat contact.**

Examples are dry heat (fire), moist heat (steam or liquid), chemicals, lightning, electricity, and radiation. Burns are usually as follows:

first-degree burns—superficial epidermal lesions, erythema, hyperesthesia, and no blisters. Sunburn is an example.

second-degree burns (partial-thickness burn injury)—epidermal and dermal lesions, erythema, blisters, and hyperesthesia (Fig. 16–7A).

third-degree burns (full-thickness burn injury)—epidermis and dermis are destroyed (necrosis of skin), and subcutaneous layer is damaged, leaving charred, white tissue (Fig. 16–7B).

cellulitis	**Diffuse, acute infection of the skin marked by local heat, redness, pain, and swelling.**

Abscess and tissue destruction can occur if antibiotics are not taken. Areas of poor lymphatic drainage are susceptible to this skin infection.

eczema	**Inflammatory skin disease with erythematous, papulovesicular lesions.**

This chronic or acute dermatitis is often accompanied by pruritus and may occur without any obvious cause. It is a common allergic reaction in children and also occurs in adults. Allergy may be to foods, dust, or pollens. Treatment depends on the cause but usually includes the use of corticosteroids.

exanthematous viral diseases	**Rash (exanthem) of the skin due to a viral infection.**

Examples are **rubella** (German measles), **rubeola** (measles), and **varicella** (chickenpox).

gangrene	**Death of tissue associated with loss of blood supply.**

In this condition, ischemia resulting from injury, inflammation, frostbite, diseases such as diabetes, or arteriosclerosis can lead to necrosis of tissue followed by bacterial invasion and putrefaction (proteins are decomposed by bacteria).

A 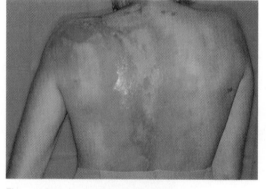 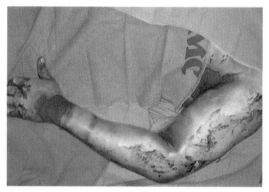 B

Figure 16–7

Burns. (A) Second-degree injury. Wound sensation is painful and very sensitive to touch and air currents. **(B) Third-degree burn** showing viable color (deep-red, white, black and brown). The wound itself is insensate (does not respond to pinprick sensation). (From Black JM, Hawks JH, Keene, AM: Medical-Surgical Nursing: Clinical Management for Positive Outcomes, 6th ed. Philadelphia, WB Saunders, 2001.)

impetigo	**Bacterial inflammatory skin disease characterized by vesicles, pustules, and crusted-over lesions.**

This is a contagious **pyoderma** (**py/o** means pus) and is usually caused by staphylococci or streptococci. Systemic use of antibiotics and proper cleansing of lesions are effective treatments.

psoriasis	**Chronic, recurrent dermatosis marked by itchy, scaly, red plaques covered by silvery gray scales** (Fig. 16–8).

Psoriasis commonly forms on the forearms, knees, legs, and scalp. It is neither infectious nor contagious but is caused by an increased rate of growth of the basal layer of the epidermis. The cause is unknown, but the condition runs in families and may be worsened by anxiety. Treatment is palliative (relieving but not curing) and includes topical lubricants, keratolytics, and steroids. Psoralen-ultraviolet A (PUVA) light therapy is also used.

scabies	**A contagious, parasitic infection of the skin with intense pruritus.**

Scabies (from *scabere,* meaning to "scratch") commonly affects areas such as the groin, nipples, and skin between the fingers. Treatment is topical medicated cream to destroy the scabies mites (tiny parasites).

scleroderma	**A chronic progressive disease of the skin with hardening and shrinking of connective tissue.**

Fibrous scar tissue infiltrates the skin, and the heart, lungs, kidneys, and esophagus may be affected as well. Skin is thick, hard, and rigid, and pigmented patches may occur. The cause is not known. Palliative treatment consists of drugs, such as immunosuppressives and anti-inflammatory agents, and physical therapy.

systemic lupus erythematosus (SLE)	**Chronic inflammatory disease of collagen in the skin, of joints, and of internal organs.**

Lupus (meaning wolf-like; physicians thought the shape and color of the skin lesions resembled the bite of a wolf) produces a characteristic "butterfly" pattern of redness over the cheeks and nose. In more severe cases, the extent of erythema increases and all exposed areas of the skin may be involved. Primarily a disease of females, lupus is an autoimmune condition. High levels of certain antibodies are found in the patient's blood. Corticosteroids and immunosuppressive drugs are used to control symptoms.

SLE should be differentiated from chronic **discoid lupus erythematosus (DLE),** which is a milder, scaling, plaque-like, superficial eruption of the skin confined to the face, scalp, ears, chest, arms, and back. The reddish patches heal and leave scars.

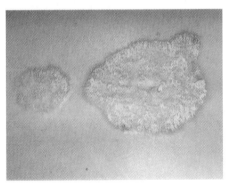

Figure 16–8

Psoriasis. Scaly erythematous plaque, with silvery scales on top. (From Jarvis C: Physical Examination and Health Assessment, 3rd ed. Philadelphia, WB Saunders, 2000.)

A

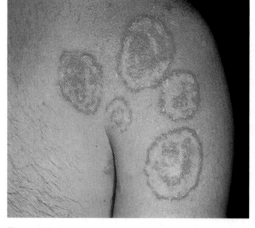

B

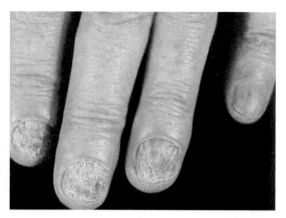

Figure 16-9

(A) Tinea corporis (ringworm). (B) Tinea unguium. Fungal infection of the nail causes the distal nail plate to turn yellow or white. Hyperkeratotic debris accumulates, causing the nail to separate from the nail bed (onycholysis). (**A** from Lewis SM, Heitkemper MM, Dirksen SR: Medical-Surgical Nursing: Assessment and Management of Clinical Pro, 5th ed. St. Louis, Mosby, 2000; **B** reprinted with permission from American Academy of Dermatology. All rights reserved. From Seidel HM: Mosby's Guide to Physical Examination, 4th ed. St. Louis, Mosby, 1998.)

tinea	**Infection of the skin caused by a fungus.**
	Tinea Corporis, or **ringworm,** so called because the infection is in a ring-like pattern (see Fig. 16–9A), is highly contagious and causes severe pruritus. Other examples are **tinea pedis** (athlete's foot), which affects the skin between the toes, **tinea capitis** (on the scalp), **tinea barbae** affecting the skin under a beard), and **tinea unguium** (affecting the nails) (Fig. 16–9B). Treatment is with antifungal agents. The word **tinea** is from Latin and means "worm."
vitiligo (vĭt-ĭl-Ĭ-gō)	**Loss of pigment (depigmentation) in areas of the skin (milk-white patches).**
	Also known as **leukoderma** (Fig. 16–10). There is an increased association of vitiligo with certain autoimmune conditions such as thyroiditis, hyperthyroidism, and diabetes mellitus.

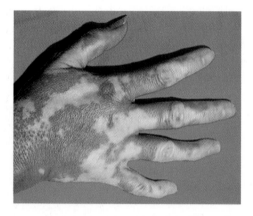

Figure 16-10

Vitiligo on the hand (Latin: *vitium* meaning "a blemish"). Epidermal melanocytes are completely lost in depigmented areas through an autoimmune process. (From Jarvis C: Physical Examination and Health Assessment, 3rd ed., Philadelphia, WB Saunders, 2000, p. 223.)

Skin Neoplasms

Benign Neoplasms

callus

Increased growth of cells in the keratin layer of the epidermis caused by pressure or friction.

The feet (Figure 16–11A) and the hands are common sites. A **corn** is a type of callus that develops a hard core (a whitish, corn-like central kernel).

keloid

Hypertrophied, thickened scar that occurs after trauma or surgical incision.

Keloids (Figure 16–11B) occur because of excessive collagen formation in the skin during connective tissue repair. The term comes from the Greek *kelis,* meaning "blemish." Surgical excision is often combined with intralesional steroid injections or low-dose radiotherapy.

A normal scar left by a healed wound is called a **cicatrix** (SĬK-ă-trĭks).

keratosis

Thickened area of the epidermis.

Some keratoses are caused by excessive exposure to light **(actinic keratosis).** **Seborrheic keratoses** are tan to black warty lesions.

leukoplakia

White, thickened patches on mucous membrane tissue of the tongue or cheek.

This precancerous lesion is common in smokers and may be caused by chronic inflammation.

Callus —

A

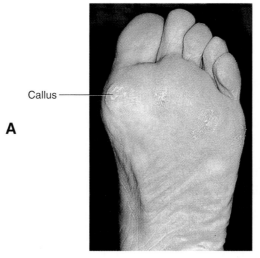
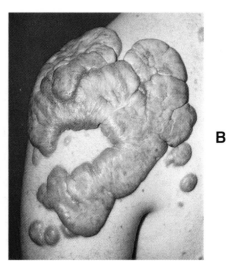

B

Figure 16–11

(A) Callus on the sole of the foot. **(B) Keloid. (A** from Mosby's Medical, Nursing, and Allied Health Dictionary, 6th ed., St. Louis, Mosby, 2002, p. 265; **B** from Ignatavicius DD, Workman ML: Medical-Surgical Nursing: Critical Thinking for Collaborative Care, 4th ed. Philadelphia, WB Saunders, 2002, p. 1544.)

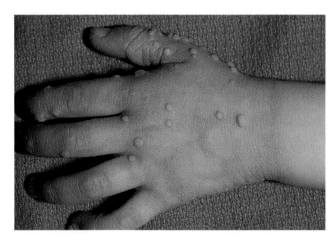

Figure 16–12

Verruca vulgaris. Warts are multiple papules with rough, pebble-like surfaces. (From Cotran RS, Kumar V, Collins T: Robbins Pathologic Basis of Disease, 6th ed. Philadelphia, WB Saunders, 1999, p. 1208.)

nevus (plural: **nevi**)	**Pigmented lesion of the skin.**

Nevi include dilated blood vessels (telangiectasis) radiating out from a point (vascular spiders), hemangiomas, and moles. Many are present at birth, but some are acquired.

Dysplastic nevi are moles that do not form properly and may progress to form a type of skin cancer called melanoma (see **malignant melanoma**).

verruca	**Epidermal growth caused by a virus (wart).**

Verruca vulgaris (common) is the most frequent type of wart (see Fig. 16–12). Plantar warts (verrucae) occur on the soles of the feet, juvenile warts occur on the hands and face of children, and venereal warts occur on the genitals and around the anus. Warts are removed with acids, electrocautery, or freezing with liquid nitrogen (cryosurgery). If the virus remains in the skin, the wart frequently regrows.

Cancerous Lesions

basal cell carcinoma	**Malignant tumor of the basal cell layer of the epidermis.**

This is the most frequent type of skin cancer. It is a slow-growing tumor that usually occurs on the face, especially near or on the nose. See Figure 16–13A. It almost never metastasizes.

Kaposi sarcoma	**Malignant, vascular, neoplastic growth characterized by cutaneous nodules. Frequently on the lower extremities** (Figure 16–13 B).

Nodules range in color from deep pink to dark blue and purple. The condition is associated with acquired immunodeficiency syndrome (AIDS).

malignant melanoma	**Cancerous growth composed of melanocytes.**

This malignancy is attributed to the intense exposure to sunlight that many people experience. Melanoma usually begins as a mottled, light brown to black, flat macule with irregular borders (Fig. 16–14). The lesions may turn shades of red, blue, and white and may crust on the surface and bleed. Melanomas often arise in preexisting moles (dysplastic nevi) and frequently appear on the upper back, lower legs, arms, head, and neck.

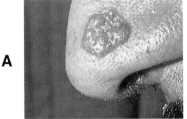

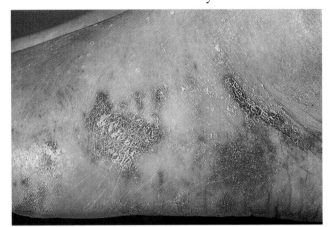

Figure 16–13

(A) Basal cell carcinoma. (B) Kaposi sarcoma. (**A** from Mosby's Medical, Nursing, and Allied Health Dictionary, 6th ed. St. Louis, Mosby, 2002, p. 184; **B** courtesy Christopher DM. Fletcher, MD, Brigham and Women's Hospital, Boston, MA from Cotran RS, Kumar V, Collins T: Robbins Pathologic Basis of Disease, 6th ed. Philadelphia, WB Saunders, 1999, p. 536.)

Biopsy is required to confirm the diagnosis of melanoma, and prognosis is commonly determined by measuring tumor thickness in millimeters.

Melanomas often metastasize to the lung, liver, bone, and brain. Treatment includes excision of the tumor, regional lymphadenectomy, chemotherapy/ immunotherapy, or radiotherapy.

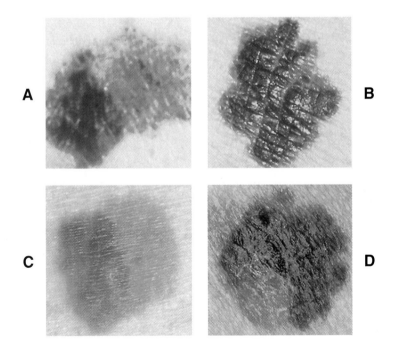

Figure 16–14

The ABCDs of melanoma. (A) Asymmetry: one half unlike the other half. **(B) Border:** irregular or poorly circumscribed border. **(C) Color:** varied from one area to another; shades of tan and brown; black; sometimes white, red or blue. **(D) Diameter:** usually larger than 6mm (diameter of a pencil eraser). (From Lewis SM, Heitkemper MM, Dirksen SR: Medical-Surgical Nursing: Assessment and Management of Clinical Problems, 5th ed. St. Louis, Mosby, 2000, p. 504.)

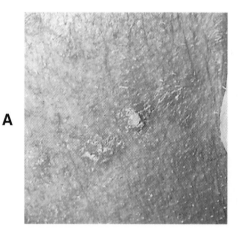

A

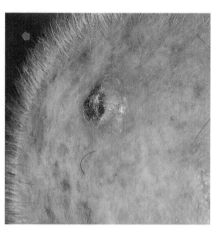

B

Figure 16–15

(A) Actinic (solar) keratosis. (B) Squamous cell carcinoma. Lesions are often nodular and ulcerated. (**A** from Ignatavicius DD, Workman ML: Medical-Surgical Nursing: Critical Thinking for Collaborative Care, 4th ed. Philadelphia, WB Saunders, 2002, p. 1502; **B** from Cotran RS, Kumar V, Collins T: Robbins Pathologic Basis of Disease, 6th ed. Philadelphia, WB Saunders, 1999, p. 1186.)

squamous cell carcinoma	**Malignant tumor of the squamous epithelial cells of the epidermis.**

This tumor may grow in places other than the skin, wherever squamous epithelium is found (mouth, larynx, bladder, esophagus, lungs). **Actinic** (sun-related) **keratoses** (Fig. 16–15A) are premalignant lesions in people with sun-damaged skin. Progression to squamous cell carcinoma (Fig. 16–15B) may occur if lesions are not removed. Treatment is surgical excision, cryotherapy, curettage and electrodesiccation, or radiotherapy.

VII. Laboratory Tests, Clinical Procedures, and Abbreviations

Laboratory Tests

bacterial analyses	**Samples of skin are sent to a laboratory to detect presence of microorganisms.**

Purulent (pus-filled) material or **exudate** (fluid that accumulates) are often taken for examination.

fungal tests	**Scrapings from skin lesions, hair specimens, or nail clippings are sent to a laboratory for culture and microscopic examination.**

The specimen may also be treated with a potassium hydroxide (KOH) preparation and examined microscopically. A positive KOH test often eliminates the need for a culture.

Clinical Procedures

cryosurgery Use of subfreezing temperature via liquid nitrogen application to destroy tissue.

curettage Use of a sharp dermal curet (curette) to scrape away a skin lesion.

A curet is shaped like a spoon or scoop. It may be blunt or sharp.

electrodesiccation Tissue is destroyed by burning with an electric spark.

This procedure is used following curettage to remove and destroy small cancerous lesions with well-defined borders.

Mohs surgery Thin layers of a malignant growth are removed, and each is examined under a microscope.

Mohs surgery is a specialized form of excision to treat basal and squamous cell carcinomas. It is also known as **microscopically controlled surgery.**

skin biopsy Suspected malignant skin lesions are removed and sent to the pathology laboratory for microscopic examination.

In a **punch biopsy,** a surgical instrument removes a core of tissue by rotation of its sharp, circular edge. In a **shave biopsy,** tissue is excised using a cut parallel to the surface of the surrounding skin.

skin test The reaction of the body to a substance by observing the results of injecting the substance intradermally or applying it topically to the skin.

Skin tests are used to diagnose allergies and disease. In the **patch test,** an allergen-treated piece of gauze or filter paper is applied to the skin. If the skin becomes red or swollen, the result is positive. In the **scratch test,** several scratches are made in the skin, and a very minute amount of test material is inserted into the scratches. The Schick test (diphtheria), Mantoux, and purified protein derivative (PPD) tests (tuberculosis) are other skin tests.

Abbreviations

ABCD	asymmetry (of shape), border (irregularity), color (variation with one lesion), diameter (greater than 6 mm); characteristics associated with skin cancer	**PPD**	purified protein derivative; skin test for tuberculosis
		PUVA	psoralen–ultraviolet A light therapy (treatment for psoriasis)
bx	biopsy	**SLE**	systemic lupus erythematosus
Derm.	dermatology	**subcut**	subcutaneous
DLE	discoid lupus erythematosus		

VIII. Practical Applications

This section contains actual medical reports using terms that you have studied in this and previous chapters. Explanations of more difficult terms are added in brackets. Answers to the questions are on page 662 after Answers to Exercises.

Disease Descriptions

1. **Candidiasis** (*Candida* is a yeast-like fungus): This fungus is normally found on mucous membranes, skin, and vaginal mucosa. Under certain circumstances (excessive warmth; administration of birth control pills, antibiotics, and corticosteroids; debilitated states; infancy), it can change to a pathogen and cause localized or generalized mucocutaneous disease. Examples are paronychial lesions, lesions in areas of the body where rubbing opposed surfaces is common (groin, perianal, axillary, inframammary, and interdigital), thrush (white plaques attached to oral or vaginal mucous membranes), and vulvovaginitis.

2. **Cellulitis:** This is a common nonsuppurative infection of connective tissue with severe inflammation of the dermal and subcutaneous layers of the skin. Cellulitis appears on an extremity as a reddish-brown area of edematous skin. A surgical wound, puncture, insect bite, skin ulcer, or patch of dermatitis is the usual means of entry for bacteria (most cases are caused by streptococci). Therapy entails rest, elevation, hot wet packs, and antibiotics. Any cellulitis on the face should be given special attention because the infection may extend directly to the brain.

3. **Mycosis fungoides:** This rare, chronic skin condition is caused by the infiltration of malignant lymphocytes. Contrary to its name (myc/o = fungus), it is not caused by a fungus but was formerly thought to be of fungal origin. It is characterized by generalized erythroderma and large, reddish, raised tumors that spread and ulcerate. In some cases, the malignant cells may involve lymph nodes and other organs. Treatment with topical nitrogen mustard and radiation can be effective in controlling the disease.

Dermatologic Write Up: Physical Examination of the Skin

A wide variety of lesions are seen on the face, shoulders, and back. The predominant lesions are pustules on an inflammatory base. Many pustules are confluent (running together) over the chin and forehead. Comedones are present on the face, especially along the nasolabial folds. Inflammatory papules are present on the lower cheeks and chin. Large abscesses and ulcerated cysts are present over the upper shoulder area. Numerous scars are present over the face and upper back.

Questions on the Dermatologic Write Up

1. **In this skin condition, the dominant damage to tissue involves:**
   (A) discolored flat lesions
   (B) grooves or crack-like sores
   (C) small elevations containing pus

2. **Comedones are:**
   (A) sebum plugs partially blocking skin pores
   (B) contagious, infectious plugs of sebum
   (C) small, pinpoint hemorrhages
3. **Papules are also known as:**
   (A) purpura
   (B) pimples
   (C) freckles
4. **In the scapular region, lesions are:**
   (A) large pigmented areas
   (B) numerous collections of blisters
   (C) large collections of sacs containing pus with erosion of skin
5. **A hypertrophied scar (cicatrix) is also known as a:**
   (A) wheal
   (B) keloid
   (C) polyp
6. **What is your diagnosis of this skin condition, based on the physical examination?**
   (A) acne vulgaris
   (B) leukoplakia
   (C) scabies

IX. Exercises

Remember to check your answers carefully with those given in Section X, Answers to Exercises.

A. Select from the following terms to complete the sentences below.

basal layer	dermis	lunula	sebum
collagen	keratin	melanin	stratum corneum
cuticle	lipocyte		

1. A fat cell is a (an) _____.

2. The half-moon–shaped white area at the base of a nail is the _____.

3. A structural protein found in skin and connective tissue is _____.

4. A black pigment found in the epidermis is _____.

5. The deepest region of the epidermis is the _____.

6. The outermost layer of the epidermis, which consists of flattened, keratinized cells, is the

   _____.

7. An oily substance secreted by sebaceous glands is _____.

8. The middle layer of the skin is the _____.

9. A hard, protein material found in epidermis, hair, and nails is _____.

10. A band of epidermis at the base and sides of the nail plate is the _____.

B. Complete the following terms based on their meanings as given below.

1. The outermost layer of skin: epi _____

2. Profuse sweating: dia _____

3. Excessive secretion from sebaceous glands: sebo _____

4. Inflammation and swelling of soft tissue around a nail: par _____

5. Fungal infections of hands and feet: dermato _____

6. Burning sensation (pain) in skin: caus _____

C. Match the term in column I with the descriptive meanings in column II. Write the letter of the answer in the space provided.

Column I

1. squamous epithelium _____

2. sebaceous gland _____

3. albinism _____

4. electrocautery _____

5. subcutaneous tissue _____

6. collagen _____

7. dermis _____

8. melanocyte _____

9. erythema _____

10. dermabrasion _____

Column II

A. middle, connective tissue layer of skin

B. surgical procedure to scrape away tissue

C. flat, scale-like cells

D. connective tissue protein

E. pigment deficiency of the skin

F. contains a dark pigment

G. redness of skin

H. contains lipocytes

I. oil-producing organ

J. knife used to burn through tissue

D. Build medical terms based on the definitions and word parts given.

1. surgical repair of the skin: dermato _____

2. pertaining to under the skin: sub _____

3. abnormal condition of lack of sweat: an _____

4. abnormal condition of proliferation of horny, keratinized cells: kerat _____

5. abnormal condition of dry, scaly skin: _____ osis

6. loosening of the epidermis: epidermo _____

7. yellow tumor (nodule under the skin): _____ oma

8. pertaining to under the nail: sub _____

9. abnormal condition of fungus in the hair: _____ mycosis

10. abnormal condition of nail fungus: onycho _____

11. removal of wrinkles _____ ectomy

E. Give the meanings for the following combining forms.

1. melan/o _____

2. adip/o _____

3. squam/o _____

4. xanth/o _____

5. myc/o _____

6. onych/o _____

7. pil/o _____

8. xer/o _____

9. trich/o _____

10. erythem/o _____

11. albin/o _____

12. ichthy/o _____

13. hidr/o _____

14. ungu/o _____

15. cauter/o _____

16. steat/o _____

17. rhytid/o _____

F. Match the cutaneous lesion with its meaning below.

cyst   macule   pustule
crust (scab)   nodule   ulcer
erosion   papule   vesicle
fissure   polyp   wheal

1. circumscribed collection of clear fluid (blister) _____

2. smooth, slightly elevated edematous area _____

3. discolored, flat lesion (freckle) _____

4. groove or crack-like sore _____

5. mushroom-like growth extending on a stalk _____

6. small elevation containing pus (small abscess) _____

7. closed sac containing fluid or semisolid material _____

8. open sore on the skin or mucous membrane _____

9. solid elevation of the skin (pimple) _____

10. solid, elevated lesion more than 1 cm in diameter _____

11. collection of dried serum and cellular debris _____

12. wearing away or loss of epidermal tissue _____

G. Give the medical terms for the following.

1. baldness _____

2. bluish-black mark (macule) caused by hemorrhages into the skin _____

3. itching _____

4. acute allergic reaction in which red, round wheals develop on the skin _____

5. merging ecchymoses over the body _____

6. blackhead _____

7. small, pinpoint hemorrhages _____

H. Match the pathological skin condition with its description below.

acne vulgaris   gangrene   scleroderma
basal cell carcinoma   impetigo   squamous cell carcinoma
decubitus ulcer   malignant melanoma   systemic lupus erythematosus
eczema   psoriasis   tinea

1. malignant neoplasm originating in scale-like cells of the epidermis _____

2. buildup of sebum and keratin in pores of the skin leading to papular and pustular eruptions

_____

3. fungal skin infection _____

4. chronic disease marked by hardening and shrinking of connective tissue in the skin

_____

5. bedsore _____

6. necrosis of skin tissue resulting from ischemia _____

7. chronic or acute inflammatory skin disease with erythematous, pustular, or papular lesions

_____

8. widespread inflammatory disease of the joints and collagen of the skin with "butterfly" rash on the

face _____

9. cancerous tumor composed of melanocytes _____

10. chronic, recurrent dermatosis marked by silvery-gray scales covering red patches on the skin

_____

11. malignant neoplasm originating in the basal layer of the epidermis _____

12. contagious, infectious pyoderma _____

I. Circle the term that best fits the definition given.

1. contagious parasitic infection with intense pruritus: **(scleroderma, scabies)**

2. measles: **(rubella, rubeola)**

3. chickenpox: **(varicella, eczema)**

4. thickened cicatrix (scar): **(tinea, keloid)**

5. white patches on mucous membrane of tongue or cheek: **(leukoplakia, albinism)**

6. characterized by a rash: **(gangrene, exanthematous)**

7. thickening of epidermis related to sunlight exposure: **(actinic keratosis, callus)**

8. small, pinpoint hemorrhages: **(psoriasis, petechiae)**

9. large blisters: **(bullae, purpura)**

10. colored pigmentation of skin (mole): **(nevus, verruca)**

11. sac of fluid and hair over sacral region: **(ecchymosis, pilonidal cyst)**

12. acute allergic reaction in which hives develop: **(vitiligo, urticaria)**

J. Describe the following types of burns.

1. second-degree burn _____

2. first-degree burn _____

3. third-degree burn _____

K. Match the following medical terms with their more common meanings below.

alopecia   exanthem   tinea pedis
comedones   nevi   urticaria
decubitus ulcer   pruritus   verrucae
ecchymosis   seborrheic dermatitis   vesicles

1. blackheads _____   7. warts _____

2. moles _____   8. athlete's foot _____

3. baldness _____   9. "black-and-blue" mark _____

4. itching _____   10. dandruff _____

5. hives _____   11. blisters _____

6. bedsore _____   12. rash _____

L. Describe how the following conditions affect the skin.

1. pyoderma _____

2. xeroderma _____

3. leukoderma _____

4. erythema _____

5. dermatomycosis _____

6. callus _____

7. keloid _____

8. purpura _____

9. telangiectasis _____

10. gangrene _____

M. Give short answers for the following.

1. Two skin tests for allergy are _____ and _____.

2. The _____ test is an intradermal test for diphtheria.

3. The _____ test or _____ test are skin tests for tuberculosis.

4. Purulent means _____.

5. A surgical procedure to core out a disk of skin for microscopic analysis is a (an) _____.

6. The procedure in which thin layers of a malignant growth are removed and each is examined under the microscope is _____.

7. A type of skin cancer associated with AIDS and marked by dark blue-purple lesions over the skin is _____.

8. Abnormal, premalignant moles are _____.

9. Removal of skin tissue using a cut parallel to the surface of the surrounding skin is called a (an) _____.

10. Destruction of tissue by use of intensely cold temperatures is _____.

11. Scraping away skin to remove acne scars and fine wrinkles on the skin is _____.

12. Removal of subcutaneous fat tissue by aspiration is _____.

13. Destruction of tissue using an electric spark is _____.

14. Use of a sharp spoon-like instrument to scrape away tissue is _____.

N. Circle the term that best completes the meaning of the sentence.

1. Since he had been a teenager, Jim had had red, scaly patches on his elbows and the backs of his knees. Dr. Horn diagnosed Jim's dermatological condition as **(vitiligo, impetigo, psoriasis)** and prescribed a special cream.

2. Clarissa noticed a rash across the bridge of her nose and aching in her joints. She saw a rheumatologist, who did some blood work and diagnosed her condition as **(rheumatoid arthritis, systemic lupus erythematosus, scleroderma)**.

3. Bea had large, red patches all over her trunk and neck after eating shrimp. The doctor prescribed hydrocortisone cream to relieve her itching **(seborrhea, acne, urticaria)**.

4. The poison ivy she touched caused incredible **(pruritus, calluses, keratosis)**, and Maggie was scratching her arms raw.

5. Kelly was fair-skinned with red hair. She had many benign nevi on her arms and legs, but Dr. Keefe was especially worried about one pigmented lesion with an irregular, raised border that he biopsied and found to be malignant **(melanoma, Kaposi sarcoma, pyoderma)**.

6. After five days of high fever, 3-year-old Sadie developed a red rash all over her body. The pediatrician described it as a viral **(eczema, purpura, exanthem)** and told her mother it was a case of **(rubeola, impetigo, scabies)**.

7. Several months after her surgery, Mabel's scar became raised and thickened. It had **(atrophied, stratified, hypertrophied)**, and her physician described it as a **(nevus, verruca, keloid)**.

8. Perry had a bad habit of biting his nails and picking the **(follicle, cuticle, subcutaneous tissue)** surrounding his nails. Often, he developed inflammation and swelling of the soft tissue around the nail, a condition known as **(onychomycosis, onycholysis, paronychia)**.

9. Brenda noticed a small papillomatous wart on her hand. Her **(oncologist, dermatologist, psychologist)** explained that it was a **(pustule, polyp, verruca)** and was caused by a **(bacterium, virus, toxin)**. The doctor suggested removing it by **(Mohs surgery, cryosurgery, curettage)**.

10. Sarah, a teenager, was self-conscious about the inflammatory lesions of papules and pustules on her face. She noticed blackheads or **(wheals, bullae, comedones)** and whiteheads (collections of pus). She was advised to begin taking antibiotics and medications to dry her **(acne vulgaris, scleroderma, gangrene)**.

X. Answers to Exercises

A

1. lipocyte
2. lunula
3. collagen
4. melanin
5. basal layer
6. stratum corneum
7. sebum
8. dermis
9. keratin
10. cuticle

B

1. epidermis
2. diaphoresis
3. seborrhea
4. paronychia
5. dermatophytosis or dermatomycosis (tinea)
6. causalgia

C

1. C
2. I
3. E
4. J
5. H
6. D
7. A
8. F
9. G
10. B

D

1. dermatoplasty
2. subcutaneous
3. anhidrosis
4. keratosis
5. ichthyosis
6. epidermolysis
7. xanthoma
8. subungual
9. trichomycosis
10. onychomycosis
11. rhytidectomy

E

1. black
2. fat
3. scale-like
4. yellow
5. fungus
6. nail
7. hair
8. dry
9. hair
10. redness
11. white
12. scaly, dry
13. sweat
14. nail
15. heat, burn
16. fat
17. wrinkle

F

1. vesicle
2. wheal
3. macule
4. fissure
5. polyp
6. pustule
7. cyst
8. ulcer
9. papule
10. nodule
11. crust
12. erosion

G

1. alopecia
2. ecchymosis
3. pruritus
4. urticaria
5. purpura
6. comedo
7. petechiae

H

1. squamous cell carcinoma
2. acne vulgaris
3. tinea
4. scleroderma
5. decubitus ulcer
6. gangrene
7. eczema
8. systemic lupus erythematosus
9. malignant melanoma
10. psoriasis
11. basal cell carcinoma
12. impetigo

I

1. scabies
2. rubeola
3. varicella
4. keloid
5. leukoplakia
6. exanthematous
7. actinic keratosis
8. petechiae
9. bullae
10. nevus
11. pilonidal cyst
12. urticaria

J

1. damage to the epidermis and dermis with blisters, erythema, and hyperesthesia
2. damage to the epidermis with erythema and hyperesthesia; no blisters
3. destruction of both epidermis and dermis and damage to subcutaneous layer

Continued on following page

K

1. comedones
2. nevi
3. alopecia
4. pruritus

5. urticaria
6. decubitus ulcer
7. verrucae
8. tinea pedis

9. ecchymosis
10. seborrheic dermatitis
11. vesicles
12. exanthem

L

1. collections of pus in the skin
2. dry skin
3. white patches of skin (vitiligo)
4. redness of skin
5. abnormal condition of fungal infection in the skin

6. increased growth of epidermal horny-layer cells due to excess pressure or friction
7. thickened, hypertrophied scar tissue
8. merging ecchymoses (purple patches) under the skin

9. abnormal dilation (-ectasis) of tiny blood vessels (angi/o) under the skin (tel- means complete)
10. necrosis (death) of skin tissue

M

1. scratch test; patch test
2. Schick
3. Mantoux; PPD
4. pus-filled
5. punch biopsy

6. Mohs surgery
7. Kaposi sarcoma
8. dysplastic nevi
9. shave biopsy
10. cryosurgery

11. dermabrasion
12. liposuction
13. electrodesiccation
14. curettage

N

1. psoriasis
2. systemic lupus erythematosus
3. urticaria
4. pruritus

5. melanoma
6. exanthem; rubeola
7. hypertrophied; keloid

8. cuticle; paronychia
9. dermatologist; verruca; cryosurgery
10. comedones; acne vulgaris

Answers to Practical Applications

1. C
2. A
3. B

4. C
5. B
6. A

XI. Pronunciation of Terms

Pronunciation Guide

ā as in āpe   ă as in ăpple
ē as in ēven   ĕ as in ĕvery
ī as in īce   ĭ as in ĭnterest
ō as in ōpen   ŏ as in pŏt
ū as in ūnit   ŭ as in ŭnder

To test your understanding of the terminology in this chapter, write the meaning of each term in the space provided. In addition, you may wish to cover the terms and write them by looking at your definitions. Make sure your spelling is correct. The page number after each term indicates where it is defined or used in the text so you can easily check your responses.

Vocabulary, Combining Forms, and Suffixes

Term	Pronunciation	Meaning
adipose (636)	ĂD-ĭ-pōs	
albinism (636)	ĂL-bĭ-nĭzm	

albino (635)	ăl-BĪ-nō	
alopecia (642)	ăl-ō-PĒ-shē-ă	
anhidrosis (637)	ăn-hī-DRŌ-sĭs	
apocrine sweat gland (635)	ĂP-ō-krĭn swĕt glănd	
basal layer (635)	BĀ-săl LĀ-ĕr	
causalgia (636)	kăw-ZĂL-jă	
collagen (635)	KŎL-ă-jĕn	
cuticle (635)	KŪ-tĭ-k'l	
dermabrasion (637)	dĕrm-ă-BRĀ-zhŭn	
dermatitis (637)	dĕr-mă-TĪ-tis	
dermatologist (637)	dĕr-mă-TŎL-ō-jĭst	
dermatomycosis (638)	dĕr-mă-tō-mī-KŌ-sĭs	
dermatophytosis (638)	dĕr-mă-tō-fī-TŌ-sĭs	
dermatoplasty (637)	DĔR-mă-tō-plăs-tē	
dermis (635)	DĔR-mĭs	
diaphoresis (637)	dī-ă-fŏr-RĒ-sĭs	
electrocautery (637)	ĕ-lĕk-trō-KĂW-tĕr-ē	
epidermis (635)	ĕp-ĭ-DĔR-mĭs	
epidermolysis (637)	ĕp-ĭ-dĕr-MŎL-ĭ-sĭs	
epithelium (635)	ĕp-ĭ-THĒL-ē-ŭm	
erythema (637)	ĕr-ĭ-THĒ-mă	
erythematous (637)	ĕr-ĭ-THĒ-mă-tŭs	
hair follicle (635)	hār FŎL-ĭ-k'l	
ichthyosis (637)	ĭk-thē-Ō-sĭs	
integumentary system (635)	ĭn-tĕg-ū-MĔN-tăr-ē SĬS-tĕm	
keratin (635)	KĔR-ă-tĭn	
keratosis (638)	kĕr-ă-TŌ-sĭs	
leukoderma (639)	lū-kō-DĔR-mă	
leukoplakia (647)	lū-kō-PLĀ-kē-ă	
lipocyte (635)	LĬP-ō-sīt	
lipoma (638)	lī-PŌ-mă or lĭ-PŌ-mă	
liposuction (638)	lī-pō-SŬK-shun	

lunula (635)	LŪ-nū-lă	_____
melanin (635)	MĔL-ă-nĭn	_____
melanocyte (638)	mĕ-LĂN-ō-sīt	_____
melanoma (648)	mĕl-ă-NŌ-mă	_____
onycholysis (638)	ŏn-ĭ-kē-ŎL-ĭ-sĭs	_____
onychomycosis (638)	ŏn-ĭ-kō-mī-KŌ-sĭs	_____
paronychia (638)	păr-ō-NĬK-ē-ă	_____
paronychium (635)	păr-ŏn-NĬK-ē-um	_____
pilosebaceous (639)	pī-lō-sĕ-BĀ-shŭs	_____
pyoderma (639)	pī-ō-DĔR-mă	_____
rhytidectomy (639)	rĭt-ĭ-DĔK-tō-mē	_____
sebaceous gland (635)	sĕ-BĀ-shŭs glănd	_____
seborrhea (639)	sĕb-ō-RĒ-ă	_____
seborrheic dermatitis (639)	sĕb-ō-RĒ-ĭk dĕr-mă-TĪ-tĭs	_____
sebum (635)	SĒ-bŭm	_____
squamous epithelium (635)	SKWĀ-mŭs ĕp-ĭ-THĒ-lē-ŭm	_____
steatoma (639)	stē-ă-TŌ-mă	_____
stratified (635)	STRĂT-ĭ-fīd	_____
stratum (plural: strata) (636)	STRĂ-tŭm (STRă-tă)	_____
stratum corneum (636)	STRĂ-tŭm KŏR-nē-ŭm	_____
subcutaneous tissue (636)	sŭb-kū-TĀ-nē-ŭs TĬSH-ū	_____
subungual (639)	sŭb-ŬNG-wăl	_____
trichomycosis (639)	trĭk-ō-mī-KŌ-sĭs	_____
xanthoma (639)	zăn-THŌ-mă	_____
xeroderma (639)	zē-rō-DĔR-mă	_____

Lesions, Symptoms, Abnormal Conditions, and Neoplasms; Laboratory Tests and Clinical Procedures

Term	Pronunciation	Meaning
abscess (641)	ĂB-sĕs	_____
acne (643)	ĂK-nē	_____
actinic keratosis (647)	ăk-TĬN-ĭk kĕr-ă-TŌ-sis	_____

alopecia areata (642)	ăl-ō-PĒ-shē-ă ăr-ē-ĂT-ă	_____
basal cell carcinoma (648)	BĀ-săl sĕl kăr-sĭ-NŌ-mă	_____
bulla (plural: bullae) (641)	BŬL-ă (BŬL-ē)	_____
burns (644)	bŭrnz	_____
callus (647)	KĂL-ŭs	_____
cellulitis (644)	sĕl-ū-LĪ-tis	_____
cicatrix (647)	SĬK-ă-trĭks	_____
comedo (plural: comedones) (643)	KŎM-ĕ-dō (kŏm-ĕ-DŌNZ)	_____
crust (640)	krŭst	_____
curettage (651)	kŭr-ĕ-TAG	_____
cyst (640)	sĭst	_____
decubitus ulcer (641)	dē-KŪ-bĭ-tŭs ŬL-sĕr	_____
dysplastic nevi (648)	dĭs-PLĂS-tik NĒ-vī	_____
ecchymosis (plural: ecchymoses) (643)	ĕk-ĭ-MŌ-sĭs (ĕk-ĭ-MŌ-sēz)	_____
eczema (644)	ĔK-zĕ-mă	_____
electrodesiccation (651)	ĕ-lĕk-trō-dĕ-sĭ-KĀ-shun	_____
erosion (641)	ĕ-RŌ-shŭn	_____
exanthematous viral disease (644)	ĕg-zăn-THĔM-ă-tŭs VĪ-răl dĭ-ZĒZ	_____
fissure (641)	FĬSH-ŭr	_____
fungal tests (650)	FŬNG-ăl tĕsts	_____
gangrene (644)	găng-GRĒN	_____
impetigo (645)	ĭm-pĕ-TĪ-gō	_____
Kaposi sarcoma (648)	KĂH-pō-sē săr-KŌ-mă	_____
keloid (647)	KĒ-lŏyd	_____
macule (641)	MĂK-ūl	_____
malignant melanoma (648)	mă-LĬG-nănt mĕ-lă-NŌ-mă	_____
Mohs surgery (651)	mōz SŬR-jĕ-rē	_____
nevus (plural: nevi) (648)	NĒ-vŭs (NĒ-vī)	_____

nodule (641)	NŎD-ūl	_____
papule (641)	PĂP-ūl	_____
petechia (plural: petechiae) (643)	pĕ-TĒ-kē-ă (pĕ-TĒ-kē-ī)	_____
pilonidal cyst (640)	pī-lō-NĪ-dăl sĭst	_____
polyp (641)	PŎL-ĭp	_____
pruritus (643)	prōō-RĪ-tŭs	_____
psoriasis (645)	sō-RĪ-ă-sĭs	_____
purpura (643)	PĔR-pĕr-ă	_____
purulent (650)	PŪ-rōō-lĕnt	_____
pustule (641)	PŬS-tūl	_____
rubella (644)	rōō-BĔL-ă	_____
rubeola (644)	rōō-bē-Ō-lă	_____
scabies (645)	SKĀ-bēz	_____
scleroderma (645)	sklĕr-ō-DĔR-mă	_____
sebaceous cyst (640)	sĕ-BĀ-shŭs sĭst	_____
skin biopsy (651)	skĭn BĪ-ŏp-sē	_____
skin test (651)	skĭn tĕst	_____
squamous cell carcinoma (650)	SKWĀ-mŭs sĕl kăr-sĭ-NŌ-mă	_____
systemic lupus erythematosus (645)	sĭs-TĔM-ĭk LŌŌ-pŭs ĕr-ĭ-thē-mă-TŌ-sĭs	_____
tinea (646)	TĬN-ē-ă	_____
ulcer (641)	ŬL-sĕr	_____
urticaria (643)	ŭr-tĭ-KĀ-rē-ă	_____
varicella (644)	văr-ĭ-SĔL-ă	_____
verruca (plural: verrucae) (648)	vĕ-RŌŌ-kă (vĕ-RŌŌ-kē)	_____
vesicle (641)	VĔS-ĭ-k'l	_____
vitiligo (646)	vĭt-ĭl-Ī-gō	_____
wheal (642)	wēl	_____

XII. Review Sheet

Write the meanings of the word parts in the spaces provided and test yourself. Check your answers with the information in the chapter or in the glossary (Medical Terms—English) at the end of the book.

COMBINING FORMS

Combining Form	Meaning	Combining Form	Meaning
adip/o	_____	melan/o	_____
albin/o	_____	myc/o	_____
caus/o	_____	onych/o	_____
cauter/o	_____	phyt/o	_____
cutane/o	_____	pil/o	_____
derm/o	_____	py/o	_____
dermat/o	_____	rhytid/o	_____
diaphor/o	_____	seb/o	_____
erythem/o	_____	sebace/o	_____
erythemat/o	_____	squam/o	_____
hidr/o	_____	steat/o	_____
hydr/o	_____	trich/o	_____
ichthy/o	_____	ungu/o	_____
kerat/o	_____	xanth/o	_____
leuk/o	_____	xer/o	_____
lip/o	_____		

Continued on following page

SUFFIXES

Suffix	Meaning	Suffix	Meaning
-algia	_____	-osis	_____
-derma	_____	-ous	_____
-esis	_____	-plakia	_____
-lysis	_____	-plasty	_____
-ose	_____	-rrhea	_____

GIVE COMBINING FORMS FOR THE FOLLOWING (FIRST LETTERS ARE GIVEN).

fat	a_____	sweat	d _____		
	l_____		h _____		
	s_____	yellow	x_____		
white	a_____	dry	x_____		
	l_____	scaly, dry	i _____		
skin	c_____	redness	e _____		
	d_____		e _____		
nail	o_____	hard, horny	k _____		
	u _____	burn, burning	c_____		
hair	p_____	black	m _____		
	t_____	fungus	m _____		
plant	p_____				

chapter

Sense Organs:
The Eye and the Ear

This chapter is divided into the following sections

In this chapter you will
- Identify locations and functions of the major parts of the eye and ear.
- Name the combining forms, prefixes, and suffixes most commonly used to describe these organs and their parts.
- Describe the pathological conditions that may affect the eye and ear.
- Identify clinical procedures that pertain to ophthalmology and otology.
- Apply your new knowledge to understanding medical terms in their proper contexts, such as medical reports and records.

I. Introduction

The **eye** and the **ear** are sense organs, like the skin, taste buds, and **olfactory** (centers of smell in the nose) regions. As such, they are receptors whose sensitive cells may be activated by a particular form of energy or stimulus in the external or internal environment. The sensitive cells in the eye and ear respond to the stimulus by initiating a series of nerve impulses along sensory nerve fibers that lead to the brain.

No matter what stimulus affects a particular receptor, the sensation felt is determined by regions in the brain connected to that receptor. Thus mechanical injury that stimulates receptor cells in the eye and ear produces sensations of vision (flashes of light) and sound (ringing in the ears). If one could make a nerve connection between the sensitive receptor cells of the ear and the area in the brain associated with sight, it would be possible to perceive, or "see," sounds.

Figure 17–1 recapitulates the general pattern of events when such stimuli as light and sound are applied to sense organs such as the eye and ear.

II. The Eye

A. Anatomy and Physiology

Label Figure 17–2 as you read the following:

Light rays enter the dark center of the eye, the **pupil** [1]. The **conjunctiva** [2] is a membrane lining the inner surfaces of the eyelids and anterior portion of the eyeball over the white of the eye. The conjunctiva is clear and colorless except when blood vessels are dilated. Dust and smoke may cause the blood vessels to dilate and give the conjunctiva a reddish appearance, commonly known as bloodshot eyes.

Before entering the eye through the pupil, light passes through the **cornea** [3]. The cornea is a fibrous, transparent tissue that extends over the pupil and colored portion of

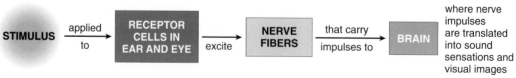

Figure 17–1

Pattern of events in the stimulation of a sense organ.

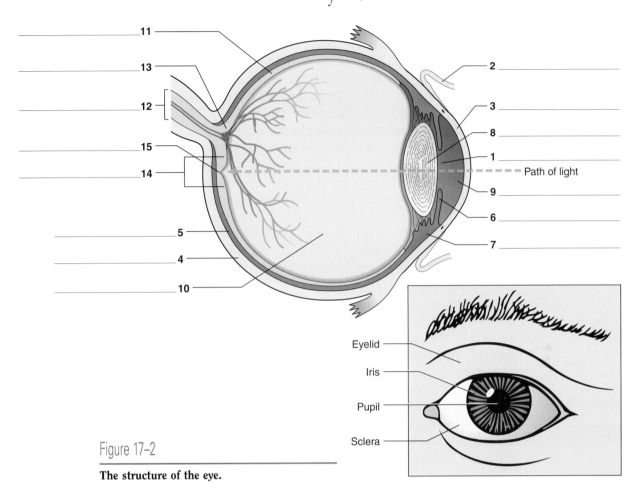

Figure 17–2

The structure of the eye.

the eye. The function of the cornea is to bend, or **refract,** the rays of light, so they are focused properly on the sensitive receptor cells in the posterior region of the eye. The normal, healthy cornea is avascular (has no blood vessels) but receives nourishment from blood vessels near its junction with the opaque white of the eye, the **sclera** [4]. Corneal transplants for people with scarred or opaque corneas are successful because antibodies responsible for rejection of foreign tissue do not reach the avascular, transplanted corneal tissue. The sclera is a tough, fibrous, supportive, connective tissue that extends from the cornea on the anterior surface of the eyeball to the optic nerve in the back of the eye.

The **choroid** [5] is a dark brown membrane inside the sclera. It contains many blood vessels that supply nutrients to the eye. The choroid is continuous with the pigment-containing **iris** [6] and the **ciliary body** [7] on the anterior surface of the eye.

The iris is the colored (it can appear blue, green, hazel, gray, or brown) portion of the eye that surrounds the pupil. Muscles of the iris constrict the pupil in bright light and dilate the pupil in dim light, thereby regulating the amount of light entering the eye. The inset in Figure 17–2 shows the iris and its relationship to the pupil.

The ciliary body, on each side of the **lens** [8], contains muscles that adjust the shape and thickness of the lens. These changes in the shape of the lens cause **refraction** of light rays. Refraction is the bending of rays as they pass through the cornea, lens, and other tissues. Muscles of the ciliary body produce flattening of the lens (for distant vision) and thickening and rounding (for close vision). This refractory adjustment is **accommodation.**

Besides regulating the shape of the lens, the ciliary body also secretes a fluid called **aqueous humor,** which is found in the **anterior chamber** [9] of the eye. Aqueous humor maintains the shape of the anterior portion of the eye and nourishes the structures in that region. The fluid is constantly produced and leaves the eye through a canal that carries it into the bloodstream. Another cavity of the eye is the **vitreous chamber,** which is a large region behind the lens filled with a soft, jelly-like material, the **vitreous humor** [10]. Vitreous humor maintains the shape of the eyeball and is not constantly reformed. Its escape may result in significant damage to the eye, leading to blindness. Both the aqueous and the vitreous humors further refract light rays.

The **retina** [11] is the thin, delicate, and sensitive nerve layer of the eye. As light energy, in the form of waves, travels through the eye, it is refracted (by the cornea, lens, and fluids), so that it focuses on sensitive receptor cells of the retina called the **rods** and **cones.** There are approximately 6.5 million cones and 120 million rods in the retina. The cones function in bright levels of light and are responsible for color and central vision. There are three types of cones, each stimulated by one of the primary colors in light (red, green, or blue). Most cases of color blindness affect either the green or the red receptors, so that the two colors cannot be distinguished from each other. Rods function at reduced levels of light and are responsible for peripheral vision.

Light energy, when focused on the retina, causes a chemical change in the rods and cones, initiating nerve impulses that then travel from the eye to the brain via the **optic nerve** [12]. The region in the eye where the optic nerve meets the retina is called the **optic disc** [13]. Because there are no light receptor cells in the optic disc, it is known as the blind spot of the eye. The **macula** [14] is a small, oval, yellowish area to the side of the optic disc. It contains a central depression called the **fovea centralis** [15], which is composed largely of cones and is the location of the sharpest vision in the eye. If a portion of the fovea or macula is damaged, vision is reduced and central-vision blindness occurs. Figure 17–3 shows the retina of a normal eye as seen through an ophthalmoscope. The **fundus** of the eye is this posterior, inner part that is visualized through the ophthalmoscope.

Fovea centralis   Macula

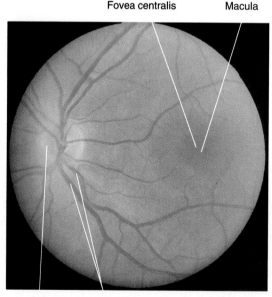

Optic disc   Retinal vessels

Figure 17-3

The posterior, inner part (fundus) of the eye, showing the retina as seen through an ophthalmoscope. (From Thibodeau GA, Patton KT: Anatomy and Physiology, 5th ed. St. Louis, Mosby, 2003, p. 466.)

Figure 17–4 illustrates the pathway of the light-stimulated nervous impulse from the sensitive cells of the retina to the visual region of the cerebral cortex in the brain. The rods and cones in the **retina** synapse (meet) with neurons that lead to the **optic nerve fibers.** As the optic nerve fibers travel into the brain, the fibers located more medially cross in an area called the **optic chiasm.** Nerve fibers from the right half of each retina (the purple lines in the figure) now form an **optic tract,** synapsing in the **thalamus** of the brain and ending in the right visual region of the **cerebral cortex.** Similarly, fibers from the left half of each retina (the orange lines in the figure) merge to form the optic tract and pass from the thalamus to the left region of the **cerebral cortex.** In the visual area of the cerebral cortex (the occipital lobe of the brain) the images (one from each eye) are fused, and a single visual sensation with a three-dimensional effect is experienced. This is called **binocular vision.**

Damage to nerve cells in the **right cerebral cortex** (such as that caused by a stroke) causes loss of vision in the left visual field. Similarly, damage in the **left cerebral cortex**

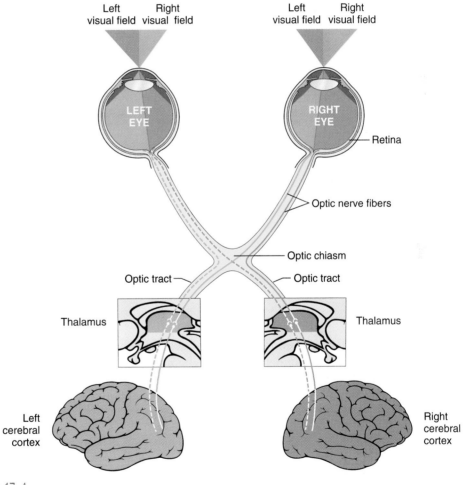

Figure 17–4

Visual pathway from the retina to the cerebral cortex (occipital lobe of the brain). Notice that one half of the visual field of each eye is projected to the other (contralateral) side of the brain.

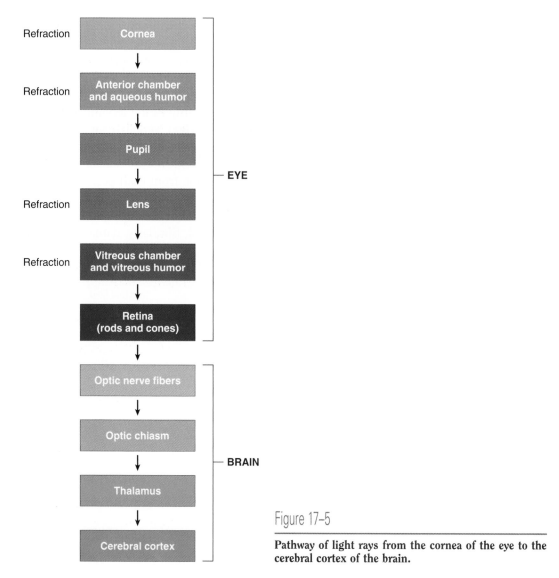

Figure 17–5

Pathway of light rays from the cornea of the eye to the cerebral cortex of the brain.

causes loss of vision in the right visual field. This loss of vision in the contralateral (opposite side) visual field is called **hemianopsia** (**hemi-** means half, **an-** means without, **-opsia** means vision).

Figure 17–5 summarizes the pathway of light rays from the cornea to the inner visual region in the cerebral cortex of the brain.

B. Vocabulary

This list reviews many new items introduced in the text. Short definitions reinforce your understanding of the terms. See Section VII of this chapter for pronunciation of more difficult terms.

accommodation

Normal adjustment of the eye for seeing objects at various distances. The ciliary body adjusts the lens (flattening or rounding it) to change refraction and bring objects into focus on the retina.

anterior chamber	Area behind the cornea and in front of the lens and iris. It contains aqueous humor.
aqueous humor	Fluid produced by the ciliary body and found in the anterior chamber.
biconvex	Having two sides that are rounded, elevated, and curved evenly, like part of a sphere. The lens of the eye is a biconvex body.
choroid	Middle, vascular layer of the eye, between the retina and the sclera.
ciliary body	Structure on each side of the lens that connects the choroid and iris. It contains ciliary muscles, which control the shape of the lens, and it secretes aqueous humor.
cone	Photoreceptor cell in the retina that transforms light energy into a nerve impulse. Cones are responsible for color and central vision.
conjunctiva	Delicate membrane lining the eyelids and covering the anterior eyeball.
cornea	Fibrous transparent layer of clear tissue that extends over the anterior portion of the eyeball.
fovea centralis	Tiny pit or depression in the retina that is the region of clearest vision.
fundus of the eye	Posterior, inner part of the eye.
iris	Colored portion of the eye.
lens	Transparent, biconvex body behind the pupil of the eye. It bends (refracts) light rays to bring them into focus on the retina.
macula	Yellowish region on the retina lateral to and slightly below the optic disc; contains the fovea centralis, which is the center depression containing only cone photoreceptors.
optic chiasm	Point at which the fibers of the optic nerve cross in the brain (**chiasm** means crossing).
optic disc	Region at the back of the eye where the optic nerve meets the retina. It is the blind spot of the eye because it contains only nerve fibers, no rods or cones, and is thus insensitive to light.
optic nerve	Cranial nerve carrying impulses from the retina to the brain (cerebral cortex).
pupil	Dark opening of the eye, surrounded by the iris, through which light rays pass.
refraction	Bending of light rays by the cornea, lens, and fluids of the eye to bring the rays into focus on the retina. **Refract** means to break (-fract) back (re-).
retina	Light-sensitive nerve cell layer of the eye containing photoreceptor cells (rods and cones).

rod	Photoreceptor cell of the retina essential for vision in dim light and for peripheral vision.
sclera	Tough, white, outer coat of the eyeball.
vitreous humor	Soft, jelly-like material behind the lens; helps maintain the shape of the eyeball.

C. Combining Forms, Suffixes, and Terminology: Structures and Fluids; Conditions

Write the meanings of the medical terms in the spaces provided.

STRUCTURES AND FLUIDS
Combining Forms

Combining Form	Meaning	Terminology	Meaning
aque/o	water	aqueous humor	_____
blephar/o	eyelid (see also **palpebr/o**)	blepharitis	_____
		blepharoptosis	_____

blef-ă-rŏp-TŌ-sĭs. *Also called ptosis. This condition may be caused by abnormalities of the eyelid muscle or by nerve damage.*

conjunctiv/o	conjunctiva	conjunctivitis	_____

Commonly called pinkeye. See Figure 17–6A.

cor/o	pupil (see also **pupill/o**)	anisocoria	_____

anis/o means unequal. Anisocoria may be an indication of neurological injury or disease. See Figure 17–6B.

A 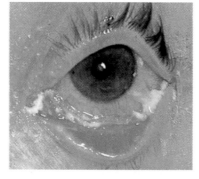 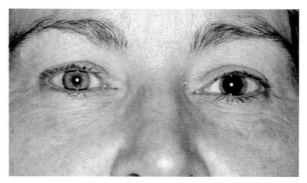 B

Figure 17-6

(A) Acute bacterial conjunctivitis. Notice the discharge of pus characteristic of this highly contagious infection of the conjunctiva. **(B) Anisocoria.** (A from Newell FW: Ophthalmology: Principles and Concepts, 7th ed. St. Louis, Mosby, 1992. B from Mosby's Medical, Nursing, and Allied Health Dictionary, 6th ed. St. Louis, Mosby, 2002, p. 101.)

corne/o	cornea (see also **kerat/o**)	corneal ulcer _____ *From the Latin corneus meaning horny. Perhaps, as it protrudes outward, the cornea was thought to resemble the bud of a growing horn.*
cycl/o	ciliary body or muscle of the eye	cycloplegic _____
dacry/o	tears, tear duct (see also **lacrim/o**)	dacryoadenitis _____ *Figure 17–7 shows the lacrimal gland and lacrimal ducts.*
ir/o **irid/o**	iris (colored portion of the eye around the pupil)	iritis _____ *Characterized by pain, sensitivity to light, and lacrimation. A corticosteroid is prescribed to reduce inflammation.* iridic _____ iridectomy _____ *A portion of the iris is removed to improve drainage of aqueous humor or remove a foreign body.*
kerat/o	cornea	keratitis _____
lacrim/o	tears	lacrimal _____ lacrimation _____
ocul/o	eye	intraocular _____

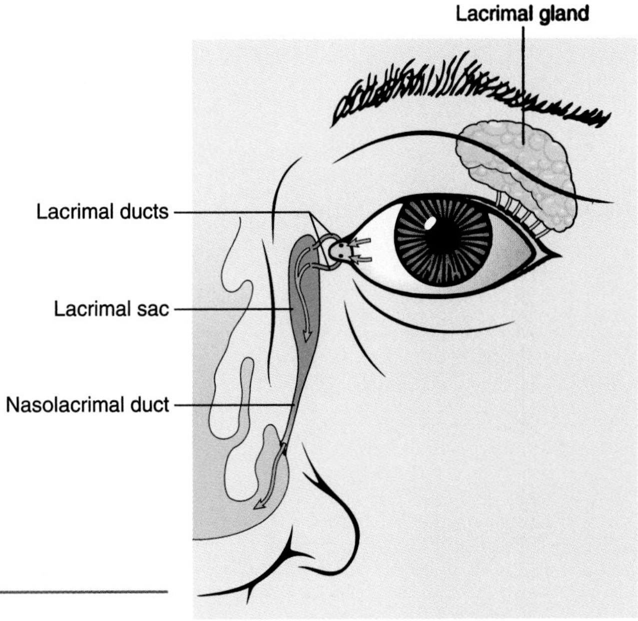

Figure 17–7

Lacrimal (tear) gland and ducts.

ophthalm/o   eye   ophthalmologist _____

A medical doctor who specializes in treating disorders of the eye.

ophthalmic _____

ophthalmoplegia _____

opt/o
optic/o   eye, vision   optic _____

optometrist _____

Nonmedical person who can examine eyes to determine vision problems and prescribe lenses (doctor of optometry; OD).

optician _____

Nonmedical person who grinds lenses and fits glasses but cannot prescribe lenses.

palpebr/o   eyelid   palpebral _____

papill/o   optic disc (disk); nipple-like   papilledema _____

-edema means swelling. This condition is associated with increased intracranial pressure and hyperemia (increased blood flow) in the region of the optic disc.

phac/o
phak/o   lens of the eye   phacoemulsification _____

Technique of cataract extraction using ultrasonic vibrations to fragment (emulsify) the lens and aspirate it from the eye.

aphakia _____

This may be congenital, but most often it is the result of extraction of a cataract (clouded lens) without placement of an artificial lens (pseudophakia).

pupill/o   pupil   pupillary _____

retin/o   retina   retinitis _____

Retinitis pigmentosa *is a genetic disorder (pigmented scar forms on the retina) that destroys retinal rods. Decreased vision and night blindness (nyctalopia) occur.*

hypertensive retinopathy _____

Lesions, such as narrowed arterioles, microaneurysms, hemorrhages, and exudates (fluid leakage) are found on examination of the fundus.

scler/o	sclera (white of the eye)	corneoscleral _____
		scleritis _____
uve/o	uvea; vascular layer of the eye (iris, ciliary body, and choroid)	uveitis _____
vitre/o	glassy	vitreous humor _____

CONDITIONS
Combining Forms

Combining Form	Meaning	Terminology	Meaning
ambly/o	dull, dim	amblyopia _____	

-opia means vision. Amblyopia is partial loss of sight and also known as lazy eye because it is associated with failure of the eyes to work together to focus on the same point.

| dipl/o | double | diplopia _____ | |
| glauc/o | gray | glaucoma _____ | |

-oma here means mass or collection of fluid (aqueous humor). The term comes from the dull gray-green gleam of the affected eye in advanced cases. See page 682, Section II (E), Pathological Conditions.

| mi/o | smaller, less | miosis _____ | |

*Contraction of the pupil. A **miotic** is a drug (such as pilocarpine) that causes the pupil to contract.*

| mydr/o | widen, enlarge | mydriasis _____ | |

Enlargement of pupils. Atropine and cocaine cause dilation, or enlargement, of pupils.

| nyct/o | night | nyctalopia _____ | |

-opia means vision; -al comes from ala meaning blindness. Night blindness is poor vision at night, but good vision on bright days. Deficiency of vitamin A leads to nyctalopia.

| phot/o | light | photophobia _____ | |

Sensitivity to light.

presby/o	old age	presbyopia _____	

See page 681, Section II (D), Errors of Refraction.

scot/o	darkness	scotoma _____

An area of depressed vision surrounded by an area of normal vision; a blind spot. This can result from damage to the retina or the optic nerve.

xer/o	dry	xerophthalmia _____

Suffixes			
Suffix	Meaning	Terminology	Meaning
-opia	vision	hyperopia _____	

Hypermetropia (farsightedness). See Section II (D), Errors of Refraction.

-opsia	vision	hemianopsia _____	

Absence of vision in half of the visual field (space of vision of each eye). Stroke victims frequently have damage to the brain on one side of the visual cortex and experience hemianopsia (the visual loss is in the right or left visual field of both eyes).

-tropia	to turn	esotropia _____	

*Inward (eso-) turning of an eye. **Exotropia** is an outward turning of an eye. These are examples of **strabismus** (defect in eye muscles so that both eyes cannot be focused on the same point at the same time).*

D. Errors of Refraction

astigmatism

Defective curvature of the cornea or lens of the eye.

This problem results from one or more abnormal curvatures of the cornea or lens. This causes light rays to be unevenly and not sharply focused on the retina, so that the image is distorted. A cylindrical lens placed in the proper position in front of the eye can correct this problem (Fig. 17–8A).

hyperopia (hypermetropia)

Farsightedness.

As Figure 17–8B illustrates, the eyeball in this condition is too short or the refractive power of the lens is too weak. Parallel rays of light tend to focus behind the retina, which results in a blurred image. A convex lens (thicker in the middle than at the sides) bends the rays inward before they reach the cornea, and thus the rays can be focused properly on the retina.

myopia

Nearsightedness.

In myopia (**my-** comes from Greek *myein,* meaning "to shut," referring to the observation that myopic persons usually peer through half-closed eyelids), the eyeball is too long or the refractive power of the lens so strong that light rays do not properly focus on the retina. The image perceived is blurred because the light rays are focused in front of the retina. Concave glasses (thicker at the periphery than in the middle) correct this condition because the lenses spread the rays out before they reach the cornea, and thus they can be properly focused directly on the retina (Fig. 17–8C).

presbyopia   **Impairment of vision as a result of old age.**

With increasing age, loss of elasticity of the ciliary body impairs its ability to adjust the lens for accommodation to near vision. The lens of the eye cannot become fat to bend the rays coming from near objects (less than 20 feet). The light rays focus behind the retina, as in hyperopia. Therefore, a convex lens is needed to refract the rays coming from objects closer than 20 feet.

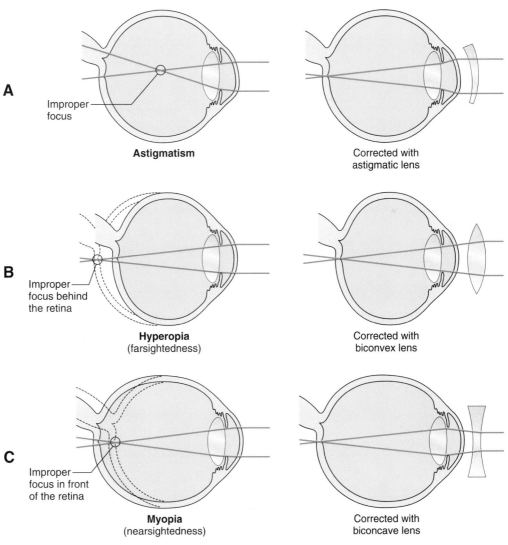

A

Improper focus

Astigmatism

Corrected with astigmatic lens

B

Improper focus behind the retina

Hyperopia
(farsightedness)

Corrected with biconvex lens

C

Improper focus in front of the retina

Myopia
(nearsightedness)

Corrected with biconcave lens

Figure 17–8

Errors of refraction. (A) Astigmatism and its correction. **(B)** Hyperopia and its correction. **(C)** Myopia and its correction. Dashed lines in B and C indicate the contour and size of the normal eye.

E. Pathological Conditions

cataract

Clouding of the lens, causing decreased vision (Fig. 17–9).

A cataract is a type of degenerative eye disease (protein in the lens aggregates and clouds vision) and is linked to the process of aging (senile cataracts). Some cataracts, however, are present at birth, and others occur with diabetes mellitus, ocular trauma, and prolonged high-dose corticosteroid administration. Vision appears blurred as the lens clouds over and becomes opaque. Lens cloudiness can be seen with an ophthalmoscope or the naked eye. Surgical removal of the lens and implantation of an artificial lens behind the iris are treatments for cataracts. If an intraocular lens cannot be inserted, the patient may wear eyeglasses or contact lenses to help refraction.

chalazion

Small, hard, cystic mass (granuloma) on the eyelid; formed as a result of chronic inflammation of a sebaceous gland (meibomian gland) along the margin of the eyelid (Fig. 17–10).

Chalazions (kă-LĀ-zē-ŏn) often require incision and drainage.

diabetic retinopathy

Retinal effects of diabetes mellitus include microaneurysms, hemorrhages, dilation of retinal veins, and neovascularization (new blood vessels form in the retina).

Edema (macular edema) occurs as fluid leaks from blood vessels into the retina and vision is blurred. **Exudates** (fluid leaking from the blood) appear in the retina as yellow-white spots. Laser photocoagulation and vitrectomy (see pages 687 and 688, Section II [F], Clinical Procedures) are helpful to patients in whom hemorrhaging has been severe.

glaucoma

Increased intraocular pressure results in damage to the retina and optic nerve.

Intraocular pressure is elevated because of the inability of aqueous humor to drain from the eye and enter the bloodstream. Normally, aqueous humor is formed by the ciliary body, flows into the anterior chamber, and leaves the eye at the angle

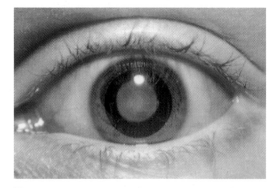

Figure 17–9

Cataract. The lens appears cloudy. (Courtesy of Ophthalmic Photography at the University of Michigan, WK Kellogg Eye Center, Ann Arbor, MI. From Black JM, Hawks JH, Keene AM: Medical-Surgical Nursing: Clinical Management for Positive Outcomes, 6th ed. Philadelphia, WB Saunders, 2001, p. 1815.)

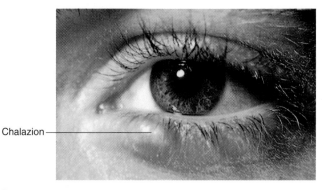

Chalazion

Figure 17–10

Chalazion. (Courtesy Ophthalmic Photography at the University of Michigan, WK Kellogg Eye Center, Ann Arbor, MI. From Black JM, Hawks JH, Keene AM: Medical-Surgical Nursing, 5th ed. Philadelphia, WB Saunders, 1997.)

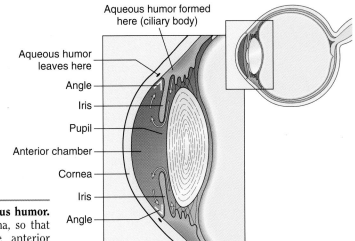

Aqueous humor formed here (ciliary body)

Aqueous humor leaves here

Angle

Iris

Pupil

Anterior chamber

Cornea

Iris

Angle

Figure 17–11

Glaucoma and circulation of aqueous humor. Circulation is impaired in glaucoma, so that aqueous fluid builds up in the anterior chamber.

where the cornea and iris meet. If fluid cannot leave or too much fluid is produced, pressure builds up in the anterior chamber (Fig. 17–11).

Glaucoma is diagnosed by means of **tonometry** (see page 686, Section II [F], Clinical Procedures), with an instrument applied externally to the eye after administration of local anesthetic. Acute glaucoma is marked by extreme ocular pain, blurred vision, redness of the eye, and dilation of the pupil. If untreated, it may cause blindness. Chronic glaucoma may produce no symptoms other than gradual loss of peripheral vision, headaches, blurred vision, and halos around bright lights.

Administration of drugs to lower intraocular pressure can control the condition. Sometimes, laser therapy is used to tighten fibers in the ciliary body or to create a hole in the periphery of the iris (iridotomy), which allows aqueous humor to flow more easily to the anterior chamber and reduces intraocular pressure.

hordeolum (stye)

Localized, purulent, inflammatory staphylococcal infection of a sebaceous gland in the eyelid.

Hot compresses may help localize the infection and promote drainage. In some cases, surgical incision may be necessary. **Hordeolum** (hŏr-DĒ-ō-lŭm) means barley corn. See Table 17–1 for a list of common eyelid abnormalities.

Table 17–1. **EYELID ABNORMALITIES**

Abnormality	Description
Blepharitis	Inflammation of eyelid; redness, crusting, and swelling along lid margins
Chalazion	Granuloma formed around an inflamed sebaceous gland
Dacryocystitis	Blockage, inflammation, and infection of a nasolacrimal duct and lacrimal sac causing redness and swelling on lower lid
Ectropion	Outward sagging and eversion of the eyelid, leading to improper lacrimation and corneal drying and ulceration
Entropion	Inversion of the eyelid, causing the lashes to rub against the eye; corneal abrasion may result
Hordeolum (sty)	Infection of a sebaceous gland producing a small, superficial white nodule along lid margin
Ptosis	Drooping of upper lid margin as a result of neuromuscular problems
Xanthelasma	Raised yellowish plaque on eyelids caused by lipid disorders (**xanth/o** = yellow, **-elasma** = plate)

macular degeneration

Progressive damage to the macula of the retina.

Macular degeneration is one of the leading causes of blindness in the elderly. It causes severe loss of central vision (Fig. 17–12). Peripheral vision (using the part of the retina that is outside the macula region) is retained.

Macular degeneration occurs in both a "dry" and "wet" form. The dry form (affecting about 85 percent of patients) is marked by atrophy and degeneration of retinal cells and deposits of clumps of extracellular debris or **drusen.** The wet form results from development of new (neovascular) and leaky (exudative) blood vessels close to the macula.

There is no treatment for dry macular degeneration. Wet macular degeneration can be treated with laser photocoagulation of the leaking vessels.

retinal detachment

Two layers of the retina separate from each other.

Trauma to the eye, head injuries, bleeding, scarring from infection, or shrinkage of the vitreous humor can produce holes or tears in the retina and result in the separation of layers. Patients often see bright flashes of light **(photopsia)** and then later notice a shadow or "curtain" falling across the field of vision. **Floaters** are black spots, usually composed of vitreous clumps that detach from the retina. In some cases, floaters may be a sign of a retinal hole, tear, or detachment caused by pigmented cells from the damaged retina or bleeding that has occurred as a result of a detachment.

Photocoagulation (making pinpoint burns to form scar tissue and seal holes) and cryotherapy (creating a "freezer burn" that forms a scar and knits a tear together) are used to repair retinal tears. A **scleral buckle** (see page 688, Section II [F], Clinical Procedures) made of silicone may be sutured to the sclera directly over the detached portion of the retina to push the two retinal layers together. In selected retinal detachments, a procedure called **pneumatic retinopexy** is performed. A gas bubble is injected into the vitreous cavity to put pressure on the area of retinal tear until the retina is reattached.

strabismus

Abnormal deviation of the eye.

A failure of the eyes to look in the same direction because of weakness of a muscle controlling the position of one eye. Different forms of strabismus include **esotropia** (one eye turns inward; cross-eyed), **exotropia** (one eye turns outward;

A 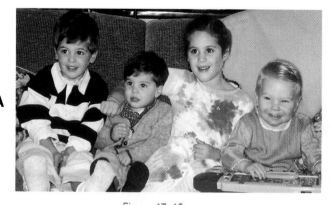 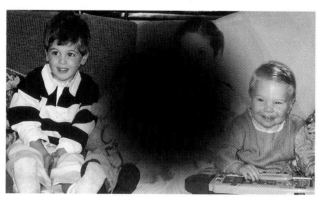 B

Figure 17–12

(A) Picture as seen with **normal vision. (B)** The same picture as it would appear to someone with **macular degeneration.** (Photograph shows the author's grandchildren: Solomon, Gus, and Bebe Thompson and Benjamin Chabner, November 2002.)

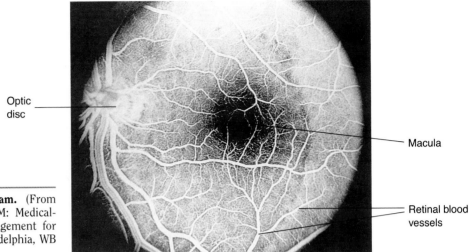

Optic disc

Macula

Retinal blood vessels

Figure 17-13

A normal fluorescein angiogram. (From Black JM, Hawks JH, Keene AM: Medical-Surgical Nursing: Clinical Management for Positive Outcomes, 6th ed. Philadelphia, WB Saunders, 2001, p. 1797.)

wall-eyed), and **hypertropia** (upward deviation of one eye). Treatment includes medications in the form of eyedrops, corrective lenses, eye exercises and patching of the normal eye, or surgery to restore muscle balance.

In children, strabismus may lead to **diplopia** and possibly **amblyopia** (partial loss of vision or lazy eye). Amblyopia is reversible until the retina is fully developed at about 7 years of age.

F. Clinical Procedures and Abbreviations

Diagnostic

fluorescein angiography

Intravenous injection of fluorescein (a dye) followed by serial photographs of the retina through dilated pupils.

This test provides diagnostic information about blood flow in the retina, detects vascular changes in diabetic and hypertensive retinopathy, and identifies lesions in the macular area of the retina (Fig. 17–13).

ophthalmoscopy

Visual examination of the interior of the eye.

The pupil is dilated and the physician holds the ophthalmoscope close to the patient's eye, shining the light into the back of the eye (Fig. 17–14).

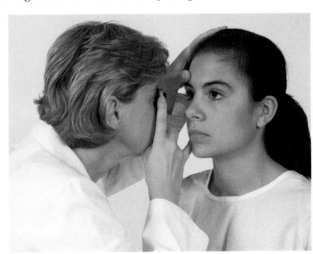

Figure 17-14

Ophthalmoscopy. In addition to examining the cornea, lens, and vitreous humor for opacities (cloudiness), the examiner can see the blood vessels at the back of the eye (fundus) and note degenerative changes in the retina. (From Jarvis C: Physical Examination and Health Assessment, 3rd ed. Philadelphia, WB Saunders, 2000, p. 318.)

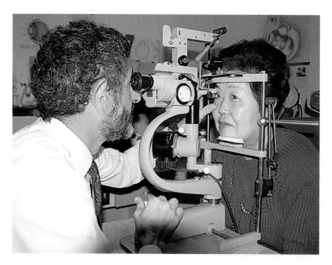

Figure 17–15

Slit lamp examination measuring intra-ocular pressure by tonometry. (From Lewis SM, Heitkemper MM, Dirksen SR: Medical-Surgical Nursing: Assessment and Management of Clinical Problems, 5th ed. St. Louis, Mosby, 2000.)

slit lamp microscopy	**Examination of anterior ocular structures under microscopic magnification.**

This procedure provides a magnified view of the conjunctiva, sclera, cornea, anterior chamber, iris, lens, and vitreous. Devices attached to a slit lamp expand the scope of the examination. **Tonometry** (ton/o = tension) measures intraocular pressure to detect glaucoma (Fig. 17–15).

visual acuity test	**Clarity of vision is assessed** (Fig. 17–16A).

A patient reads from a Snellen chart at 20 ft (distance vision test). Visual acuity is expressed as a ratio, such as 20/20. The first number is the distance the patient is standing from the chart. The second number is the distance at which a person with normal vision could have read the same line of the chart. If the best a patient can see is the 20/200 line, then at 20 feet the patient can see what a "healthy eye" sees at 200 feet.

Mirrors are used so that measurements can be taken at less than 20 feet and still are equivalent to vision measured at 20 feet.

visual field test	**Measures the area within which objects are seen when the eyes are fixed, looking straight ahead without moving the head** (Fig. 17–16B).

A 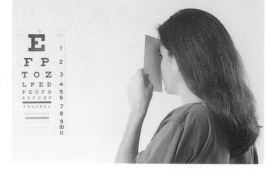 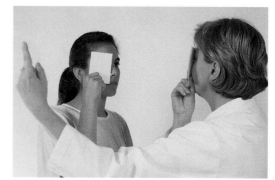 B

Figure 17–16

(A) The Snellen chart assesses visual acuity. **(B) Visual fields** are examined by comparing the patient's field of vision with that of the examiner's (assuming the examiner's is normal). (From Jarvis C: Physical Examination and Health Assessment, 3rd ed. Philadelphia, WB Saunders, 2000, pp. 307 and 309.)

Treatment

enucleation

Removal of the entire eyeball.

This surgery is necessary to treat tumors, such as ocular melanoma (malignant tumor of pigmented cells in the choroid layer) or if an eye has become blind and painful from trauma or disease, such as glaucoma.

keratoplasty

Surgical repair of the cornea.

Also known as **corneal transplant** (penetrating keratoplasty), the ophthalmic surgeon removes the patient's scarred or opaque cornea and replaces it with a donor cornea ("button" or graft), which is sutured into place (Fig. 17–17).

laser photocoagulation

Intense, precisely focused light beam (argon laser) creates an inflammatory reaction that seals retinal tears and leaky retinal blood vessels.

This procedure is useful to treat retinal detachment, diabetic retinopathy, and macular degeneration. Laser is an acronym for <u>l</u>ight <u>a</u>mplification by <u>s</u>timulated <u>e</u>mission of <u>r</u>adiation.

LASIK

Use of an eximer laser to correct errors of refraction (myopia, hyperopia, and astigmatism).

Performed as an outpatient, under local anesthesia, the surgeon lifts the top layer of the cornea (a flap is made) and uses a laser to sculpt the cornea. The corneal flap is then repositioned. LASIK is an acronym for laser *in situ* keratomileusis (shaping the cornea).

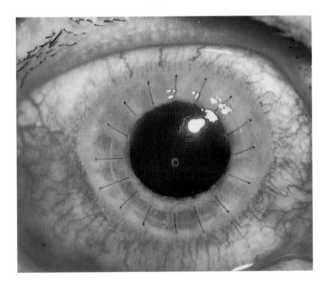

Figure 17-17

Clinical appearance of the eye after keratoplasty. (Courtesy of Ophthalmic Photography at the University of Michigan, WK Kellogg Eye Center, Ann Arbor, MI. From Black JM, Hawks JH, Keene AM: Medical-Surgical Nursing: Clinical Management for Positive Outcomes, 6th ed. Philadelphia, WB Saunders, 2001, p. 1822.)

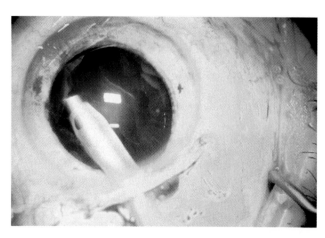

Figure 17–18

Phacoemulsification of a cataractous lens through a small, self-sealing, scleral-tunnel incision. (From Lewis SM, Heitkemper MM, Dirksen SR: Medical-Surgical Nursing: Assessment and Management of Clinical Problems, 5th ed. Mosby, St. Louis, 2000, p. 454.)

phacoemulsification

Ultrasonic vibrations break up the lens, which is then aspirated through the ultrasonic probe (Fig. 17–18).

This is the typical surgery for cataract removal. The ophthalmic surgeon uses a small, self-sealing scleral-tunnel incision (Fig. 17–18). In most patients, an intraocular lens (IOL) is implanted at the time of surgery.

scleral buckle

Suture of a silicone band to the sclera over a detached portion of the retina.

The band pushes the two parts of the retina against each other to bring together the two layers of the detached retina (Fig. 17–19).

vitrectomy

Removal of the vitreous humor.

The vitreous is replaced with a clear solution. This is necessary when blood and scar tissue accumulate in the vitreous humor (a complication of diabetic retinopathy).

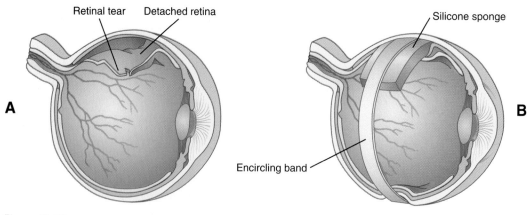

Figure 17–19

(A) Detached retina. (B) Scleral buckling procedure to repair retinal detachment. (From Ignatavicius DD, Workman ML: Medical-Surgical Nursing: Critical Thinking for Collaborative Care, 4th ed. Philadelphia, WB Saunders, 2002, p. 1041.)

Abbreviations

AMD	age-related macular degeneration	**OU**	both eyes (Latin, *oculus uterque*)
IOL	intraocular lens	**PERRLA**	pupils equal, round, reactive to light and accommodation
IOP	intraocular pressure	**POAG**	primary open-angle glaucoma
LASIK	laser *in situ* keratomileusis	**VA**	visual acuity
OD	right eye (Latin, *oculus dexter*); doctor of optometry (optometrist)	**VF**	visual field
OS	left eye (Latin, *oculus sinister*)		

III. The Ear

A. Anatomy and Physiology

Sound waves are received by the outer ear, conducted to special receptor cells within the ear, and transmitted by those cells to nerve fibers that lead to the auditory region of the brain in the cerebral cortex. Sensations of sound are perceived within the nerve fibers of the cerebral cortex.

Label Figure 17–20 as you read the following paragraphs describing the anatomy and physiology of the ear.

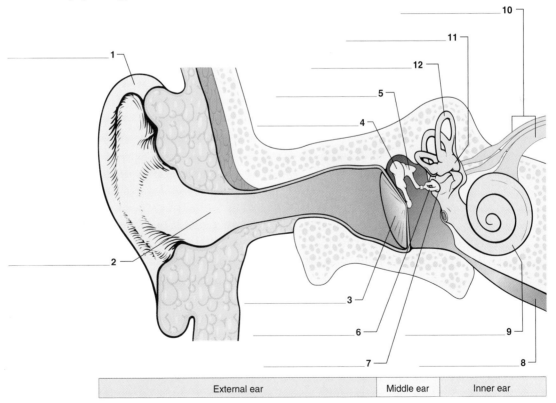

Figure 17-20

Anatomy of the ear.

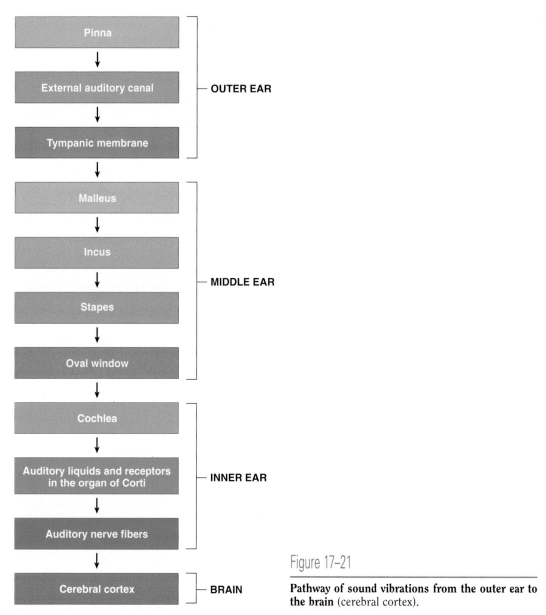

Figure 17–21

Pathway of sound vibrations from the outer ear to the brain (cerebral cortex).

The ear can be divided into three separate regions: outer ear, middle ear, and inner ear. The outer and middle ears function in the conduction of sound waves through the ear, and the inner ear contains structures that receive the auditory waves and relay them to the brain.

Outer Ear

Sound waves enter the ear through the **pinna,** or **auricle** [1], which is the projecting part, or flap, of the ear. The **external auditory meatus (auditory canal)** [2] leads from the pinna and is lined with numerous glands that secrete a yellowish-brown, waxy substance called **cerumen.** Cerumen lubricates and protects the ear.

Middle Ear

Sound waves travel through the auditory canal and strike a membrane between the outer and the middle ear. This is the **tympanic membrane,** or **eardrum** [3]. As the eardrum vibrates, it moves three small bones, or **ossicles,** that conduct the sound waves through the middle ear. These bones, in the order of their vibration, are the **malleus** [4], the **incus** [5], and the **stapes** [6]. As the stapes moves, it touches a membrane called the **oval window** [7], which separates the middle from the inner ear.

Before proceeding with the pathway of sound conduction and reception into the inner ear, an additional structure that affects the middle ear should be mentioned. The **auditory** or **eustachian tube** [8] is a canal leading from the middle ear to the pharynx. It is normally closed but opens upon swallowing. In an efficient way, this tube can prevent damage to the eardrum and shock to the middle and inner ears. Normally the pressure of air in the middle ear is equal to the pressure of air in the external environment; however, if you ascend in the atmosphere, as in flying in an airplane, climbing a high mountain, or riding a fast elevator, the atmospheric pressure, and that in the outer ear, drops, while the pressure in the middle ear remains the same—greater than that in the outer ear. This inequality of air pressure on the inside and outside of the eardrum forces the eardrum to bulge outward and eventually to burst. Swallowing opens the eustachian tube so that air can leave the middle ear and enter the throat until the atmospheric and middle ear pressures are balanced. The eardrum then relaxes, and the danger of its bursting is averted.

Inner Ear

Sound vibrations, having been transmitted by the movement of the eardrum to the bones of the middle ear, reach the inner ear via the fluctuations of the oval window that separates the middle and inner ears. The inner ear is also called the **labyrinth** because of its circular, maze-like structure. The part of the labyrinth that leads from the oval window is a bony, snail-shaped structure called the **cochlea** [9]. The cochlea contains special auditory liquids called **perilymph** and **endolymph** through which the vibrations travel. Also present in the cochlea is a sensitive auditory receptor area called the **organ of Corti.** In the organ of Corti, tiny hair cells receive vibrations from the auditory liquids and relay the sound waves to **auditory nerve fibers** [10], which end in the auditory center of the cerebral cortex, where these impulses are interpreted and "heard."

Study Figure 17–21, which is a schematic representation of the pathway of sound vibrations from the outer ear to the brain.

The ear is an important organ of equilibrium (balance), as well as an organ for hearing. Refer back to Figure 17–20. The **vestibule** [11] connects the cochlea (for hearing) to three **semicircular canals** [12] for balance. The semicircular canals (containing two membranous sacs called the saccule and utricle) contain a fluid, endolymph, as well as sensitive hair cells. In an intricate manner, the fluid and hair cells fluctuate in response to the movement of the head. This sets up impulses in nerve fibers that lead to the brain. Messages are then sent to muscles in all parts of the body to assure that equilibrium is maintained.

B. Vocabulary

This list reviews many new terms introduced in the text. Short definitions reinforce your understanding of the terms. See Section VII of this chapter for pronunciation of terms.

auditory canal	Channel that leads from the pinna to the eardrum.
auditory meatus	Auditory canal.
auditory nerve fibers	Carry impulses from the inner ear to the brain (cerebral cortex). These fibers compose the vestibulocochlear nerve (cranial nerve VIII).
auditory tube	Channel between the middle ear and the nasopharynx; **eustachian tube.**
auricle	Flap of the ear; the protruding part of the external ear, or **pinna.**
cerumen	Waxy substance secreted by the external ear; also called **ear wax.**
cochlea	Snail-shaped, spirally wound tube in the inner ear; contains hearing-sensitive receptor cells.
endolymph	Fluid within the labyrinth of the inner ear.
eustachian tube	Auditory tube.
incus	Second ossicle (bone) of the middle ear; incus means **anvil.**
labyrinth	Maze-like series of canals of the inner ear. This includes the cochlea, vestibule, and semicircular canals.
malleus	First ossicle of the middle ear; malleus means hammer.
organ of Corti	Sensitive auditory receptor area found in the cochlea of the inner ear.
ossicle	Small bone of the ear; includes the malleus, incus, and stapes.
oval window	Membrane between the middle and the inner ears.
perilymph	Fluid contained in the labyrinth of the inner ear.
pinna	Auricle; flap of the ear.
semicircular canals	Passages in the inner ear associated with maintaining equilibrium.
stapes	Third ossicle of the middle ear. Stapes means stirrup.
tympanic membrane	Membrane between the outer and the middle ear; also called the **eardrum.**
vestibule	Central cavity of the labyrinth, connecting the semicircular canals and the cochlea. The vestibule contains two structures, the saccule and utricle, that help to maintain equilibrium.

C. Combining Forms, Suffixes, and Terminology

Write the meaning of the medical term in the space provided.

Combining Forms

Combining Form	Meaning	Terminology	Meaning
acous/o	hearing	acoustic _____	
audi/o	hearing, the sense of hearing	audiometer _____	
		audiogram _____	
audit/o	hearing	auditory _____	
aur/o **auricul/o**	ear (see also **ot/o**)	aural _____	
		postauricular _____	
cochle/o	cochlea	cochlear _____	
mastoid/o	mastoid process	mastoiditis _____	

The mastoid process is the posterior portion of the temporal bone extending downward behind the external auditory meatus. Mastoiditis, caused by bacterial infection, spreads from the middle ear.

myring/o	eardrum, tympanic membrane (see also **tympan/o**)	myringotomy _____	
		myringitis _____	
ossicul/o	ossicle	ossiculoplasty _____	
ot/o	ear	otic _____	
		otomycosis _____	
		otopyorrhea _____	
		otolaryngologist _____	
salping/o	eustachian tube, auditory tube	salpingopharyngeal _____	

In the context of female anatomy, salping/o means the fallopian tubes.

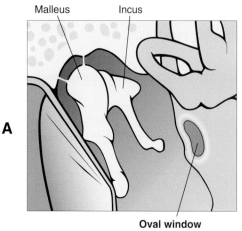
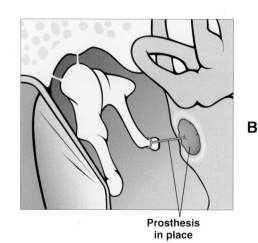

Malleus   Incus

A

B

Oval window
(stapes — separating the incus and
oval window — has been removed)

**Prosthesis
in place**

Figure 17–22

(A) Stapedectomy. Using microsurgical technique and a laser, the stapes bone is removed from the middle ear.
(B) A prosthetic device (wire, Teflon, or metal) is placed into the incus and attached to a hole in the oval window.

staped/o	stapes (third bone of the middle ear)	stapedectomy _____ *After stapedectomy a prosthetic device is used to connect the incus and the oval window (Fig. 17–22). See otosclerosis, page 696.*
tympan/o	eardrum, tympanic membrane	tympanoplasty _____ *Surgical reconstruction of the bones of the middle ear with reconnection of the eardrum to the oval window. Figure 17–23A shows a normal tympanic membrane (eardrum).*
vestibul/o	vestibule	vestibulocochlear _____

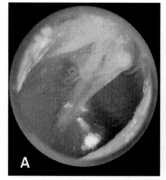
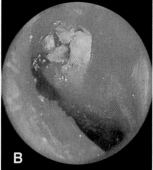
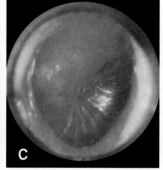
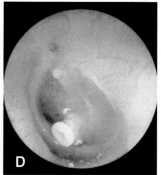

Figure 17–23

(A) Healthy tympanic membrane. (B) Tympanic membrane with cholesteatoma. (C) Tympanic membrane with acute otitis media. (D) Myringotomy with tympanostomy tube. (A-C Courtesy Richard A. Buckingham, Clinical Professor, Otolaryngology, Abraham Lincoln School of Medicine, University of Illinois, Chicago. From Barkauskas VH, et al: Health and Physical Assessment, 3rd ed. St. Louis, Mosby, 2002, pp. 278 and 290; **D** from Mosby's Medical, Nursing, and Allied Health Dictionary, 6th ed. St. Louis, Mosby, 2002, p. 1148.)

| Suffixes | | | |
Suffix	Meaning	Terminology	Meaning
-acusis or -cusis	hearing	hyper<u>acusis</u> _____	
		Abnormally acute sensitivity to sounds.	
		presby<u>cusis</u> _____	
		This type of nerve deafness occurs with the process of aging.	
-otia	ear condition	mac<u>rotia</u> _____	
		Abnormally large ears; congenital anomaly.	
		mic<u>rotia</u> _____	
		Abnormally small ears; congenital anomaly.	

D. Symptoms and Pathological Conditions

acoustic neuroma

Benign tumor arising from the acoustic vestibulocochlear nerve (8th cranial nerve) in the brain.

This tumor causes tinnitus (ringing in the ears), vertigo (dizziness), and decreased hearing as its initial symptoms. Small tumors are resected by microsurgical techniques or ablated (removed) by radiosurgery (using powerful and precise x-ray beams rather than a surgical incision).

cholesteatoma

Collection of skin cells and cholesterol in a sac within the middle ear.

These cyst-like masses produce a foul-smelling discharge and are most often the result of chronic otitis media. They are associated with perforations of the tympanic membrane (Fig. 17–23B).

deafness

Loss of the ability to hear.

Nerve deafness (sensorineural hearing loss) results from impairment of the cochlea or auditory (acoustic) nerve. **Conductive deafness** results from impairment of the middle ear ossicles and membranes transmitting sound waves into the cochlea.

Ménière disease

Disorder of the labyrinth of the inner ear marked by elevated endolymph pressure within the cochlea (cochlear hydrops) and semicircular canals (vestibular hydrops).

Symptoms are tinnitus, heightening sensitivity to loud sounds, progressive loss of hearing, headache, nausea, and vertigo. Attacks last minutes or continue for hours. The cause is unknown, and treatment is bed rest, sedation, and drugs to combat nausea and vertigo. Surgery may be necessary to relieve accumulation of fluid from the inner ear.

otitis media	**Inflammation of the middle ear.**

Acute otitis media is infection of the middle ear often following an upper respiratory infection (URI). Pain and fever with redness and loss of mobility of the tympanic membrane are symptoms (Fig. 17–23C). As bacteria invade the middle ear, pus formation occurs **(suppurative otitis media)**. It is treated with antibiotics, but if the condition becomes chronic, myringotomy may be required to ventilate the middle ear.

Serous otitis media is a noninfectious inflammation with accumulation of serous fluid. It often results from a dysfunctional or obstructed auditory tube. Treatment includes myringotomy to aspirate fluid and tympanostomy tubes placed in the eardrum to allow ventilation of the middle ear. See Figure 17–23D.

otosclerosis	**Hardening of the bony tissue of the labyrinth of the ear.**

The result of this condition is that bone forms around the oval window and causes fixation or **ankylosis** (stiffening) of the stapes bone (ossicle). Conduction deafness occurs as the ossicles cannot pass on vibrations when sound enters the ear. Stapedectomy with replacement by a **prosthesis** (artificial part) is effective in restoring hearing (see Fig. 17–22). In order to perform this operation, the oval window must be **fenestrated** (opened) using a laser.

tinnitus	**Sensation of noises (ringing, buzzing, whistling, booming) in the ears.**

Caused by irritation of delicate hair cells in the inner ear, this disease symptom may be associated with presbycusis, Ménière disease, otosclerosis, chronic otitis, labyrinthitis, and other disorders. Tinnitus can be persistent and severe and can interfere with a patient's daily life. Treatment includes biofeedback to help the patient relax and exert control over stress and anxiety if these are contributing factors.

Tinnitus, a Latin-derived term, means tinkling.

vertigo	**Sensation of irregular or whirling motion either of oneself or of external objects.**

Vertigo can result from disease in the labyrinth of the inner ear or in the nerve that carries messages from the semicircular canals to the brain. Equilibrium and balance are affected, and nausea may occur as well.

E. Clinical Procedures

audiometry	**Testing the sense of hearing.**

An **audiometer** is an electric device that delivers acoustic stimuli of specific frequencies to determine a patient's hearing loss for each frequency. See Figure 17–24. Results are shown on a chart or **audiogram.**

cochlear implant	**Surgically implanted device allowing sensorineural hearing-impaired persons to understand speech.**

A small computer converts sound waves into electronic impulses. Electrodes are placed in the internal ear with the computer attached to the external ear. The electronic impulses then directly stimulate nerve fibers.

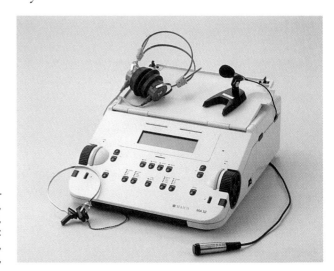

Figure 17-24

Pure-tone audiometer. (Courtesy Maico, Minneapolis, MN. In Ignatavicius DD, Workman ML: Medical-Surgical Nursing: Critical Thinking for Collaborative Care, 4th ed. Philadelphia, WB Saunders, 2002, p. 1057.)

ear thermometry	**Measurement of the temperature of the tympanic membrane by detection of infrared radiation from the eardrum.**

A device is inserted into the auditory canal, and results, which reflect the body's temperature, are obtained within 2 seconds. See Figure 17–25.

otoscopy — **Visual examination of the ear with an otoscope.** (See Fig. 17–26).

tuning fork test — **Test of ear conduction using a vibration source (tuning fork).**

To perform the **Rinne test,** the examiner places the base of the vibrating fork against the patient's mastoid bone (bone conduction) and in front of the auditory meatus (air conduction). In the **Weber test,** the tuning fork is placed on the center of the forehead. The loudness of sound is equal in both ears if hearing is normal.

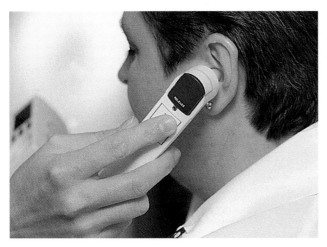

Figure 17-25

Ear thermometry using a tympanic membrane thermometer. (From Mosby's Medical, Nursing, and Allied Health Dictionary, 6th ed. St. Louis, Mosby, 2002, p. 1766.)

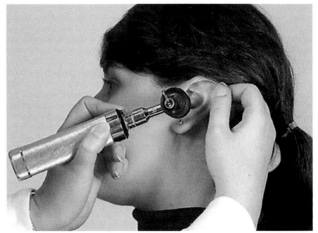

Figure 17-26

Otoscopic examination. The auricle is pulled up and back. The hand holding the otoscope is braced against the face for stabilization. (From Lewis SM, Heitkemper MM, Dirksen SR: Medical-Surgical Nursing: Assessment and Management of Clinical Problems, 5th ed. Mosby, St. Louis, 2000, p. 436.)

Abbreviations

AD	right ear (Latin, *auris dextra*)		assessing eye movements (**nystagmus** is rapidly twitching eye movement)
AOM	acute otitis media		
AS	left ear (Latin, *auris sinistra*)	**ENT**	ears, nose, and throat
EENT	eyes, ears, nose, and throat	**PE tube**	pressure equalizing tube; a polyethylene ventilating tube placed in the eardrum
ENG	electronystagmography; a test of the balance mechanism of the inner ear by	**SOM**	serous otitis media

IV. Practical Applications

This section contains two listings of services and diagnoses and a medical report using terms that you have studied in this and previous chapters. Explanations of more difficult terms are added in brackets. Answers to the questions are on page 710 after Answers to Exercises.

Operating Schedule and Diagnoses: Eye and Ear Hospital

Match the operation in column I with a diagnosis in column II.

Operation—Column I

1. phacoemulsification with IOL; OS _____

2. blepharoplasty _____

3. scleral buckle _____

4. vitrectomy _____

5. radical mastoidectomy _____

6. keratoplasty _____

7. cochlear implant _____

8. laser photocoagulation of the macula _____

9. incision and drainage of hordeolum _____

Diagnosis—Column II

A. scarred and torn cornea
B. ptosis of eyelid skin
C. retinal detachment
D. diabetic retinopathy
E. macular degeneration
F. chronic stye
G. chronic infection of a bone behind the ear
H. severe deafness
I. senile cataract; left eye

Operative Report

Preoperative Diagnosis. Bilateral chronic serous otitis media; tonsilloadenoiditis.
Operation. Bilateral myringotomies and ventilation tube insertion; T and A.
Procedure. With the patient in the supine position and under general endotracheal anesthesia, inspection of AD was made under the operating microscope. The external canal was clear, tympanic membrane was divided. A purulent discharge appeared to be present. This drainage was suctioned out and the ear thoroughly lavaged [washed out]. A ventilating tube was put in place and otic drops were administered. Same procedure for AS.

The patient was placed in the Rose position [supine with the head over the table edge in full extension] and the adenoids removed with adenoid curettes and adenoid biopsy forceps. A nasopharyngeal sponge was put in place. The right tonsil was then grasped with tonsil forceps, dissected free, and removed with snare. Bleeding was controlled with suction cautery. The nasopharyngeal sponge was removed and no further bleeding noted. The patient tolerated the procedure well and left the OR in good condition.

V. Exercises

Remember to check your answers carefully with those given in Section VI, Answers to Exercises.

A. *Match the structure of the eye with its description below. Write the letter of the description in the space provided.*

Column I

1. pupil _____

2. conjunctiva _____

3. cornea _____

4. sclera _____

5. choroid _____

6. iris _____

7. ciliary body _____

8. lens _____

9. retina _____

10. vitreous humor _____

Column II

A. contains sensitive cells called rods and cones that transform light energy into nerve impulses

B. contains muscles that control the shape of the lens and secretes aqueous humor

C. transparent structure behind the iris and in front of the vitreous humor; it refracts light rays onto the retina

D. jelly-like material behind the lens that helps to maintain the shape of the eyeball

E. dark center of the eye through which light rays enter

F. vascular layer of the eyeball that is continuous with the iris

G. delicate membrane lining the eyelids and covering the anterior eyeball

H. fibrous layer of clear tissue that extends over the anterior portion of the eyeball

I. colored portion of the eye; surrounds the pupil

J. tough, white, outer coat of the eye

B. Supply the terms that complete the following sentences.

1. The region at the back of the eye where the optic nerve meets the retina is the

     _____.

2. The normal adjustment of the lens (becoming fatter or thinner) to bring an object into focus on the

   retina is _____.

3. A yellowish region on the retina lateral to the optic disc is the _____.

4. The tiny pit or depression in the retina that is the region of clearest vision is the

     _____.

5. The bending of light rays by the cornea, lens, and fluids of the eye is _____.

6. The point at which the fibers of the optic nerve cross in the brain is the _____.

7. The photoreceptor cells in the retina that make the perception of color possible are the

     _____.

8. The photoreceptor cells in the retina that make vision in dim light possible are the

     _____.

9. The _____ is the area behind the cornea and in front of the lens and iris. It
   contains aqueous humor.

10. The posterior, inner part of the eye is the _____.

C. Give the meanings of the following terms.

1. optic nerve _____

2. biconvex _____

3. anisocoria _____

4. cycloplegic _____

5. palpebral _____

6. mydriasis _____

7. miosis _____

8. papilledema _____

9. photophobia _____

10. scotoma _____

D. Complete the medical terms based on their meanings and the word parts given.

1. inflammation of an eyelid: _____ itis

2. inflammation of the conjunctiva: _____ itis

3. inflammation of a tear gland: _____ itis

4. inflammation of the iris: _____ itis

5. inflammation of the cornea: _____ itis

6. inflammation of the white of the eye: _____ itis

7. inflammation of the retina: _____ itis

8. prolapse of the eyelid: blephar _____

9. pertaining to tears: _____ al

10. pertaining to within the eye: intra _____

N. Give the meanings of the following medical terms.

1. labyrinth _____

2. semicircular canals _____

3. auditory (eustachian) tube _____

4. stapes _____

5. organ of Corti _____

6. perilymph and endolymph _____

7. cerumen _____

8. vestibule _____

9. oval window _____

10. tympanic membrane _____

O. Complete the following terms based on their definitions.

1. instrument to examine the ear: _____ scope

2. removal of the third bone of the middle ear: _____ ectomy

3. pertaining to the auditory tube and throat: _____ pharyngeal

4. flow of pus from the ear: oto _____

5. instrument to measure hearing: _____ meter

6. incision of the eardrum: _____ tomy

7. surgical repair of the eardrum: _____ plasty

8. deafness due to old age: _____ cusis

9. small ear: micr _____

10. inflammation of the middle ear: ot _____

P. Give the meanings of the following medical terms.

1. vertigo _____

2. Ménière disease _____

3. otosclerosis _____

4. tinnitus _____

5. labyrinthitis _____

6. cholesteatoma _____

7. suppurative otitis media _____

8. acoustic neuroma _____

9. mastoiditis _____

10. myringitis _____

Q. Give the meanings of the following abbreviations relating to otology.

1. ENG _____

2. AS _____

3. AD _____

4. EENT _____

5. ENT _____

6. PE tube _____

R. Circle the correct term to complete each sentence.

1. Dr. Jones specializes in pediatric ophthalmology. His examination of children with poor vision often leads to the diagnosis of (**cataract, amblyopia, glaucoma**), or lazy eye.

2. Stella's near vision became progressively worse as she aged. Her physician told her that she had a common condition called (**presbyopia, detached retina, anisocoria**), which many elderly patients develop.

3. Matthew rubbed his itchy eyes constantly and thus spread his "pinkeye" or (**conjunctivitis, blepharitis, myringitis**) from one eye to the other. Dr. Chang prescribed antibiotics for this common condition.

4. As Paul's (**mastoiditis, otitis media, tinnitus**) became progressively worse, his doctor worried that this ringing in his ears might be caused by a benign brain tumor, a(an) (**cholesteatoma, acoustic neuroma, glaucoma**).

5. Before her second birthday, Sally had so many episodes of (**vertigo, otosclerosis, suppurative otitis media**) that Dr. Sills recommended the placement of PE tubes.

6. Sixty-eight-year-old Bob experienced blurred vision in the central portion of his visual field. After careful examination of his **(cornea, sclera, retina)**, his **(ophthalmologist, optician, optometrist)** told him his condition was **(glaucoma, iritis, macular degeneration)**. The doctor explained that the form of this condition was atrophic or **(dry, wet)**, causing photoreceptor rods and cones to die.

7. If Bob's condition had been diagnosed as the **(dry, wet)** form, it might have been treated with **(cryotherapy, intraocular lenses, laser photocoagulation)** to seal leaky blood vessels.

8. Sarah suddenly experienced bright flashes of light in her right eye. She also told her physician that she had a sensation of a curtain being pulled over part of the visual field in that eye. Her doctor examined her eye with **(keratoplasty, ophthalmoscopy, tonometry)** and determined that she had **(retinal refraction, retinal detachment, diabetic retinopathy)**. Surgery, known as **(enucleation, vitrectomy, scleral buckling)**, was recommended.

9. Carol awakened with a sensation of dizziness or **(vertigo, tinnitus, presbycusis)** as she tried to get out of bed. She was totally incapacitated for several days and noticed hearing loss in her left ear. Her physician explained that fluid called **(pus, endolymph, mucus)** had accumulated in her **(auditory tube, middle ear, cochlea)** and her condition was **(otosclerosis, cholesteatoma, Ménière disease)**. He prescribed drugs to control her dizziness and nausea.

10. Patients with conductive hearing loss are helped by reconstruction of the **(labyrinth, tympanic membrane, auditory tube)**, a procedure known as **(myringoplasty, audiometry, otoscopy)**. Patients with sensorineural hearing loss may be helped by a **(hearing aid, cochlear implant, stapedectomy)**.

VI. Answers to Exercises

A

1. E	5. F	8. C
2. G	6. I	9. A
3. H	7. B	10. D
4. J		

B

1. optic disc (disk)	5. refraction	8. rods
2. accommodation	6. optic chiasm	9. anterior chamber
3. macula	7. cones	10. fundus
4. fovea centralis		

C

1. cranial nerve that carries impulses from the retina to the brain	4. pertaining to paralysis of the ciliary muscles	9. condition of sensitivity to ("fear of") light
2. having two sides that are rounded, elevated, and curved evenly	5. pertaining to the eyelid	10. blind spot; area of darkened (diminished) vision surrounded by clear vision
3. condition of pupils of unequal (anis/o) size	6. condition of enlargement of the pupil	
	7. condition of narrowing of the pupil	
	8. swelling in the region of the optic disc	

D

1. blepharitis	5. keratitis	8. blepharoptosis
2. conjunctivitis	6. scleritis	9. lacrimal
3. dacryoadenitis	7. retinitis	10. intraocular
4. iritis		

E

1. corneal ulcer
2. uveitis
3. xerophthalmia
4. hemianopsia

5. exotropia
6. ophthalmologist
7. optometrist

8. optician
9. aphakia
10. esotropia

F

1. dimness of vision; lazy eye (resulting from strabismus and diplopia)
2. farsightedness
3. decreased vision at near resulting from old age

4. nearsightedness
5. night blindness; decreased vision at night

6. double vision
7. defective curvature of the lens and cornea leading to blurred vision

G

1. retina; long; strong; front; concave
2. short; weak; back; convex

3. constricts
4. dilates

H

1. diabetic retinopathy
2. retinal detachment
3. strabismus

4. cataract
5. macular degeneration
6. hordeolum (stye)

7. chalazion
8. glaucoma
9. retinitis pigmentosa

I

3. stroke (hemianopsia)—loss of half of the visual field caused by a stroke occurring in the left visual cortex.

Glaucoma would cause loss of peripheral vision first (darkness around the edges of the picture). A cataract

would cause blurred vision. Macular degeneration would produce loss of central vision.

J

1. tears
2. tears
3. cornea
4. cornea
5. eyelid

6. eyelid
7. pupil
8. pupil
9. lens
10. lens

11. eye
12. eye
13. eye
14. darkness

K

1. phacoemulsification
2. visual acuity test
3. tonometry
4. laser photocoagulation

5. LASIK
6. fluorescein angiography
7. scleral buckle
8. visual field examination

9. vitrectomy
10. ophthalmoscopy
11. slit lamp ocular examination
12. keratoplasty

L

1. both eyes
2. visual acuity
3. right eye

4. left eye
5. visual field
6. intraocular lens

7. intraocular pressure
8. pupils equal, round, reactive to light and accommodation

M

1. pinna (auricle)
2. external auditory canal
3. tympanic membrane
4. malleus

5. incus
6. stapes
7. oval window
8. cochlea

9. auditory liquids and receptors
10. auditory nerve fibers
11. cerebral cortex

Continued on following page

N

1. cochlea and organs of equilibrium (semicircular canals and vestibule)
2. organ of equilibrium in the inner ear
3. passageway between the middle ear and the throat
4. third ossicle (little bone) of the middle ear

5. region in the cochlea that contains auditory receptors
6. auditory fluids circulating within the inner ear
7. wax in the external auditory meatus

8. central cavity of the inner ear that connects the semicircular canals and the cochlea
9. delicate membrane between the middle and the inner ears
10. eardrum

O

1. otoscope
2. stapedectomy
3. salpingopharyngeal
4. otopyorrhea

5. audiometer
6. myringotomy (tympanotomy)
7. tympanoplasty (myringoplasty)

8. presbycusis
9. microtia
10. otitis media

P

1. sensation of irregular or whirling motion either of oneself or of external objects
2. disorder of the labyrinth marked by elevation of ear fluids and pressure within the cochlea (tinnitus, vertigo, and nausea result)

3. hardening of the bony tissue of the labyrinth of the inner ear
4. noise (ringing, buzzing) in the ears
5. inflammation of the labyrinth of the inner ear
6. collection of skin cells and cholesterol in a sac within the middle ear

7. inflammation of the middle ear with bacterial infection and pus collection
8. benign tumor arising from the acoustic nerve in the brain
9. inflammation of the mastoid process (behind the ear)
10. inflammation of the eardrum

Q

1. electronystagmography; a test of balance
2. left ear

3. right ear
4. eyes, ears, nose, and throat
5. ears, nose, and throat

6. pressure equalizing tube; ventilating tube placed in the eardrum

R

1. amblyopia
2. presbyopia
3. conjunctivitis
4. tinnitus; acoustic neuroma
5. suppurative otitis media

6. retina; ophthalmologist; macular degeneration; dry
7. wet; laser photocoagulation
8. ophthalmoscopy; retinal detachment; scleral buckling

9. vertigo; endolymph; cochlea; Ménière disease
10. tympanic membrane; myringoplasty; cochlear implant

Answers to Practical Applications

1. I
2. B
3. C

4. D
5. G
6. A

7. H
8. E
9. F

VII. Pronunciation of Terms

Pronunciation Guide

To test your understanding of the terminology in this chapter, write the meaning of each term in the space provided. In addition, you may wish to cover the terms and write them by looking at your definitions. Make sure your spelling is correct. The page number after each term indicates where it is defined or used in the text so you can easily check your responses.

ā as in āpe   ă as in ăpple
ē as in ēven   ĕ as in ĕvery
ī as in īce   ĭ as in ĭnterest
ō as in ōpen   ŏ as in pŏt
ū as in ūnit   ŭ as in ŭnder

Vocabulary and Terminology

Eye

Term	Pronunciation	Meaning
accommodation (674)	ă-kŏm-ō-DĀ-shŭn	_____
amblyopia (679)	ăm-blē-Ō-pē-ă	_____
anisocoria (676)	ăn-ī-sō-KŌ-rē-ă	_____
anterior chamber (675)	ăn-TĒ-rē-ŏr CHĀM-bĕr	_____
aphakia (678)	ă-FĀ-kē-ă	_____
aqueous humor (675)	ĂK-wē-ŭs or Ā-kwē-ŭs HŪ-mĕr	_____
astigmatism (680)	ă-STĬG-mă-tĭsm	_____
biconvex (675)	bī-KŎN-vĕks	_____
blepharitis (676)	blĕf-ă-RĪ-tĭs	_____
blepharoptosis (676)	blĕf-ă-rŏp-TŌ-sĭs	_____
cataract (682)	KĂT-ă-răkt	_____
chalazion (675)	kă-LĀ-zē-ŏn	_____
choroid (675)	KŎR-oyd	_____
ciliary body (675)	SĬL-ē-ăr-ē BŎD-ē	_____

cone (675)	kōn	
conjunctiva (675)	kŏn-jŭnk-TĪ-vă	
conjunctivitis (676)	kŏn-jŭnk-tĭ-VĪ-tĭs	
cornea (675)	KŎR-nē-ă	
corneal ulcer (677)	KŎR-nē-ăl ŬL-sĕr	
corneoscleral (679)	kŏr-nē-ō-SKLĔ-răl	
cycloplegic (677)	sī-klō-PLĒ-jĭk	
dacryoadenitis (677)	dăk-rē-ō-ăd-ĕ-NĪ-tĭs	
diabetic retinopathy (682)	dī-ă-BĔT-ĭk rĕ-tĭn-NŎP-ă-thē	
diplopia (679)	dĭp-LŌ-pē-ă	
enucleation (687)	ē-nū-klē-Ā-shun	
esotropia (680)	ĕs-ō-TRŌP-pē-ă	
exotropia (680)	ĕk-sō-TRŌ-pē-ă	
fluorescein angiography (685)	flōō-ō-RĔS-ē-ĭn ăn-jē-ŎG-ră-fē	
fovea centralis (675)	FŌ-vē-ă sĕn-TRĂ-lĭs	
fundus (675)	FŬN-dŭs	
glaucoma (682)	glăw-KŌ-mă	
hemianopsia (680)	hĕ-mē-ă-NŎP-sē-ă	
hordeolum (683)	hŏr-DĒ-ō-lŭm	
hyperopia (680)	hī-pĕr-Ō-pē-ă	
hypertensive retinopathy (678)	hī-pĕr-TĔN-sĭv rĕ-tĭ-NŎP-ă-thē	
intraocular (677)	ĭn-tră-ŎK-ū-lăr	
iridectomy (677)	ĭr-ĭ-DĔK-tō-mē	
iridic (677)	ĭ-RĬD-ĭk	
iris (675)	Ī-rĭs	
iritis (677)	ī-RĪ-tĭs	

keratitis (677)   kĕr-ă-TĪ-tĭs   _____

keratoplasty (687)   kĕr-ă-tō-PLĂS-tē   _____

lacrimal (677)   LĂK-rĭ-măl   _____

lacrimation (677)   lă-krĭ-MĀ-shŭn   _____

laser photocoagulation (687)   LĀ-zĕr fō-tō-kō-ăg-ū-LĀ-shŭn   _____

lens (675)   lĕnz   _____

macula (675)   MĂK-ū-lă   _____

macular degeneration (684)   MĂK-ū-lăr dē-jĕn-ĕ-RĀ-shŭn   _____

miosis (679)   mī-Ō-sĭs   _____

miotic (679)   mī-ŎT-ĭk   _____

mydriasis (679)   mĭ-DRĪ-ă-sĭs   _____

myopia (680)   mī-Ō-pē-ă   _____

nyctalopia (679)   nĭk-tă-LŌ-pē-ă   _____

ophthalmic (678)   ŏf-THĂL-mĭk   _____

ophthalmologist (678)   ŏf-thăl-MŎL-ō-jĭst   _____

ophthalmoplegia (678)   ŏf-thăl-mō-PLĒ-jă   _____

ophthalmoscopy (685)   ŏf-thăl-MŎS-kō-pē   _____

optic chiasm (675)   ŎP-tĭk KĪ-ăzm   _____

optic disc (675)   ŎP-tĭk dĭsk   _____

optician (678)   ŏp-TĬSH-ăn   _____

optic nerve (675)   ŎP-tĭk nĕrv   _____

optometrist (678)   ŏp-TŎM-ĕ-trĭst   _____

palpebral (678)   PĂL-pĕ-brăl   _____

papilledema (678)   păp-ĕ-lĕ-DĒ-mă   _____

phacoemulsification (688)   făk-ō-ĕ-mŭl-sĭ-fĭ-KĀ-shŭn   _____

photophobia (679)   fō-tō-FŌ-bē-ă   _____

presbyopia (681)   prĕz-bē-Ō-pē-ă   _____ pupil (675)   PŪ-pĭl   _____

pupillary (678)   PŪ-pĭ-lăr-ē   _____

refraction (675)   rē-FRĂK-shŭn   _____

retina (675)   RĔT-ĭ-nă   _____

retinal detachment (684)   RĔ-tĭ-năl dē-TĂCH-mĕnt   _____

retinitis pigmentosa (678)   rĕt-ĭ-NĪ-tĭs pĭg-mĕn-TŌ-să   _____

rod (676)   rŏd   _____

sclera (676)   SKLĔ-ră   _____

scleral buckle (688)   SKLĔ-răl BŬK'l   _____

scleritis (679)   sklĕ-RĪ-tĭs   _____

scotoma (680)   skō-TŌ-mă   _____

slit lamp   slĭt lămp   _____
    microscopy (686)   mī-KRŎS-kō-pē

strabismus (684)   stră-BĬZ-mŭs   _____

tonometry (686)   tō-NŎM-ĕ-trē   _____

uveitis (679)   ū-vē-Ī-tĭs   _____

visual acuity test (686)   VĬZ-ū-ăl ă-KŪ-ĭ-tē tĕst   _____

visual field test (686)   VĬZ-ū-ăl fēld tĕst   _____

vitrectomy (688)   vĭ-TRĔK-tō-mē   _____

vitreous humor (676)   VĬT-rē-ŭs HŪ-mŏr   _____

xerophthalmia (680)   zĕr-ŏf-THĂL-mē-ă   _____

Ear

Term	Pronunciation	Meaning
acoustic (693)	ă-KOOS-tĭk	_____
acoustic neuroma (695)	ă-KOOS-tĭk nū-RŌ-mă	_____
audiogram (696)	ĂW-dē-ō-grăm	_____
audiometer (696)	ăw-dē-ŎM-ĕ-tĕr	_____

audiometry (696)	ăw-dē-ŎM-ĕ-trē	_____
auditory canal (692)	ăw-dĭ-TŌ-rē kă-NĂL	_____
auditory meatus (692)	ăw-dĭ-TŌ-rē mē-Ā-tŭs	_____
auditory nerve fibers (692)	ăw-dĭ-TŌ-re nĕrv FĪ-bĕrz	_____
auditory tube (692)	ăw-dĭ-TŌ-rē toob	_____
aural (693)	ĂW-răl	_____
auricle (692)	ĂW-rĭ-k'l	_____
cerumen (692)	sĕ-ROO-mĕn	_____
cholesteatoma (695)	kō-lē-stē-ă-TŌ-mă	_____
cochlea (692)	KŎK-lē-ă	_____
cochlear (693)	KŎK-lē-ăr	_____
deafness (695)	DĔF-nĕs	_____
ear thermometry (697)	ear thĕr-MŎM-ĕ-trē	_____
endolymph (692)	ĔN-dō-lĭmf	_____
eustachian tube (692)	ū-STĀ-shŭn or ū-STĀ-kē-ăn	_____
hyperacusis (695)	hī-pĕr-ă-kū-sis	_____
incus (692)	ĬNG-kŭs	_____
labyrinth (692)	LĂB-ĭ-rĭnth	_____
macrotia (695)	măk-RŌ-shē-ă	_____
malleus (692)	MĂL-ē-ŭs	_____
mastoiditis (693)	măs-toy-DĪ-tĭs	_____
Ménière disease (695)	mĕn-ē-ĀR dĭ-ZĒZ	_____
microtia (695)	mī-KRŌ-shē-ă	_____
myringitis (693)	mĭr-ĭn-JĪ-tĭs	_____
myringotomy (693)	mĭr-ĭn-GŎT-ō-mē	_____
ossicle (692)	ŎS-ĭ-k'l	_____
ossiculoplasty (693)	ŏs-ĭ-kū-lō-PLĂS-tē	_____

otic (693)   Ō-tĭk   _____

otolaryngologist (693) ō-tō-lă-rĭn-GŎL-ō-jĭst   _____

otomycosis (693)   ō-tō-mī-KŌ-sĭs   _____

otopyorrhea (693)   ō-tō-pī-ō-RĒ-ă   _____

otosclerosis (696)   ō-tō-sklĕ-RŌ-sĭs   _____

otoscopy (697)   ō-TŎS-kō-pē   _____

oval window (692)   Ō-văl WĬN-dō   _____

perilymph (692)   PĔR-ĭ-lĭmf   _____

pinna (692)   PĬN-ă   _____

postauricular (693)   pōst-ăw-RĬK-ū-lăr   _____

presbycusis (695)   prĕz-bē-KŪ-sĭs   _____

salpingopharyngeal (693) săl-pĭng-gō-fă-RĬN-gē-ăl   _____

semicircular canals (692) sĕ-mē-SĔR-kū-lăr kă-NĂLZ   _____

serous otitis media (696) SĔR-ŭs ō-TĪ-tĭs MĒ-dē-ă   _____

stapedectomy (694)   stā-pĕ-DĔK-tō-mē   _____

stapes (692)   STĀ-pēz   _____

suppurative otitis   SŪ-pĕr-ă-tĭv ō-TĪ-tĭs   _____
  media (696)   MĒ-dē-ă

tinnitus (696)   tĭ-NĪ-tĭs   _____

tuning fork tests (697) TŌŌ-nĭng fŏrk tĕsts   _____

tympanic membrane (692) tĭm-PĂN-ĭk MĔM-brān   _____

tympanoplasty (694)   tĭm-pă-nō-PLĂS-tē   _____

vertigo (696)   VĔR-tĭ-gō   _____

vestibule (692)   VĔS-tĭ-būl   _____

vestibulocochlear (694) vĕs-tĭb-ū-lō-KŌK-lē-ăr   _____

VIII. Review Sheet

Write the meaning of the word parts in the spaces provided and test yourself. Check your answers with the information in the chapter or in the glossary (Medical Terms—English) at the end of the book.

COMBINING FORMS

Combining Form	Meaning	Combining Form	Meaning
acous/o	_____	lacrim/o	_____
ambly/o	_____	mastoid/o	_____
anis/o	_____	mi/o	_____
aque/o	_____	myc/o	_____
audi/o	_____	mydr/o	_____
audit/o	_____	myring/o	_____
aur/o	_____	nyct/o	_____
auricul/o	_____	ocul/o	_____
blephar/o	_____	ophthalm/o	_____
cochle/o	_____	opt/o	_____
conjunctiv/o	_____	optic/o	_____
cor/o	_____	ossicul/o	_____
corne/o	_____	ot/o	_____
cycl/o	_____	palpebr/o	_____
dacry/o	_____	papill/o	_____
dipl/o	_____	phac/o	_____
glauc/o	_____	phak/o	_____
ir/o	_____	phot/o	_____
irid/o	_____	presby/o	_____
kerat/o	_____	pupill/o	_____

Continued on following page

retin/o _____ tympan/o _____

salping/o _____ uve/o _____

scler/o _____ vestibul/o _____

scot/o _____ vitre/o _____

staped/o _____ xer/o _____

SUFFIXES

Suffix	**Meaning**	**Suffix**	**Meaning**
-acusis	_____	-otia	_____
-cusis	_____	-phobia	_____
-opia	_____	-plegic	_____
-opsia	_____	-tropia	_____

chapter

Endocrine System

This chapter is divided into the following sections

In this chapter you will

- Identify the endocrine glands and their hormones.
- Gain an understanding of the functions of these hormones in the body.
- Analyze medical terms related to the endocrine glands and their hormones.
- Describe the abnormal conditions resulting from excessive and deficient secretions of the endocrine glands.
- Identify laboratory tests, clinical procedures, and abbreviations related to endocrinology.
- Apply your new knowledge to understanding medical terms in their proper contexts, such as medical reports and records.

I. Introduction

The endocrine system is an information signaling system much like the nervous system. However, the nervous system uses nerves to conduct information, whereas the endocrine system uses blood vessels as information channels. **Glands** located in many regions of the body release into the bloodstream specific chemical messengers called **hormones** (from the Greek word *hormōn*, meaning "urging on"), which regulate the many and varied functions of an organism. For example, one hormone stimulates the growth of bones, another causes the maturation of sex organs and reproductive cells, and another controls the metabolic rate (metabolism) within all the individual cells of the body. In addition, one powerful endocrine gland below the brain secretes a wide variety of different hormones that travel through the bloodstream and regulate the activities of other endocrine glands.

Hormones produce their effects by binding to **receptors,** which are recognition sites in the various **target tissues** on which the hormones act. The receptors initiate specific biological effects when the hormones bind to them. Each hormone has its own receptor, and binding of a receptor by a hormone is much like the interaction of a key and a lock.

All of the **endocrine glands,** no matter which hormones they produce, secrete their hormones directly into the bloodstream rather than into ducts leading to the exterior of the body. Those glands that send their chemical substances into ducts and out of the body are called **exocrine glands.** Examples of exocrine glands are sweat, mammary, mucous, salivary, and lacrimal (tear) glands.

The ductless, internally secreting **endocrine glands** are listed as follows. Locate these glands on Figure 18–1.

[1] thyroid gland
[2] parathyroid glands (four glands)
[3] adrenal glands (one pair)
[4] pancreas (islets of Langerhans)
[5] pituitary gland

[6] ovaries in female (one pair)
[7] testes in male (one pair)
[8] pineal gland
[9] thymus gland

The last two glands on this list, the pineal and the thymus glands, are included as endocrine glands because they are ductless, although little is known about their endocrine function in the human body. The **pineal gland,** located in the central portion of the brain, secretes melatonin. **Melatonin** functions to support the body's "biological clock" and is thought to induce sleep. The pineal gland has been linked to a mental condition, seasonal affective disorder (SAD), in which a person suffers depression in winter months. Melatonin secretion increases with deprivation of light and is inhibited by sunlight. Calcification of the pineal gland can occur and can be an important radiological landmark when x-rays of the brain are examined.

The **thymus gland,** located behind the sternum in the mediastinum, resembles a lymph gland in structure. It contains lymphatic tissue and T-cell lymphocytes. The gland produces a hormone, **thymosin,** and is important in the development of immune responses in newborns (it is large in childhood but shrinks in adulthood). Removal of the thymus gland is helpful in treating a muscular-neurological disorder called myasthenia gravis.

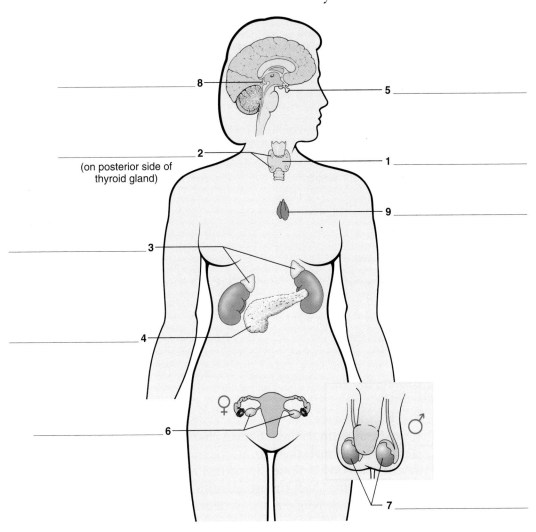

8

5

2
(on posterior side of
thyroid gland)

1

9

3

4

6

7

Figure 18–1

The endocrine system.

Table 18–1. ENDOCRINE TISSUE (APART FROM MAJOR GLANDS): LOCATION, SECRETION, AND ACTION

Location	Secretion	Action
Body cells	Prostaglandins	Aggregation of platelets Contract uterus Lower acid secretion in stomach Lower blood pressure
Gastrointestinal tract	Cholecystokinin Gastrin Secretin	Contracts gallbladder Stimulates gastric secretion Stimulates pancreatic enzymes
Kidney	Erythropoietin	Stimulates erythrocyte production
Pineal gland	Melatonin	Induces sleep and affects mood
Placenta	hCG	Sustains pregnancy
Skin	Vitamin D	Affects absorption of calcium
Thymus gland	Thymosin	Affects immune response

Hormones are also secreted by endocrine tissue apart from the major glands. Examples are **erythropoietin** (kidney), **human chorionic gonadotropin** (placenta), and **cholecystokinin** (gallbladder). **Prostaglandins** are hormone-like substances that affect the body in many ways. First found in semen (produced by the prostate gland) but now recognized in cells throughout the body, prostaglandins (1) stimulate the contraction of the uterus; (2) regulate body temperature, platelet aggregation, and acid secretion in the stomach; and (3) have the ability to lower blood pressure.

Endocrine tissue (apart from the major glands) is reviewed in Table 18–1. Use it as a reference.

II. Thyroid Gland

A. Location and Structure

Label Figure 18–2.

The **thyroid gland** [1] is composed of a right and a left lobe on either side of the **trachea** [2], just below a large piece of cartilage called the **thyroid cartilage** [3]. The thyroid cartilage covers the larynx and produces the prominence on the neck known as the "Adam's apple." The **isthmus** [4] of the thyroid gland is a narrow strip of glandular tissue that connects the two lobes on the ventral (anterior) surface of the trachea.

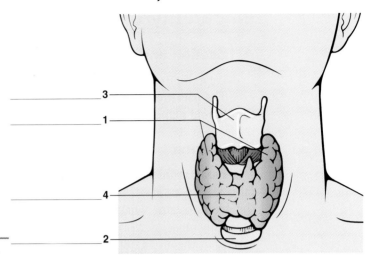

Figure 18–2

The thyroid gland, anterior view.

B. Function

Two of the hormones secreted by the thyroid gland are **thyroxine** or **tetraiodothyronine (T₄)** and **triiodothyronine (T₃).** These hormones are synthesized in the thyroid gland from **iodine,** which is picked up from the blood circulating through the gland, and from an amino acid called tyrosine. T_4 (containing four atoms of iodine) is much more concentrated in the blood, whereas T_3 (containing three atoms of iodine) is far more potent in affecting the metabolism of cells. Most thyroid hormone is bound to protein molecules as it travels in the bloodstream.

T_4 and T_3 are necessary in the body to maintain a normal level of metabolism in all body cells. Cells need oxygen to carry on metabolic processes, one aspect of which is burning food to release the energy stored within it. Thyroid hormone aids cells in their uptake of oxygen and thus supports the metabolic rate in the body. Injections of thyroid hormone raise the metabolic rate, whereas removal of the thyroid gland, diminishing thyroid hormone content in the body, results in a lower metabolic rate, heat loss, and poor physical and mental development.

A more recently discovered hormone produced by the thyroid gland is **calcitonin.** Calcitonin is secreted when calcium levels in the blood are high. It stimulates calcium to leave the blood and enter the bones, thus lowering blood calcium back to normal. Calcitonin contained in a nasal spray can be used for treatment of osteoporosis (loss of bone density). By increasing calcium storage in bone, calcitonin can strengthen weakened bone tissue and prevent spontaneous bone fractures. Figure 18–3 summarizes the hormones secreted by the thyroid gland.

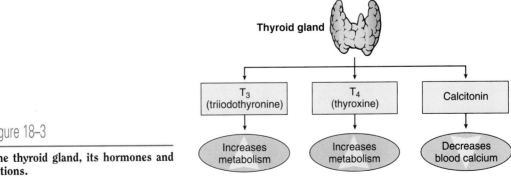

Figure 18–3

The thyroid gland, its hormones and actions.

III. Parathyroid Glands

A. Location and Structure

Label Figure 18–4.

The **parathyroid glands** [1] are four small, oval bodies located on the dorsal aspect of the **thyroid gland** [2].

B. Function

Parathyroid hormone (PTH) is secreted by the parathyroid glands. This hormone (also known as **parathormone**) mobilizes **calcium** (a mineral substance) from bones into the bloodstream, where calcium is necessary for proper functioning of body tissues, especially muscles. Normally, calcium in the food we eat is absorbed from the intestine and carried by the blood to the bones, where it is stored. The adjustment of the level of calcium in the blood is a good example of the way hormones in general control the **homeostasis** (equilibrium or constancy in the internal environment) of the body. If blood calcium decreases (as in pregnancy or in a condition of vitamin D deficiency), parathyroid hormone secretion increases to cause calcium to leave the bones and enter the bloodstream. Thus blood calcium levels are brought back to normal (Fig. 18–5). Conversely, a situation of too much calcium in the bloodstream causes decreased PTH secretion (calcium leaves the blood to enter bones), decreasing blood calcium, so that homeostasis is achieved again.

IV. Adrenal Glands

A. Location and Structure

Label Figure 18–6.

The **adrenal glands,** or **suprarenal glands,** are two small glands; one is situated on top of each **kidney** [1]. Each gland consists of two parts: an outer portion, the **adrenal cortex** [2], and an inner portion, the **adrenal medulla** [3]. The cortex and medulla are two glands in one, each secreting its own different endocrine hormones. The cortex secretes steroid hormones or **corticosteroids** (complex chemicals derived from cholesterol), and the medulla secretes **catecholamines** (chemicals derived from amino acids).

B. Function

The **adrenal cortex** secretes three types of **corticosteroids.**

1. **Glucocorticoids**—These steroid hormones have an important influence on the metabolism of sugars, fats, and proteins within all body cells and have a powerful anti-inflammatory effect.

   Cortisol (also called **hydrocortisone**) is the most important glucocorticoid hormone. Cortisol increases the ability of cells to make new sugars out of fats and proteins (gluconeogenesis) and regulates the quantity of sugars, fats, and proteins in the blood and cells.

   Cortisone is a hormone very similar to cortisol and can be prepared synthetically. Cortisone is useful in treating inflammatory conditions such as rheumatoid arthritis.

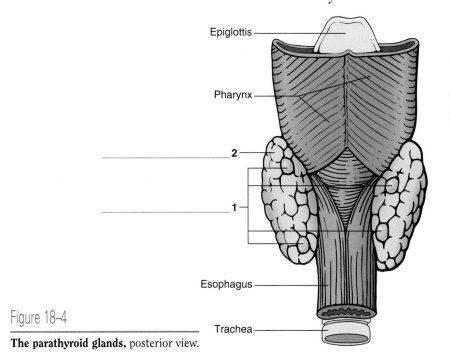

Epiglottis

Pharynx

2

1

Esophagus

Trachea

Figure 18–4

The parathyroid glands, posterior view.

Parathyroid glands

↓

Parathyroid hormone (PTH)

↓

Increases blood calcium

Figure 18–5

The parathyroid glands, their hormone and action.

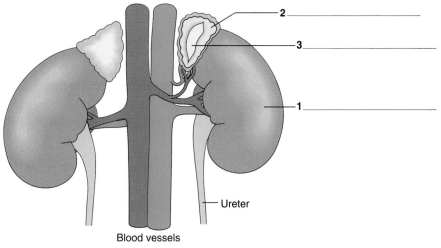

2

3

1

Ureter

Blood vessels

Figure 18–6

The adrenal (suprarenal) glands.

2. **Mineralocorticoids**—These hormones are essential to life because they regulate the amounts of mineral salts (also called **electrolytes**) that are retained in the body. A proper balance of water and salts in the blood and tissues is essential to the normal functioning of the body.

 Aldosterone is a mineralocorticoid hormone. The secretion of aldosterone by the adrenal cortex increases the reabsorption into the bloodstream of **sodium** (a mineral electrolyte commonly found in salts) by the kidney tubules. At the same time, aldosterone stimulates the excretion of another electrolyte called **potassium.**

 The secretion of aldosterone increases manyfold in the face of a severely sodium-restricted diet, thereby enabling the body to hold needed salt in the bloodstream.

3. **Gonadocorticoids**—These are sex hormones, **androgen** (male hormone) and **estrogen** (female hormone), that influence secondary sex characteristics, such as pubic and axillary hair in both boys and girls. Excess adrenal androgen secretion in females leads to **virilism** (development of male characteristics).

The **adrenal medulla** secretes two types of **catecholamine** hormones:

1. **Epinephrine (adrenaline)**—This hormone increases cardiac rate, dilates bronchial tubes, and stimulates the production of glucose from a storage substance called glycogen when glucose is needed by the body.
2. **Norepinephrine (noradrenaline)**—This hormone constricts vessels and raises blood pressure.

 Both epinephrine and norepinephrine are **sympathomimetic** agents because they mimic, or copy, the actions of the sympathetic nervous system. During times of stress, these hormones are secreted by the adrenal medulla in response to nervous stimulation. They help the body respond to crisis situations by raising blood pressure, increasing heartbeat and respiration, and bringing sugar out of storage in the cells.

 Figure 18–7 summarizes the hormones that are secreted by the adrenal glands and notes their actions.

V. Pancreas

A. Location and Structure

 Label Figure 18–8.

 The **pancreas** [1] is located near and partially behind the **stomach** [2] in the region of the first and second lumbar vertebrae. The endocrine tissue of the pancreas consists of specialized hormone-producing cells called the **islets of Langerhans** [3]. More than 98 percent of the pancreas consists of exocrine cells (glands and ducts). These cells secrete digestive enzymes into the gastrointestinal tract.

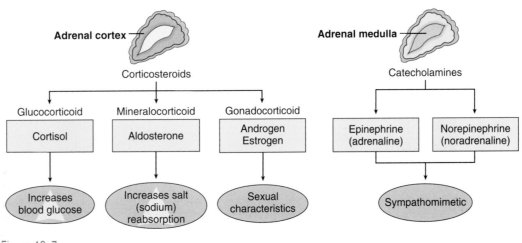

Figure 18–7

The adrenal cortex and adrenal medulla, their hormones and actions.

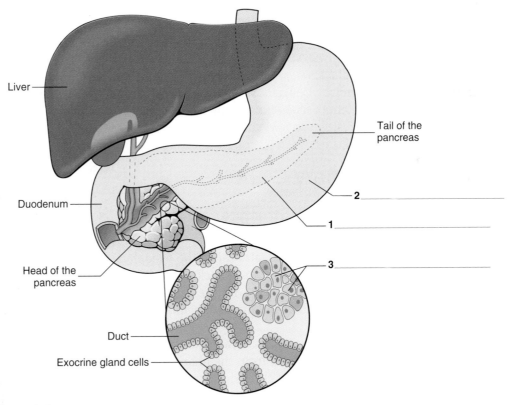

Figure 18–8

The pancreas and surrounding organs.

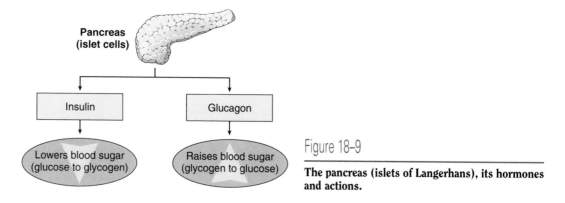

Figure 18–9

The pancreas (islets of Langerhans), its hormones and actions.

B. Function

The islets of Langerhans produce **insulin** (produced by beta cells) and **glucagon** (produced by alpha cells). Both play a role in proper metabolism of sugars and starches in the body. Insulin promotes the movement of **glucose** (sugar) and other nutrients out of the blood and into cells. When blood glucose rises, insulin, released from the beta islet cells, causes glucose to enter body cells to be used for energy. Also, it stimulates conversion of **glucose** to **glycogen** (a starch-storage form of sugar) in the liver. Another pancreatic hormone, glucagon, promotes the movement of glucose into the blood when glucose levels are below normal. It causes the breakdown of stored liver **glycogen** to **glucose,** so that the sugar content of blood leaving the liver rises.

Figure 18–9 reviews the secretions of the islet cells and their actions.

VI. Pituitary Gland

A. Location and Structure

Label Figure 18–10.

The **pituitary gland,** also called the **hypophysis,** is a small, pea-sized gland located at the base of the brain in a small, pocket-like depression of the skull called the **sella turcica.** It is a well-protected gland, with the entire mass of the brain above it and the nasal cavity below. The ancient Greeks incorrectly imagined that its function was to produce *pituita* or nasal secretion.

The pituitary consists of two distinct parts: an **anterior lobe** or **adenohypophysis** [1], formed by an upgrowth from the pharynx and glandular in nature; and a **posterior lobe** or **neurohypophysis** [2], derived from a downgrowth at the base of the brain. The **hypothalamus** [3] is a region of the brain that is close to the pituitary gland. Signals transmitted from the hypothalamus control the secretions by the pituitary gland. Special secretory neurons in the hypothalamus send releasing and inhibiting factors (hormones) via capillaries to the anterior pituitary gland. These factors stimulate or inhibit secretion of hormones from the anterior pituitary (Fig. 18–11A). The hypothalamus also produces and secretes hormones directly to the posterior pituitary gland, where the hormones are stored and then released (Fig. 18–11B).

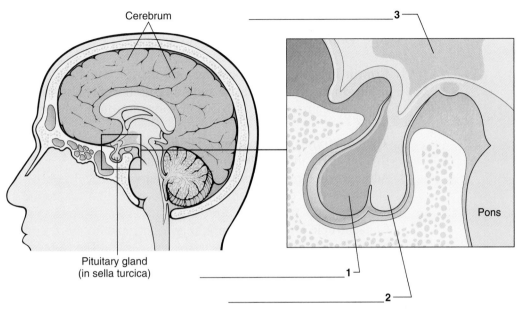

Cerebrum

Pons

Pituitary gland
(in sella turcica)

Figure 18–10

The pituitary gland.

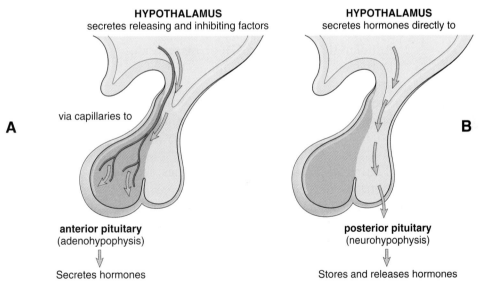

HYPOTHALAMUS
secretes releasing and inhibiting factors

HYPOTHALAMUS
secretes hormones directly to

via capillaries to

A

B

anterior pituitary
(adenohypophysis)

↓

Secretes hormones

posterior pituitary
(neurohypophysis)

↓

Stores and releases hormones

Figure 18–11

(A) The relationship of the **hypothalamus** to the **anterior pituitary gland** and **(B)** its relationship to the **posterior pituitary gland.**

B. Function

The hormones of the **anterior pituitary gland** are as follows:

1. **Growth hormone (GH)** or **somatotropin (STH)**—Promotes protein synthesis that results in the growth of bone and other tissues. GH also stimulates the liver to make insulin-like growth factor (IGF1) or somatomedin C, which stimulates the growth of bones.
2. **Thyroid-stimulating hormone (TSH; thyrotropin)**—Stimulates the growth of the thyroid gland and its secretion of its hormones.
3. **Adrenocorticotropic hormone (ACTH; adrenocorticotropin)**—Stimulates the growth of the adrenal cortex and increases its secretion of steroid hormones (primarily cortisol).
4. **Gonadotropic hormones**—Several gonadotropic hormones influence the growth and hormone secretion of the ovaries in females and the testes in males. In the female, **follicle-stimulating hormone (FSH)** and **luteinizing hormone (LH)** stimulate the growth of eggs in the ovaries, the production of hormones, and ovulation.

    In the male, FSH influences the production of sperm and LH (as interstitial cell–stimulating hormone) stimulates the testes to produce testosterone.
5. **Prolactin (PRL)**—Stimulates breast development during pregnancy and sustains milk production after birth.

The **posterior pituitary gland** stores and releases two important hormones that are synthesized in the hypothalamus:

1. **Antidiuretic hormone (ADH; or vasopressin)**—Stimulates the reabsorption of water by the kidney tubules. In addition, ADH also increases blood pressure by constricting arterioles.
2. **Oxytocin (OT)**—Stimulates the uterus to contract during childbirth and maintains labor during childbirth. Oxytocin is also secreted during suckling and causes the production of milk from the mammary glands.

Figure 18–12 reviews the hormones secreted by the pituitary gland and their functions.

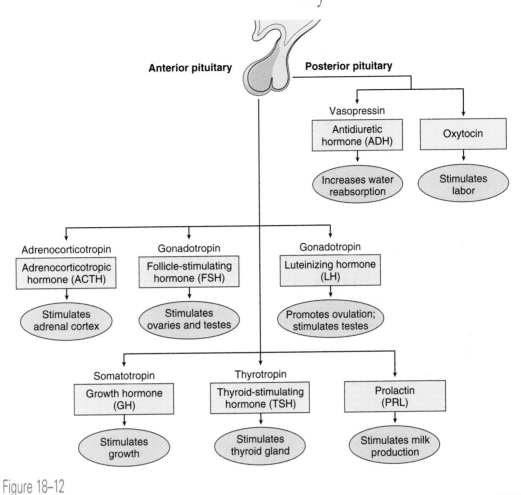

Figure 18–12

The pituitary gland, its hormones and actions.

VII. Ovaries

A. Location and Structure

The **ovaries** are two small glands located in the lower abdominal region of the female. The ovaries produce the female gamete, the ovum, as well as hormones that are responsible for female sex characteristics and regulation of the menstrual cycle.

B. Function

The ovarian hormones are **estrogens** (**estradiol** and estrone) and **progesterone.** Estrogens are responsible for development and maintenance of secondary sex characteristics, such as hair and breast development. Progesterone is responsible for the preparation and maintenance of the uterus in pregnancy.

VIII. Testes

A. Location and Structure

The **testes** are two small, ovoid glands suspended from the inguinal region of the male by the spermatic cord and surrounded by the scrotal sac. The testes produce the male gametes, spermatozoa, as well as the male hormone called **testosterone.**

B. Function

Testosterone is an **androgen** (male steroid hormone) that stimulates and promotes the growth of secondary sex characteristics in the male (development of beard and pubic hair, deepening of voice, and distribution of fat).

Figure 18–13 reviews the hormones secreted by the ovaries and testes.

Table 18–2 lists the major endocrine glands, their hormones, and the actions they produce.

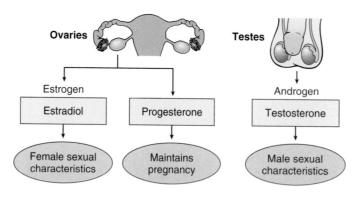

Figure 18–13

The ovaries and testes, their hormones and actions.

Table 18–2. MAJOR ENDOCRINE GLANDS, THE HORMONES THEY PRODUCE, AND THEIR ACTIONS

Endocrine Gland	Hormone	Action
Thyroid	Thyroxine; triiodothyronine	Increases metabolism in body cells
	Calcitonin	Lowers blood calcium
Parathyroids	Parathyroid hormone	Increases blood calcium
Adrenals		
Cortex	Cortisol (glucocorticoid)	Increases blood sugar
	Aldosterone (mineralocorticoid)	Increases reabsorption of sodium
	Sex hormones: androgens, estrogens (gonadocorticoids)	Maintain secondary sex characteristics
Medulla	Epinephrine (adrenaline)	Sympathomimetic
	Norepinephrine (noradrenaline)	Sympathomimetic
Pancreas		
Islet cells	Insulin	Decreases blood sugar (glucose to glycogen)
	Glucagon	Increases blood sugar (glycogen to glucose)
Pituitary		
Anterior lobe	Growth hormone (GH; somatotropin)	Increases bone and tissue growth
	Thyroid-stimulating hormone (TSH)	Stimulates production of thyroxine and growth of the thyroid gland
	Adrenocorticotropic hormone (ACTH)	Stimulates secretion of hormones from the adrenal cortex, especially cortisol
	Gonadotropins	
	Follicle-stimulating hormone (FSH)	Oogenesis and spermatogenesis
	Luteinizing hormone (LH)	Promotes ovulation; testosterone secretion
	Prolactin (PRL)	Promotes growth of breast tissue and milk secretion
Posterior lobe	Antidiuretic hormone (ADH; vasopressin)	Stimulates reabsorption of water by kidney tubules
	Oxytocin	Stimulates contraction of the uterus during labor and childbirth
Ovaries	Estrogens	Develops and maintains secondary sex characteristics in the female
	Progesterone	Prepares and maintains the uterus in pregnancy
Testes	Testosterone	Promotes growth and maintenance of secondary sex characteristics in the male

IX. Vocabulary

This list reviews many new terms introduced in the text. Short definitions reinforce your understanding of the terms. See Section XVIII of this chapter for pronunciation of more difficult terms.

Major Glands

adrenal cortex
Outer section of each adrenal gland.

adrenal medulla
Inner section of each adrenal gland.

ovaries
Two endocrine glands in a female's lower abdomen; responsible for egg production and estrogen and progesterone secretion.

pancreas
Endocrine gland behind the stomach. Islet cells (islets of Langerhans) secrete hormones from the pancreas.

parathyroid glands
Four small endocrine glands on the posterior side of the thyroid gland.

pituitary gland (hypophysis)
Endocrine gland at the base of the brain; composed of an anterior lobe (**adenohypophysis**) and a posterior lobe (**neurohypophysis**). It weighs only 1/16th of an ounce and is a half inch across.

testes
Two endocrine glands enclosed in the scrotal sac of a male; responsible for sperm production and testosterone secretion.

thyroid gland
Endocrine gland in the neck.

Hormones

adrenaline
Produced by the adrenal medulla; also called **epinephrine.** Adrenaline increases heart rate and blood pressure.

adrenocorticotropic hormone (ACTH)
Produced by the anterior lobe of the pituitary gland (adenohypophysis); also called **adrenocorticotropin.** ACTH stimulates the adrenal cortex.

aldosterone
Produced by the adrenal cortex; increases salt (sodium) reabsorption.

androgen
Male hormone produced by the testes and to a lesser extent by the adrenal cortex; testosterone is an example.

antidiuretic hormone (ADH)
Secreted by the posterior lobe of the pituitary gland (neurohypophysis). ADH (**vasopressin**) increases reabsorption of water by the kidney.

calcitonin
Produced by the thyroid gland. Calcitonin lowers blood calcium.

cortisol
Produced by the adrenal cortex; increases blood sugar.

epinephrine	Produced by the adrenal medulla; also called **adrenaline.** Epinephrine (a sympathomimetic) increases heart rate and blood pressure and dilates airways.
estradiol	An estrogen (female hormone) produced by the ovaries.
estrogen	Female hormone produced by the ovaries and to a lesser extent by the adrenal cortex. Examples are estradiol and estrone.
follicle-stimulating hormone (FSH)	Produced by the anterior lobe of the pituitary gland (adenohypophysis). FSH stimulates hormone secretion and egg production by the ovaries and sperm production by the testes.
glucagon	Hormone produced by the alpha islet cells of the pancreas; increases blood sugar by conversion of glycogen (starch) to glucose.
growth hormone (GH)	Produced by the anterior lobe of the pituitary gland (adenohypophysis); also called **somatotropin.** GH stimulates the growth of bones and tissues.
insulin	Produced by the beta islet cells (*insula* means "island") of the pancreas. Insulin lowers blood sugar by transport and conversion of glucose to glycogen (starch).
luteinizing hormone (LH)	Produced by the anterior lobe of the pituitary gland (adenohypophysis). LH stimulates ovulation in females and testosterone secretion in males.
norepinephrine	Produced by the adrenal medulla and as a sympathomimetic increases heart rate and blood pressure. Nor- in chemistry means a parent compound from which another is derived.
oxytocin (OT)	Secreted by the posterior lobe of the pituitary gland (neurohypophysis); stimulates contraction of the uterus during labor and childbirth.
parathormone (PTH)	Produced by the parathyroid glands; increases blood calcium.
progesterone	Produced by the ovaries; prepares the uterus for pregnancy.
prolactin (PRL)	Produced by the anterior lobe of the pituitary gland (adenohypophysis); promotes milk secretion.
somatotropin (STH)	Produced by the anterior lobe of the pituitary gland (adenohypophysis); also called **growth hormone.**
testosterone	Male hormone produced by the testes.
thyroid-stimulating hormone (TSH)	Produced by the anterior lobe of the pituitary gland (adenohypophysis). TSH acts on the thyroid gland to promote its functioning; also called **thyrotropin.**

thyroxine (T₄)	Produced by the thyroid gland; also called **tetraiodothyronine.** T_4 increases metabolism in cells.
triiodothyronine (T₃)	Produced by the thyroid gland; T_3 increases metabolism in cells.
vasopressin	Secreted by the posterior lobe of the pituitary gland (neurohypophysis); also called **antidiuretic hormone.**

Related Terms

catecholamines	Hormones derived from an amino acid and secreted by the adrenal medulla. Epinephrine is a catecholamine.
corticosteroids	Hormones (steroid) produced by the adrenal cortex. Glucocorticoids, mineralocorticoids, and gonadocorticoids are examples.
electrolyte	Mineral salt found in the blood and tissues and necessary for proper functioning of cells; potassium, sodium, and calcium are examples.
glucocorticoid	Hormone secreted by the adrenal cortex; necessary for use of sugars, fats, and proteins by the body and for the body's normal response to stress. Cortisol is an example.
gonadocorticoid	Sex hormone secreted by the adrenal cortex.
homeostasis	Tendency of an organism to maintain a constant internal environment.
hormone	Substance, produced by an endocrine gland, that travels through the blood to a distant organ or gland where it influences the structure or function of that organ or gland.
hypothalamus	Region of the brain lying below the thalamus and above the pituitary gland. It produces releasing factors and hormones that affect the pituitary gland.
mineralocorticoid	Steroid hormone produced by the adrenal cortex to regulate mineral salts (electrolytes) and water balance in the body. Aldosterone is an example.
receptor	Cellular protein that binds to a hormone so that a response can be elicited.
sella turcica	Cavity in the skull that contains the pituitary gland.
steroid	Complex substance related to fats (derived from a sterol, such as cholesterol) and of which many hormones are made. Examples of steroids are estrogens, androgens, glucocorticoids, and mineralocorticoids. **Ster/o** means solid, **-ol** means oil.
sympathomimetic	Pertaining to mimicking or copying the effect of the sympathetic nervous system. Adrenaline is a sympathomimetic hormone (raises blood pressure and heart rate and dilates airways).
target tissue	Cells of an organ that are affected by specific hormones.

X. Combining Forms, Suffixes, Prefixes, and Terminology: Glands and Related Terms

Write the meanings of the medical terms in the spaces provided.

Glands

Combining Forms

Combining Form	Meaning	Terminology	Meaning
aden/o	gland	adenectomy	_____
adren/o	adrenal glands	adrenopathy	_____
adrenal/o	adrenal glands	adrenalectomy	_____
gonad/o	sex glands (ovaries and testes)	gonadotropin	_____
		-tropin means to act upon, to turn. A gonadotropin acts on (stimulates) the gonads. Examples are FSH and LH.	
		hypogonadism	_____
		Deficiency of gonadotropins can produce hypogonadism.	
pancreat/o	pancreas	pancreatectomy	_____
parathyroid/o	parathyroid gland	parathyroidectomy	_____
pituitar/o	pituitary gland, hypophysis	hypopituitarism	_____
		Pituitary dwarfism (see page 748, Section XI, Abnormal Conditions) is caused by hypopituitarism.	
thyr/o	thyroid gland	thyrotropin hormone	_____
		Thyroid-stimulating hormone (TSH).	
thyroid/o	thyroid gland	thyroiditis	_____
		*May result from bacterial or viral infection, or an autoimmune reaction. Symptoms are throat pain, swelling, tenderness, and signs of hyperthyroidism. The condition may progress to destruction of the thyroid gland and hypothyroidism. In **Hashimoto disease** or autoimmune thyroiditis antibodies trigger lymphocytes to destroy follicular cells in the thyroid gland producing hypothyroidism.*	

Related Terms

Combining Forms			
Combining Form	Meaning	Terminology	Meaning
andr/o	male	androgen _____	
		Androgens are produced by the testes in males and by the adrenal cortex in males and females.	
calc/o	calcium	hypercalcemia _____	
		hypocalcemia _____	
cortic/o	cortex, outer region	corticosteroid _____	
		Cortisol is an example of a corticosteroid.	
crin/o	secrete	endocrinologist _____	
dips/o	thirst	polydipsia _____	
		Symptom associated with both diabetes mellitus and diabetes insipidus (see page 745, Section XI, Abnormal Conditions).	
estr/o	female	estrogenic _____	
gluc/o	sugar	glucagon _____	
		-agon means to assemble or gather together. Glucagon raises blood sugar by stimulating its release from glycogen into the bloodstream.	
glyc/o	sugar	hyperglycemia _____	
		glycemic _____	
		A patient with diabetes mellitus requires glycemic control.	
		glycogen _____	
		Glycogen is animal starch that is converted to glucose by the hormone glucagon.	
home/o	sameness	homeostasis _____	
		-stasis means to control.	

hormon/o	hormone	hormonal _____
insulin/o	insulin	hypoinsulinism _____
kal/i	potassium (an electrolyte)	hypokalemia _____

This condition can occur in dehydration and with excessive vomiting and diarrhea. The heart is particularly sensitive to potassium loss.

lact/o	milk	prolactin _____

-in means a substance.

myx/o	mucus	myxedema _____

Mucus-like material accumulates under the skin. See page 742, Section XI, Abnormal Conditions, under hypothyroidism.

natr/o	sodium (an electrolyte)	hyponatremia _____

Occurs with hyposecretion of the adrenal cortex as salts and water leave the body.

phys/o	growing	hypophysectomy _____

The hypophysis is the pituitary gland, which is so named because it grows from the undersurface (hypo-) of the brain.

somat/o	body	somatotropin _____

Growth hormone.

ster/o	solid structure	steroid _____

This complex, solid, ring-shaped molecule resembles a sterol (such as cholesterol); many hormones (androgens, estrogens, glucocorticoids, and mineralocorticoids) are steroids.

toc/o	childbirth	oxytocin _____

oxy- means swift, rapid.

toxic/o	poison	thyrotoxicosis _____

Condition caused by excessive thyroid gland activity and oversecretion of thyroid hormone. Symptoms are sweating, weight loss, tachycardia, and nervousness.

ur/o	urine	antidiuretic hormone _____

Posterior pituitary hormone that affects the kidneys and reduces water loss.

Suffixes			
Suffix	Meaning	Terminology	Meaning
-agon	assemble, gather together	gluc<u>agon</u>	_____
-in, -ine	a substance	epineph<u>rine</u>	_____
-tropin	stimulating the function of (to turn or act upon)	adrenocortico<u>tropin</u>	_____
		-tropic is the adjective form (adrenocorticotropic hormone).	
-uria	urine condition	glycos<u>uria</u>	_____
		Symptom of diabetes mellitus.	

Prefixes			
Prefix	Meaning	Terminology	Meaning
eu-	good, normal	<u>eu</u>thyroid	_____
oxy-	rapid, sharp, acid	<u>oxy</u>tocin	_____
pan-	all	<u>pan</u>hypopituitarism	_____
tetra-	four	<u>tetra</u>iodothyronine	_____
		iod/o means iodine.	
tri-	three	<u>tri</u>iodothyronine	_____

XI. Abnormal Conditions

Thyroid Gland

Enlargement of the thyroid gland is **goiter** (Fig. 18–14A). **Endemic** (**en-** means in; **dem/o** means people) **goiter** occurs in certain regions and peoples where there is a lack of **iodine** in the diet. Goiter occurs when low iodine levels lead to low T_3 and T_4 levels. This causes feedback to the hypothalamus and adenohypophysis, stimulating them to secrete releasing factors and TSH. TSH then promotes the thyroid gland to secrete T_3 and T_4, but because there is no iodine available, the only effect is to increase the size of the gland (goiter). Treatment is to increase the supply of iodine (as iodized salt) in the diet.

Another type of goiter is **nodular** or **adenomatous goiter,** in which hyperplasia occurs as well as nodules and adenomas. Some patients with nodular goiter develop hyperthyroidism and symptoms such as rapid pulse, tremors, nervousness, and excessive sweating. Treatment is thyroid-blocking drugs or radioactive iodine to suppress thyroid functioning.

Hypersecretion

hyperthyroidism

Overactivity of the thyroid gland.

The most common form of this condition is **thyrotoxicosis** or **Graves disease** (resulting from autoimmune processes). Hyperplasia of the thyroid parenchyma (glandular cells) occurs, so that excessive hormone is produced. The metabolic rate in cells is increased, leading to sweating, weight loss, rapid and irregular heartbeat, diarrhea, and warm and moist skin. In addition, **exophthalmos** (protrusion of the eyeballs) occurs as a result of swelling of tissue behind the eyeball, pushing it forward. Treatment of Graves disease includes management with antithyroid drugs to reduce the amount of thyroid hormone produced by the gland and administration of radioactive iodine, which destroys the overactive glandular tissue. Figure 18–14B shows a patient with Graves disease and exophthalmos.

A 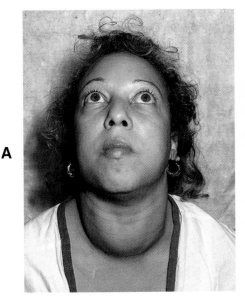 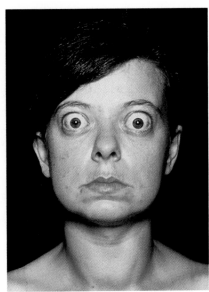 B

Figure 18–14

(A) Goiter. Notice the wide neck, indicating enlargement of the thyroid gland. Goiter comes from the Latin *guttur,* meaning "throat." **(B) Exophthalmos** in Graves disease. Note the staring or startled expression. (**A** from Swartz M: Textbook of Physical Diagnosis, 4th ed. Philadelphia, WB Saunders, 2002. **B** from Seidel H et al: Mosby's Guide to Physical Examination, 4th ed. St. Louis, Mosby, 1998, p. 264.)

Hyposecretion

hypothyroidism

Underactivity of the thyroid gland.

Any one of several conditions can produce hypothyroidism (thyroidectomy, thyroiditis, endemic goiter, destruction of the gland by irradiation), but all have similar physiological effects. These include fatigue, muscular and mental sluggishness, weight gain, fluid retention, slow heart rate, low body temperature, and constipation. Two examples of hypothyroidism are as follows:

Myxedema—This is advanced hypothyroidism in adulthood. Atrophy of the thyroid gland occurs, and practically no hormone is produced. The skin becomes dry and puffy (edema) because of the collection of mucus-like (**myx/o** means mucus) material under the skin. Many patients also develop atherosclerosis because lack of thyroid hormone increases the quantity of blood lipids (fats). Recovery may be complete if thyroid hormone is given soon after symptoms appear. Figure 18–15A shows a patient with myxedema.

Cretinism—Extreme hypothyroidism during infancy and childhood leads to a lack of normal physical and mental growth. Skeletal growth is more inhibited than soft tissue growth, so the **cretin** has the appearance of an obese, short, and stocky child. Treatment consists of administration of thyroid hormone, which may be able to reverse some of the hypothyroid effects.

Neoplasms

thyroid carcinoma

Cancer of the thyroid gland.

Some tumors (follicular carcinomas) are slow growing, and others (anaplastic) may metastasize widely. Adenomas (benign growths) are distinguished from carcinomas (malignant growths) by radioactive iodine tracer scans. "Hot" tumor areas (those collecting more radioactivity than surrounding tissues) usually

A 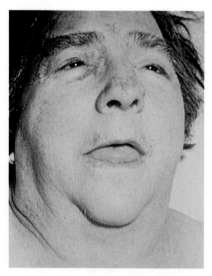 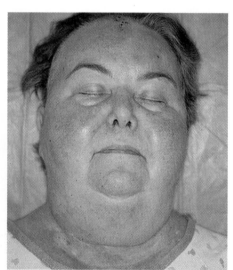 B

Figure 18–15

(A) Myxedema. Note the dull, puffy, yellowed skin; course, sparse hair; periorbital (around the orbits of the eyes) edema; prominent tongue. **(B) Cushing syndrome.** Facial features include a rounded, or moon-shaped, face with thin, erythematous skin. Hirsutism may also be present. (**A** courtesy Paul W Ladenson, MD, The Johns Hopkins University and Hospital, Baltimore, MD; **A** and **B** from Seidel HM et al: Mosby's Guide to Physical Examination, 5th ed. St. Louis, Mosby, 2003, p. 270.)

indicate hyperthyroidism and benign growth; "cold," nonfunctional nodules can be either benign or malignant. Ultimately, fine-needle aspiration, surgical biopsy, or excision is required to make the diagnosis. Thyroidectomy with lymph node removal is required for most thyroid carcinomas. Postsurgical treatment with radioactive iodine to destroy remaining tissue may be necessary.

Parathyroid Glands

Hypersecretion

hyperparathyroidism

Excessive production of parathormone.

Hypercalcemia occurs as calcium leaves the bones and enters the bloodstream, where it can produce damage to the kidneys and heart. Bones become decalcified with generalized loss of bone density (osteoporosis) and susceptibility to fractures and cysts. Kidney stones can occur as a result of hypercalcemia. The cause is parathyroid hyperplasia or a parathyroid tumor. Treatment is resection of the overactive tissue.

Hyposecretion

hypoparathyroidism

Deficient production of parathyroid hormone.

Hypocalcemia results as calcium remains in bones and is unable to enter the bloodstream. This leads to muscle and nerve weakness with spasms of muscles, a condition called **tetany** (constant muscle contraction). Administration of calcium plus large quantities of vitamin D (to promote absorption of calcium) can control the calcium level in the bloodstream.

Adrenal Cortex

Hypersecretion

adrenal virilism

Excessive output of adrenal androgens.

Adrenal hyperplasia or more commonly adrenal adenomas or carcinomas can cause **virilization** in adult women. Symptoms include amenorrhea, **hirsutism** (excessive hair on the face and body), acne, and deepening of the voice. Drug therapy to suppress androgen production and adrenalectomy are possible treatments.

Cushing syndrome

A group of symptoms produced by excess cortisol from the adrenal cortex.

A number of signs and symptoms occur as a result of increased glucocorticoids, including obesity, moon-like fullness of the face, excess deposition of fat in the thoracic region of the back (so-called buffalo hump), hyperglycemia, hypernatremia, hypokalemia, osteoporosis, virilization, and hypertension. The cause may be excess ACTH secretion (called Cushing syndrome) or tumor of the adrenal cortex. Tumors and disseminated cancers can be associated with ectopic secretion of hormone, such as ectopic ACTH produced by nonendocrine neoplasms (lung and thyroid tumors). Figure 18–15B shows a woman with Cushing syndrome.

In clinical practice, most cases of Cushing syndrome are caused by the administration of exogenous (from outside the body) glucocorticoids in the treatment of immune disorders, such as rheumatoid arthritis, lupus erythematosus, asthma, and renal and skin conditions.

Hyposecretion

Addison disease

Hypofunctioning of the adrenal cortex.

Mineralocorticoids and glucocorticoids are produced in deficient amounts. Hypoglycemia (from deficient glucocorticoids), hyponatremia (due to excessive loss of sodium in urine), fatigue, weakness, weight loss, salt craving, low blood pressure, and darker pigmentation of the skin are symptoms of the condition. Some cases are caused by an autoimmune adrenalitis; others by infection or surgical resection. Treatment consists of daily cortisone administration and intake of salts or administration of a synthetic form of aldosterone.

Adrenal Medulla

Hypersecretion

pheochromocytoma

Benign tumor of the adrenal medulla (tumor cells stain a dark or dusky [phe/o] color [chrom/o]).

The tumor cells produce excess secretion of epinephrine and norepinephrine. Symptoms are hypertension, palpitations, severe headaches, sweating, flushing of the face, and muscle spasms. Surgery to remove the tumor and administration of antihypertensive drugs are possible treatments.

Pancreas

Hypersecretion

hyperinsulinism

Excess secretion of insulin causing hypoglycemia.

The cause may be a tumor of the pancreas (benign adenoma or carcinoma) or an overdose of insulin. Hypoglycemia occurs as insulin draws sugar out of the bloodstream. Fainting spells, convulsions, and loss of consciousness are common because a minimal level of blood sugar is necessary for proper mental functioning.

Hyposecretion

diabetes mellitus

Lack of insulin secretion or resistance of insulin in promoting sugar, starch, and fat metabolism in cells.

In diabetes mellitus (mellitus means sweet or sugary), insulin insufficiency or ineffectiveness prevents sugar from leaving the blood and entering the body cells, where it is normally used to produce energy. There are two major types of diabetes mellitus.

Type 1 diabetes, with onset usually in childhood, involves destruction of the beta islet cells of the pancreas and complete deficiency of insulin in the body. Patients are usually thin and require frequent injections of insulin to maintain a normal level of glucose in the blood. It is also possible to administer insulin through a portable pump, which infuses the drug continuously through a needle indwelling under the skin (Fig. 18–16).

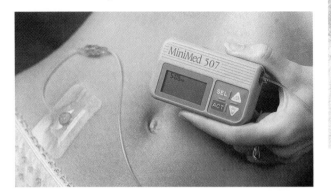

Figure 18-16

Insulin pump. It can be programmed to deliver doses of insulin according to varying body needs. (Courtesy MiniMed Technologies, Sylmar, California in Mosby's Medical, Nursing, and Allied Health Dictionary, 6th ed. St. Louis, Mosby, 2002, p. 903.)

Type 2 diabetes is a separate disease from Type 1 and has a different inheritance pattern. Patients are usually older, and obesity is very common. The islet cells are not destroyed, and there is a relative deficiency of insulin secretion with a resistance by target tissues to the action of insulin. Treatment is with diet, weight reduction, exercise, and, if necessary, insulin or oral hypoglycemic agents. The oral hypoglycemic agents can stimulate the release of insulin from the pancreas and improve the body's sensitivity to insulin.

Table 18-3 compares the features, symptoms, and treatments of Type 1 and Type 2 diabetes.

Both Type 1 and Type 2 diabetes are associated with primary and secondary complications. **Primary complications** of Type 1 include **ketoacidosis** (fats are improperly burned, leading to an accumulation of ketones and acids in the body) and **coma** when blood sugar concentration gets too high or the patient receives an insufficient amount of insulin. **Hypoglycemia** occurs when too much insulin is taken by the patient. **Insulin shock** is severe hypoglycemia caused by an overdose of insulin, decreased intake of food, or excessive exercise. Symptoms are sweating, trembling, nervousness, irritability, and numbness. Treatment requires an immediate dose of glucose orally or parenterally (other than through the gastrointestinal tract). Convulsions, coma, and death can result if the diabetic person is not treated.

Table 18-3. **COMPARISON OF TYPE 1 AND TYPE 2 DIABETES MELLITUS**

	Type 1	Type 2
FEATURES	Usually occurs **before age 30** **Abrupt, rapid onset** **Little or no insulin** production **Thin** or **normal** body weight at onset **Ketoacidosis** often occurs	Usually occurs **after age 30** **Gradual onset;** asymptomatic **Insulin usually present** 85% are **obese** **Ketoacidosis** seldom occurs
SYMPTOMS	Polyuria (glycosuria promotes loss of water) Polydipsia (dehydration causes thirst) Polyphagia (tissue breakdown causes hunger)	**Polyuria** sometimes seen **Polydipsia** sometimes seen **Polyphagia** sometimes seen
TREATMENT	**Insulin**	**Diet; oral hypoglycemics** or **insulin**

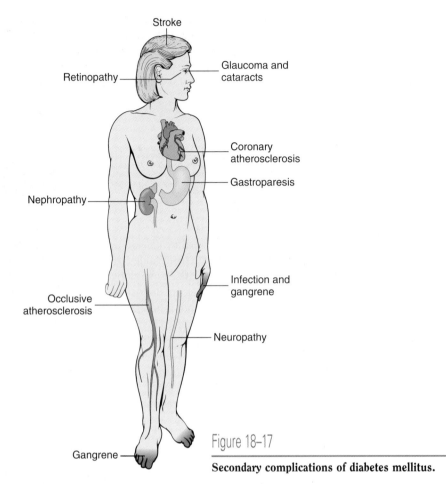

Figure 18–17

Secondary complications of diabetes mellitus.

Secondary (long-term) **complications** appear many years after the patient develops diabetes. These include eye disorders such as glaucoma and cataract and destruction of the blood vessels of the retina **(diabetic retinopathy),** causing visual loss and blindness; destruction of the kidneys **(diabetic nephropathy),** causing renal insufficiency and often requiring hemodialysis or renal transplantation; destruction of blood vessels, with **atherosclerosis** leading to stroke, heart disease, and peripherovascular ischemia (gangrene, infection, and loss of limbs); and destruction of nerves **(diabetic neuropathy)** involving pain or loss of sensation, most commonly in the extremities. Loss of gastric motility **(gastroparesis)** also occurs. Figure 18–17 reviews the secondary complications of diabetes mellitus.

As a result of hormonal changes during pregnancy, **gestational diabetes** can occur in women with a predisposition to diabetes during the second or third trimester of pregnancy. After delivery, blood glucose usually returns to normal. Type 2 diabetes may develop in these women later in life.

Pituitary Gland (Anterior Lobe)

Hypersecretion

acromegaly

Enlargement of the extremities (acr/o means extremities) **caused by hypersecretion of the anterior pituitary *after* puberty.**

An excess of growth hormone (GH) is produced by adenomas of the pituitary gland that occur during adulthood. This excess GH stimulates the liver to secrete a hormone (somatomedin C, or IGF) that causes the clinical manifestations of acromegaly. Bones in the hands, feet, face, and jaw grow abnormally large, producing a characteristic Frankenstein-type facial appearance. The pituitary adenoma can be irradiated or surgically removed. Figure 18–18 shows a woman with acromegaly. Measurement of blood levels of somatomedin C as GH fluctuates is a test for acromegaly.

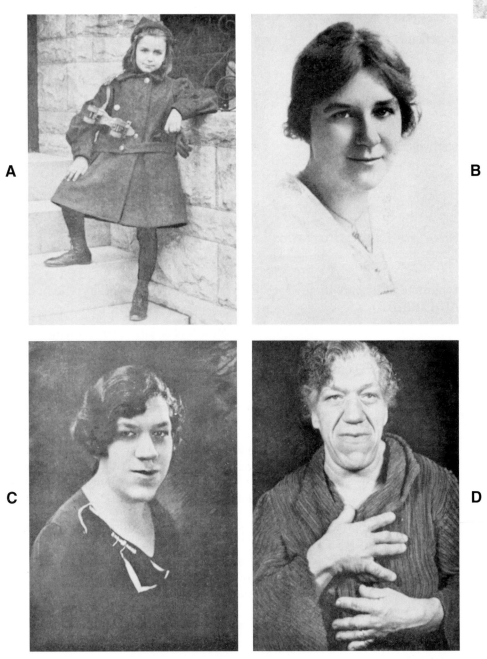

Figure 18–18

Progression of acromegaly: (A) patient at age 9; **(B)** age 16, with possible early features of acromegaly; **(C)** age 33, well-established acromegaly; **(D)** age 52, end-stage acromegaly. **(A-D** reprinted from Clinical Pathological Conference, Am J Med 1956; 20:133, with permission from Excerpta Medica, Inc.)

gigantism

Hyperfunctioning of the pituitary gland *before* puberty, leading to abnormal overgrowth of the body.

Benign adenomas of the pituitary gland that occur before a child reaches puberty produce an excess of growth hormone. Gigantism can be corrected by early diagnosis in childhood, followed by resection of the tumor or irradiation of the pituitary.

Hyposecretion

dwarfism

Congenital hyposecretion of growth hormone; hypopituitary dwarfism.

The children affected are normal mentally, but their bones remain small. Treatment consists of administration of growth hormone. Achondroplastic dwarfs differ from hypopituitary dwarfs in that they have a genetic defect in cartilage formation that limits the growth of long bones.

panhypopituitarism

All pituitary hormones are deficient.

Tumors of the sella turcica as well as arterial aneurysms may be etiological factors, causing a failure of the pituitary to secrete hormones that stimulate major glands in the body.

Pituitary Gland (Posterior Lobe)

Hypersecretion

syndrome of inappropriate ADH (SIADH)

Excessive secretion of antidiuretic hormone (ADH).

Hypersecretion of ADH produces excess water retention in the body. Treatment consists of dietary water restriction. Tumor, drug reactions, and head injury are some of the possible causes.

Hyposecretion

diabetes insipidus

Insufficient secretion of antidiuretic hormone (vasopressin).

Deficient antidiuretic hormone causes the kidney tubules to fail to hold back (reabsorb) needed water and salts. Clinical symptoms include polyuria and polydipsia. Synthetic preparations of ADH are administered with nasal sprays or intramuscularly as treatment. **Insipidus** means tasteless, reflecting the condition of dilute urine.

Table 18–4 reviews the abnormal conditions associated with hypersecretions and hyposecretions of the endocrine glands.

Table 18-4. ABNORMAL CONDITIONS OF ENDOCRINE GLANDS

Endocrine Gland	Hypersecretion	Hyposecretion
Adrenal cortex	Adrenal virilism Cushing syndrome	Addison disease
Adrenal medulla	Pheochromocytoma	
Pancreas	Hyperinsulinism	Diabetes mellitus
Parathyroid glands	Hyperparathyroidism (osteoporosis, kidney stones)	Hypoparathyroidism (tetany, hypocalcemia)
Pituitary (anterior lobe)	Acromegaly Gigantism	Dwarfism Panhypopituitarism
Pituitary (posterior lobe)	Syndrome of inappropriate antidiuretic hormone	Diabetes insipidus
Thyroid gland	Exophthalmic goiter (Graves disease, thyrotoxicosis) Nodular (adenomatous) goiter	Cretinism (children) Endemic goiter Myxedema (adults)

XII. Laboratory Tests

fasting blood sugar (FBS)

Measures circulating glucose level in a patient who has fasted at least 4 hours.

This test can diagnose diabetes mellitus. A nonfasting test is the **oral glucose tolerance test,** in which the patient drinks 75 grams of glucose and samples for glucose are drawn immediately at 30, 60, 90, and 120 minutes. This test is also used to diagnose gestational diabetes.

The **glycosylated hemoglobin test** measures long-term glucose control. A high level indicates poor glucose control in diabetic patients.

serum and urine tests

Measurement of hormones, electrolytes, glucose, and other substances in serum (blood) and urine as indicators of endocrine function.

Serum studies include growth hormone, somatomedin C (insulin-like growth factor 1), prolactin level, gonadotropin levels, parathyroid hormone, calcium, and cortisol.

Urine studies include glucose (Clinistix, Labstix), ketone (Acetest, Ketostix), and 17-ketosteroids (adrenal and gonadal function). A **urinary microalbumin test** measures small quantities of albumin in urine as a marker or harbinger of diabetic nephropathy.

thyroid function tests

Measurement of T_3, T_4, and TSH in the bloodstream.

XIII. Clinical Procedures

exophthalmometry	Measurement of eyeball protrusion (as in Graves disease) with an exophthalmometer.
computed tomography (CT) scan	Transverse x-ray views of endocrine glands to assess size and infiltration by tumor.
magnetic resonance imaging (MRI) of the head	Magnetic and radiofrequency pulses produce images of the hypothalamus and pituitary gland to locate abnormalities.
radioactive iodine uptake	Radioactive iodine is administered orally, and its uptake into the thyroid gland is measured as evidence of thyroid function.
thyroid scan	A scanner detects radioactivity and visualizes the thyroid gland after intravenous administration of a radioactive (technetium) compound.

Nodules and tumors can be evaluated.

Abbreviations

ACTH	adrenocorticotropic hormone		**ICSH**	interstitial cell–stimulating hormone
ADH	antidiuretic hormone (vasopressin)		**IDDM**	insulin-dependent diabetes mellitus; type 1 diabetes
BGM	blood glucose monitoring		**IGF**	insulin-like growth factor; also called somatomedin (produced in the liver, it stimulates the growth of bones)
BMR	basal metabolic rate (an indicator of thyroid function, but not in current use)			
DI	diabetes insipidus		**K**	potassium
DM	diabetes mellitus		**LH**	luteinizing hormone
FBG	fasting blood glucose		**MEN**	multiple endocrine neoplasia; hereditary hormonal disorder marked by adenomas and carcinomas
FBS	fasting blood sugar			
FSH	follicle-stimulating hormone		**Na**	sodium
GH	growth hormone		**NIDDM**	non insulin–dependent diabetes mellitus; type 2 diabetes
GTT	glucose tolerance test; ability to respond to a glucose load. This is a test for diabetes.		**17-OH**	17-hydroxycorticosteroids
			OT	oxytocin
HbA1C	test for the presence of glucose attached to hemoglobin (glycosylated hemoglobin test). A high level indicates poor glucose control in diabetic patients.		**PRL**	prolactin
			PTH	parathyroid hormone (parathormone)

RAI	radioactive iodine; treatment for Graves disease	T₃	triiodothyronine
RIA	radioimmunoassay; measures hormone levels in plasma	T₄	thyroxine
		TFT	thyroid function test
SIADH	syndrome of inappropriate ADH	TSH	thyroid-stimulating hormone
STH	somatotropin		

XIV. Practical Applications

Answers to the questions in each case report are on page 761 after Answers to Exercises.

Case Report 1

A 24-year-old college student, known diabetic, was admitted for treatment of ketoacidosis. He had a several-year history of diabetes and had been taking insulin in the morning and in the evening. After the history was pieced together from the patient and his friends, it appeared that he had been getting progressively ill over several days following a flu-like episode and may well not have taken his insulin on the day of admission. He was found, slightly drowsy and confused, by classmates. His respirations were rapid, his pulse was 126, and he offered no sensible answers to questions. Blood sugar level was elevated at 728 mg/dL [100 mg/dL is normal], and blood ketones were positive. The patient was treated with insulin intravenously, and over the course of the next 24 hours the ketoacidosis cleared.

Questions

1. **Ketoacidosis is a complication of**
   (A) diabetes insipidus
   (B) diabetes mellitus
   (C) both A and B
2. **A symptom of ketoacidosis is**
   (A) tachypnea
   (B) bradycardia
   (C) hypoglycemia
3. **Ketoacidosis occurs when**
   (A) insulin blood levels are high
   (B) sugar is not transported to cells and fats are burned improperly
   (C) insulin is given intravenously

B. Give the meanings of the following abbreviations for hormones.

1. ADH _____

2. ACTH _____

3. LH _____

4. FSH _____

5. TSH _____

6. PTH _____

7. GH _____

8. PRL _____

9. T_4 _____

10. T_3 _____

11. OT _____

12. STH _____

C. Match the following hormones with their actions.

ACTH	epinephrine	parathyroid hormone
ADH	estradiol	testosterone
aldosterone	insulin	thyroxine
cortisol		

1. sympathomimetic; raises heart rate and blood pressure _____

2. promotes growth and maintenance of male sex characteristics _____

3. stimulates water reabsorption by kidney tubules; decreases urine output _____

4. increases metabolism in body cells _____

5. raises blood calcium _____

6. increases reabsorption of sodium by kidney tubules _____

7. stimulates secretion of hormones from the adrenal cortex _____

8. increases blood sugar _____

9. helps transport glucose to cells and decreases blood sugar _____

10. develops and maintains female sex characteristics _____

D. Indicate whether the following conditions are related to hypersecretion or hyposecretion. Also, select from the following the endocrine gland and hormone involved in each disease.

Glands

		Hormones	
adenohypophysis	pancreas	ADH	GH
adrenal cortex	parathyroid gland	aldosterone	insulin
adrenal medulla	testes	cortisol	parathyroid hormone
neurohypophysis	thyroid	epinephrine	thyroxine
ovaries			

Condition	*Hypo or Hyper*	*Gland and Hormone*
1. Cushing syndrome	_____	_____
2. tetany	_____	_____
3. Graves disease	_____	_____
4. diabetes insipidus	_____	_____
5. acromegaly	_____	_____
6. myxedema	_____	_____
7. diabetes mellitus	_____	_____
8. Addison disease	_____	_____
9. gigantism	_____	_____
10. endemic goiter	_____	_____
11. cretinism	_____	_____
12. pheochromocytoma	_____	_____

E. Build medical terms based on the definitions and word parts given.

1. abnormal condition (poison) of the thyroid gland: thyro _____

2. removal of the pancreas: _____ ectomy

3. condition of deficiency or underdevelopment of the sex organs: hypo _____

4. pertaining to producing female (characteristics): _____ genic

5. removal of the pituitary gland: _____ ectomy

6. deficiency of calcium in the blood: hypo _____

7. excessive sugar in the blood: _____ emia

8. inflammation of the thyroid gland: _____ itis

9. specialist in the study of hormone disorders: _____ ist

10. disease condition of the adrenal glands: adren _____

F. Give the meanings of the following conditions.

1. hyponatremia _____

2. polydipsia _____

3. hyperkalemia _____

4. hypercalcemia _____

5. hypoglycemia _____

6. glycosuria _____

7. euthyroid _____

8. hyperthyroidism _____

9. tetany _____

10. ketoacidosis _____

G. The following hormones are all produced by the anterior lobe of the pituitary gland (note that they all have the same suffix, -tropin). Name the target tissue they act on or stimulate in the body.

1. gonadotropins _____

2. somatotropin _____

3. thyrotropin _____

4. adrenocorticotropin _____

H. Give the meanings of the following medical terms.

1. steroids _____

2. catecholamines _____

3. adenohypophysis _____

4. tetany _____

5. exophthalmos _____

6. mineralocorticoids _____

7. homeostasis _____

8. sympathomimetic _____

9. glucocorticoids _____

10. epinephrine _____

11. glycogen _____

12. androgen _____

13. corticosteroid _____

14. oxytocin _____

15. tetraiodothyronine _____

16. adrenal virilism _____

17. thyroid carcinoma _____

18. hirsutism _____

19. acromegaly _____

20. estradiol _____

I. Give the meanings of the following terms related to diabetes mellitus.

1. Type 1 _____

2. diabetic neuropathy _____

3. ketoacidosis _____

4. hypoglycemia _____

5. Type 2 _____

6. diabetic retinopathy _____

7. diabetic coma _____

8. diabetic nephropathy _____

9. atherosclerosis _____

10. hyperglycemia _____

11. gastroparesis _____

12. insulin shock _____

J. Explain the following laboratory tests or clinical procedures related to the endocrine system.

1. thyroid scan _____

2. fasting blood sugar _____

3. radioactive iodine uptake _____

4. exophthalmometry _____

K. Circle the term that best fits the meaning of the sentence.

1. Phyllis was diagnosed with Graves disease when her husband noticed her **(panhypopituitarism, hirsutism, exophthalmos)**. Her eyes seemed to be bulging out of their sockets.

2. Helen had a primary brain tumor called a **(pituitary, thyroid, adrenal)** adenoma. Her entire endocrine system was disrupted, and her physician recommended surgery and radiation to help relieve her symptoms.

3. Bessie's facial features gradually became "rough" in her late thirties and forties. By the time she was 50, her children noticed her very large hands and recommended that she see an endocrinologist, who diagnosed her chronically progressive condition as **(hyperinsulism, gigantism, acromegaly)**.

4. Bobby was brought into the emergency room because he was found passed out in the kitchen. He had forgotten his insulin and had developed **(Cushing disease, hyperparathyroidism, diabetic ketoacidosis)**.

5. Because her 1-hour test of blood sugar was slightly abnormal, Selma's obstetrician ordered a **(glucose tolerance test, thyroid function test, Pap smear)** to rule out gestational **(hyperthyroidism, chlamydial infection, diabetes)**.

6. Bill noticed that he was passing his urine more frequently **(polyphagia, polyuria, hyperglycemia)** and experiencing increased thirst **(polydipsia, hypernatremia, polyphagia)**. His wife urged him to see a physician, who performed a **(serum calcium test, urinalysis, serum sodium test)** that revealed inappropriately dilute **(blood, sweat, urine)**. Measurement of a hormone **(PTH, ADH, STH)** in his blood showed low levels. His diagnosis was **(DI, DM, SIADH)**. Treatment with **(oxytocin, cortisol, vasopressin)** was prescribed via nasal spray, and his condition improved.

7. Mary noticed that she had gained weight recently and that her face had a moon-like fullness with new heavy hair growth. Blood and urine tests showed excessive secretion of adrenal **(mineralocorticoids, catecholamines, glucocorticoids)**. **(CT scan of the abdomen, MRI of the head, chest x-ray)** revealed enlargement of both **(kidneys, adrenal glands, lobes of the brain)**. Her doctor made the diagnosis of **(Graves disease, Cushing syndrome, Addison disease)**.

8. Jack had several fractures of ribs and vertebrae in a skiing accident. X-rays of his bones revealed a generalized decrease in bone density **(osteoporosis, tetany, acromegaly)**. A blood test showed an elevated level of high serum **(sodium, calcium, growth hormone)** and high levels of **(mineralocorticoids, somatotropin, parathyroid hormone)**. A CT scan of the neck revealed a **(thymus, parathyroid, thyroid)** adenoma, which was removed surgically, and he recovered fully. His bone disease and symptoms were all related to **(hypoparathyroidism, hyperparathyroidism, hypothyroidism)**.

XVI. Answers to Exercises

A

1. anterior lobe of the pituitary gland (adenohypophysis)
2. posterior lobe of the pituitary gland (neurohypophysis)
3. adrenal cortex
4. islet cells of the pancreas
5. thyroid gland
6. adrenal cortex
7. anterior lobe of the pituitary gland; these hormones are FSH and LH
8. adrenal medulla
9. posterior lobe of the pituitary gland
10. anterior lobe of the pituitary gland
11. anterior lobe of the pituitary gland
12. islet cells of the pancreas
13. anterior lobe of the pituitary gland
14. ovaries
15. ovaries
16. testes

B

1. antidiuretic hormone
2. adrenocorticotropic hormone
3. luteinizing hormone
4. follicle-stimulating hormone
5. thyroid-stimulating hormone
6. parathyroid hormone
7. growth hormone
8. prolactin
9. thyroxine; tetraiodothyronine
10. triiodothyronine
11. oxytocin
12. somatotropin

C

1. epinephrine
2. testosterone
3. ADH
4. thyroxine
5. parathyroid hormone
6. aldosterone
7. ACTH
8. cortisol
9. insulin
10. estradiol

Continued on following page

adrenocorticotropic hormone (734)   ă-drē-nō-kŏr-tĭ-kō-TRŌP-ĭk HŎR-mōn   _____

adrenocorticotropin (734)   ă-drē-nō-kŏr-tĭ-kō-TRŌ-pĭn   _____

adrenopathy (737)   ă-drē-NŎP-ă-thē   _____

aldosterone (734)   ăl-DŎS-tě-rōn or ăl-dō-STĔR-ŏn   _____

androgen (734)   ĂN-drō-jěn   _____

antidiuretic hormone (734)   ăn-tĭ-dī-ū-RĔT-ĭk HŎR-mōn   _____

calcitonin (734)   kăl-sĭ-TŌ-nĭn   _____

catecholamines (736)   kăt-ě-KŌL-ă-mēnz   _____

corticosteroid (736)   kŏr-tĭ-kō-STĔ-royd   _____

cortisol (734)   KŎR-tĭ-sōl   _____

electrolyte (736)   ě-LĔK-trō-līt   _____

endocrinologist (738)   ěn-dō-krĭ-NŎL-ō-jĭst   _____

epinephrine (735)   ěp-ĭ-NĔF-rĭn   _____

estradiol (735)   ěs-tră-DĪ-ŏl   _____

estrogen (735)   ĔS-trō-jěn   _____

estrogenic (738)   ěs-trō-JĔN-ĭk   _____

euthyroid (740)   ū-THĪ-royd   _____

follicle-stimulating hormone (735)   FŎL-ĭ-k'l STĬM-ū-lā-ting HŎR-mōn   _____

glucagon (735)   GLOO-kă-gŏn   _____

glucocorticoid (736)   gloo-kō-KŎR-tĭ-koyd   _____

glycemic (738)   glī-SĒ-mĭk   _____

glycogen (738)   GLĪ-kō-jěn   _____

glycosuria (740)   glī-kōs-Ū-rē-ă   _____

gonadocorticoid (736)   gō-năd-ō-KŎR-tĭ-koyd   _____

gonadotropin (737)   gō-năd-ō-TRŌ-pĭn   _____

growth hormone (735)   GRŌ-TH HŎR-mōn   _____

homeostasis (736)	hō-mē-ō-STĀ-sĭs	
hormonal (739)	hŏr-MŎ-năl	
hormone (736)	HŎR-mōn	
hypercalcemia (738)	hī-pĕr-kăl-SĒ-mē-ă	
hyperglycemia (738)	hī-pĕr-glī-SĒ-mē-ă	
hypocalcemia (738)	hī-pō-kăl-SĒ-mē-ă	
hypogonadism (737)	hī-pō-GŌ-năd-ĭzm	
hypoinsulinism (739)	hī-pō-ĬN-sū-lĭn-ĭzm	
hypokalemia (739)	hī-pō-kā-LĒ-mē-ă	
hyponatremia (739)	hī-pō-nā-TRĒ-mē-ă	
hypophysectomy (739)	hī-pō-fĭ-SĔK-tō-mē	
hypophysis (734)	hī-PŎF-ĭ-sĭs	
hypopituitarism (737)	hī-pō-pĭ-TOO-ĭ-tă-rĭzm	
hypothalamus (736)	hī-pō-THĂL-ă-mŭs	
insulin (735)	ĬN-sū-lĭn	
luteinizing hormone (735)	LŪ-tē-ĭn-īz-ĭng HŎR-mōn	
mineralocorticoid (736)	mĭn-ĕr-ăl-ō-KŎR-tĭ-koyd	
neurohypophysis (734)	nū-rō-hī-PŎF-ĭ-sĭs	
norepinephrine (735)	nŏr-ĕp-ĭ-NĔF-rĭn	
oxytocin (735)	ŏk-sĕ-TŌ-sĭn	
pancreas (734)	PĂN-krē-ăs	
pancreatectomy (737)	păn-krē-ă-TĔK-tō-mē	
parathormone (735)	păr-ă-THŎR-mōn	
parathyroidectomy (737)	păr-ă-thī-roy-DĔK-tō-mē	
parathyroid glands (734)	păr-ă-THĪ-royd glănz	
pineal gland (720)	pī-NĒ-ăl glănd	
pituitary gland (734)	pĭ-TOO-ĭ-tĕr-ē glănd	

polydipsia (738)   pŏl-ē-DĬP-sē-ă   _____

progesterone (735)   prō-JĔS-tĕ-rōn   _____

prolactin (735)   prō-LĂK-tĭn   _____

sella turcica (736)   SĔL-ă TŬR-sĭ-kă   _____

somatotropin (735)   sō-mă-tō-TRŌ-pĭn   _____

steroid (736)   STĔR-oyd   _____

sympathomimetic (736) sĭm-pă-thō-mĭ-MĔT-ĭk _____

testosterone (735)   tĕs-TŎS-tĕ-rōn   _____

tetraiodothyronine (736) tĕ-tră-ī-ō-dō-THĪ-rō-nēn _____

thyroid gland (734)   THĪ-royd glănd   _____

thyroiditis (737)   thī-royd-Ī-tĭs   _____

thyrotropin (735)   thī-rō-TRŌ-pĭn   _____

thyroxine (736)   thī-RŎK-sĭn   _____

triiodothyronine (736) trī-ī-ō-dō-THĪ-rō-nĕn _____

vasopressin (736)   văz-ō-PRĔS-ĭn   _____

Abnormal Conditions, Laboratory Tests, and Clinical Procedures

Term	Pronunciation	Meaning
acromegaly (746)	ăk-rō-MĔG-ă-lē	_____
Addison disease (744)	ĂD-ĭ-sŏn dĭ-ZĒZ	_____
adrenal virilism (743)	ă-DRĒ-năl VĬR-ĭ-lĭzm	_____
cretinism (742)	KRĒ-tĭn-ĭzm	_____
Cushing syndrome (743)	KŬSH-ĭng SĬN-drōm	_____
diabetes insipidus (748)	dī-ă-BĒ-tēz ĭn-SĬP-ĭ-dŭs	_____
diabetes mellitus (744)	dī-ă-BĒ-tēz MĔL-ĭ-tŭs or mĕ-LĪ-tŭs	_____
dwarfism (748)	DWARF-ĭzm	_____
endemic goiter (741)	ĕn-DĔM-ĭk GOY-tĕr	_____

exophthalmos (741)	ĕk-sŏf-THĂL-mōs	_____
exophthalmometry (750)	ĕk-sŏf-thăl-MŎM-ĕ-trē	_____
fasting blood sugar (749)	FĂS-tĭng blŭd SŬG-ăr	_____
gastroparesis (746)	găs-trō-păr-Ē-sĭs	_____
gigantism (748)	JĪ-găn-tĭzm	_____
glucose tolerance test (749)	GLŪ-kōs TŎL-ĕr-ăns test	_____
goiter (741)	GOY-tĕr	_____
Graves disease (741)	GRĀVZ dĭ-ZĒZ	_____
hirsutism (743)	HĔR-soo t-ĭzm	_____
hyperinsulinism (744)	hī-pĕr-ĬN-sū-lĭn-ĭzm	_____
hyperparathyroidism (743)	hī-pĕr-pă-ră-THĪ-royd-ĭzm	_____
hyperthyroidism (741)	hī-pĕr-THĪ-royd-ĭsm	_____
hypoparathyroidism (743)	hī-pō-pă-ră-THĪ-royd-ĭzm	_____
hypothyroidism (742)	hī-pō-THĪ-royd-ĭzm	_____
ketoacidosis (745)	kē-tō-ă-sĭ-DŌ-sĭs	_____
myxedema (742)	mĭk-sĕ-DĒ-mă	_____
nodular goiter (741)	NŎD-ū-lăr GOY-tĕr	_____
panhypopituitarism (748)	păn-hī-pō-pĭ-TŪ-ĭ-tăr-ĭzm	_____
pheochromocytoma (744)	fē-ō-krō-mō-sī-TŌ-mă	_____
radioactive iodine uptake (750)	rā-dē-ō-ĂK-tĭv Ī-ō-dīn ŬP-tāk	_____
syndrome of inappropriate ADH (748)	SĬN-drōm of ĭn-ă-PRŌ-prē-ĭt ADH	_____
tetany (743)	TĔT-ă-nē	_____
thyroid carcinoma (742)	THĪ-royd kăr-sĭ-NŌ-mă	_____
thyroid function tests (749)	THĪ-royd FŬNK-shŭn tĕsts	_____
thyroid scan (750)	THĪ-royd skăn	_____
thyrotoxicosis (741)	thī-rō-tŏk-sĭ-KŌ-sĭs	_____

III. Carcinogenesis

What Causes Cancer?

The process of transformation from a normal cell to a cancerous one **(carcinogenesis)** is only partially understood at the present time. What is clear is that malignant transformation results from damage to the genetic material, or **DNA (deoxyribonucleic acid),** of the cell. Strands of DNA in the cell nucleus form **chromosomes,** which become readily visible under a microscope when a cell is preparing to divide into two (daughter) cells. In order to understand what causes cancer, it is necessary to learn more about DNA and its functions in a normal cell.

DNA has two main functions in a normal cell. First, DNA controls the production of new cells (cell division). When a cell divides, the DNA material in each chromosome copies itself so that exactly the same DNA is passed to the two new daughter cells that are formed. This process of cell division is called **mitosis** (Fig. 19–4A).

Second, between cycles of mitosis, DNA controls the production of new proteins **(protein synthesis)** in the cell. DNA contains about 40,000 separate and distinct **genes** that direct the process of protein synthesis. Genes are made up of an arrangement of units called **nucleotides** (containing a sugar, phosphate, and base, such as adenine, guanine, thymine, or cytosine). DNA (as coded nucleotides) sends a molecular message outside the nucleus to the cytoplasm of the cell, directing the synthesis of specific proteins (such as hormones and enzymes) essential for normal cell function and growth. This message is transmitted in the following way. In the nucleus, the coded message with instructions for making a specific protein is copied from DNA onto another molecule called **RNA (ribonucleic acid).** Then RNA travels from the nucleus to the cytoplasm of the cell, carrying the coded message to direct the formation of specific proteins (Fig. 19–4B).

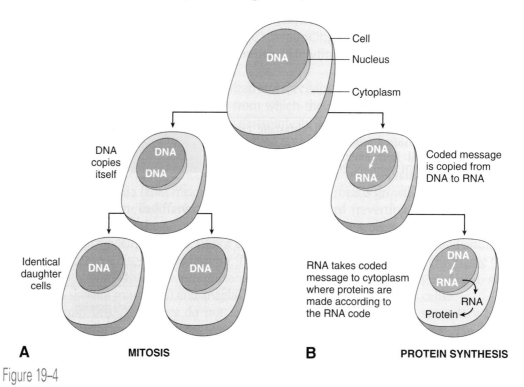

A   **MITOSIS**   **B**   **PROTEIN SYNTHESIS**

Figure 19–4

Two functions of DNA. (A) Mitosis (the process of cell division). **(B)** Protein synthesis (creating new proteins for cellular growth).

When a cell becomes malignant, however, the processes of mitosis and protein synthesis are disturbed. Cancer cells reproduce almost continuously, and abnormal proteins are made. Malignant cells are anaplastic; that is, their DNA stops making codes that allow the cells to carry on the function of mature cells. Instead, altered DNA and altered cellular programs make new signals that lead to cell proliferation, movement of cells, invasion of adjacent tissue, and metastasis.

The damage to DNA that results in malignancy may be caused by environmental factors, such as toxic chemicals, sunlight, tobacco smoke, and viruses. The specific damage usually involves chemical changes in the nucleotide components of DNA. These changes interfere with the accurate coding for new protein synthesis. Once these changes are established in a cell, they are passed on to daughter cells. Such an inheritable change in DNA is called a **mutation.** Mutations, particularly those that affect cell growth or DNA repair, lead to malignant growths.

Although most DNA changes, or mutations, lead to higher-than-normal rates of growth, some mutations found in cancer cells actually prevent the cells from dying. In recent years, scientists have recognized that some types of cancers have lost the normal blueprints that direct aging or damaged cells to die. Normal cells undergo spontaneous disintegration by a process known as **apoptosis,** or programmed cell death. Some cancer cells have lost elements of this program and thus can live indefinitely.

Environmental Agents

Agents from the environment, such as chemicals, drugs, tobacco smoke, radiation, and viruses, can cause damage to DNA and thus produce cancer. These environmental agents are called **carcinogens.**

Chemical carcinogens are found in a variety of products and drugs, including **hydrocarbons** (in cigarette, cigar, and pipe smoke and automobile exhaust), insecticides, dyes, industrial chemicals, insulation, and hormones. For example, the hormone diethylstilbestrol (DES) causes a malignant tumor, carcinoma of the vagina, in daughters of women treated with DES during pregnancy. Drugs such as estrogens can cause cancer by stimulating the proliferation of cells in target organs such as the lining of the uterus.

Radiation, whatever its source—sunlight, x-rays, radioactive substances, nuclear fission—is a wave of energy. When this energy interacts with DNA, it causes DNA damage and mutations that lead to cancer. Thus, leukemia (a cancerous condition of white blood cells) may be an occupational hazard of radiologists, who are routinely exposed to x-rays. There is a high incidence of leukemia and other cancers among survivors of atomic bomb explosions, as at Hiroshima and Nagasaki. Ultraviolet radiation given off by the sun can cause skin cancer, especially in persons with lightly pigmented, or fair, skin.

Some **viruses** are carcinogenic. For example, the human T-cell leukemia virus (HTLV) causes a form of leukemia in adults. Kaposi sarcoma is caused by another virus, herpes type VIII. Other viruses are known to cause cervical cancer (papilloma virus) and a tumor of lymph nodes called Burkitt lymphoma (Epstein-Barr virus). These tumor-producing viruses, called **oncogenic viruses,** fall into two categories: **RNA viruses** (composed of RNA and known as retroviruses) and **DNA viruses** (composed of DNA).

In addition to transmission of cancer by whole viruses, pieces of normal DNA called **oncogenes** can cause normal cells to become malignant if they are activated by mutations. An oncogene (cancer-causing gene) is a piece of DNA whose activation is associated with the conversion of a normal cell into a cancerous cell. Some examples of

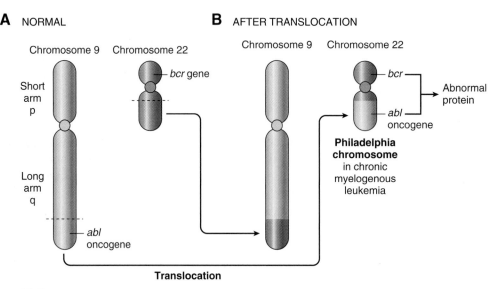

A NORMAL

B AFTER TRANSLOCATION

Figure 19–5

Chromosomal (oncogene) translocation leading to the Philadelphia chromosome and chronic myelogenous leukemia (CML). **(A)** Normal chromosomes 9 and 22. **(B)** Translocation of the *abl* oncogene from the long arm (q) of chromosome 9 to the long arm of chromosome 22 (next to the *bcr* gene). This forms a combination oncogene *bcr-abl* that produces an abnormal protein (tyrosine kinase), which leads to malignant transformation (CML).

oncogenes are *ras* (colon cancer), *myc* (lymphoma), and *bcr-abl* (chronic myelogenous leukemia).

In chronic myelogenous leukemia, the oncogene *bcr-abl* is activated when pieces from two different chromosomes switch locations. This genetic change (mutation) is called a **translocation.** The oncogene *abl* on chromosome 9 moves to a new location on the base of chromosome 22, close to a gene called *bcr.* When these two genes are located near each other, they cause the production of an abnormal protein that makes the leukocyte divide and causes a malignancy (chronic myelogenous leukemia). The new chromosome formed from the translocation is called the **Philadelphia chromosome** (it was discovered in 1970 in Philadelphia) (Fig. 19–5).

Heredity

Cancer may be caused not only by environmental factors, but also by inherited factors. Susceptibility to some forms of cancer is transmitted from parents to offspring through defects in the DNA of the egg or sperm cells. Examples of known inherited cancers are **retinoblastoma** (tumor of the retina of the eye), **polyposis coli syndrome** (polyps that grow in the colon and rectum), and certain other inherited forms of colon, breast, and kidney cancer.

Each of these diseases is caused by loss of a segment of DNA or by a change in the coding sequence of DNA. Detection of these changes in the DNA code is possible by analysis of genes on a chromosome. This is accomplished through DNA sequencing, a step-by-step analysis of the nucleotide sequence of the affected gene, or by small DNA probes that test the overall fit of a person's gene to a normal gene sequence.

In many cases, it is believed that these tumors arise because of inherited or acquired abnormalities in certain genes called **suppressor genes.** In normal individuals, these

Table 19–1. GENES IMPLICATED IN HEREDITARY CANCERS

Cancer	Gene	Chromosomal Location*
Breast; ovarian	*BRCA1*	17q21
Breast; ovarian	*BRCA2*	13q12-13
Polyposis coli syndrome	*APC*	5q21
Li-Fraumeni (multiple cancers)	*p53*	17p13
Retinoblastoma	*Rb1*	13q14
Wilms tumor	*WT1*	11p13
Renal cell carcinoma	*VHL*	3p21-26

*The first number is the chromosome; p is the short arm of the chromosome, and q is the long arm of the chromosome. The second number is the region (band) of the chromosome.

suppressor genes regulate growth, promote differentiation, and suppress oncogenes from causing cancer. Loss of a normal suppressor gene takes the brake off the process of cell division and leads to cancer. Examples of suppressor genes are the **retinoblastoma gene (Rb-1)** and the **p53** gene (named after the molecular weight of the protein that it codes for). A loss or mutation of the p53 gene (located on chromosome 17) can lead to numerous human cancers, such as colon and breast cancer.

Because inherited changes can be detected in all tissues of the body, not simply cancerous cells, blood cells from family members may be tested to determine whether a person has inherited the cancer-causing gene. This is known as **genetic screening.** Affected individuals may be watched carefully to detect tumors at an early stage. Table 19–1 lists several hereditary cancers and the name of the responsible gene. Figure 19–6 reviews the role of environmental agents and heredity in carcinogenesis.

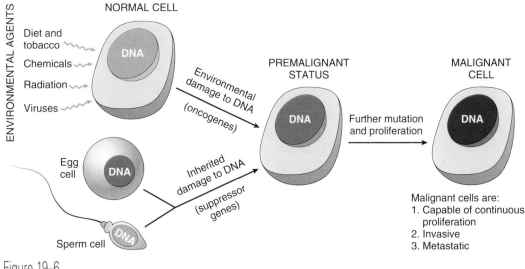

Figure 19–6

The role of environmental agents and heredity in carcinogenesis (transformation of a normal to malignant cell).

IV. Classification of Cancerous Tumors

Almost half of all cancer deaths are caused by malignancies that originate in lung, breast, or colon; however, in all there are more than 100 distinct types of cancer, each having a unique set of symptoms and requiring a specific type of therapy. It is possible to divide these types of cancer into three broad groups on the basis of **histogenesis**—that is, by identifying the particular type of tissue **(hist/o)** from which the tumor cells arise **(-genesis).** These major groups are **carcinomas, sarcomas,** and **mixed-tissue tumors.**

Carcinomas

Carcinomas, the largest group, are solid tumors that are derived from epithelial tissue that lines external and internal body surfaces, including skin, glands, and digestive, urinary, and reproductive organs. Approximately 90 percent of all malignancies are carcinomas.

Table 19–2 gives examples of specific carcinomas and the epithelial tissue from which they derive. Benign tumors of epithelial origin are usually designated by the term **adenoma,** which indicates that the tumor is of epithelial or glandular **(aden/o)** origin. For

Table 19–2. CARCINOMAS AND THE EPITHELIAL TISSUES FROM WHICH THEY DERIVE

Type of Epithelial Tissue	Malignant Tumor (Carcinomas)
GASTROINTESTINAL TRACT	
Colon	Adenocarcinoma of the colon
Esophagus	Esophageal carcinoma
Liver	Hepatocellular carcinoma (hepatoma)
Stomach	Gastric adenocarcinoma
GLANDULAR TISSUE	
Adrenal glands	Carcinoma of the adrenals
Breast	Carcinoma of the breast
Pancreas	Carcinoma of the pancreas (pancreatic adenocarcinoma)
Prostate	Carcinoma of the prostate
Thyroid	Carcinoma of the thyroid
KIDNEY AND BLADDER	
	Renal cell carcinoma (hypernephroma)
	Transitional cell carcinoma of the bladder
LUNG	
	Adenocarcinoma (bronchioloalveolar)
	Large cell carcinoma
	Small (oat) cell carcinoma
	Squamous cell (epidermoid)
REPRODUCTIVE ORGANS	
	Adenocarcinoma of the uterus
	Carcinoma of the penis
	Choriocarcinoma of the uterus or testes
	Cystadenocarcinoma (mucinous or serous) of the ovaries
	Seminoma and embryonal cell carcinoma (testes)
	Squamous cell (epidermoid) carcinoma of the vagina or cervix
SKIN	
Basal cell layer	Basal cell carcinoma
Melanocyte	Malignant melanoma
Squamous cell layer	Squamous cell carcinoma

example, a gastric adenoma is a benign tumor of the glandular epithelial cells lining the stomach. Malignant tumors of epithelial origin are named by using the term **carcinoma** and adding the type of tissue in which the tumor occurs. Thus, a **gastric adenocarcinoma** is a cancerous tumor arising from glandular cells lining the stomach.

Sarcomas

Sarcomas are less common than carcinomas, comprising less than 5 percent of all malignant tumors. They derive from connective tissues in the body, such as bone, fat, muscle, cartilage, and bone marrow and from cells of the lymphatic system. Often, the term **mesenchymal tissue** is used to describe embryonic connective tissue from which sarcomas are derived. The middle, or mesodermal, layer of the embryo gives rise to the connective tissues of the body as well as to blood and lymphatic vessels.

Table 19–3 gives examples of specific types of sarcomas and the connective tissues from which they derive. Benign tumors of connective tissue origin are named by adding the suffix **-oma** to the type of tissue in which the tumor occurs. For example, a benign tumor of bone is called an **osteoma.** Malignant tumors of connective tissue origin are frequently named by using the term **sarcoma** (**sarc/o** means flesh). For example, an **osteosarcoma** is a malignant tumor of bone.

Table 19–3. **SARCOMAS AND THE CONNECTIVE TISSUES FROM WHICH THEY DERIVE**

Type of Connective Tissue	Malignant Tumor
BONE	
	Osteosarcoma (osteogenic sarcoma)
	Ewing sarcoma
MUSCLE	
Smooth (visceral) muscle	Leiomyosarcoma
Striated (skeletal) muscle	Rhabdomyosarcoma
CARTILAGE	
	Chondrosarcoma
FAT	
	Liposarcoma
FIBROUS TISSUE	
	Fibrosarcoma
BLOOD VESSEL TISSUE	
	Angiosarcoma
BLOOD-FORMING TISSUE	
All leukocytes	Leukemias
Lymphocytes	Hodgkin disease
	Non-Hodgkin lymphomas
	Burkitt lymphoma
Plasma cells	Multiple myeloma
NERVE TISSUE	
Embryonic nerve tissue	Neuroblastoma
Glial tissue	Astrocytoma (tumor of glial cells called astrocytes)
	Glioblastoma multiforme

Table 19-4. MIXED-TISSUE TUMORS

Type of Tissue	Malignant Tumor
Kidney	Wilms tumor (embryonal adenosarcoma)
Ovaries and testes	Teratoma (tumor composed of bone, muscle, skin, gland cells, cartilage, etc.)

In addition to the solid tumors of connective tissue origin, sarcomas include tumors arising from blood-forming tissue. **Leukemias** are tumors derived from bone marrow, whereas **lymphomas** are derived from immune cells of the lymphatic system. Connective tissue within the brain (glial cells) and embryonic tissue of the nervous system give rise to **gliomas** (such as astrocytomas of the brain) and **neuroblastomas.**

Mixed-tissue Tumors

Mixed-tissue tumors are derived from tissue that is capable of differentiating into both epithelial and connective tissue. These uncommon tumors are thus composed of several different types of cells. Examples of mixed-tissue tumors (Table 19–4) can be found in the kidney, ovaries, and testes.

V. Pathological Descriptions

The following terms are used to describe the appearance of a malignant tumor, on either gross (visual) or on microscopic examination.

Gross Descriptions

cystic	Forming large open spaces filled with fluid. **Mucinous** tumors are filled with mucus (thick, sticky fluid), and **serous** tumors are filled with a thin, watery fluid resembling serum. The most common site of cystic tumors is in ovaries.
fungating	Mushrooming pattern of growth in which tumor cells pile one on top of another and project from a tissue surface. Tumors found in the colon are often of this type.
inflammatory	Having the features of inflammation; that is, redness, swelling, and heat. Inflammatory changes result from tumor blockage of the lymphatic drainage of the skin, as in breast cancer.
medullary	Pertaining to large, soft, fleshy tumors. Thyroid and breast tumors may be medullary.
necrotic	Containing dead tissue. Any type of tumor can outgrow its blood supply and undergo necrosis.

polypoid	Growths that are like projections extending outward from a base. **Sessile** polypoid tumors extend from a broad base, and **pedunculated** polypoid tumors extend from a stem or stalk. Both benign and malignant tumors of the colon may grow as polyps.
ulcerating	Characterized by an open, exposed surface resulting from the death of overlying tissue. Ulcerating tumors are often found in the stomach, breast, colon, and skin.
verrucous	Resembling a wart-like growth. Tumors of the gingiva (gum) are frequently verrucous.

Microscopic Descriptions

alveolar	Tumor cells form patterns resembling small, microscopic sacs; commonly found in tumors of muscle, bone, fat, and cartilage.
carcinoma *in situ*	Referring to localized tumor cells that have not invaded adjacent structures. Cancer of the cervix may begin as carcinoma *in situ.*
diffuse	Spreading evenly throughout the affected tissue. Malignant lymphomas may display diffuse involvement of lymph nodes.
dysplastic	Pertaining to abnormal formation of cells. These tumors display a highly abnormal but not clearly cancerous appearance. Dysplastic nevi (moles on skin) are an example.
epidermoid	Resembling squamous epithelial cells (thin, plate-like), often occurring in the respiratory tract.
follicular	Forming small, microscopic, gland-type sacs. Thyroid gland cancer is an example.
nodular	Forming multiple areas of tightly packed clusters of cells with lightly populated areas in between. Malignant lymphomas may display a nodular pattern of lymph node involvement.
papillary	Forming small, finger-like or nipple-like projections of cells. Bladder or thyroid gland cancer may be described as papillary.
pleomorphic	Composed of a variety of types of cells. Mixed-cell tumors are examples.
scirrhous	Densely packed (scirrhous means hard) tumors, containing dense bands of fibrous tissue; commonly found in breast or stomach cancers.
undifferentiated	Lacking microscopic structures typical of normal mature cells.

VI. Grading and Staging Systems

Tumors are classified on the basis of their location, microscopic appearance, and extent of spread. Of particular importance are the tumor's **grade** (its degree of maturity or differentiation under the microscope) and its **stage** (its extent of spread within the body). These two properties influence the prognosis (the chances of successful treatment and survival) and determine the specific treatment to be used.

When grading a tumor, the pathologist is concerned with the microscopic appearance of the tumor cells, specifically with their degree of maturation or differentiation. Often, three or four grades are used. **Grade I** tumors are very well differentiated, so that they closely resemble cells from the normal parent tissue of their origin. **Grade IV** tumors are so undifferentiated or anaplastic that even recognition of the tumor's tissue of origin may be difficult. **Grades II** and **III** are intermediate in appearance, moderately or poorly differentiated, as opposed to well differentiated (grade I) and undifferentiated (grade IV).

Grading is often of value in determining the prognosis of certain types of cancers, such as cancer of the urinary bladder, prostate gland, ovary, and brain tumors (astrocytomas). Patients with grade I tumors have a high survival rate, and patients with grades II, III, and IV tumors have an increasingly poorer survival rate. Grading is also used in evaluating cells obtained from body fluids in preventive screening tests, such as **Papanicolaou (Pap) smears** of the uterine cervix, tracheal secretions, or stomach secretions.

The staging of cancerous tumors is based on the extent of spread of the tumor. An example of a staging system is the **TNM/International Staging System.** It has been applied to malignancies such as lung cancer, as well as to many other tumors. **T** refers to the size and degree of local extension of the **tumor; N** refers to the number of regional lymph **nodes** that have been invaded by tumor; and **M** refers to the presence or absence of **metastases** (spreads to distant sites) of the tumor cells. Numbers denote size and degree of involvement: For example, 0 indicates undetectable, and 1, 2, 3, and 4 a progressive increase in size or involvement. TNM may be based on clinical data (physical examination and radiological assessment) or actual pathologic evaluation of the tumor and adjacent lymph nodes. In some cases, bone marrow, liver, or other tissues are biopsied to confirm metastases. Table 19–5 presents the TNM staging system for lung cancer.

Other staging systems use letters such as A, B, C, and D or numbers such as I, II, III, and IV to indicate the extent of spread of tumor in the body. For example, in the Duke staging system for colon cancer, A = disease confined to the colon; B = penetration of the muscle lining in the wall of the colon; C = involvement of lymph nodes; D = metastasis.

Table 19-5. **INTERNATIONAL TNM STAGING SYSTEM FOR LUNG CANCER**

Stage	TNM Description	5-Year Survival, %
I	T1-T2, N0, M0	60–80
II	T1-2, N1, M0	25–50
III A	T3, N0-1, M0	25–40
	T1-3, N2, M0	10–30
III B	Any T4 or N3, M0	<5
IV	Any M1	<5

Primary Tumor (T)

T1	Tumor <3 cm diameter
T2	Tumor >3 cm diameter or has associated atelectasis-obstructive pneumonitis extending to the hilar region
T3	Tumor with direct extension into the chest wall, diaphragm, mediastinum, pleura, or pericardium
T4	Tumor invades the mediastinum or presence of a malignant pleural effusion

Regional Lymph Nodes (N)

N0	No node involvement
N1	Metastasis to lymph nodes in the peribronchial and ipsilateral (same side as the primary tumor) hilar region
N2	Metastasis to ipsilateral hilar and subcarinal (under the bifurcation of the trachea into the lungs) lymph nodes
N3	Metastasis to contralateral mediastinal or hilar nodes or any nodes near the clavicular (collar) bone

Distant Metastasis (M)

M0	No known metastasis
M1	Distant metastasis present with site specified (e.g., brain, liver)

Source: Modified from *Harrison's Manual of Medicine,* 15th ed. New York: McGraw-Hill Professional, 2002, p. 284.

VII. Cancer Treatment

Four major approaches to cancer treatment are **surgery, radiation therapy, chemotherapy,** and **biological therapy.** Each method **(modality)** may be used alone, but often they are used together in combined-modality programs to improve the overall treatment result.

Surgery

In many patients with cancer, the tumor is discovered before it has spread, and it may be cured by surgical excision. Some common cancers in which surgery may be curative are those of the stomach, breast, colon, lung, and uterus (endometrium). Often, surgical removal of the primary tumor prevents local spread or complications, even in the presence of distant disease. A **debulking procedure** may be used if the tumor is attached to a vital organ and cannot be completely removed. As much tissue as possible is removed and the patient receives **adjuvant** (assisting) radiation or chemotherapy.

The following is a list of terms that describe surgical procedures used in treating cancer.

cryosurgery	Malignant tissue is frozen and thus destroyed. This procedure is occasionally used to treat bladder and prostate tumors.
electrocauterization	Malignant tissue is destroyed by burning. Electrocauterization is used in treating tumors of the rectum and colon, when surgical removal is not possible.
en bloc resection	Tumor is removed along with a large area of surrounding tissue containing lymph nodes. Modified radical mastectomy, colectomy, and gastrectomy are examples.
excisional biopsy	Removal of tumor and a margin of normal tissue. This procedure provides a specimen for diagnosis and may be curative for small tumors.
exenteration	Wide resection involving removal of the tumor, its organ of origin, and all surrounding tissue in the body space. Pelvic exenteration may be performed to treat large primary tumors of the uterus.
fulguration	Destruction of tissue by electric sparks generated by a high-frequency current.
incisional biopsy	Piece of tumor is removed for examination to establish a diagnosis. More extensive surgical procedure or other forms of treatment, such as chemotherapy or x-ray, then are used to treat the bulk of the tumor.

Radiation Therapy (Radiation Oncology)

The goal of radiation therapy is to deliver a maximal dose of ionizing radiation (irradiation) to the tumor tissue and a minimal dose to the surrounding normal tissue. In reality, this goal is difficult to achieve, and usually one accepts a degree of residual normal cell damage (**morbidity**) as a side effect of the destruction of the tumor. High-dose radiation produces damage to DNA. Newer techniques of radiation utilize high-energy beams of **protons** (atomic particles) to improve the focus of the beam and limit damage to normal tissues.

Terms used in the field of radiation therapy for cancer are as follows:

brachytherapy	Implantation of small, scaled containers or **seeds** of radioactive material directly into the tumor **(interstitial therapy);** or in close proximity to the tumor **(intracavitary therapy).** An implant may be temporary (as in tumors of the head and neck or gynecologic malignancies) or permanent with prostatic implants (seeds) into tumors.
electron beams	Low-energy beams for treatment of skin or surface tumors.
external beam radiation (teletherapy)	Radiation applied to a tumor from a distant source (linear accelerator).
fields	Defined areas that are bombarded by radiation.
fractionation	A method of dividing radiation into small, repeated doses rather than providing fewer large doses. Fractionation allows larger total doses to be given while causing less damage to normal tissue.
gray (Gy)	Unit of radiation equal to 100 rad (radiation dose absorbed by the tissue).
linear accelerator	A large electronic device that produces high-energy x-ray (or photon) beams for the treatment of deep-seated tumors. (See Figure 19–7.)

Figure 19–7

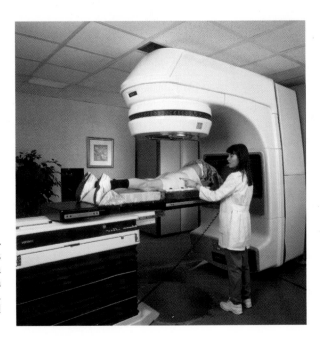

Linear accelerator. Radiation therapy is delivered to a patient positioned under a linear accelerator to receive treatment for a lesion in the posterior portion of his hip. (Courtesy Dr. Arthur Brimberg, Riverhill Radiation Oncology, Yonkers, New York.)

proton therapy

Highly focused, high-energy irradiation. This treatment requires large machinery such as a cyclotron to generate particles.

rad

Radiation absorbed dose.

radiocurable tumor

Tumor that can be completely eradicated by radiation therapy. Usually, this is a localized tumor with no evidence of metastasis. Lymphomas and Hodgkin disease are examples. (See Figure 19–8.)

radioresistant tumor

Tumor that requires large doses of radiation to produce death of the cells. Connective tissue tumors are the most radioresistant.

radiosensitive tumor

Tumor in which irradiation can cause the death of cells without serious damage to surrounding tissue. Tumors of hematopoietic (blood-forming) and lymphatic origins are radiosensitive.

radiosensitizers

Drugs that increase the sensitivity of tumors to x-rays. Many cancer chemotherapy drugs, especially 5-fluorouracil and cisplatin, sensitize tumors and normal tissue to radiation and improve the outcome of treatment.

A 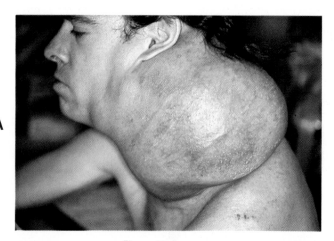 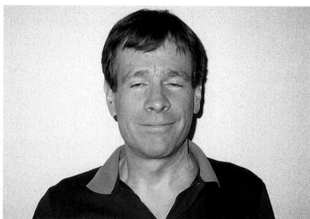 B

Figure 19–8

(A) Patient with Hodgkin disease before radiation therapy. **(B)** Patient 6 years after radiation therapy. (From Lewis SM, Heitkemper MM, Dirksen SR: Medical-Surgical Nursing: Assessment and Management of Clinical Problems, 5th ed. St. Louis, Mosby, 2000, p. 287.)

Radiotherapy, although it may be either a **palliative** (relieving symptoms) or curative agent, can produce undesirable side effects on normal body tissues that are incidentally irradiated. Some complications are reversible with time, and recovery takes place soon after radiotherapy is completed. Side effects include the following:

Alopecia (baldness); usually permanent with radiation
Fibrosis (increase in connective tissue) in the lungs
Mucositis (inflammation and ulceration of mucous membranes); in the mouth, pharynx, vagina, bladder, large or small intestine
Myelosuppression (bone marrow depression); anemia, leukopenia, and thrombocytopenia
Nausea and vomiting; as reaction to radiation to the brain (vomiting center is located in the brain) or gastrointestinal tract (loss of epithelial lining tissue)
Pneumonitis (inflammation of the lungs)
Xerostomia (dryness of the mouth); occurs after radiation to the salivary glands

Chemotherapy, Biological Therapy, and Differentiating Agents

Chemotherapy

Cancer chemotherapy is the treatment of cancer using chemicals (drugs). It is the standard treatment for many types of cancer, and it produces cures in most patients who have choriocarcinoma, testicular cancer, acute lymphocytic leukemia, and Hodgkin disease. Chemotherapy may be used alone or in combination with surgery and radiation to improve cure rates.

The field of **pharmacokinetics** (**-kinetic** means pertaining to movement) is concerned with measuring the amount of drug that is present over time in various body compartments (such as blood, urine, and spinal fluid). These measurements require specialized analytical equipment.

The ideal is to develop drugs that kill large numbers of tumor cells without harming normal cells. Because normal cells, such as bone marrow and gastrointestinal lining cells, have a rapidly dividing cell population, they suffer considerable damage from antitumor drugs. Scientists working in the field of pharmacokinetics use information from research to design better routes (oral, intravenous) and schedules of administration to achieve the greatest tumor kill with the least toxicity (harm) to normal cells.

Combination chemotherapy is the use of two or more antitumor drugs together to kill a specific type of malignant growth. In chemotherapy, drugs are given according to a written **protocol,** or plan, that details the route, schedule, and frequency of doses administered. Usually, drug therapy is continued until the patient achieves a complete **remission,** the absence of all signs of disease. At times, chemotherapy is an **adjuvant** (aid) to surgery. Drugs are used to kill possible hidden disease in patients who, after surgery, are otherwise free of any evidence of malignancy.

Drugs cause tumor cells to die by damaging their DNA. Tumor cells with damaged DNA undergo **apoptosis,** or self-destruction. They have impaired capacity to repair their DNA and, in general, are less able than normal cells to survive DNA damage due to drugs and radiation.

The following are categories of cancer chemotherapeutic agents. Table 19–6 lists the specific drugs in each of these categories and the particular cancers they are used to treat.

1. **Alkylating agents.** These are synthetic compounds containing one or two alkyl groups. The chemicals interfere with the process of DNA synthesis by attaching to DNA molecules. Toxic side effects include nausea and vomiting, diarrhea, bone marrow depression (myelosuppression), and alopecia (hair loss). These are common side effects because cells in the gastrointestinal tract, bone marrow, and scalp are rapidly dividing cells, which along with tumor cells, are susceptible to the lethal effects of chemotherapeutic drugs. Most side effects disappear after treatment is suspended.

2. **Antibiotics.** These drugs are produced by bacteria or fungi. They act by binding to DNA in the cell, thus promoting DNA strand breaks and preventing the replication or copying of DNA. Toxic side effects include alopecia, stomatitis (inflammation of the mouth), myelosuppression, and gastrointestinal disturbances.

3. **Antimetabolites.** These drugs inhibit the synthesis of nucleotide components of DNA, or they may act as fraudulent copies of normal nucleotides and become incorporated into the DNA strand, where they directly block the replication of DNA. Toxic side effects are myelosuppression with leukopenia, thrombocytopenia, and anemia; and damage to cells that line the mouth and digestive tract leading to stomatitis, nausea, and vomiting.

4. **Antimitotics.** These chemicals are derived from bacteria, fungi, or plants or from animals found on coral reefs or in the ocean. **Taxol,** and the vinca alkaloids, are isolated from plants and block the function of the cell structural protein, the microtubule, which is essential for mitosis. They are used frequently in combination with other chemotherapeutic agents. Side effects include myelosuppression, alopecia, and nerve damage.

5. **Hormonal agents.** Hormones are a class of chemicals made by endocrine glands in the body. Examples are estrogens made in the ovaries and androgens made in the testes and adrenal glands. Hormones attach to receptor proteins in target tissues. The hormone-receptor complex stimulates certain normal tissues, such as breast or uterine lining cells, to divide and grow. Some tumors, such as prostate cancers, depend on the presence of a hormone (in this case, androgens) to grow, and hormone removal (orchiectomy) leads to tumor regression. Steroid (cholesterol-derived) hormones, such as prednisone, have growth-inhibiting effects on leukemias and breast cancer. Other compounds, called hormone antagonists, are designed to block the growth-promoting effects of estrogens or androgens, and are used in breast cancer and prostate cancer, respectively.

Breast cancers have **estrogen receptors.** These tumors respond to the removal of estrogen by oophorectomy or the use of antiestrogen drugs such as **tamoxifen,** which block estrogenic effects. **Flutamide** blocks androgen action and causes regression of prostate cancer.

Table 19–6. SELECTED CANCER CHEMOTHERAPEUTIC AGENTS AND THE CANCERS THEY TREAT

Chemotherapeutic Agent	Type of Cancer
ALKYLATING AGENTS	
Carmustine (BCNU)	Brain
Carboplatin (Paraplatin)	Ovarian
Chlorambucil (Leukeran)	Chronic lymphocytic leukemia (CLL)
Cisplatin (Platinol)	Testicular; ovarian
Cyclophosphamide (Cytoxan)	Lymphoma
Dacarbazine (DTIC-Dome)	Hodgkin lymphoma
Mechlorethamine, nitrogen mustard (Mustargen)	Lymphoma
Melphalan (Alkeran)	Multiple myeloma
ANTIBIOTICS	
Bleomycin (Blenoxane)	Testicular
Daunorubicin (Cerubidine)	Acute myelogenous leukemia (AML)
Doxorubicin (Adriamycin, Doxil)	Breast
Idarubicin (Idamycin)	Acute myelogenous leukemia (AML)
Mitomycin-C (Mutamycin)	Lung
ANTIMETABOLITES	
Cladribine (Leustatin)	Hairy cell leukemia
Cytarabine (ara-C, Cytosar-U)	Acute myelogenous leukemia (AML)
Fludarabine (Fludara)	Chronic lymphocytic leukemia (CLL)
5-Fluorouracil, 5-FU (various)	Colon
Methotrexate, MTX (Folex, Mexate)	Acute lymphocytic leukemia (ALL)
Pentostatin, DCF (Nipent)	Hairy cell leukemia
ANTIMITOTICS	
Docetaxel (Taxotere)	Breast
Paclitaxel (Taxol)	Breast, ovary
Vinca alkaloids	Lymphoma
Vinblastine (Velban)	
Vincristine (Oncovin)	
Vinorelbine (Navelbine)	Breast
HORMONES AND HORMONE ANTAGONISTS	
Dexamethasone (Decadron)	Lymphoma
Flutamide (Eulexin)	Prostate
Leuprolide (Lupron)	Prostate
Prednisone (various)	Acute lymphocytic leukemia (ALL)
Tamoxifen (Nolvadex)	Breast
Anastrozole (Arimedex)	Breast

Note: Brand names are in parentheses.

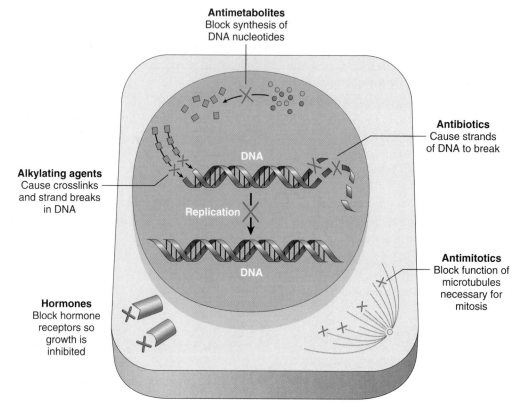

Antimetabolites
Block synthesis of
DNA nucleotides

Antibiotics
Cause strands
of DNA to break

Alkylating agents
Cause crosslinks
and strand breaks
in DNA

DNA

Replication

DNA

Antimitotics
Block function of
microtubules
necessary for
mitosis

Hormones
Block hormone
receptors so
growth is
inhibited

Figure 19–9

Mechanisms of action of cancer chemotherapeutic agents.

Table 19–7. CANCERS AND CHEMOTHERAPEUTIC REGIMENS

Type of Cancer	Combination Regimen	
Breast	AC	**A**driamycin (doxorubicin)
		Cyclophosphamide
Bladder	M-VAC	**M**ethotrexate
		Vinblastine
		Adriamycin (doxorubicin)
		Cisplatin
Hodgkin disease	ABVD	**A**driamycin (doxorubicin)
		Bleomycin
		Vinblastine
		Dacarbazine
Ovarian	Carbo-Tax	**Carbo**platin
		Taxol (paclitaxel)

Note: Generic names are in parentheses.

Figure 19–9 illustrates the mechanisms of action of cancer chemotherapeutic agents. Often, drugs are administered in combination, according to carefully planned regimens. Table 19–7 gives examples of drug combination regimens (protocols).

Tumor cells grow by establishing a new blood supply via **angiogenesis** (growth of new blood vessels). Tumors secrete specific proteins, such as vascular endothelial growth factor (VEGF), which stimulates the formation of new vessels. **Antiangiogenic drugs** interfere with angiogenesis. Examples of these drugs are **endostatin** and **angiostatin,** which prevent tumor growth (in mice) by inhibiting the growth of new blood vessels. Other new drugs directly bind to, and inactivate, VEGF-receptors on new blood vessels. Thalomid (thalidomide) is believed to act as an antiangiogenic agent and is useful in treating multiple myeloma, a plasma cell tumor.

The newest class of anticancer drugs are **molecularly targeted drugs.** These drugs are designed to block the function of growth factors, their receptors, and signaling pathways in tumor cells. Gleevec (imatinib mesylate), which blocks the *bcr-abl* tyrosine kinase in CML cells (see Figure 19–5), is the first drug of this type approved for use in cancer.

Biological Therapy

Another approach to cancer treatment is to use the body's own defenses to fight tumor cells. Investigators are exploring how the elements of the immune system can be restored, enhanced, mimicked, and manipulated to destroy cancer cells. Substances produced by normal cells that directly block tumor growth or that stimulate the immune system and other body defenses are called **biological response modifiers.** Examples of these substances are **interferons** (made by lymphocytes), **monoclonal antibodies** (made by mouse cells and capable of binding to human tumors), **colony-stimulating factors (CSFs)** that stimulate blood-forming cells to combat the myelosuppressive side effects of chemotherapy, and **interleukins** that stimulate the immune system to destroy tumors. Table 19–8 lists various biological agents and their modes of action.

Table 19–8. BIOLOGICAL AGENTS AND THEIR MODES OF ACTION

Biological Agent	Mode of Action
Darbepoietin alfa (Aranesp)	Long-acting erythropoietin
Erythropoietin (Epogen, Procrit)	Promotes growth of red blood cells
Filgrastim (Neupogen)	Colony-stimulating factor; promotes the growth of white blood cells (leukocytes)
Gemtuzimab ozogamicin (Mylotarg)	Monoclonal antibody with an attached toxic; binds specifically to leukemia cells and allows the toxin to enter and kill cells
Interferons (Roferon, Intron)	Promote broad immune response
Interleukin 2, IL-2 (Interleukin-2)	Promotes immune response of T lymphocytes
Pegfilgrastim (Neulasta)	Long-acting filgrastim (Neupogen)
Rituximab (Rituxan)	Monoclonal antibody binding to cell surface receptor; induces apoptosis
Trastuzumab (Herceptin)	Monoclonal antibody binding to cell surface; blocks growth-signaling pathways in a cell; induces apoptosis

Note: Brand names are in parentheses.

Table 19–9. **NEWEST ANTICANCER DRUGS AND THEIR MODES OF ACTION**

Drug	Mode of Action
All-trans retinoic acid or ATRA	Differentiating agent; useful in acute promyelocytic leukemia (APL)
Arsenic trioxide (Trisenox)	Differentiating agent; useful in acute promyelocytic leukemia (APL)
Imatinib mesylate (Gleevec)	Molecularly targeted drug; useful in chronic myelogenous leukemia (CML)
Thalidomide (Thalomid)	Antiangiogenic drug; useful in multiple myeloma

Note: Brand names are in parentheses.

Differentiating Agents

Some new drugs cause tumor cells to differentiate, stop growing, and die. These include ATRA (all-trans retinoic acid), a vitamin A derivative, which is highly active against acute promyelocytic leukemia (APL), and arsenic trioxide (Trisenox), which has similar effects on APL. Table 19–9 lists the newest anticancer drugs with their modes of action.

VIII. Vocabulary

This list reviews many of the new terms introduced in the text. Short definitions reinforce your understanding of the terms. See Section XVI of this chapter for help in pronouncing the more difficult terms.

adjuvant therapy	Assisting primary treatment. Drugs are given early in the course of treatment, along with surgery or radiation to attack cancer cells that may be too small to be detected by diagnostic techniques.
alkylating agents	Synthetic chemicals containing alkyl groups that interfere with DNA synthesis.
anaplasia	Loss of differentiation of cells; reversion to a more primitive cell type.
antibiotics	Chemical substances, produced by bacteria, that inhibit the growth of cells; used in cancer chemotherapy.
antimetabolites	Chemicals that prevent cell division by inhibiting the formation of substances necessary to make DNA; used in cancer chemotherapy.
antimitotics	Drugs that block mitosis (replication) in cells. Taxol is an antimitotic used to treat breast and ovarian cancers.
apoptosis	Programmed cell death. Apo- means off, away, and -ptosis means to fall. Normal cells undergo apoptosis when damaged or aging. Some cancer cells have lost the ability to undergo apoptosis, and they live forever.
benign tumor	Noncancerous.

biological response modifiers	Substances produced by normal cells that either directly block tumor growth or stimulate the immune system.
biological therapy	Use of the body's own defense mechanisms to fight tumor cells.
carcinogens	Agents that cause cancer; chemicals and drugs, radiation, and viruses.
carcinoma	Cancerous tumor made up of cells of epithelial origin.
cellular oncogenes	Pieces of DNA that, when broken or dislocated, can cause a normal cell to become malignant.
chemotherapy	Treatment with drugs.
combination chemotherapy	Use of several chemotherapeutic agents together for the treatment of tumors.
dedifferentiation	Loss of differentiation of cells; reversion to a more primitive, embryonic cell type; anaplasia or undifferentiation.
deoxyribonucleic acid (DNA)	Genetic material within the nucleus of a cell; controls cell division and protein synthesis.
differentiating agents	Drugs that promote tumor cells to differentiate, stop growing, and die.
differentiation	Specialization of cells.
electron beams	Low-energy beams of radiation for treatment of skin or surface tumors.
encapsulated	Surrounded by a capsule; benign tumors are encapsulated.
external beam radiation	Radiation applied to a tumor from a distant source.
fractionation	Giving radiation in small, repeated doses.
genetic screening	Family members are tested to determine whether they have inherited a cancer-causing gene.
grading of tumors	Evaluating the degree of maturity of tumor cells.
gray (Gy)	Unit of radiation equal to 100 rad (absorbed dose of radiation).
gross description of tumors	Visual appearance of tumors: cystic, fungating, inflammatory, medullary, necrotic, polypoid, ulcerating, and verrucous.
infiltrative	Extending beyond normal tissue boundaries.
invasive	Having the ability to enter and destroy surrounding tissue.
linear accelerator	Device that produces high-energy x-ray beams for treatment of deep-seated tumors.

malignant tumor	Tending to become worse and result in death; having the characteristics of invasiveness, anaplasia, and metastasis.
mesenchymal	Embryonic connective tissue; mes = middle, enchym/o = to pour.
metastasis	Spread of a malignant tumor to a secondary site; literally, beyond (meta-) control (-stasis).
microscopic description (of tumors)	The appearance of tumors when viewed under a microscope: alveolar, carcinoma *in situ,* diffuse, dysplastic, epidermoid, follicular, nodular, papillary, pleomorphic, scirrhous, undifferentiated.
mitosis	Replication of cells; a stage in a cell's life cycle involving the production of two identical cells from a parent cell.
mixed-tissue tumors	Tumors composed of different types of tissue (epithelial as well as connective tissue).
modality	Method of treatment, such as surgery, chemotherapy, or radiation.
molecularly targeted drugs	Anticancer drugs designed to block the function of growth factors, their receptors, and signaling pathways in tumor cells.
morbidity	The condition of being diseased.
mucinous	Containing mucus.
mutation	Change in the genetic material (DNA) of a cell; may be caused by chemicals, radiation, or viruses or may occur spontaneously.
neoplasm	New growth; benign or malignant tumors.
nucleotide	Unit of DNA (gene) composed of a sugar, phosphate and base. The sequence or arrangement of nucleotides on a gene is the genetic code.
oncogene	A region of DNA (genetic material) found in tumor cells (cellular oncogene) or in viruses that cause cancer (viral oncogene). Oncogenes are designated by a three-letter word, such as *abl, erb, jun, myc, ras,* and *src.*
palliative	Relieving, but not curing symptoms.
pedunculated	Possessing a stem or stalk (peduncle); characteristic of some polypoid tumors.
pharmacokinetics	Study of the distribution in and removal of drugs from the body over a period of time.
protocol	An explicit, detailed plan for treatment.

rad	Unit of absorbed radiation dose.
radiation	Energy carried by a stream of particles. Various forms of radiation can cause cancer.
radiocurable tumor	Cells that are eradicated by radiation therapy.
radioresistant tumor	Cells that require large doses of radiation to be destroyed.
radiosensitive tumor	A tumor in which radiation can cause the death of cells.
radiosensitizers	Drugs that increase the sensitivity of tumors to x-rays.
radiotherapy	Treatment using radiation; radiation oncology.
relapse	Return of symptoms of disease.
remission	Absence of symptoms of disease.
ribonucleic acid (RNA)	Cellular substance (located within and outside the nucleus) that, along with DNA, plays an important role in the synthesis of proteins in a cell.
sarcoma	Cancerous tumor derived from connective tissue.
serous	Pertaining to a thin, watery fluid (serum).
sessile	Having no stem; characteristic of some polypoid tumors.
solid tumor	Tumor composed of a mass of cells.
staging of tumors	System of evaluating the extent of spread of tumors. An example is the TNM system (tumor, nodes, and metastasis).
steroids	Complex, naturally occurring chemicals, such as hormones, that are used as chemotherapeutic agents.
surgical procedures to treat cancer	Methods of removing cancerous tissue: cryosurgery, electrocauterization, en bloc resection, excisional biopsy, exenteration, fulguration, incisional biopsy.
ultraviolet radiation	Rays given off by the sun.
viral oncogenes	Pieces of DNA from viruses that infect a normal cell and cause it to become malignant.
virus	An infectious agent that reproduces by entering a host cell and using the host's genetic material to make copies of itself.

IX. Combining Forms, Suffixes, Prefixes, and Terminology

Write the meanings of the medical terms in the spaces provided.

Combining Forms

Combining Form	Meaning	Terminology	Meaning
alveol/o	small sac	alveolar _____	

Microscopic description of tumor cell arrangement (found in connective tissue tumors).

cac/o	bad	cachexia _____	

General ill health and malnutrition associated with chronic disease (-hexia means habit).

carcin/o	cancer, cancerous	carcinoma *in situ* _____	

Localized cancer; confined to the site of origin.

cauter/o	burn, heat	electrocauterization _____	
chem/o	chemical, drug	chemotherapy _____	
cry/o	cold	cryosurgery _____	
cyst/o	sac of fluid	cystic tumor _____	
fibr/o	fibers	fibrosarcoma _____	
follicul/o	small glandular sacs	follicular _____	

A microscopic description of cellular arrangement in glandular tumors.

fung/i	fungus, mushroom	fungating tumor _____	
medull/o	soft, inner part	medullary tumor _____	
mucos/o	mucous membrane	mucositis _____	
mut/a	genetic change	mutation _____	

-ation means process.

mutagen/o	causing genetic change	mutagenic _____	
onc/o	tumor	oncology _____	

papill/o	nipple-like	papillary _____

A microscopic description of tumor cell growth.

pharmac/o	chemical, drug	pharmacokinetics _____

-kinetic means pertaining to movement.

plas/o	formation	dysplastic _____

Microscopic description of cells that are highly abnormal but not clearly cancerous.

ple/o	many, more	pleomorphic _____

Microscopic description of tumors that are composed of a variety of cells.

polyp/o	polyp	polypoid tumor _____

-oid means resembling.

radi/o	rays, x-rays	radiotherapy _____

sarc/o	flesh, connective tissue	osteosarcoma _____

scirrh/o	hard	scirrhous _____

Microscopic description of densely packed, fibrous tumor cell composition.

xer/o	dry	xerostomia _____

Suffixes

Suffix	Meaning	Terminology	Meaning
-blastoma	immature tumor	retinoblastoma _____	
		neuroblastoma _____	

This sarcoma of nervous system origin affects infants and children up to the age of 10 years, usually arising in the autonomic nervous system or adrenal medulla.

-genesis	formation	angiogenesis _____	
-oma	mass, tumor	adenocarcinoma _____	
-plasia	formation, growth	hyperplasia _____	
-plasm	formation, growth	neoplasm _____	

| -suppression | to stop | myelo<u>suppression</u> | _____ |
| -therapy | treatment | biological <u>therapy</u> | _____ |

Prefixes

Prefix	Meaning	Terminology	Meaning
ana-	backward	<u>ana</u>plasia	_____
apo-	off, away	<u>apo</u>ptosis	_____
brachy-	near	<u>brachy</u>therapy	_____
epi-	upon	<u>epi</u>dermoid	_____

Microscopic description of tumor cells that resemble epidermal tissue.

meta-	beyond; change	<u>meta</u>stasis	_____
		<u>meta</u>plasia	_____

The abnormal transformation of adult differentiated cells to differentiated tissue of another kind. This change is reversible. An example is the change (from columnar epithelial cells to squamous epithelial cells) that occurs in the respiratory epithelium of habitual cigarette smokers.

tele-	far	<u>tele</u>therapy	_____

X. Laboratory Tests

protein marker tests

Measure the level of proteins in the blood or on the surface of tumor cells.

These tests diagnose cancer or detect its recurrence after treatment. Examples are:

Protein	Measured Where	Type of Cancer
acid phosphatase	blood	prostate
alpha-fetoprotein	blood	liver and testicular
beta-HCG	blood	choriocarcinoma and testicular
CA-125	blood	ovarian
CEA (carcinoembryonic antigen)	blood	colorectal and GI
estrogen receptor	tumor cells	breast
PSA (prostate-specific antigen	blood	prostate
15.3 and 29.7	blood	breast
19.9	blood	pancreatic

XI. Clinical Procedures

The following are specialized procedures used to detect or treat malignancies. X-rays, CT scans, MRI, and ultrasound (described throughout the text and specifically in Chapter 20) are also important diagnostic procedures in oncology.

bone marrow biopsy

Aspiration of bone marrow tissue and examination under a microscope for evidence of malignant cells.

bone marrow or stem cell transplant

Bone marrow or stem cells infused intravenously into a patient.

In an **autologous transplant,** marrow previously obtained from the patient and stored is reinfused when needed. In an **allogeneic transplant** (all/o means other), marrow is obtained from a living donor other than the recipient. In a **stem cell transplant,** undifferentiated blood cells called stem cells are harvested from the peripheral blood of a patient instead of from the bone marrow. After receiving chemotherapy, the patient gets a reinfusion of the stem cells to repopulate the bone marrow with blood cells.

fiberoptic colonoscopy

Visual examination of the colon using a fiberoptic instrument.

This is an important screening procedure to detect cancer and remove premalignant polyps.

exfoliative cytology

Cells are scraped from the region of suspected disease and examined under a microscope.

The Pap test (smear) to detect carcinoma of the cervix and vagina is an example (Fig. 19–10).

laparoscopy

Visual examination of the abdominal cavity using small incisions and a laparoscope. Also known as peritoneoscopy.

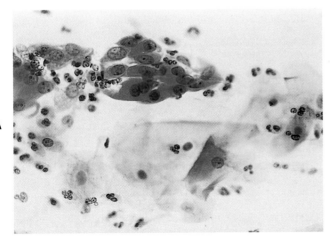
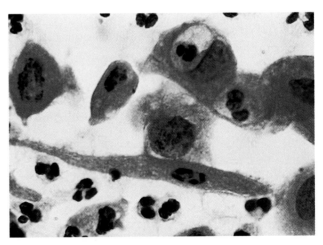

A   B

Figure 19–10

(A) Normal exfoliative cytological smear (Pap smear) from the cervicovaginal region. It shows flattened squamous cells and some neutrophils as well. **(B) Abnormal cervicovaginal smear** shows numerous malignant cells that have pleomorphic (irregularly shaped) and hyperchromatic (stained) nuclei. (Courtesy Dr. PK Gupta, Department of Pathology and Laboratory Medicine, University of Pennsylvania Medical Center, Philadelphia, Penn.)

mammography	**X-ray examination of the breast to detect breast cancer.**
needle biopsy	**Insertion of a needle into a tissue to remove a core of tissue.**
	A physician uses **needle aspiration** to withdraw free cells from a fluid-filled cavity (cystic areas of the breast), or from a solid mass of tumor.
radionuclide scans	**Radioactive substances (radionuclides) are injected intravenously and scans (images) are taken of organs.**
	These tests detect tumor and metastases. Examples of radionuclides are gallium-67 (whole body scan), rose Bengal (liver), and technetium-99m (liver and spleen).

Abbreviations

BMT	bone marrow transplantation		**mets**	metastases
bx	biopsy		**MoAb**	monoclonal antibody
Ca	cancer		**NED**	no evidence of disease
CEA	carcinoembryonic antigen		**NHL**	non-Hodgkin lymphoma
cGy	centigray (one hundredth of a gray) or rad		**Pap smear**	Papanicolaou smear
chemo	chemotherapy		**PD**	progressive disease (tumor increases in size)
CR	complete response (disappearance of all tumor)		**PR**	partial response (tumor is one-half of its original size)
CSF	colony-stimulating factor; examples are G-CSF (granulocyte colony-stimulating factor) and GM-CSF (granulocyte-macrophage colony-stimulating factor)		**prot.**	protocol
			PSA	prostate-specific antigen
			PSCT	peripheral stem cell transplant
DES	diethylstilbestrol		**rad**	radiation absorbed dose
DNA	deoxyribonucleic acid			
ER	estrogen receptor		**RNA**	ribonucleic acid
EPO	erythropoietin; promotes growth of red blood cells		**SD**	stable disease (tumor does not shrink but does not grow)
5-FU	5-fluorouracil		**TNM**	tumor, nodes, metastases
Ga	gallium		**VEGF**	vascular endothelial growth factor
Gy	gray (unit of radiation equal to 100 rads)		**XRT, RT**	radiation therapy

XII. Practical Applications

This section contains a FYI (for your information) exercise followed by an actual medical report and chart rounds using terms that you have studied in this and previous chapters. Answers to questions are on page 809 after Answers to Exercises.

FYI   Malignant tumors whose names do not contain the combining forms carcin/o or sarc/o

---

Malignant tumor	*Description*
Glioma	Primary brain tumor
Hepatoma	Liver tumor (hepatocellular carcinoma)
Hypernephroma	Kidney tumor
Lymphoma	Lymph node tumor
Melanoma	Tumor of pigmented skin cells
Mesothelioma	Tumor of cells within the pleura
Multiple myeloma	Bone marrow cell tumor
Thymoma	Thymus gland tumor

Questions

1. Which tumor develops from a dysplastic nevus? _____

2. Which tumor arises from an organ located within the mediastinum?

   _____

3. Which tumor arises from an organ in the RUQ of the abdomen?

   _____

4. Which tumor has types called astrocytoma, ependymoma, glioblastoma

   multiforme? _____

5. Which tumor is also known as a renal cell carcinoma?

   _____

6. Which tumor is characterized by large numbers of plasma cells (bone marrow

   antibody-producing cells)? _____

7. Which tumor arises from membrane cells surrounding the lungs?

   _____

8. Which tumor has a type known as Hodgkin disease?

   _____

B. Match the following terms or abbreviations with their meanings below.

chemical carcinogen   mitosis   RNA
DNA   mutation   ultraviolet radiation
ionizing radiation   oncogene   virus

1. replication of cells; two identical cells are produced from a parent cell _____

2. change in the genetic material of a cell _____

3. genetic material within the nucleus that controls replication and protein synthesis

   _____

4. cellular substance (ribonucleic acid) that is important in protein synthesis _____

5. rays given off by the sun; can be carcinogenic _____

6. energy carried by a stream of particles; can be carcinogenic _____

7. infectious agent that reproduces by entering a host cell and using the host's genetic material to

   make copies of itself _____

8. a region of genetic material found in tumor cells and in viruses that cause cancer

   _____

9. an agent (hydrocarbon, insecticide, hormone) that causes cancer _____

C. Give the meanings of the following terms.

1. solid tumor _____

2. adenoma _____

3. adenocarcinoma _____

4. osteoma _____

5. osteosarcoma _____

6. mixed-tissue tumor _____

7. neoplasm _____

8. pharmacokinetics _____

9. benign _____

10. differentiation _____

D. Name the terms that describe microscopic tumor growth. Definitions and word parts are given.

1. small nipple-like projections: pap _____

2. abnormal formation of cells: dys _____

3. localized growth of cells: carcin _____

4. densely packed; containing fibrous tissue: _____ ous

5. patterns resembling small, microscopic sacs: alv _____

6. small, gland-type sacs: foll _____

7. variety of cell types: pleo _____

8. lacking structures typical of mature cells: un _____

9. spreading evenly throughout the tissue: di _____

10. many areas of tightly packed clusters of cells: nod _____

11. resembling epithelial cells: epiderm _____

E. Match the following gross descriptions of tumors with their meanings as given below.

cystic	medullary	ulcerating
fungating	necrotic	verrucous
inflammatory	polypoid	

1. containing dead tissue _____

2. mushrooming pattern of growth: tumor cells pile on top of each other _____

3. characterized by large, open, exposed surfaces _____

4. characterized by redness, swelling, and heat _____

5. growths are projections from a base; sessile and pedunculated tumors are examples

_____

6. tumors from large, open spaces filled with fluid; serous and mucinous tumors are examples

_____

7. tumors resemble wart-like growths _____

8. tumors are large, soft, and fleshy _____

F. Circle or supply the appropriate medical terms.

1. A **(carcinoma/sarcoma)** is a cancerous tumor composed of cells of epithelial tissue. An example of such a cancerous tumor is a (an) _____.

2. A **(carcinoma/sarcoma)** is a cancerous tumor composed of connective tissue. An example of such a cancerous tumor is a (an) _____.

3. Retinoblastoma and polyposis coli syndrome are examples of **(chemical carcinogens/inherited cancers)**.

4. The assessment of a tumor's degree of maturity or microscopic differentiation is **(grading/staging)** of the tumor.

5. The assessment of a tumor's extent of spread within the body is known as **(grading/staging)**.

6. In the TNM staging system, T stands for **(tissue/tumor)**, N stands for (node/necrotic), and M stands for **(mitotic/metastasis)**.

7. The transformation of adult, differentiated tissue to differentiated tissue of another type is called **(metaplasia/anaplasia)**.

8. The formation of new blood vessels is known as **(apoptosis/angiogenesis)**.

G. Match the surgical procedure in column I with its meaning in column II. Write the letter of the meaning in the space provided.

Column I

1. fulguration _____

2. en bloc resection _____

3. incisional biopsy _____

4. excisional biopsy _____

5. cryosurgery _____

6. electrocauterization _____

7. exenteration _____

Column II

A. removal of tumor and a margin of normal tissue for diagnosis and possible cure of small tumors

B. burning a lesion to destroy tumor cells

C. wide resection involving removal of tumor, its organ of origin, and surrounding tissue in the body space

D. destruction of tissue by electric sparks generated by a high-frequency current

E. removal of entire tumor and regional lymph nodes

F. freezing a lesion to kill tumor cells

G. cutting into a tumor and removing a piece to establish a diagnosis

H. Give medical terms for the following.

1. The method of treating cancer using high-energy radiation is _____.

2. If tumor tissue requires large doses of radiation to kill cells, it is a (an) _____ tumor.

3. If radiation can cause loss of tumor cells without serious damage to surrounding regions, the

   tumor is _____.

4. A tumor that can be completely eradicated by irradiation is a (an) _____ tumor.

5. The method of giving radiation in small, repeated doses is _____.

6. Drugs that increase the sensitivity of tumors to x-rays are _____.

7. Treatment of cancerous tumors with drugs is _____.

8. The study of the distribution and disappearance of drugs in the body is _____.

9. The use of two or more drugs to kill tumor cells is _____.

10. A large electronic device that produces high-energy x-ray beams for treatment of deep-seated

    tumors is a (an) _____.

11. Alkylating agents, antimetabolites, hormones, antibiotics, and antimitotics are all types of

    _____ agents.

12. Implantation of seeds of radioactive material directly into a tumor is _____.

13. Unit of radiation equal to 100 rad _____.

14. Radiation applied to a tumor from a distant source is _____.

15. Highly focused, high-energy radiation requiring a cyclotron machine is _____.

16. Defined areas that are bombarded by radiation are _____.

I. Match the following side effects of radiotherapy and chemotherapy with its description or treatment described below:

alopecia   nausea   pneumonitis
fibrosis   oral mucositis   xerostomia
myelosuppression

1. Ulceration of lining cells in the mouth caused by radiation to the jaw _____.

2. Drug treatment for breast cancer destroys epithelial cells in the stomach and causes a sensation

   leading to vomiting _____.

3. Radiation to the lungs causes inflammation of the lungs _____.

4. Chemotherapy for ovarian cancer causes loss of hair on the head _____.

5. Bone marrow destruction with leukopenia, anemia, and thrombocytopenia _____.

6. Radiation to the lungs causes increase in connective tissue _____.

7. Radiation of salivary glands causes dryness of the mouth _____.

J. Give the meanings of the following medical terms.

1. modality _____

2. adjuvant therapy _____

3. protocol _____

4. remission _____

5. relapse _____

6. morbidity _____

7. biological therapy _____

8. biological response modifiers _____

9. interferon _____

10. monoclonal antibodies _____

11. apoptosis _____

12. cachexia _____

13. differentiating agents _____

14. molecularly targeted drugs _____

15. nucleotide _____

K. Match the test or procedure with its description below.

beta-HCG test	estrogen receptor assay	needle biopsy
bone marrow biopsy	exfoliative cytology	PSA test
CA-125	laparoscopy	stem cell transplant
CEA test		

1. test for the presence of a portion of human chorionic gonadotropin hormone (a marker for

   testicular cancer) _____

2. protein marker for ovarian cancer detected in the blood _____

3. visual examination of the abdominal cavity; peritoneoscopy _____

4. test for the presence of a hormone receptor on breast cancer cells _____

5. removal and microscopic examination of bone marrow tissue _____

6. aspiration of tissue for microscopic examination _____

7. blood test for the presence of an antigen related to prostate cancer _____

8. blood test for carcinoembryonic antigen (marker for GI cancer) _____

9. cells are scraped off tissue and microscopically examined _____

10. blood-forming cells are infused intravenously _____

L. Circle the correct term to complete each sentence.

1. Pauline was diagnosed with a meningioma, which is usually a (an) **(benign, anaplastic, necrotic)** tumor. The doctor told her that it was not malignant, but that it should be removed because of the pressure it was causing on the surrounding tissues.

2. Marlene underwent surgical resection of her breast mass. Dr. Smith recommended **(dedifferentiated, modality, adjuvant)** therapy because her tumor was large and she had one positive lymph node.

3. Unfortunately, at the time of diagnosis, the tumor had spread to distant sites because it was **(pleomorphic, metastatic, mutagenic)**. The oncologist recommended beginning chemotherapy as soon as possible.

4. The polyp in Lisa's colon was *not* pedunculated, and Dr. Sidney described it as flat and **(fungating, scirrhous, sessile)**.

gray (791)	grā	_____
hyperplasia (795)	hī-pĕr-PLĀ-zē-ă	_____
incisional biopsy (782)	ĭn-SĪZH-ŭn-ăl BĪ-ŏp-sē	_____
infiltrative (791)	ĬN-fĭl-trā-tĭv	_____
invasive (791)	ĭn-VĀ-sĭv	_____
laparoscopy (797)	lă-păr-ŎS-kō-pē	_____
malignant (792)	mă-LĬG-nănt	_____
mammography (798)	mă-MŎG-ră-fē	_____
medullary tumor (794)	MĔD-ū-lār-ē TOO-mŏr	_____
metaplasia (796)	mĕ-tă-PLĀ-zē-ă	_____
metastasis (792)	mĕ-TĂS-tă-sĭs	_____
mitosis (792)	mī-TŌ-sĭs	_____
modality (792)	mō-DĂL-ĭ-tē	_____
molecularly targeted drugs (792)	mō-LĔK-kū-lăr-lē TĂR-gĕt-ĕd drŭgz	_____
morbidity (792)	mŏr-BĬD-ĭ-tē	_____
mucinous (792)	MŪ-sĭ-nŭs	_____
mucositis (794)	mū-kō-SĪ-tĭs	_____
mutagenic (794)	mū-tă-JĔN-ĭk	_____
mutation (792)	mū-TĀ-shŭn	_____
myelosuppression (796)	mī-ĕ-lō-sū-PRĔ-shŭn	_____
necrotic tumor (778)	nĕ-KRŎT-ĭk TOO-mŏr	_____
needle biopsy (798)	NĒ-dl BĪ-ŏp-sē	_____
neoplasm (792)	NĒ-ō-plăzm	_____
neuroblastoma (795)	nŭ-rō-blăs-TŌ-mă	_____
nodular (779)	NŎD-ū-lăr	_____
nucleotide (792)	NŪ-klē-ō-tīd	_____
oncogene (792)	ŎNGK-ō-jēn	_____

oncology (794)   ŏn-KŎL-ō-jē   _____

osteosarcoma (795)   ŏs-tē-ō-săr-KŌ-mă   _____

palliative (792)   PĂL-ē-ă-tĭv   _____

papillary (795)   PĂP-ĭ-lăr-ē   _____

pedunculated (792)   pĕ-DŬNG-kū-lāt-ĕd   _____

pharmacokinetics (792)   făr-mă-kō-kĭ-NĔT-ĭks   _____

pleomorphic (795)   plē-ō-MŎR-fĭk   _____

pneumonitis (785)   nū-mō-NĪ-tĭs   _____

polypoid tumor (795)   PŎL-ĭ-poyd TOO-mŏr   _____

protein marker test (796)   PRŌ-tēn MĂRK-ĕr tĕst   _____

protocol (792)   PRŌ-tō-kŏl   _____

rad (792)   răd   _____

radiation (793)   rā-dē-Ā-shŭn   _____

radiocurable tumor (793)   rā-dē-ō-KŪR-ă-b'l TOO-mŏr _____

radionuclide scans (798)   rā-dē-ō-NŪ-klīd skănz   _____

radioresistant tumor (793) rā-dē-ō-rĕ-ZĬS-tănt TOO-mŏr _____

radiosensitive tumor (793) rā-dē-ō-SĔN-sĭ-tĭv TOO-mŏr _____

radiosensitizer (793)   rā-dē-ō-SĔN-sĭ-tī-zĕr   _____

radiotherapy (793)   rā-dē-ō-THĔR-ă-pē   _____

relapse (793)   rē-LĂPS   _____

remission (793)   rē-MĬSH-ŭn   _____

retinoblastoma (795)   rĕt-ĭ-nō-blăs-TŌ-mă   _____

ribonucleic acid (793)   rī-bō-nū-KLĒ-ik ĂS-ĭd   _____

sarcoma (793)   săr-KŌ-mă   _____

scirrhous (795)   SKĬR-ŭs   _____

serous (793)   SĒ-rŭs   _____

sessile (793)   SĔS-ĭl   _____

solid tumor (793)   SŎL-ĭd TOO-mŏr   _____

staging of tumors (793)   STĀ-jĭng of TOO-mŏrz   _____

stem cell transplant (797) stĕm sĕl TRĂNZ-plănt   _____

steroids (793)   STĔR-oydz   _____

teletherapy (796)   tĕl-ē-THĔ-ră-pē   _____

ulcerating tumor (779)   ŬL-sĕ-rā-tĭng TOO-mŏr   _____

verrucous   vĕ-ROO-kŭs or VĔR-oo-kŭs _____
  tumor (779)   TOO-mŏr

viral oncogenes (793)   VĪ-răl ŎNGK-ō-jĕnz   _____

virus (793)   VĪ-rŭs   _____

xerostomia (795)   zĕr-ō-STŌ-mē-ă   _____

XVI. Review Sheet

Write the meanings of the combining forms in the spaces provided and test yourself. Check your answers with the information in the chapter or in the glossary (Medical Terms—English) at the back of the book.

COMBINING FORMS

Combining Form	Meaning	Combining Form	Meaning
aden/o		mut/a	
alveol/o		mutagen/o	
cac/o		onc/o	
carcin/o		papill/o	
cauter/o		pharmac/o	
chem/o		plas/o	
cry/o		ple/o	
cyst/o		polyp/o	
fibr/o		radi/o	
follicul/o		sarc/o	
fung/i		scirrh/o	
medull/o		xer/o	
mucos/o			

Continued on following page

SUFFIXES

Suffix	Meaning	Suffix	Meaning
-ary	_____	-ptosis	_____
-blastoma	_____	-stasis	_____
-oid	_____	-stomia	_____
-oma	_____	-suppression	_____
-plasia	_____	-therapy	_____
-plasm	_____		

PREFIXES

Prefix	Meaning	Prefix	Meaning
ana-	_____	epi-	_____
anti-	_____	hyper-	_____
apo-	_____	meta-	_____
brachy-	_____	tele-	_____
dys-	_____		

chapter

Radiology and Nuclear Medicine

This chapter is divided into the following sections

In this chapter you will

- ■ Learn the physical properties of x-rays.
- ■ Become familiar with diagnostic techniques used by radiologists and nuclear physicians.
- ■ Identify the x-ray views and patient positions used in x-ray examinations.
- ■ Learn about the role of radioactivity in the diagnosis of disease.
- ■ Become familiar with medical terms used in the specialties of radiology and nuclear medicine.
- ■ Apply your new knowledge to understanding medical terms in their proper contexts, such as medical reports and records.

I. Introduction

Radiology (also called **roentgenology** after its discoverer, Wilhelm Conrad Röentgen) is the medical specialty concerned with the study of x-rays. **X-rays** are invisible waves of energy that are produced by an energy source (x-ray machine, cathode ray tube) and are useful in the diagnosis and treatment of disease.

Nuclear medicine is the medical specialty that studies the characteristics and uses of **radioactive substances** in the diagnosis of disease. Radioactive substances are materials that emit high-speed particles and energy-containing rays from the interior of their matter. The emitted particles and rays are called **radioactivity** and can be of three types: **alpha particles, beta particles,** and **gamma rays. Gamma rays** are similar to x-rays in that they have no mass and are used effectively as a diagnostic label to trace the path and uptake of chemical substances in the body.

The personnel involved in these medical fields are varied. A **radiologist** is a physician who specializes in the practice of diagnostic radiology. A **nuclear physician** is a physician who specializes in the practice of administering diagnostic nuclear medicine procedures.

Allied health care professionals who work with physicians in the fields of radiology and nuclear medicine are **radiologic technologists.** Types of radiologic technologists are: **radiographers** (aid physicians in administering diagnostic x-ray procedures), **nuclear medicine technologists** (attend to patients undergoing nuclear medicine procedures and operate devices under the direction of a nuclear physician), and **sonographers** (aid physicians in performing ultrasound procedures).

II. Radiology

A. Characteristics of X-Rays

Several characteristics of x-rays are useful to physicians in the diagnosis and treatment of disease. Some of these characteristics are the following:

1. **Ability to cause exposure of a photographic plate.** If a photographic plate is placed in front of a beam of x-rays, the x-rays, traveling unimpeded through the air, will expose the silver coating of the plate and cause it to blacken.
2. **Ability to penetrate different substances to varying degrees.** X-rays pass through the different types of substances in the human body (air in the lungs, water in blood vessels and lymph, fat around muscles, and metal such as calcium in bones) with varying ease. Air is the least dense substance and exhibits the greatest transmission. Fat is denser, water is next, followed by metal, which is the densest and transmits least. If the x-rays are absorbed (stopped) by the denser body substance (e.g., calcium in bones), they do not reach the photographic plate held behind the patient, and white areas are left in the x-ray film (plate). Figure 20–1 is an example of an x-ray photograph.

   A substance is said to be **radiolucent** if it permits passage of most of the x-rays. Lung tissue (containing air) is an example of a radiolucent substance, and it appears black on an x-ray image. **Radiopaque** substances (bones) are those that absorb most of the x-rays they are exposed to, allowing only a small fraction of the x-rays to reach the x-ray plate. Thus, normally radiopaque, calcium-containing bone appears white on an x-ray image.

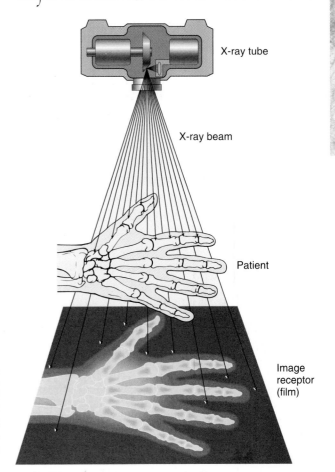

X-ray tube

X-ray beam

Patient

Image
receptor
(film)

Figure 20-1

X-ray photograph (radiograph) of the hand.
Relative position of x-ray tube, patient
(hand), and film necessary to make the x-ray
photograph is shown. Bones tend to stop
diagnostic x-rays, but soft tissue does not.
This results in the light and dark regions
that form the image.

3. **Invisibility.** X-rays cannot be detected by sight, sound, or touch. Workers exposed to x-rays must wear a **film badge** to detect and record the amount of radiation to which they have been exposed. The film badge contains a special film that is exposed by x-rays. The amount of blackness on the film is an indication of the amount of x-rays or gamma rays received by the wearer.

4. **Travel in straight lines.** This property allows the formation of precise shadow images on the x-ray plate and also permits x-ray beams to be directed accurately at a tissue site during radiotherapy.

5. **Scattering of radiation.** Scattering occurs when x-rays come in contact with any material. Greater scatter occurs with dense objects and less scatter with those substances that are radiolucent. In addition, because scatter can blur images and expose areas of film that otherwise would be in shadow, a grid (containing thin lead strips arranged parallel to the x-ray beams) is placed in front of the film to absorb scattered radiation before it strikes the x-ray film.

6. **Ionization.** X-rays have the ability to ionize substances through which they pass. Ionization is a chemical process in which the energy of an x-ray beam causes rearrangement and disruption within a substance, so that previously neutral particles are changed to charged particles called **ions.** This strongly ionizing ability of x-rays is a double-edged sword. In x-ray therapy, the ionizing effect of x-rays can help kill cancerous cells and stop tumor growth; however, ionizing x-rays in small doses can

affect normal body cells, leading to tissue damage and malignant changes. Thus, persons exposed to high doses of x-rays are at risk of developing leukemia, thyroid tumors, breast cancer, or other malignancies.

B. Diagnostic Techniques

X-Rays

X-rays are used in a variety of ways to detect pathological conditions. The most common use of the diagnostic x-ray is dental, to locate cavities (caries) in teeth. Other areas examined include the digestive, nervous, reproductive, and endocrine systems and the chest and bones. Some special diagnostic x-ray techniques are the following:

Computed Tomography or Computerized Axial Tomography (CT, CAT). Machines called **CT scanners** beam x-rays at multiple angles through a section of a patient's body. The absorption of all these x-rays, after they pass through the body, is detected and used by a computer to create a cross-sectional picture of the body section examined (Figure 20–2). The ability of (sensitivity) CT scanners to detect abnormalities is increased by the use of iodine-containing contrast agents, which outline blood vessels and enhance soft tissues.

The CT scanners are highly sensitive in detecting disease in bony structures and can actually provide images of internal organs that are impossible to visualize with ordinary x-ray technique. Figure 20–3 shows a series of CT scans through various regions of the body.

Contrast Studies. In x-ray film, the natural differences in the density of body tissues (e.g., air in lung, calcium in bone) produce contrasting shadow images on the x-ray film; however, when x-rays pass through two adjacent body parts composed of substances of the same density (e.g., the digestive organs in the abdomen), their images cannot be distinguished on the film or on the screen. It is necessary, then, to inject a **contrast medium** into the structure or fluid to be visualized so that the specific part, organ, tube, or liquid can be visualized as a negative imprint on the dense contrast agent.

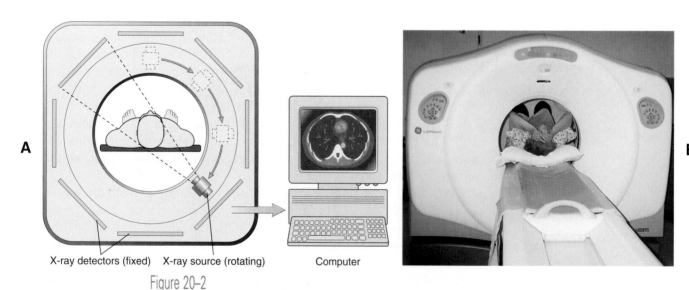

A   B

X-ray detectors (fixed)   X-ray source (rotating)   Computer

Figure 20–2

(A) A **CT scanner** has a rotating x-ray source and a fixed ring of detectors. (B) **A patient in a CT scanner.** This patient has arms above her head during a chest CT.

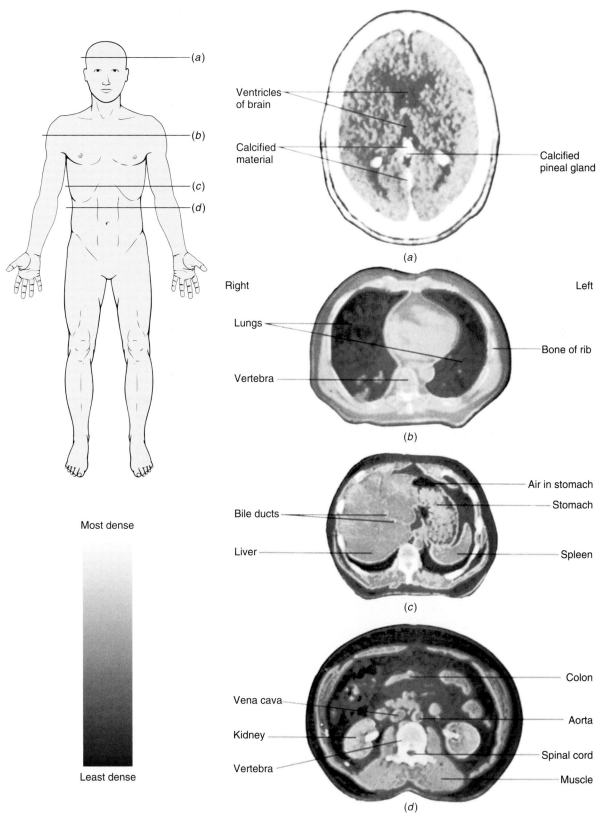

Ventricles of brain

Calcified material

Calcified pineal gland

(a)

Right

Left

Lungs

Bone of rib

Vertebra

(b)

Bile ducts

Air in stomach

Stomach

Liver

Spleen

(c)

Most dense

Least dense

Colon

Vena cava

Aorta

Kidney

Spinal cord

Vertebra

Muscle

(d)

Figure 20–3

CT scans through various regions of the body. The level of the scan is indicated on the figure of the body. The bar below the figure indicates the gradient of structure density as represented by black (least dense, such as air) and white (most dense, such as bone). (CT scan courtesy Professor Jan H. Ehringer.)

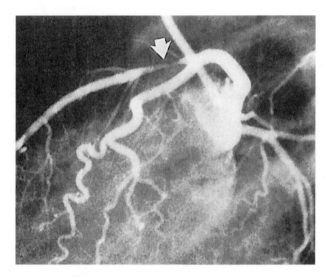

Figure 20–4

Coronary angiography shows stenosis (see arrow) of the left anterior descending coronary artery. (From Braunwald E: Heart Disease: A Textbook of Cardiovascular Medicine, 4th ed. Philadelphia, WB Saunders, 1992.)

The following are artificial contrast materials used in diagnostic radiological studies:

Barium Sulfate. Barium sulfate is a metallic powder that is mixed in water and used for examination of the upper and lower GI (gastrointestinal) tract. An **upper GI series** involves oral ingestion of barium sulfate so that the esophagus, stomach, and duodenum can be visualized. A **small bowel follow-through** traces the passage of barium in a sequential manner as it passes through the small intestine. A **barium enema (lower GI series)** opacifies the lumen (passageway) of the large intestine using an enema containing barium sulfate.

A **double-contrast study** uses both a radiopaque and a radiolucent contrast medium. For example, the walls of the stomach or intestine are coated with barium and the lumen is filled with air. The radiographs show the pattern of mucosal ridges (see Fig. 6–1A).

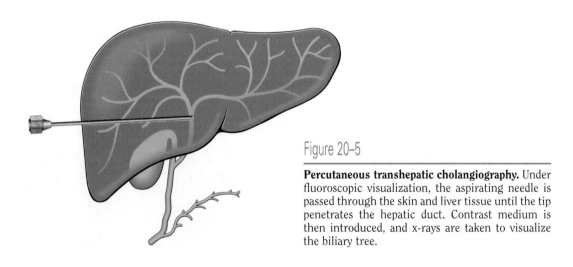

Figure 20–5

Percutaneous transhepatic cholangiography. Under fluoroscopic visualization, the aspirating needle is passed through the skin and liver tissue until the tip penetrates the hepatic duct. Contrast medium is then introduced, and x-rays are taken to visualize the biliary tree.

Iodine Compounds. Radiopaque fluids containing up to 50 percent iodine are used in the following tests:

angiography	An x-ray image (angiogram) of blood vessels and heart chambers is obtained after injecting a water-soluble dye through a catheter (tube) into the appropriate blood vessel or heart chamber. In clinical practice, the terms angiogram and arteriogram are used interchangeably. Figure 20–4 shows coronary angiography, which determines the degree of obstruction of the arteries that supply blood to the heart.
arthrography	Contrast or air, or both, is injected into a joint, and x-rays are taken of the joint.
cholangiography	X-ray images are taken after injecting contrast into the bile ducts intravenously or after surgery of the gallbladder and biliary tract (directly into the tube left in the tract since surgery). An alternative route for injection of contrast is via a needle through the skin and into the liver. This is **percutaneous transhepatic cholangiography** (Fig. 20–5).
digital subtraction angiography (DSA)	An x-ray image of contrast-injected blood vessels is produced by taking two x-rays (the first without contrast) and using a computer to subtract obscuring shadows from the image.
hysterosalpingography	An x-ray record of the endometrial cavity and fallopian tubes after injecting contrast material through a catheter inserted through the vagina and into the endocervical canal. This procedure determines the patency of the fallopian tubes.
myelography	An x-ray of the spinal cord (myel/o) after injecting contrast agent into the subarachnoid space surrounding the spinal cord. It is usually performed in patients who cannot have an MRI (magnetic resonance imaging). After injection of contrast, x-ray films and a CT scan are taken. The procedure is called **CT myelography.**
pyelography	X-ray images are made of the renal pelvis and urinary tract after contrast is injected into a vein **(intravenous pyelogram)** or after dye is injected directly into the urethra, bladder, and ureters **(retrograde pyelogram).** **Urography** is another term used to describe the process of recording x-ray images of the urinary tract after the introduction of contrast.

Some individuals experience side effects caused by the iodine-containing contrast substances. These effects can range from mild reactions such as flushing, nausea, warmth, or tingling sensations to severe, life-threatening reactions characterized by airway spasm, hives, laryngeal edema (swelling of the larynx), vasodilation, and tachycardia. Treatment involves immediate establishment of an airway and ventilation followed by injections of epinephrine (adrenaline), corticosteroids, or antihistamines.

Fluoroscopy. This x-ray procedure uses a fluorescent screen instead of a photographic plate to derive a visual image from the x-rays that pass through the patient. The fact that ionizing radiation such as x-rays can produce **fluorescence** (rays of light energy emitted as a result of exposure to and absorption of radiation from another source) is the basis for fluoroscopy. The fluorescent screen glows when it is struck by the x-rays. Opaque tissue such as bone appears as a dark shadow image on the fluorescent screen.

A major advantage of fluoroscopy over normal radiography is that internal organs, such as the heart and digestive tract organs, can be observed in motion. In addition, the patient's position can be changed constantly to provide the right view at the right time so that the most useful diagnostic information can be obtained.

Digital computerized imaging techniques can be used to enhance conventional and fluoroscopic x-ray images. A lower dose of x-ray is used to achieve higher quality images, and computerized digital images can be sent via networks to other locations and computer monitors so that many people can share information and assist in diagnoses.

Image-intensifier systems for fluoroscopy can brighten fluoroscopic images and can be combined with television and movie cameras and videotape recorders to obtain a permanent record of either a fluoroscopic or an x-ray examination. This procedure is called **cineradiography** (cine- means motion).

Interventional Radiology. Interventional radiologists perform invasive procedures (therapeutic or diagnostic) under fluoroscopic, CT, and more recently MR (magnetic resonance) guidance. Procedures include placement of drainage catheters, drainage of abscesses, occlusion of bleeding vessels, and instillation of antibiotics or chemotherapy through catheters. In addition, interventional radiologists are performing thermal (heating or freezing), radiofrequency, and ultrasound ablation (destruction) of benign and malignant lesions.

Ultrasound

This technique employs high-frequency, inaudible sound waves that bounce off body tissues and are then recorded to give information about the anatomy of an internal organ. An instrument called a **transducer** or **probe** is placed near or on the skin, which is covered with a thin coating of gel to assure good transmission of sound waves. The transducer

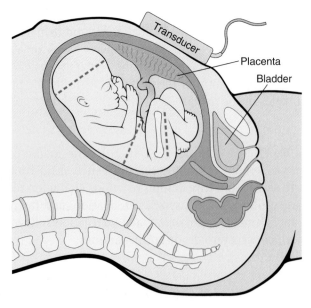

Figure 20–6

Fetal measurements taken with ultrasound imaging. Dashed lines indicate the image planes for measurements of the fetal head, abdomen, and femur.

Figure 20-7

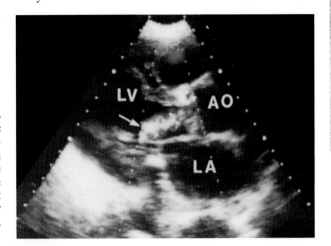

Color-flow imaging in a patient with aortic regurgitation. The brightly colored, high-velocity jet *(arrow)* can be seen passing from the aorta (AO) to the left ventricle (LV). The center of the jet is white, and the edges are shades of blue. (From Braunwald E: Heart Disease: A Textbook of Cardiovascular Medicine, 5th ed. Philadelphia, WB Saunders, 1997.)

emits sound waves in short, repetitive pulses. The ultrasound waves move with different speeds through body tissues and detect interfaces between tissues of different densities. An echo reflection of the sound waves is formed as the waves hit the various body tissues and pass back to the transducer.

These ultrasonic echoes are then recorded as a composite picture of the area of the body over which the instrument has passed. The record produced by ultrasound is called a **sonogram.**

Ultrasound is used as a diagnostic tool not only by radiologists but also by neurosurgeons and ophthalmologists to detect intracranial and ophthalmic lesions, by cardiologists to detect heart valve and blood vessel disorders **(echocardiography),** by gastroenterologists to locate abdominal masses outside the digestive organs, and by obstetricians and gynecologists to differentiate single and multiple pregnancies as well as to help in performing amniocentesis and in locating tumors or cysts. Fetal size and age can also be measured using ultrasound. The measurements are made of the head, abdomen, and femur based on ultrasound images taken in various fetal planes (Fig. 20–6).

Ultrasound has several advantages in that the sound waves are nonionizing and noninjurious to tissues at the energy ranges utilized for diagnostic purposes. Because water is an excellent conductor of the ultrasonic beams, patients are requested to drink large quantities of water before examination so that the urinary bladder will be distended and enable better viewing of pelvic and abdominal organs.

Two ultrasound techniques, **Doppler ultrasound** and **color-flow imaging,** make it possible to record blood velocity (in diagnosing vascular disease) and to image major blood vessels in patients at risk for stroke. Figure 20–7 shows color-flow imaging in a patient with aortic regurgitation (blood flowing backward from the aorta into the left ventricle).

Ultrasound, like fluoroscopy, has also been used in interventional radiology to guide needle biopsies for the puncture of cysts and for the placement of needles for amniocentesis.

Magnetic Imaging or Magnetic Resonance Imaging (MRI or MR)

This is a type of diagnostic radiography that uses electromagnetic energy rather than x-rays. The technique produces sagittal, coronal (frontal), and axial (cross-sectional) images. MRI is based on the fact that the nuclei of some atoms behave like little magnets when a larger magnetic field is applied. The nuclei spin and emit radio waves that create an image as the nuclei move back to an equilibrium position. Hydrogen nuclei, present in water and abundant in living tissue, are the nuclei used to create the image.

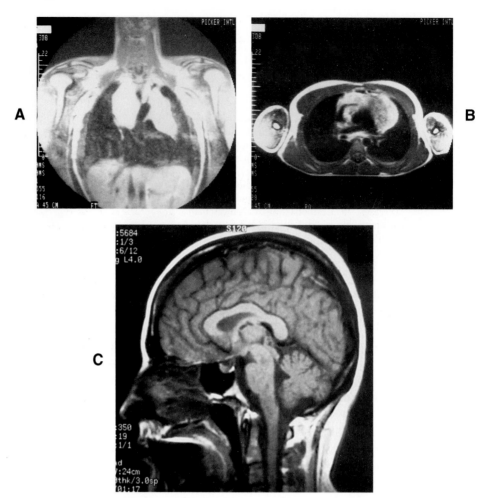

Figure 20–8

Magnetic resonance images. (A) Frontal (coronal) view of the upper body. White masses in the chest are Hodgkin disease lesions. **(B) Transverse view** of the same patient with chest mass. **(C) Sagittal view** of the head (normal magnetic resonance image) showing cerebrum, ventricles, cerebellum, and medulla oblongata. (**C** From Black JM, Hawks JH, Keene AM: Medical-Surgical Nursing: Clinical Management for Positive Outcomes, 6th ed. Philadelphia, WB Saunders, 2001, p. 1985.)

MR examinations are performed with and without contrast. The contrast agent most commonly used for MRI is gadolinium (Gd). As iodine contrast does with CT, gadolinium enhances vessels and tissues, increases the sensitivity for lesion detection, and helps differentiate between normal and abnormal tissues and structures. MRI is useful for providing soft-tissue images, detecting edema in the brain, projecting a direct image of the spinal cord, detecting tumors in the chest and abdomen, and visualizing the cardiovascular system. Figure 20–8 shows three different MR images (coronal, axial, and sagittal).

MRI is not used for patients with pacemakers or metallic implants because the powerful MR magnet can interfere with the position and functioning of such devices. The sounds (loud tapping) heard during the test are caused by the pulsing of the magnetic field as it scans the body.

Figure 20–9 summarizes radiological diagnostic techniques.

C. X-Ray Positioning

In order to take the best view of the part of the body being radiographed, the patient, film, and x-ray tube must be positioned in the most favorable alignment possible. There are

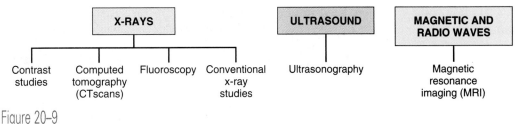

Figure 20–9

Summary of radiological diagnostic techniques.

special terms used by radiologists to refer to the direction of travel of the x-ray through the patient. X-ray terms describing the direction of the x-ray beam follow and are illustrated in Figure 20–10:

1. **Posteroanterior (PA) view.** In this most commonly requested chest x-ray view, x-rays travel from a posteriorly placed source to an anteriorly placed detector.
2. **Anteroposterior (AP) view.** X-rays travel from an anteriorly placed source to a posteriorly placed detector.
3. **Lateral view.** In a left lateral view, x-rays travel from a source located to the right of the patient to a detector placed to the left of the patient.
4. **Oblique view.** X-rays travel in a slanting direction at an angle from the perpendicular plane. Oblique views show regions ordinarily hidden and superimposed in routine PA and AP views.

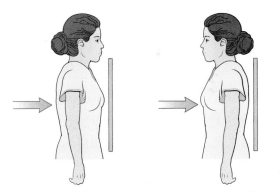

1. Posteroanterior (PA) view   2. Anteroposterior (AP) view

Figure 20–10

Positions for x-ray views. The arrow denotes the direction of the x-ray beam through the patient.

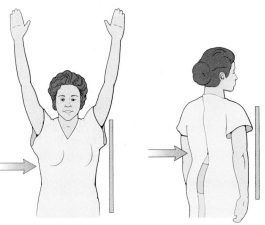

3. Left lateral view   4. Oblique view

The following terms are used to describe the position of the patient or part of the body in the x-ray examination:

abduction	Moving the part of the body away from the midline of the body or away from the body.
adduction	Moving the part of the body toward the midline of the body or toward the body.
eversion	Turning outward.
extension	Lengthening or straightening a flexed limb.
flexion	Bending a part of the body.
inversion	Turning inward.
lateral decubitus	Lying down on the side with the x-ray beam horizontally positioned.
prone	Lying on the belly (face down).
recumbent	Lying down (may be prone or supine).
supine	Lying on the back (face up).

III. Nuclear Medicine

A. Radioactivity and Radionuclides

The emission of energy in the form of particles or rays coming from the interior of a substance is called **radioactivity.** A **radionuclide** (or **radioisotope**) is a substance that gives off high-energy particles or rays as it disintegrates. Radionuclides are produced in either a nuclear reactor or a charged-particle accelerator (cyclotron) or by irradiating stable substances, causing disruption and instability. **Half-life** is the time required for a radio-active substance (radionuclide) to lose half of its radioactivity by disintegration. Knowledge of a radionuclide's half-life is important in determining how long the radioactive substance will emit radioactivity when in the body. The half-life must be long enough to allow for diagnostic imaging but as short as possible to minimize patient exposure to radiation.

Radionuclides emit three types of radioactivity: **alpha particles, beta particles,** and **gamma rays.** Gamma rays, which have greater penetrating ability than alpha and beta particles, and more ionizing power, are especially useful to physicians in both the diagnosis and the treatment of disease. Technetium-99m (^{99m}Tc) is essentially a pure gamma emitter with a half-life of 6 hours. Its properties make it the most frequently used radionuclide in diagnostic imaging.

B. Nuclear Medicine Tests: *In Vitro* and *In Vivo* Procedures

Nuclear medicine physicians use two types of tests in the diagnosis of disease: ***in vitro*** (in the test tube) procedures and ***in vivo*** (in the body) procedures. ***In vitro*** procedures involve analysis of blood and urine specimens using radioactive chemicals. For example, a **radioimmunoassay (RIA)** is an *in vitro* procedure that combines the use of radioactive chemicals and antibodies to detect hormones and drugs in a patient's blood. The test allows the detection of minute amounts of substances or compounds. RIA is used to monitor the amount of digitalis, a drug used to treat heart disease, in a patient's bloodstream and can detect hypothyroidism in newborn infants.

In vivo tests trace the amounts of radioactive substances within the body. They are given directly to a patient to evaluate the function of an organ or to image it. For example, in **tracer studies** a specific radionuclide is incorporated into a chemical substance and administered to a patient. The combination of the radionuclide and a drug or chemical is called a **radiopharmaceutical** (or **labeled compound**). Each radiopharmaceutical is designed to concentrate in a certain organ. The organ can then be imaged with the radiation given off by the radionuclide.

A sensitive, external detection instrument called a **gamma camera (scintiscanner)** is used to determine the distribution and localization of the radiopharmaceutical in various organs, tissues, and fluids. See Figure 20–11. The amount of radiopharmaceutical at a given location is proportional to the rate at which the gamma rays are emitted. Nuclear medicine studies depict the physiological behavior (how the organ works) rather than the specific anatomy of an organ.

The procedure of making an image to follow the distribution of radioactive substance in the body is called **scintigraphy (radionuclide scanning),** and the image produced is called a **scintiscan. Uptake** refers to the rate of absorption of the radiopharmaceutical into an organ or tissue.

Radiopharmaceuticals may be administered by many different routes to obtain a scan of a specific organ in the body. For example, in the case of a **lung scan,** the radiopharmaceutical can be given intravenously (**perfusion studies,** which rely on passage of the radioactive compound through the capillaries of the lungs) or by inhalation of a gas or aerosol (**ventilation studies**), which fills the air sacs (alveoli). The combination of these tests permits sensitive and specific diagnosis of clots in the lung (pulmonary emboli).

A 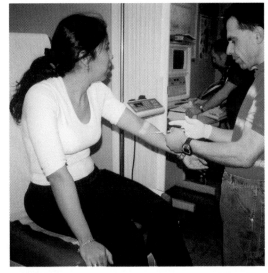   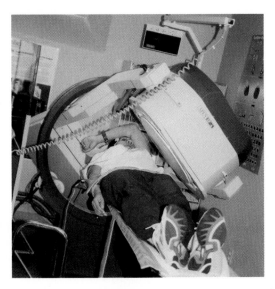 **B**

Figure 20–11

(A) Patient receiving intravenous injection of radionuclide for detection of heart function. **(B) Gamma camera** moves around patient, detecting radioactivity in heart muscle.

Other examples of diagnostic procedures that utilize radionuclides are as follows:

1. **Bone scan.** ^{99m}Tc (technetium) is used to label phosphate substances and is injected intravenously. The phosphate compound is taken up preferentially by bone, and the skeleton can be imaged in 2 or 3 hours by use of a scintiscanner. Waiting 2 to 3 hours allows much of the radiopharmaceutical to be excreted in urine and allows for better visualization of the skeleton. The scan is useful in demonstrating malignant metastases to the skeleton, which appear as areas of high uptake ("hot spots") on the scan.

2. **Gallium scan.** The radioisotope gallium-67 is injected intravenously and has an affinity for tumors and non-neoplastic lesions such as abscesses. Gallium also has an affinity for areas of inflammation as occurs in pneumonitis.

3. **Liver and spleen scans.** To visualize the liver and spleen, a radiopharmaceutical (^{99m}Tc and sulfur colloid) is injected intravenously, and images are taken with a scintiscanner (gamma camera). Areas of tumor or abscess are shown as **photopenic** areas (regions of reduced uptake). Abnormalities such as cirrhosis, abscesses, tumor, hepatomegaly, and hepatitis can be detected by liver scanning, and splenomegaly due to tumor, cyst, abscess, or rupture can be diagnosed with spleen scanning.

4. **Positron emission tomography (PET scan).** This radionuclide technique produces images of the distribution of radioactivity (through emission of positrons) in a region of the body. It is similar to the CT scan, but radioisotopes are used instead of contrast and x-rays. The radionuclides are incorporated (by intravenous injection) into the tissues to be scanned, and an image is made showing where the radionuclide (18F-FDG, a radioactive glucose molecule) is or is not being metabolized. For example, PET scanning has determined that schizophrenics do not metabolize glucose equally in all parts of the brain and that drug treatment can bring improvement to these regions. Thus, areas of metabolic deficiency can be pinpointed by PET, making it helpful in diagnosing and treating other neurological disorders such as stroke, epilepsy, Alzheimer disease, and brain tumors, as well as abdominal and pulmonary malignancies. See Figure 20–12.

5. **Single-photon emission computed tomography (SPECT).** This technique involves an intravenous injection of radioactive tracer (such as Technetium 99m) and the computer reconstruction of a three-dimensional image based on a composite of many views. Clinical applications include detecting liver tumors, detecting cardiac ischemia, and evaluating bone disease of the spine.

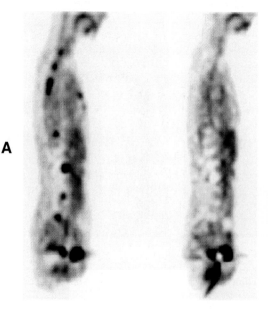

A

B

Figure 20–12

Whole-body PET images. (A) 18F-FDG sagittal image of patient with breast cancer metastases. Numerous tumors (dark spots) are seen along the spine and sternum. **(B) Image obtained after chemotherapy** shows regression of the cancer. (From Ballinger PW, Frank ED: Merrill's Atlas of Radiographic Positions and Radiologic Procedures, 10th ed. St. Louis, Mosby, 2003, vol. 3, p. 549.)

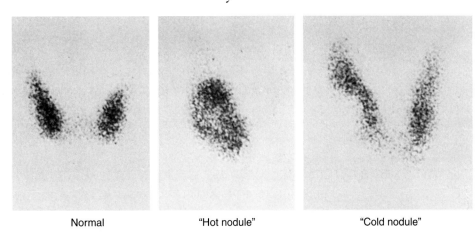

Normal   "Hot nodule"   "Cold nodule"

Figure 20–13

Thyroid scans. The scan of a "hot nodule" shows a darkened area of increased uptake, which indicates a diseased thyroid gland. The scan of a "cold nodule" shows an area of decreased uptake, which indicates a non-functioning region, a common occurrence when normal tissue is replaced by malignancy. (From Beare PG, Myers JL: Adult Health Nursing, 3rd ed. St. Louis, Mosby, 1998.)

6. **^{99m}Technetium sestamibi (Cardiolite) scan.** This radiopharmaceutical is injected intravenously and traced to heart muscle. An exercise tolerance test is used with it for an ETT-MIBI scan. In a **mu**ltiple **g**ated **a**cquisition **(MUGA)** scan, technetium-99m is injected intravenously to study the motion of the heart wall muscle and the ventricle's ability to eject blood (ejection fraction).

7. **Thallium (Tl) scan.** Thallium 201(^{201}Tl) is injected intravenously to allow for myocardial perfusion. A high concentration of thallium 201 is present in well-perfused heart muscle cells, but infarcted or scarred myocardium does not extract any Tl, showing up as "cold spots." If the defective area is ischemic, the cold spots fill in (become "warm") on delayed images.

8. **Thyroid scan.** Radionuclide is administered intravenously. The scan produced can help determine the size and shape of the thyroid gland. Hyperfunctioning thyroid nodules (adenomas) accumulate higher amounts of ^{131}I radioactivity and are termed "hot." Thyroid carcinoma does not concentrate radioiodine well and, therefore, is seen as a "cold" spot on the scan. Figure 20–13 shows thyroid scans.

Figure 20–14 reviews *in vitro* and *in vivo* nuclear medicine diagnostic tests.

NUCLEAR MEDICINE TESTS

IN VITRO	**Radioimmunoassay**

IN VIVO	**Tracer Studies:** Bone scan Gallium scan Liver/spleen scan Lung scan (ventilation/perfusion) Positron emission tomography (PET) Single-photon emission computed tomography (SPECT) ^{99m}Technetium-sestamibi scan ^{201}Thallium scan Thyroid scan

Figure 20–14

In vitro and *in vivo* nuclear medicine diagnostic tests.

IV. Vocabulary

This list reviews many of the new terms introduced in the text. Short definitions reinforce your understanding of the terms. See Section XI of this chapter for help in pronouncing the more difficult terms.

cineradiography	Use of motion picture techniques to record a series of x-ray images during fluoroscopy.
computed tomography (CT)	Diagnostic x-ray procedure whereby a cross-section image of a specific body segment is produced; also known as computed axial tomography (CAT).
contrast studies	Materials (contrast media) are injected to obtain contrast with surrounding tissue when shown on the x-ray film.
fluorescence	Emission of glowing light that results from exposure to and absorption of radiation from x-rays.
fluoroscopy	Process of using x-rays to produce a fluorescent image on an image intensifier.
gamma camera	Machine to detect radiopharmaceuticals in the body for diagnostic purposes (scintiscanner).
gamma rays	High-energy rays emitted by radioactive substances.
half-life	Time required for a radioactive substance to lose half its radioactivity by disintegration.
interventional radiology	Therapeutic procedures that are performed by a radiologist.
in vitro	A process, test, or procedure in which something is measured or observed *outside* a living organism.
in vivo	A process, test, or procedure in which something is measured or observed *in* a living organism.
ionization	Transformation of electrically neutral substances into electrically charged ones.
labeled compound	Radiopharmaceutical.
magnetic resonance (MR)	A magnetic field and radio waves are used to form sagittal, coronal, and axial images of the body.
nuclear medicine	Medical specialty that studies the uses of radioactive substances (radionuclides) in diagnosis of disease.
positron emission tomography (PET)	Radioactive substances are given intravenously and then emit positrons, which create a cross-sectional image of the metabolism of the body, representing local concentration of the radioactive substance.

radioimmunoassay	Test that combines the use of radioactive chemicals and antibodies to detect minute quantities of substances in a patient's blood.
radioisotope	Radioactive form of a substance; radionuclide.
radiology	Medical specialty concerned with the study of x-rays and their use in the diagnosis of disease; includes other forms of energy, such as ultrasound and magnetic waves.
radiolucent	Permitting the passage of most x-rays. Radiolucent structures appear black on x-ray film.
radionuclide	Radioactive chemical element that gives off energy in the form of radiation; radioisotope.
radiopaque	Obstructing the passage of x-rays. Radiopaque structures appear white on the x-ray film.
radiopharmaceutical	Radioactive drug (radionuclide plus chemical) that is administered safely for diagnostic purposes.
roentgenology	Study of x-rays; radiology.
scan	General term for images of organs, parts, or transverse sections of the body produced in various ways. Most frequently used to describe images obtained from ultrasound, radioactive tracer studies, or computed tomography.
scintigraphy	Production of two-dimensional images of the distribution of radioactivity in tissues after the administration of a radiopharmaceutical imaging agent.
single-photon emission computed tomography (SPECT)	Radioactive tracer substance is injected intravenously and a computer is used to create a three-dimensional image.
tagging	Attaching a radionuclide to a chemical and following its course in the body.
tracer studies	Radionuclides are used as tags, or labels, attached to chemicals and followed as they migrate through the body.
transducer	Handheld device that sends and receives ultrasound signals.
ultrasound (US, U/S)	Diagnostic technique that projects and retrieves high-frequency sound waves as they echo off parts the body.
uptake	Rate of absorption of a radionuclide into an organ or tissue.
ventilation/perfusion studies	Radiopharmaceutical is inhaled (ventilation) and injected (perfusion) and its passage through the respiratory tract is imaged.

V. Combining Forms, Suffixes, Prefixes, and Terminology

Write the meanings of the medical terms in the spaces provided.

Combining Forms

Combining Form	Meaning	Terminology	Meaning
fluor/o	luminous, fluorescence	fluoroscopy _____	

In this term, -scopy does not refer to visual examination with an endoscope. In fluoroscopy, x-rays can be viewed directly, without taking and developing x-ray photographs. Light is emitted from the image intensifier when it is exposed to x-rays.

is/o	same	radioisotope _____	

top/o means place; radioisotopes of an element have similar structures but different weights and electric charges. A radioisotope (radionuclide) is an unstable form of an element that emits radioactivity.

pharmaceut/o	drug	radiopharmaceutical _____	

In this term, radi/o stands for radioisotope (radionuclide).

radi/o	x-rays	radiography _____	
roentgen/o	x-rays	roentgenology _____	
scint/i	spark	scintigraphy _____	
son/o	sound	hysterosonogram _____	

Saline solution is injected through a catheter inserted into the vagina and into the endocervical canal to distend the uterine cavity, which is then examined by ultrasound.

therapeut/o	treatment	therapeutic _____	
tom/o	to cut	tomography _____	

A series of x-ray images (taken as if to make slices or cuts) are made of the body to show an organ in depth. Changing the depth of focus allows each tomogram to focus on the one slice that is to be viewed.

| vitr/o | glass | *in vitro* |
| viv/o | life | *in vivo* |

Suffixes

Suffix	Meaning	Terminology	Meaning
-gram	record	angiogram	
		hysterosalpingogram	
		pyelogram	
-graphy	process of recording	computed tomography	
-lucent	to shine	radiolucent	

Radiolucent (indicating that x-rays pass through easily) areas on x-ray film appear dark on the exposed film.

| **-opaque** | obscure | radiopaque | |

Radiopaque (indicating that x-rays do not penetrate) areas on x-ray film appear white or light on exposed film.

Prefixes

Prefix	Meaning	Terminology	Meaning
cine-	movement	cineradiography	
echo-	a repeated sound	echocardiography	
ultra-	beyond	ultrasonography	

Sound waves are beyond the normal range of those that a human can hear.

VI. *Abbreviations*

Angio	angiography		**LAT**	lateral
AP	anteroposterior		**LS Films**	lumbosacral spine films
Ba	barium		**MR or MRI**	magnetic resonance; magnetic resonance imaging
CAT	computerized axial tomography		**MRA**	magnetic resonance angiography
C-spine	cervical spine films		**MUGA**	multiple-gated acquisitions scan (radioactive test to show heart function)
CT	computed tomography			
CXR	chest x-ray		**PA**	posteroanterior
Decub	decubitus (lying down)		**PACS**	picture archival and communications system; replacement of traditional films with digital equivalents that can be accessed from several places and retrieved more rapidly
DICOM	digital image communication in medicine. Standard protocol for transmission between imaging devices (i.e., CT scans and PACS workstations)			
			PET	positron emission tomography
DI	diagnostic imaging		**SPECT**	single-photon emission computed tomography; radioactive substances and a computer are used to create three-dimensional images
DSA	digital subtraction angiography			
FDG	fluorodeoxyglucose (radiopharmaceutical used in PET scanning)			
^{99m}Tc	radioactive technetium (used in heart, brain, skull, thyroid, liver, spleen, bone, and lung scans)			
^{67}Ga	radioactive gallium (used in whole-body scans)			
^{131}I	radioactive iodine (used in thyroid, liver, and kidney scans and treatment of malignant and nonmalignant conditions of the thyroid)		^{201}Tl	radioisotope (thallium) used in scanning heart muscle
			UGI	upper gastrointestinal (series)
IVP	intravenous pyelogram		**US, U/S**	ultrasound
KUB	kidneys, ureters, bladder (x-ray without contrast medium)		**VQ scan**	ventilation-perfusion scan of the lungs

VII. Practical Applications

Answers to the Case Study questions are found on page 844.

Case Study

Bill Smith, a 51-year-old sales representative, was initially diagnosed with stage III melanoma 4 years ago. He underwent surgery and interferon treatment at that time. At his three-month follow-up CT scan last year, Mr. Smith received bad news. The CT scan indicated a small 1-cm nodule, which could be a melanoma metastasis. To confirm the diagnosis, Mr. Smith underwent a PET scan.

He was admitted to the nuclear medicine unit of the hospital in the morning of the scan. He had been informed to fast (no food or beverage 12 hours before the scan). The nuclear physician had told him especially not to eat any type of sugar, which would compete with the radiopharmaceutical (18F-FDG or fluoro-deoxyglucose), which is a radioactive glucose molecule that travels to every cell in the body.

The PET scan began with an injection of a trace amount of 18F-FDG by a nuclear physician. Bill was asked to lie still for about an hour in a dark, quiet room and to avoid talking to prevent the compound from concentrating in the tongue and vocal cords. The waiting time allowed the 18F-FDG to be absorbed and released from normal tissue. After emptying his bladder, Bill reclined on a bed that moved slowly and quietly through a PET scanner, a tube similar to a CT scanner. The radioactive glucose emits charged particles called positrons, which, along with gamma rays, are detected by the scanner. Color-coded images indicate the intensity of metabolic activity throughout the body. Cancerous cells rapidly divide and hence absorb more radioactive glucose than noncancerous cells. The malignant cells show up brighter on the PET scan.

Bill's PET scan proved the CT wrong. His melanoma had not metastasized. He returned home quite relieved.

Questions

1. **In CT scanning**
   (A) a radioactive tracer is used
   (B) x-ray images reveal images in all three planes of the body
   (C) a nuclear physician performs the ultrasound procedure
   (D) images reveal anatomic structures in the axial plane

2. **In PET scanning**
   (A) a radioactive tracer is used
   (B) x-ray images reveal images in all three planes of the body
   (C) a nuclear physician performs the ultrasound procedure
   (D) images reveal anatomic structures in the axial plane

3. **Bill's case showed that**
   (A) CT scanning and PET scanning are equally effective in diagnosis of metastases
   (B) PET scanning is useful in cancer diagnosis and staging
   (C) melanoma never progresses to stage IV
   (D) a diet high in glucose helps concentrate the radioactive 18F-DFG before the PET scan

CT Upper Abdomen Using IV Contrast

Comparison was also made with prior examination. The extensive retroperitoneal and mesenteric lymphadenopathy has shown marked reduction in size. The celiac lymph nodes are also reduced, and the outlines of the lymph nodes are in the top limits of normal at this point. In images 8 and 9 the celiac lymph nodes are no longer visible. Previously described right pleural effusion is also not present. The obstructed right kidney shows atrophy and now measures approximately 7-8 cm in size. The left kidney remains much the same as before. The adrenal glands are symmetrical with normal aorta and inferior vena cava as well as abdominal wall.

General Hospital—Nuclear Medicine Dept.—Radionuclides Available

Radionuclide	Radiopharmaceutical	Admission Route	Target Organ
^{133}Xe	xenon gas	inhaled	lungs
^{99m}Tc	albumin microspheres	IV	lungs
^{87m}Sr (strontium)	solution	IV	bone
^{99m}Tc	diphosphonate	IV	bone
^{99m}Tc	pertechnetate	IV	brain
^{99m}Tc	sulfur colloid	IV	liver/spleen
^{99m}Tc	HIDA*	IV	gallbladder
^{198}Au	colloid	IV	liver
^{199}Au	colloid	IV	spleen
^{131}I	rose bengal	IV	colon
^{99m}Tc	DTPA†	IV	kidney
^{99m}TC	DMSA‡	IV	kidney
^{131}I	Hippuran	IV	kidney
^{131}I	iodide	IV	thyroid
^{201}Tl (thallium)	thallium chloride	IV	heart
^{99m}Tc	sestamibi	IV	heart
^{67}Ga (gallium)	citrate	IV	tumors and abscesses

*HIDA = *N*-(2.6-dimethyl)iminodiacetic acid
†DTPA = diethylenetriamine pentaacetic acid
‡dimercaptosuccinic acid

VIII. Exercises

Remember to check your answers carefully with those given in Section IX, Answers to Exercises.

A. *Complete the medical terms based on the definitions and word parts given.*

1. obstructing the passage of x-rays: radio _____

2. permitting the passage of x-rays: radio _____

3. aids physicians in performing ultrasound procedures: _____ grapher

4. transformation of stable substances into charged particles: _____ ization

5. radioactive drug administered for diagnostic purposes: radio _____

6. radioactive chemical that gives off energy in the form of radiation: radio _____

7. a physician who specializes in diagnostic radiology: radi _____

8. study of the uses of radioactive substances in the diagnosis of disease: _____

   medicine

B. *Match the special diagnostic techniques below with their definitions.*

cineradiography   fluoroscopy   tomography
computed tomography   interventional radiology   ultrasonography
contrast studies   magnetic resonance imaging

1. radiopaque substances are given and conventional x-rays taken _____

2. use of motion picture techniques to record x-ray images _____

3. series of x-rays are taken at different depths of an organ _____

4. use of echoes of high-frequency sound waves to diagnose disease _____

5. x-ray beams are focused from the body onto an image intensifier that glows as a result of the

   ionizing effect of x-rays _____

6. a magnetic field and radio waves are used to form images of the body _____

7. x-ray pictures are taken circularly around an area of the body, and a computer synthesizes the

   information into a composite cross-section picture _____

8. therapeutic procedures are performed by a radiologist under the guidance of fluoroscopy or

   ultrasound _____

C. *Match the diagnostic x-ray test in column I with the part of the body that is imaged in column II.*

Column I

1. myelography   _____

2. intravenous pyelography _____

3. angiography   _____

4. arthrography   _____

5. upper GI series   _____

6. cholangiography   _____

7. barium enema   _____

8. hysterosalpingography _____

Column II

A. joints
B. spinal cord
C. uterus and fallopian tubes
D. blood vessels
E. esophagus, stomach and small intestine
F. lower gastrointestinal tract
G. renal pelvis of kidney and urinary tract
H. bile vessels (ducts)

D. Match the following x-ray views or positions in column I with their meanings in column II. Write the letter of the answer in the space provided.

Column I

1. PA _____

2. supine _____

3. prone _____

4. AP _____

5. lateral _____

6. oblique _____

7. lateral decubitus _____

8. adduction _____

9. inversion _____

10. abduction _____

11. recumbent _____

12. eversion _____

13. flexion _____

14. extension _____

Column II

A. on the side
B. turned inward
C. movement away from the midline
D. lying on the belly
E. x-ray tube positioned on an angle
F. bending a part
G. straightening a limb
H. lying on the back
I. lying down on the side
J. lying down; prone or supine
K. anterior to posterior view
L. turning outward
M. posterior to anterior view
N. movement toward the midline

E. Give the meanings of the following medical terms.

1. *in vitro* _____

2. *in vivo* _____

3. radiopharmaceutical _____

4. tracer studies _____

5. uptake _____

6. perfusion lung scan _____

7. ventilation lung scan _____

8. bone scan _____

9. gallium scan _____

10. thyroid scan _____

11. ^{99m}Tc-sestamibi scan _____

F. Give the meanings of the following terms.

1. gamma camera _____

2. positron emission tomography (PET) _____

3. radioisotope _____

4. transducer _____

5. uptake _____

6. echocardiography _____

7. roentgenology _____

G. Give the meanings of the following word parts.

1. -gram _____   6. viv/o _____

2. ultra- _____   7. pharmaceut/o _____

3. fluor/o _____   8. son/o _____

4. tom/o _____   9. cine- _____

5. vitr/o _____   10. therapeut/o _____

H. Give the meanings of the following abbreviations and then select from the sentences that follow the best association for each.

Column I

1. MR _____ ____

2. SPECT _____ ____

3. PACS _____ ____

4. UGI _____ ____

5. CXR _____ ____

6. DSA _____ ____

7. IVP _____ ____

8. LAT _____ ____

9. U/S _____ ____

10. ^{99m}Tc _____ ____

Column II

A. X-ray examination of the kidney after injection of contrast.

B. Diagnostic procedure frequently used to assess fetal size and development.

C. X-ray examination of the esophagus, stomach, and intestines.

D. X-ray of blood vessels made by taking two images (with and without contrast) and subtracting one from the other.

E. Radioisotope used in nuclear medicine (tracer studies).

F. Radioactive substances and a computer are used to create three-dimensional images.

G. This diagnostic procedure produces images of all three planes of the body and visualizes soft tissue in the nervous and musculoskeletal systems.

H. Replacement of traditional films with digital equivalents.

I. X-ray position (side view).

J. Diagnostic procedure (x-rays are used) necessary to investigate thoracic disease.

I. Circle the correct term to complete each sentence.

1. Mr. Jones was scheduled for ultrasound-guided removal of his pleural effusion. He was sent to the **(interventional radiology, radiation oncology, nuclear medicine)** department for the procedure.

2. In order to better visualize Mr. Smith's colon, Dr. Wong ordered a **(perfusion study, hysterosalpingography, barium enema)**. She hoped to determine why he was having blood in his stools.

3. After the head-on collision, Sam was taken to the emergency room in an unconscious state. The paramedics suspected head trauma, and the doctors ordered an emergency **(PET scan, U/S, CT scan)** of his head.

4. In light of Sue's symptoms of fever, cough, and malaise, the doctors thought that the consolidated, hazy **(radioisotope, radiolucent, radiopaque)** area on the chest x-ray represented a pneumonia.

5. Fred, a lung cancer patient, experienced a seizure recently. His oncologist ordered a brain **(ultrasound, pulmonary angiogram, MRI)** that showed a tumor involving the left frontal lobe of the brain. Fred was treated with **(gamma camera, gamma knife, gallium)** irradiation, and the tumor decreased in size. He has had no further seizures.

6. Tom recently developed a cough and fever. A chest x-ray and **(CT, myelogram, IVP)** of the chest shows a **(pelvic, spinal, mediastinal)** mass is present. **(Mediastinoscopy, Cystoscopy, Lumbar puncture)** and biopsy of the mass reveals Hodgkin disease on pathological examination. He is treated with chemotherapy, and his symptoms disappear. A repeat x-ray shows that the mass has decreased remarkably, but a **(SPECT, MR, PET)** scan shows no uptake of 18F-FDG in the chest, indicating that the mass is fibrosis and not tumor.

7. Paola, a 50-year-old diabetic, experiences chest pain during a stress test, and her **(U/S, ECG, EEG)** shows evidence of ischemia. A **(contrast agent, transducer, radiopharmaceutical)** called ^{99m}Tc sestamibi (Cardiolite) is injected IV, and uptake is assessed with a **(probe, CT scanner, gamma camera)**, which shows an area of poor perfusion in the left ventricle.

8. Sally has a routine pelvic examination, and her **(neurologist, gynecologist, urologist)** feels an irregular area of enlargement in the anterior wall of the uterus. A pelvic **(angiogram, U/S, PET scan)** is performed, which demonstrates the presence of fibroids in the uterine wall. The exam involves placing a gel over her abdominopelvic area and a **(transducer, radionuclide, probe)** sends into and receives sound vibrations from the pelvic region.

IX. Answers to Exercises

A

1. radiopaque
2. radiolucent
3. sonographer
4. ionization
5. radiopharmaceutical
6. radioisotope or radionuclide
7. radiologist
8. nuclear medicine

B

1. contrast studies
2. cineradiography; a type of fluoroscopy
3. tomography
4. ultrasonography
5. fluoroscopy
6. magnetic resonance imaging
7. computed tomography
8. interventional radiology

C

1. B
2. G
3. D
4. A
5. E
6. H
7. F
8. C

D

1. M
2. H
3. D
4. K
5. A
6. E
7. I
8. N
9. B
10. C
11. J
12. L
13. F
14. G

E

1. Process, test, or procedure in which something is measured or observed outside a living organism.
2. Process, test, or procedure in which something is measured or observed in a living organism.
3. Radioactive drug (radionuclide plus chemical) that is given for diagnostic or therapeutic purposes.
4. Tests in which radioactive substance (radioisotopes) are used with chemicals and followed as they travel throughout the body.
5. The rate of absorption of a radionuclide into an organ or tissue.
6. A radiopharmaceutical is injected intravenously and traced within the blood vessels of the lung.
7. A radiopharmaceutical is inhaled, and its passage through the respiratory tract is imaged.
8. A radiopharmaceutical is given intravenously and taken up by bone tissue. An image allows the radioactive substance to be traced in the bone.
9. The radioisotope gallium 67 is injected intravenously, and the body is scanned.
10. Radioactive substance is given intravenously, and a scan (image) is made of its uptake in the thyroid gland.
11. Test of heart muscle function.

Continued on following page

F

1. machine that detects rays emitted by radioactive substances
2. radioactive glucose is injected and traced to body cells
3. a radioactive form (radionuclide) of a substance; gives off radiation

4. handheld device that sends and receives ultrasound signals
5. rate of absorption of a radionuclide into an organ or tissue

6. ultrasound used to create an image of the heart
7. study of x-rays; radiology

G

1. record
2. beyond
3. luminous, fluorescence
4. to cut

5. glass
6. life
7. drug

8. sound
9. motion
10. treatment

H

1. Magnetic resonance. G
2. Single-photon emission computed tomography. F
3. Picture archival and communications system. H

4. Upper gastrointestinal (series). C
5. Chest x-ray. J
6. Digital subtraction angiography. D
7. Intravenous pyelogram. A

8. Lateral. I
9. Ultrasound. B
10. Radioactive technetium. E

I

1. interventional radiology
2. barium enema

3. CT scan
4. radiopaque

Answers to Practical Applications

1. D
2. A
3. C

4. B
5. MRI, gamma knife
6. CT, mediastinal, mediastinoscopy, PET

7. ECG, radiopharmaceutical, gamma camera
8. gynecologist, U/S, transducer

X. Pronunciation of Terms

Pronunciation Guide

To test your understanding of the terminology in this chapter, write the meaning of each term in the space provided. In addition, you may wish to cover the terms and write them by looking at your definitions. Make sure your spelling is correct. The page number after each term indicates where it is defined or used in the text so you can easily check your responses.

ā as in āpe   ă as in ăpple
ē as in ēven   ĕ as in ĕvery
ī as in īce   ĭ as in ĭnterest
ō as in ōpen   ŏ as in pŏt
ū as in ūnit   ŭ as in ŭnder

Term	Pronunciation	Meaning
abduction (828)	ăb-DŬK-shŭn	_____
adduction (828)	ă-DŬK-shŭn	_____
angiogram (835)	ĂN-jē-ō-grăm	_____

anteroposterior (827)   ăn-tĕr-ō-pōs-TĔ-rē-ŏr   _____

arthrography (823)   ăr-THRŎG-ră-fē   _____

cholangiography (823)   kō-lăn-jē-ŎG-ră-fē   _____

cineradiography (832)   sĭn-ĕ-rā-dē-ŎG-ră-fē   _____

computed tomography (832)   kŏm-PŪ-tĕd tō-MŎG-ră-fē   _____

echocardiography (835)   ĕk-ō-kăr-dē-ŎG-ră-fē   _____

eversion (828)   ē-VĔR-zhŭn   _____

extension (828)   ĕk-STĔN-shŭn   _____

flexion (828)   FLĔK-shŭn   _____

fluorescence (832)   flū-RĔS-ĕns   _____

fluoroscopy (832)   flū-RŎS-kō-pē   _____

gallium scan (830)   GĂ-lē-ŭm skăn   _____

hysterosalpingogram (835)   hĭs-tĕr-ō-săl-PĬNG-gō-grăm   _____

hysterosonogram (834)   hĭs-tĕr-ō-SŎN-ō-grăm   _____

interventional radiology (832)   ĭn-tĕr-VĔN-shŭn-ăl rā-dē-ŎL-ō-jē   _____

inversion (828)   ĭn-VĔR-zhŭn   _____

in vitro (832)   in VĒ-trō   _____

in vivo (832)   in VĒ-vō   _____

labeled compound (832)   LĀ-bĕld KŎM-pŏwnd   _____

lateral decubitus (828)   LĂ-tĕr-ăl de-KŪ-bĭ-tus   _____

magnetic resonance (832)   măg-NĔT-ĭk RĔZ-ō-nans   _____

myelography (823)   mī-ĕ-LŎG-ră-fē   _____

nuclear medicine (832)   NU-klē-ar MĔD-ĭ-sĭn   _____

oblique (827)   ŏ-BLĒK   _____

photopenic (830)   fō-tō-PĒ-nĭk   _____

positron emission tomography (832)   pŏs-ĭ-trŏn ē-MĬSH-ŭn tō-MŎG-ră-fē   _____

posteroanterior (827)   pōs-tĕr-ō-ăn-TĒ-rē-ŏr   _____

prone (828)	prōn	
pyelogram (835)	PĪ-ē-lō-grăm	
radiography (834)	rā-dē-ŎG-ră-fē	
radioimmunoassay (833)	rā-dē-ō-ĭ-mū-nō-ĂS-ā	
radioisotope (833)	rā-dē-ō-Ī-sō-tōp	
radiolucent (833)	rā-dē-ō-LŪ-sĕnt	
radionuclide (833)	rā-dē-ō-NŪ-klīd	
radiopaque (833)	rā-dē-ō-PĀK	
radiopharmaceutical (833)	rā-dē-ō-făr-mă-SŪ-tĭ-kăl	
recumbent (828)	rē-KŬM-bĕnt	
roentgenology (833)	rĕnt-gĕ-NŎL-ō-jĕ	
scintigraphy (833)	sin-TĬG-ră-fē	
single photon emission computed tomography (833)	SĬNG-'l PHŌ-tŏn ē-MĬ-shŭn kŏm-PŪ-tĕd tō-MŎG-ră-fē	
sonogram (825)	SŎN-ō-grăm	
supine (828)	SŪ-pīn	
99mTechnetium sestamibi scan (831)	tĕk-NĒ-shē-ŭm sĕs-tă-MĬ-bē skăn	
thallium scan (831)	THĂL-ē-ŭm skăn	
therapeutic (834)	thĕr-ă-PŪ-tik	
thyroid scan (831)	THĪ-rŏyd skăn	
tomography (834)	tō-MŎG-ră-fē	
tracer studies (833)	TRĀ-sĕr STŬ-dēz	
transducer (833)	trănz-DŪ-sĕr	
ultrasound (833)	ŬL-tră-sownd	
uptake (833)	ŬP-tāk	
urography (823)	ū-RŎG-ră-fē	
ventilation/perfusion studies (833)	vĕn-tĭ-LĀ-shŭn/pĕr-FŪ-shŭn STŬ-dēz	

XI. Review Sheet

Write the meanings of the combining forms in the spaces provided and test yourself. Check your answers with the information in the text or in the glossary (Medical Terms—English) at the back of the book.

COMBINING FORMS

Combining Form	Meaning	Combining Form	Meaning
fluor/o		scint/i	
ion/o		son/o	
is/o		therapeut/o	
myel/o		tom/o	
pharmaceut/o		vitr/o	
radi/o		viv/o	
roentgen/o			

SUFFIXES

Suffix	Meaning	Suffix	Meaning
-gram		-lucent	
-graphy		-opaque	

PREFIXES

Prefix	Meaning	Prefix	Meaning
cine-		ultra-	
echo-			

chapter

Pharmacology

This chapter is divided into the following sections

In this chapter you will

- Learn of the various subspecialty areas of pharmacology.
- Identify the various routes of drug administration.
- Differentiate among the various classes of drugs and learn their actions and side effects.
- Define medical terms using combining forms, prefixes, and suffixes that relate to pharmacology.
- Apply your new knowledge to understanding medical terms in their proper contexts, such as medical reports and records.

Standards

The U.S. **Food and Drug Administration (FDA)** has the legal responsibility for deciding whether a drug may be distributed and sold. It sets rigorous standards for efficacy (effectiveness) and purity and requires extensive experimental testing in animals and people before it approves a new drug for sale in the United States. An independent committee of physicians, pharmacologists, pharmacists, and manufacturers, called the **United States Pharmacopeia (U.S.P.),** reviews the available commercial drugs and continually reappraises their effectiveness. Two important standards of the U.S.P. are that the drug be clinically useful (useful for patients) and available in pure form (made by good manufacturing methods). If a drug has U.S.P. after its name, it has met with the standards of the Pharmacopeia.

References

Libraries and hospitals have two large reference listings of drugs. The most complete and up-to-date is the **Hospital Formulary,** which gives information about the characteristics of drugs and their clinical usage (application to patient care) as approved by that particular hospital.

The **Physicians' Desk Reference (PDR)** is published by a private firm, and drug manufacturers pay to have their products listed. The PDR is a useful reference with several different indices to identify drugs, along with precautions, warnings about side effects, and information about the recommended dosage and administration of each drug.

III. Administration of Drugs

The route of administration of a drug (how it is introduced into the body) determines its rate and completeness of absorption into the blood, and its speed and duration of action.

Various methods of administering drugs are:

Oral Administration. Drugs given by mouth are slowly absorbed into the bloodstream through the stomach or intestinal wall. This method, although convenient for the patient, has several disadvantages. If the drug is destroyed in the digestive tract by digestive juices, or if the drug is unable to pass through the intestinal mucosa, it will be ineffective. Oral administration is also disadvantageous if time is a factor in therapy.

Sublingual Administration. Drugs placed under the tongue dissolve in the saliva. For some agents, absorption may be rapid. Nitroglycerin tablets are administered in this way to treat attacks of angina (chest pain).

Rectal Administration. Suppositories (cone-shaped objects containing drugs) and aqueous solutions are inserted into the rectum. Drugs are given by rectum when oral administration presents difficulties, as when the patient is nauseated and vomiting.

Parenteral Administration. Injection of drug from a **syringe** (tube) through a hollow needle placed under the skin, into a muscle, vein, or body cavity. There are several types of parenteral injections:

1. **Intracavitary injection.** This injection is made into a body cavity, such as the peritoneal or pleural cavity. For example, nitrogen mustard is injected into the pleural cavity in people who have pleural effusions due to malignant disease. The drug causes the pleural surfaces to adhere, thus obliterating the pleural space and preventing the accumulation of fluid.
2. **Intradermal injection.** This shallow injection is made into the upper layers of the skin and is used chiefly in skin testing for allergic reactions.

Table 21-1. **ROUTES OF DRUG ADMINISTRATION**

Oral	Sublingual	Rectal	Parenteral	Inhalation	Topical
Capsules Tablets	Tablets	Suppositories	Injections Intracavitary Intradermal Intramuscular Intrathecal Intravenous Subcutaneous	Aerosols	Lotions Creams Ointments Transdermal patches

3. **Intramuscular injection (IM).** The buttock or upper arm is usually the site for this injection into muscle. When drugs are irritating to the skin or when a large volume of a long-acting drug is needed, IM injections are advisable.
4. **Intrathecal injection.** This injection is made into the space under the membranes (meninges) surrounding the spinal cord and brain. Methotrexate (a cancer chemotherapeutic drug) is injected intrathecally for treatment of leukemia.
5. **Intravenous injection (IV).** This injection is given directly into a vein. It is used when an immediate effect from the drug is desired or when the drug cannot be safely introduced into other tissues. Good technical skill is needed to administer this injection because leakage of a drug into surrounding tissues may result in irritation and inflammation.
6. **Subcutaneous injection (SC).** Introduction of a hypodermic needle into the subcutaneous tissue under the skin, usually on the upper arm, thigh, or abdomen.

Inhalation. Vapors, or gases, taken into the nose or mouth are absorbed into the bloodstream through the thin walls of air sacs in the lungs. **Aerosols** (particles of drug suspended in air) are administered by inhalation, as are many anesthetics. Examples of aerosols are pentamidine, used to treat a form of pneumonia associated with acquired immunodeficiency syndrome (AIDS), and various aerosolized medicines used to treat asthma (spasm of the lung airways).

Topical Application. Drugs are locally applied on the skin or mucous membranes of the body. **Antiseptics** (against infection) and **antipruritics** (against itching) are commonly used as ointments, creams, and lotions. **Transdermal patches** are used to deliver drugs (such as estrogen, pain medications, and nicotine) continuously through the skin.

Table 21–1 summarizes the various routes of drug administration.

IV. Terminology of Drug Action

When a drug enters the body, the target substance with which the drug interacts to produce its effects is called a **receptor.** A drug may cross the cell membrane to reach its intracellular receptor or may react with a receptor on the cell's surface.

The following terms describe the action and interaction of drugs in the body after they have been absorbed into the bloodstream:

Additive Action. If the combination of two similar drugs is equal to the **sum** of the effects of each, then the drugs are called additive. For example, if drug A gives 10 percent tumor kill as a chemotherapeutic agent and drug B gives 20 percent tumor kill, using A and B together would give 30 percent tumor kill.

If two drugs give less than an additive effect, they are called **antagonistic.** If they produce greater than additive effects, they are **synergistic** (see **Synergism** below).

Synergism. A combination of two drugs can sometimes cause an effect that is **greater** than the sum of the individual effects of each drug given alone. For example, penicillin and streptomycin, two antibiotic drugs, are given together in the treatment of bacterial endocarditis because of their synergistic effect.

Tolerance. The effects of a given dose diminish as treatment goes on, and increasing amounts are needed to produce the same effect. Tolerance is a feature of addiction to drugs such as morphine and meperidine hydrochloride (Demerol). **Addiction** is the physical and psychological dependence on and craving for a drug and the presence of clear effects when that drug or other agent is withdrawn.

V. Drug Toxicity

Drug toxicity is the poisonous and potentially dangerous effects of some drugs. **Idiosyncrasy** is an example of an unpredictable type of drug toxicity. This is any unexpected effect that appears in the patient following administration of a drug. For example, in some individuals penicillin causes an idiosyncratic reaction, such as **anaphylaxis** (acute hypersensitivity with asthma and shock).

Other types of drug toxicity are more predictable and are based on the dosage of the drug given. Physicians are trained to be aware of the potential toxic effects of all drugs that they prescribe. **Iatrogenic** (produced by treatment) disorders can occur, however, as a result of mistakes in drug use or of individual sensitivity to a given agent.

Side effects are toxic effects that routinely result from the use of a drug. They often occur with the usual therapeutic dosage of a drug and are generally tolerable. For example, nausea, vomiting, and alopecia are common side effects of the chemotherapeutic drugs used to treat cancer.

Contraindications are factors in a patient's condition that make the use of a drug dangerous and ill advised. For example, in the presence of renal failure, it is unwise to administer a drug that is normally eliminated by the kidneys because excess drug will accumulate in the body and cause side effects.

VI. Classes of Drugs

The following are major classes of drugs with explanations of their use in the body. Specific drugs are included in tables for your reference (brand names are capitalized; generic names begin with a small letter). Appendix IV is a complete list of these drugs and their class or type.

Analgesics

An analgesic (alges/o means sensitivity to pain) is a drug that lessens pain. Mild analgesics relieve mild to moderate pain, such as myalgias, headaches, and toothaches. More potent analgesics are **narcotics** or **opioids,** which contain or are derived from opium. These drugs induce stupor (a condition of near unconsciousness and reduced mental and physical activity). They are used only to relieve severe pain because they may produce dependence (habit formation) and tolerance.

Some non-narcotic analgesics reduce fever, pain, and inflammation and are used for joint disorders (osteoarthritis and rheumatoid arthritis), painful menstruation, and acute

Table 21–2. ANALGESICS AND ANESTHETICS

Analgesics	Anesthetics
MILD	**GENERAL**
acetaminophen (Tylenol)	ether
aspirin	halothane (Fluothane)
tramadol (Ultram)	nitrous oxide
	thiopental (Pentothal)
NARCOTIC (OPIOID)	
codeine	**LOCAL**
hydrocodone w/APAP*	lidocaine (Xylocaine)
hydromorphone (Dilaudid)	lidocaine-prilocaine (EMLA-eutectic mixture of
meperidine (Demerol)	local anesthetics)
morphine	procaine (Novocaine)
oxycodone (Oxycontin)	
propoxyphene HC (Darvon)	
NONSTEROIDAL ANTI-INFLAMMATORY DRUG (NSAID)	
celecoxib (Celebrex)	
diclofenac (Voltaren)	
ibuprofen (Motrin, Advil)	
naproxen (Naprosyn, Aleve)	
rofecoxib (Vioxx)	

*Acetaminophen (Tylenol)
Note: Brand names are in parentheses.

pain. These agents are not steroid hormones (such as cortisone) and are known as **nonsteroidal anti-inflammatory drugs (NSAIDs).** NSAIDs act on tissues to inhibit prostaglandins (hormone-like substances that sensitize peripheral pain receptors). A newer class of NSAIDs are COX-2 inhibitors. They block the effects of an enzyme that activates prostaglandins. They relieve pain and inflammation as do traditional NSAIDs, but produce fewer gastrointestinal side effects. Examples are Celebrex and Vioxx, which are listed in Table 21–2 with other analgesics.

Anesthetics

An anesthetic is an agent that reduces or eliminates sensation. This affects the whole body **(general anesthetic)** or a particular region **(local anesthetic).** General anesthetics are used for surgical procedures; they depress the activity of the central nervous system, producing loss of consciousness. Local anesthetics inhibit the conduction of impulses in sensory nerves in the region in which they are injected or applied.

Table 21–2 gives examples of specific anesthetics.

Antibiotics and Antivirals

An antibiotic is a chemical substance produced by a microorganism (bacterium, yeast, or mold) that inhibits **(bacteriostatic)** or kills **(bactericidal)** bacteria, fungi, or parasites. The use of antibiotics (penicillin was first in general use in 1945) has largely controlled many conditions such as pneumonia, urinary tract infection, and streptococcal pharyngitis. Caution about the use of antibiotics is warranted because they are powerful agents. With indiscriminate use, pathogenic organisms can develop resistance to the antibiotic and destroy the antibiotic's disease-fighting capability.

Antifungal medications treat fungal infections of the skin (ringworm), vagina, mouth, central nervous system, and blood. Antitubercular drugs treat tuberculosis. Antiviral drugs

reduce the production of glucose by the liver), **alpha-glucosidase inhibitors** (temporarily block enzymes that digest sugars), **thiazolidinediones** (enhance glucose uptake into tissues), and **meglitinides** (stimulate the beta cells in the pancreas to produce insulin).

An **insulin pump** is a device strapped to the patient's waist that periodically delivers (via needle) the desired amount of insulin.

Table 21–4 lists antidiabetic drugs.

Antihistamines

These drugs block the action of histamine, which is normally released in the body in allergic reactions. Histamine causes allergic symptoms such as hives, bronchial asthma, hay fever, and in severe cases **anaphylactic shock** (dyspnea, hypotension, and loss of consciousness). Antihistamines cannot cure the allergic reaction, but they relieve its symptoms. Many antihistamines have strong **antiemetic** (prevention of nausea) activity and are used to prevent motion sickness. The most common side effects of antihistamines are drowsiness, blurred vision, tremors, digestive upset, and lack of motor coordination.

Table 21–5 lists common antihistamines.

Antiosteoporosis Drugs

Osteoporosis is a disorder marked by abnormal loss of bone density. Calcium, vitamin D, and estrogen are prescribed to increase calcium deposition in bone. Several different drugs are used to treat osteoporosis. **Bisphosphonates** prevent bone loss, and hormone-like drugs, selective estrogen receptor modulators **(SERMs),** increase bone formation. See Table 21–5.

Cardiovascular Drugs

Cardiovascular drugs act on the heart or the blood vessels to treat hypertension, angina (pain due to decreased oxygen delivery to heart muscle), heart attack, congestive heart failure, and arrhythmias. Often, before other drugs are used, daily aspirin therapy (to prevent clots in blood vessels) and sublingual **nitroglycerin** (to dilate coronary blood vessels) are prescribed. **Digoxin (Lanoxin)** helps the heart pump more forcefully in heart failure. Other cardiovascular drugs include:

Angiotensin-Converting Enzyme (ACE) Inhibitors. Dilate blood vessels to lower blood pressure, improve the performance of the heart, and reduce its workload. They prevent the conversion of angiotensin I into angiotensin II, which is a powerful vasopressor

Table 21–5. ANTIHISTAMINES AND ANTIOSTEOPOROSIS

ANTIHISTAMINES	ANTIOSTEOPOROSIS DRUGS
cetirizine (Zyrtec)	**Bisphosphonates**
chlorpheniramine maleate (Chlor-Trimeton)	alendronate (Fosamax)
diphenhydramine (Benadryl)	pamidronate disodium (Aredia)
fexofenadine (Allegra)	zoledronic acid (Zometa)
loratadine (Claritin)	
meclizine (Antivert)	**SERM**
phenergan (Promethazine)	raloxifene (Evista)

Note: Brand names are in parentheses.

(vasoconstrictor). ACE inhibitors reduce the risk of future heart attack, stroke, and death even if a patient is not hypertensive.

Angiotensin II receptor antagonists. Lower blood pressure by preventing angiotensin from acting on receptors in blood vessels. They are used in patients who do not tolerate ACE inhibitors because of cough or angioedema (swelling of tissues).

Antiarrhythmics. Reverse abnormal heart rhythms. They slow the response of heart muscle to nervous system stimulation or slow the rate at which nervous system impulses are carried through the heart.

Beta-Blockers. Decrease muscular tone in blood vessels (vasodilation), decrease output of the heart, and reduce blood pressure by blocking the action of epinephrine at receptor sites in the heart muscle and in blood vessels. Beta-blockers are prescribed for angina, hypertension, and arrhythmias and prevention of a second heart attack.

Calcium Antagonists or Calcium Channel Blockers. Dilate blood vessels and lower blood pressure; and are used to treat angina and arrhythmias. They inhibit the entry of calcium (necessary for blood vessel contraction) into the muscles of the heart and blood vessels.

Cholesterol-Lowering Drugs. Reduce hypercholesterolemia (high levels of cholesterol in the blood), which is a major factor in the development of heart disease. **Cholestyramine (Questran)** lowers cholesterol by promoting its excretion in feces. Other drugs, called **statins** or **HMG-CoA reductase inhibitors,** lower cholesterol by reducing its production in the liver.

Diuretics. Reduce the volume of blood in the body by promoting the kidney to remove water and salt through urine. They treat hypertension (high blood pressure) and congestive heart failure.

Table 21–6 reviews and gives examples of cardiovascular drugs.

Table 21–6. CARDIOVASCULAR DRUGS

ANGIOTENSIN-CONVERTING ENZYME (ACE) INHIBITORS	CHOLESTEROL-LOWERING DRUGS
enalapril maleate (Vasotec)	atorvastatin calcium (Lipitor)
lisinopril (Prinivil, Zestril)	cholestyramine (Questran)
quinapril (Accupril)	fluvastatin (Lescol)
ramipril (Altace)	lovastatin (Mevacor)
	pravastatin (Pravachol)
BETA-BLOCKERS	simvastatin sodium (Zocor)
atenolol (Tenormin)	
metoprolol (Lopressor, Toprol-XL)	**DIURETICS**
sotalol (Betapace)	furosemide (Lasix)
propranolol (Inderal)	hydrochlorothiazide (Diuril)
	spironolactone (Aldactone)
CALCIUM ANTAGONISTS	triamterene (Dyazide)
amlodipine (Norvasc)	
diltiazem (Cardizem CD)	**ANGIOTENSIN II RECEPTOR ANTAGONISTS**
nifedipine (Adalat CC, Procardia)	irbesartan (Avapro)
	losartan potassium (Cozaar)
	ANTIARRHYTHMICS
	amiodarone (Cordarone)
	flecainide (Tambocor)
	procainamide (Pronestyl)

Note: Brand names are in parentheses.

Endocrine Drugs

These drugs act in much the same manner as the naturally occurring (endogenous) hormones discussed in Chapter 19. **Androgens,** made by the testes and adrenal glands, are used for male hormone replacement and to treat endometriosis and breast cancer in women. **Antiandrogens** slow the uptake of androgens or interfere with their binding in tissues. They are prescribed for prostate cancer. **Estrogens** are female hormones, normally produced by the ovaries, that are used for symptoms associated with menopause (estrogen replacement therapy) and to prevent postmenopausal osteoporosis. They are also used as chemotherapy for some types of cancer (e.g., prostate cancer). An important **antiestrogen** drug is **tamoxifen (Nolvadex),** which is used to prevent recurrence of breast cancer and to treat metastatic breast cancer. **Aromatase inhibitors** also reduce the amount of estrogen (estradiol) in the blood.

A **selective estrogen receptor modulator (SERM)** has estrogen-like effects on bone (increase in bone mineral density) and on lipid (decrease in cholesterol levels) metabolism; however, it lacks estrogenic effects on uterus and breast tissue. **Progestins** are prescribed for abnormal uterine bleeding caused by hormonal imbalance and, together with estrogen, in hormone replacement therapy and oral contraceptives.

Thyroid hormone is administered when there is a low output of hormone from the thyroid gland. **Glucocorticoids** (adrenal corticosteroids) are prescribed for reduction of inflammation and a wide range of other disorders, including arthritis, severe skin and allergic conditions, respiratory and blood disorders, gastrointestinal ailments, and malignant conditions.

Table 21–7 gives examples of endocrine drugs.

Table 21–7. ENDOCRINE DRUGS

ANDROGEN fluoxymesterone (Halotestin) methyltestosterone (Virilon)	**GLUCOCORTICOID** dexamethasone (Decadron) prednisone (Deltasone)
ANTIANDROGEN flutamide (Eulexin) nilutamide (Casodex)	**PROGESTIN** medroxyprogesterone acetate (Cycrin, Provera) megestrol (Megace)
ESTROGEN estrogens (Premarin, Prempro, Estradiol)	**SERM** raloxifene (Evista)
ANTIESTROGEN tamoxifen (Nolvadex)	**THYROID HORMONE** levothyroxine (Levothroid, Levoxyl, Synthroid) liothyronine (Cytomel) liotrix (Thyrolar)
AROMATASE INHIBITOR anastrozole (Arimidex) fulvestrant (Faslodex) letrozole (Femara)	

Note: Brand names are in parentheses.

Gastrointestinal Drugs

These drugs are often used to relieve uncomfortable and potentially dangerous symptoms, rather than as cures for specific diseases. **Antacids** neutralize the hydrochloric acid in the stomach to relieve symptoms of peptic ulcer, esophagitis, and epigastric discomfort. **Antiulcer** drugs block secretion of acid by cells in the lining of the stomach and are prescribed for patients with gastric and duodenal ulcers and gastroesophageal reflux disease **(GERD)**. Histamine H$_2$-receptor antagonists such as **ranitidine (Zantac)** and **cimetidine (Tagamet)** turn off the system (histamine) that produces stomach acid. Another drug, **omeprazole (Prilosec)** works by stopping acid production by a different method (proton-pump inhibition).

Antidiarrheal drugs relieve diarrhea and decrease the rapid movement of the walls of the colon. **Cathartics** relieve constipation and promote defecation for diagnostic and operative procedures and are used to treat disorders of the gastrointestinal tract. Some cathartics increase the intestinal salt content to cause fluid to fill the intestines; others increase the bulk of the feces to promote peristalsis (movement of the intestinal wall). Another type of cathartic lubricates the intestinal tract to produce soft stools. **Laxatives** are mild cathartics, and **purgatives** are strong cathartics.

Antinauseants (antiemetics) relieve nausea and vomiting and also overcome vertigo, dizziness, motion sickness, and labyrinthitis (inflammation of the inner ear).

Table 21–8 lists the various types of gastrointestinal drugs and examples of each.

Table 21–8. GASTROINTESTINAL DRUGS

ANTACID

aluminum and magnesium antacid (Gaviscon)
magnesium antacid (milk of magnesia)
aluminum antacid (Rolaids)

ANTIDIARRHEAL

diphenoxylate and atropine (Lomotil)
loperamide (Imodium)
paregoric

ANTINAUSEANT (ANTIEMETIC)

metoclopramide (Reglan)
ondansetron (Zofran)
phenergan (Promethazine)
prochlorperazine maleate (Compazine)

ANTIULCER AND ANTI-GERD

cimetidine (Tagamet)
cisapride (Propulsid)
famotidine (Pepcid)
lansoprazole (Prevacid)
omeprazole (Prilosec)
ranitidine (Zantac)

CATHARTIC

casanthranol and docusate sodium (Peri-Colace)

Note: Brand names are in parentheses.

Table 21–9. RESPIRATORY DRUGS

BRONCHODILATORS
albuterol (Proventil)
epinephrine
ipratropium bromide and albuterol (Atrovent)
metaproterenol (Alupent)
salmeterol (Serevent)
theophylline (Theo-Dur)

LEUKOTRIENE MODIFIERS
montelukast (Singulair)
zafirlukast (Accolate)
zileuton (Zyflo Filmtab)

STEROIDS—INHALERS
beclomethasone (Vanceril)
flunisolide (AeroBid)
fluticasone propionate (Flovent)
triamcinolone (Azmacort)

STEROIDS—IV OR ORAL
methylprednisolone (Medrol)
prednisone

Note: Brand names are in parentheses.

Respiratory Drugs

These drugs are prescribed for the treatment of asthma, emphysema, chronic bronchitis, and bronchospasm. **Bronchodilators** open bronchial tubes and are administered by injection or aerosol inhalers. **Steroid drugs** are inhaled or given intravenously and orally to reduce chronic inflammation in respiratory passageways. **Leukotriene modifiers** are recent additions to the anti-inflammatory therapy of asthma. They prevent asthma attacks by blocking leukotriene (a bronchoconstrictor) from binding to receptors in respiratory tissues. Table 21–9 gives examples of respiratory drugs.

Sedatives and Hypnotics

Sedatives and hypnotics are medications that depress the central nervous system and promote drowsiness and sleep. They are prescribed for insomnia and sleep disorders. These products have a very high abuse potential and should be used only for short periods of time and under close supervision.

Low doses of **benzodiazepines** (that influence the part of the brain responsible for emotions) may act as sedatives and, in higher doses, as hypnotics (to promote sleep).

Table 21–10 gives examples of sedatives/hypnotics.

Stimulants

These drugs act on the brain to speed up vital processes (heart and respiration) in cases of shock and collapse. They also increase alertness and inhibit hyperactive behavior in children. High doses can produce restlessness, insomnia, and hypertension. Examples of stimulants are **amphetamines**—used to prevent narcolepsy (seizures of sleep), to suppress appetite, and to calm hyperkinetic children. **Caffeine** is also a cerebral stimulant. It is used in drugs to relieve certain types of headache by constricting cerebral blood vessels. Table 21–10 lists examples of stimulants.

Tranquilizers

These drugs are useful for controlling anxiety. Minor tranquilizers **(benzodiazepines)** control minor symptoms of anxiety. Major tranquilizers **(phenothiazines)** control more severe disturbances of behavior. Table 21–10 lists examples of minor and major tranquilizers.

Table 21-10. SEDATIVES/HYPNOTICS, STIMULANTS, TRANQUILIZERS

SEDATIVES/HYPNOTICS	TRANQUILIZERS
butabarbital (Butisol)	**Minor**
phenobarbital	*alprazolam (Xanax)
*temazepam (Restoril)	buspirone (BuSpar)
*triazolam (Halcion)	*diazepam (Valium)
zolpidem tartrate (Ambien)	*lorazepam (Ativan)
STIMULANTS	**Major**
caffeine	†chlorpromazine (Thorazine)
dextroamphetamine sulfate (Dexedrine)	lithium carbonate (Eskalith)
methylphenidate (Ritalin)	olanzapine (Zyprexa)
modafinil (Provigil)	†thioridazine (Mellaril)
	†trifluoperazine (Stelazine)

*benzodiazepine
†phenothiazine
Note: Brand names are in parentheses.

VII. Vocabulary

This list reviews many of the new terms introduced in the text. Short definitions reinforce your understanding of the terms. See Section XIII of this chapter for help in pronouncing the more difficult terms.

General Terms

addiction	Physical and psychological dependence on and craving for a drug.
additive action	Drug action in which the combination of two similar drugs is equal to the sum of the effects of each.
aerosol	Particles of drug suspended in air.
anaphylaxis	Exaggerated hypersensitivity reaction to a drug or foreign organism.
antagonistic action	Combination of two drugs gives less than an additive effect (action).
antidote	Agent given to counteract an unwanted effect of a drug.
brand name	Commercial name for a drug; trademark.
chemical name	Chemical formula for a drug.
contraindications	Factors in the patient's condition that prevent the use of a particular drug or treatment.
Food and Drug Administration (FDA)	Governmental agency having the legal responsibility for enforcing proper drug manufacture and clinical use.
generic name	Legal noncommercial name for a drug.

iatrogenic	Condition caused by treatment (drugs or procedures) given by medical personnel.
idiosyncrasy	Unexpected effect produced in a particularly sensitive individual but not seen in most patients.
inhalation	Administration of drugs in gaseous or vapor form through the nose or mouth.
medicinal chemistry	Study of new drug synthesis; relationship between chemical structure and biological effects.
molecular pharmacology	Study of interaction of drugs and subcellular entities such as DNA, RNA, and enzymes.
oral administration	Drugs are given by mouth.
parenteral administration	Drugs are given by injection into the skin, muscles, or veins (any route other than through the digestive tract). Examples are subcutaneous, intradermal, intramuscular, intravenous, intrathecal, and intracavitary injections.
pharmacist	Prepares and dispenses drugs.
pharmacy	Location for preparing and dispensing drugs; also the study of preparing and dispensing drugs.
pharmacodynamics	Study of the effects of a drug within the body.
pharmacokinetics	Calculation of drug concentration in tissues and blood over a period of time.
pharmacologist	Specialist in the properties, uses, and actions of drugs.
pharmacology	Study of the preparation, properties, uses, and actions of drugs.
Physicians' Desk Reference (PDR)	Reference book that lists drug products.
receptor	Target substance with which a drug interacts in the body.
rectal administration	Drugs are inserted through the anus into the rectum.
side effect	Toxic effect that routinely results from the use of a drug.
sublingual administration	Drugs are given by placement under the tongue.
synergism	Combination of two drugs causes an effect that is greater than the sum of the individual effects of each drug alone.

syringe	Instrument (tube) for introducing or withdrawing fluids from the body.
tolerance	Larger and larger drug doses must be given to achieve the desired effect. The patient becomes resistant to the action of a drug as treatment progresses.
topical application	Drugs are applied locally on the skin or mucous membranes of the body; ointments, creams, and lotions are applied topically.
toxicity	Harmful effects of a drug.
toxicology	Study of harmful chemicals and their effects on the body.
transport	Movement of a drug across a cell membrane into body cells.
United States Pharmacopeia (U.S.P.)	Authoritative list of drugs, formulas, and preparations that sets a standard for drug manufacturing and dispensing.
vitamin	Substance found in foods and essential in small quantities for growth and good health.

Classes of Drugs and Related Terms

ACE inhibitor	Lowers blood pressure. Angiotensin-converting enzyme (ACE) inhibitors block the conversion of angiotensin I to angiotensin II (a powerful vasoconstrictor).
amphetamine	Central nervous system stimulant.
analgesic	Relieves pain.
androgen	Male hormone.
anesthetic	Reduces or eliminates sensation; general and local.
angiotensin II receptor antagonist	Lowers blood pressure by preventing angiotensin from acting on receptors in blood vessels.
antacid	Neutralizes acid in the stomach.
antiandrogen	Slows the uptake of androgens or interferes with their binding in tissues.
antiarrhythmic	Treats abnormal heart rhythms.
antibiotic	Chemical substance, produced by a plant or microorganism, that has the ability to inhibit or kill foreign organisms in the body. Examples are antifungals, cephalosporins, erythromycin, tetracycline, antituberculars, penicillins, quinolones, and sulfonamides.

anticoagulant	Prevents blood clotting.
anticonvulsant	Prevents convulsions (abnormal brain activity).
antidepressant	Relieves symptoms of depression.
antidiabetic	Drug given to prevent or alleviate diabetes mellitus.
antidiarrheal	Prevents diarrhea.
antiemetic	Prevents nausea and vomiting.
antihistamine	Blocks the action of histamine and helps prevent symptoms of allergy.
antinauseant	Relieves nausea and vomiting; antiemetic.
antiplatelet	Reduces the tendency of platelets to stick together.
antiulcer	Inhibits the secretion of acid by cells of the lining of the stomach.
antiviral	Acts against viruses such as the herpesvirus and HIV.
aromatase inhibitor	Reduces the amount of estrogen in the blood.
bactericidal	Kills bacteria (-cidal means to kill).
bacteriostatic	Inhibits bacterial growth (-static means to stop or control).
beta-blocker	Blocks the action of epinephrine at sites on receptors of heart muscle cells, the muscle lining of blood vessels, and bronchial tubes; antiarrhythmic, antianginal, and antihypertensive.
bisphosphonate	Prevents bone loss in osteoporosis.
caffeine	Central nervous system stimulant.
calcium antagonist	Blocks the entrance of calcium into heart muscle and muscle lining of blood vessels; used as an antiarrhythmic, antianginal, and antihypertensive; **calcium channel blocker.**
cardiovascular	Acts on the heart and blood vessels. This category of drug includes ACE inhibitors, beta-blockers, calcium antagonists, cholesterol-lowering drugs, and diuretics.
cathartic	Relieves constipation.

diuretic	Increases the production of urine and thus reduces the volume of fluid in the body; antihypertensive.
emetic	Promotes vomiting.
endocrine	A hormone or hormone-like drug. Examples are androgens, estrogens, progestins, SERMs, thyroid hormone, and glucocorticoids.
estrogen	Female hormone responsible for secondary sex characteristics.
gastrointestinal	Relieves symptoms of diseases in the gastrointestinal tract. Examples are antacids, antiulcer drugs, antidiarrheal drugs, cathartics, laxatives, purgatives, and antinauseants (antiemetics).
glucocorticoid	Hormone from the adrenal cortex that raises blood sugar and reduces inflammation.
hypnotic	Produces sleep.
laxative	Weak cathartic.
narcotic	Habit-forming drug (potent analgesic) that relieves pain by producing stupor or insensibility.
progestin	Female hormone that affects the lining of the uterus during pregnancy.
purgative	Strong cathartic.
respiratory	Treats asthma, emphysema, and infections of the respiratory system. Bronchodilators are examples.
sedative	A mildly hypnotic drug that relaxes without necessarily producing sleep. Benzodiazepines are examples.
SERM	Selective estrogen modulator with estrogen-like effect on bones and fat metabolism.
stimulant	Excites and promotes activity. Caffeine and amphetamines are examples.
thyroid hormone	Stimulates cellular metabolism.
tranquilizer	Controls anxiety and severe disturbances of behavior.

VIII. Combining Forms, Prefixes, and Terminology

Write the meaning of the medical term in the space provided.

Combining Forms

Combining Form	Meaning	Terminology	Meaning
aer/o	air	aerosol _____	

-sol means solution.

alges/o	sensitivity to pain	analgesic _____	
bronch/o	bronchial tube	bronchodilator _____	

Theophylline is a smooth-muscle relaxant used to treat asthma, emphysema, and chronic bronchitis.

chem/o	drug	chemotherapy _____	
cras/o	mixture	idiosyncrasy _____	

idi/o means individual, peculiar; syn- means together. An idiosyncrasy is an abnormal, unexpected effect of a drug that is peculiar to an individual.

cutane/o	skin	subcutaneous _____	
derm/o	skin	hypodermic _____	
erg/o	work	synergism _____	
esthes/o	feeling, sensation	anesthesia _____	
hist/o	tissue	antihistamine _____	

-amine indicates a nitrogen-containing compound. Histamine is a substance found in all body tissues (it causes capillary dilation and gastric acid secretion and constricts bronchial tube smooth muscle); an excess of histamine is released when the body comes in contact with substances to which it is sensitive.

hypn/o	sleep	hypnotic _____	
iatr/o	treatment	iatrogenic _____	

lingu/o	tongue	sublingual	_____
myc/o	mold, fungus	erythromycin	_____
narc/o	stupor	narcotic	_____
or/o	mouth	oral	_____
pharmac/o	drug	pharmacology	_____
prurit/o	itching	antipruritic	_____
pyret/o	fever	antipyretic	_____
thec/o	sheath (of brain and spinal cord)	intrathecal	_____
tox/o	poison	toxic	_____
toxic/o	poison	toxicology	_____
vas/o	vessel	vasodilator	_____
ven/o	vein	intravenous	_____
vit/o	life	vitamin	_____

The first vitamins discovered were nitrogen-containing substances called amines. Table 21–11 lists vitamins, their medical names, and foods that are a major source of each.

Table 21–11. VITAMINS

Vitamin	Name	Food Source
Vitamin A	Retinol; dehydroretinol	Green, leafy and yellow vegetables; liver, eggs, cod liver oil
Vitamin B_1	Thiamine	Yeast, ham, liver, peanuts, milk
Vitamin B_2	Riboflavin	Milk, liver, green vegetables
Niacin	Nicotinic acid	Yeast, liver, peanuts, fish, poultry
Vitamin B_6	Pyridoxine	Liver, fish, yeast
Vitamin B_{12}	Cyanocobalamin	Milk, eggs, liver
Vitamin C	Ascorbic acid	Citrus fruits, vegetables
Vitamin D	Calciferol	Cod liver oil, milk, egg yolk
Vitamin E	α-Tocopherol	Wheat germ oil, cereals, egg yolk
Vitamin K	Phytonadione; menaquinone; menadione	Alfalfa, spinach, cabbage

Prefixes

Prefix	Meaning	Terminology	Meaning
ana-	upward, excessive, again	anaphylaxis	_____
		-phylaxis means protection.	
anti-	against	antidote	_____
		-dote comes from Greek, meaning what is given.	
		antibiotic	_____
contra-	against, opposite	contraindication	_____
par-	other than, apart from	parenteral	_____
		enter/o means intestine.	
syn-	together, with	synergistic	_____

IX. Abbreviations

a.c.	before meals *(ante cibum)*
ACE	angiotensin-converting enzyme
ad lib	freely as desired *(ad libitum)*
APAP	acetaminophen (Tylenol)
b.i.d.	two times a day *(bis in die)*
c̄	with
caps	capsule
cc	cubic centimeter
FDA	Food and Drug Administration
gm	gram
gt, gtt	drops *(gutta)*
h	hour *(hora)*
h.s.	at bedtime
H₂ blocker	histamine H_2-receptor antagonist
HRT	hormone replacement therapy

IM	intramuscular
INH	isoniazid (antitubercular agent)
IV	intravenous
MAOI	monoamine oxidase inhibitor; antidepressant
mg	milligram
NPO	nothing by mouth *(nil per os)*
NSAID	nonsteroidal anti-inflammatory drug
oz.	ounce
p.c.	after meals *(post cibum)*
PCA	patient-controlled administration
PDR	Physicians' Desk Reference
p.o.	by mouth *(per os)*
p.r.n.	when requested; *pro re nata* (required)
pt	patient

Q(q)	every *(quaque)*	**SERM**	selective estrogen receptor modulator
q.d.	every day *(quaque die)*	**sig.**	let it be labeled *(signetur)*
q.h.	every hour *(quaque hora)*	**SL**	sublingual
q.h.s.	every bedtime *(quaque hora somni)*	**s.o.s.**	if necessary *(si opus sit)*
q.i.d.	four times a day *(quater in die)*	**SSRI**	selective serotonin reuptake inhibitor; antidepressant
qns	quantity not sufficient	**sc, subcut**	subcutaneous
q.s.	sufficient quantity *(quantum satis)*	**tab**	tablet
qAM	every morning	**TCA**	tricyclic antidepressant
qPM	every evening	**t.i.d.**	three times daily *(ter in die)*
s̄	without *(sine)*		

X. Practical Applications

The following are the top 30 prescription drugs dispensed in U.S. community pharmacies, new and refill prescriptions, in 2001 Internet Drug Index (from NDC Health).

Top 30 Prescription Drugs—2001

Drug (Trade Name)	*Generic Name*	*Type/Use*
1. Hydrocodone w/APAP	hydrocodone w/APAP	Analgesic (narcotic)
2. Lipitor	atorvastatin	Cholesterol-lowering agent
3. Premarin	estrogen	Hormone (HRT)
4. Tenormin	atenolol	Beta-blocker
5. Synthroid	levothyroxine	Hormone (thyroid gland)
6. Zithromax	azithromycin	Antibiotic (erythromycin-type)
7. Lasix	furosemide	Diuretic
8. Amoxil	amoxicillin	Antibiotic (penicillin-type)
9. Norvasc	amlodipine	Antihypertensive (calcium channel blocker)
10. Xanax	alprazolam	Tranquilizer
11. Albuterol aerosol	albuterol	Bronchodilator
12. Claritin	loratadine	Antihistamine-decongestant
13. Diuril	chlorothiazide	Diuretic
14. Prilosec	omeprazole	Gastric acid pump inhibitor
15. Zoloft	sertraline	Antidepressant (SSRI)

Continued on following page

16.	Paxil	paroxetine	Antidepressant (SSRI)
17.	Triamterene/HCTZ	triamterene/HCTZ	Diuretic
18.	Prevacid	lansoprazole	Antiulcer/AntiGERD
19.	Ibuprofen	ibuprofen	Analgesic/NSAID
20.	Celebrex	celecoxib	NSAID
21.	Zocor	simvastatin	Cholesterol-lowering agent
22.	Cephalexin	cephalexin	Antibiotic (cephalosporin-type)
23.	Glucophage	metformin	Antidiabetic (biguanide antihyperglycemic)
24.	Vioxx	rofecoxib	NSAID
25.	Zestril	lisinopril	Antihypertensive (ACE inhibitor)
26.	Augmentin	amoxicillin/clavulanate	Antibiotic (penicillin-type)
27.	Darvocet N	propoxyphene N/APAP	Narcotic analgesic
28.	Prempro	conjugated estrogen-medroxyprogesterone	Hormone (HRT)
29.	Prednisone	prednisone	Steroid/anti-inflammatory
30.	Ortho-Cyclen 21	norgestimate/ethinyl estradiol	oral contraceptive

Prescriptions

The usual order of drug prescription is name of the drug, dosage, route of administration, time of administration. At times the physician will include a qualifying phrase to indicate why the prescription is being written. Not all information is listed with every prescription. Consider the following:

1. Fluoxetine (Prozac) 20 mg p.o. b.i.d.
2. Lisinopril (Zestril) 20 mg 1 cap q.d.
3. Ondansetron (Zofran) 4 mg 1 tab/cap t.i.d. p.r.n. for nausea
4. Ranitidine (Zantac) 300 mg 1 tab p.c. q.d.
5. Olanzapine (Zyprexa) 5 mg 1 tab q.d.
6. Acetaminophen (300 mg) & codeine (30 mg) 1 tab q.i.d. p.r.n. for pain

Questions: Match the prescriptions above with an explanation below.

A. _____ Anti-GERD drug taken after meals every day.

B. _____ Tylenol with a narcotic taken 4 times a day as needed.

C. _____ Antidepressant taken by mouth twice a day.

D. _____ Antiemetic taken 3 times a day as needed.

E. _____ Antihypertensive taken every day.

F. _____ Antipsychotic, one tablet every day.

XI. Exercises

Remember to check your answers carefully with those given in Section XII, Answers to Exercises.

A. *Match the pharmacological specialty with its description below.*

1. use of drugs in the treatment of disease _____

2. study of new drug synthesis _____

3. study of how drugs interact with subcellular parts _____

4. study of the harmful effects of drugs _____

5. study of drug effects in the body _____

6. measurement of drug concentrations in tissues and in blood over a period of time

_____

B. *Match the following terms with their meanings below.*

antidote   pharmacist   toxicologist
chemical name   pharmacologist   trade (brand) name
Food and Drug Administration   *Physicians' Desk Reference*   United States Pharmacopeia
generic name

1. Specialist in the study of the harmful effects of drugs on the body is a (an) _____.

2. Agent given to counteract harmful effects of a drug is a (an) _____.

3. Governmental agency with legal responsibility for enforcing proper drug manufacture and clinical

   use is _____.

4. The _____ is the commercial name for a drug.

5. The _____ is the complicated chemical formula for a drug.

6. The _____ is the legal noncommercial name for a drug.

7. Professional who prepares and dispenses drugs is a (an) _____.

8. Specialist (M.D. or Ph.D.) in the properties, uses, and actions of drugs is a (an)

   _____.

9. Reference book listing drug products is _____.

10. Authoritative list of drugs, formulas, and preparations that sets a standard for drug manufacturing

    and dispensing is _____.

C. *Name the route of drug administration based on its description as given below.*

1. Administered via suppository or fluid into the anus. _____

2. Administered via vapor or gas into the nose or mouth. _____

3. Administered under the tongue. _____

4. Applied locally on skin or mucous membrane. _____

5. Injected via syringe under the skin or into a vein, muscle, or body cavity. _____

6. Given by mouth and absorbed through the stomach or intestinal wall. _____

D. *Give the meanings of the following terms.*

1. intravenous _____

2. intrathecal _____

3. antiseptic _____

4. antipruritic _____

5. aerosol _____

6. intramuscular _____

7. subcutaneous _____

8. intracavitary _____

9. addiction _____

E. *Match the routes of drug administration in column I with the medications or procedures in column II. Write the letter of the answer in the space provided.*

Column I

1. intravenous _____

2. rectal _____

3. oral _____

4. topical _____

5. inhalation _____

Column II

A. lotions, creams, ointments
B. tablets and capsules
C. skin testing for allergy
D. lumbar puncture
E. deep injection, usually in buttock
F. suppositories
G. blood transfusions
H. aerosol medications

6. intrathecal _____

7. intramuscular _____

8. intradermal _____

F. *The following are descriptions of drug actions. Supply the word that fits the description.*

1. combination of two drugs is greater than the total effects of each drug by itself

    _____

2. combination of two drugs that is equal to the sum of the effects of each _____

3. effects of a given drug dose become less as treatment continues, and larger and larger doses must be

    given to achieve the desired effect _____

4. an unexpected effect that may appear in a patient following administration of a drug

    _____

5. two drugs give less than an additive effect (action) _____

G. *Give the meanings of the following terms that describe classes of drugs.*

1. antibiotic _____

2. antidepressant _____

3. antihistamine _____

4. analgesic _____

5. anticoagulant _____

6. anesthetic _____

7. antidiabetic _____

8. sedative _____

9. stimulant _____

10. tranquilizer _____

H. Match the term in column I with the associated term in column II. Write the letter of the answer in the space provided.

Column I

1. antihistamine _____
2. analgesic _____
3. antidiabetic _____
4. anticoagulant _____
5. antibiotic _____
6. stimulant _____
7. sedative/hypnotic _____
8. tranquilizer _____

Column II

A. caffeine or amphetamines
B. penicillin or erythromycin
C. insulin
D. benzodiazepine
E. heparin
F. nonsteroidal anti-inflammatory drug
G. phenothiazine
H. anaphylactic shock

I. Give the meanings of the following terms.

1. beta-blocker _____

2. androgen _____

3. glucocorticoid _____

4. calcium antagonist _____

5. estrogen _____

6. antacid _____

7. cathartic _____

8. antiemetic _____

9. bronchodilator _____

10. hypnotic _____

11. diuretic _____

12. cholesterol-lowering drug _____

J. Match the type of drug in column I with the condition it treats in column II. Write the letter of the answer in the space provided.

Column I

1. anticonvulsant _____

2. anticoagulant _____

3. antacid _____

4. progestins _____

5. antibiotic _____

6. ACE inhibitor _____

7. bronchodilator _____

8. antihistamine _____

9. tranquilizer _____

10. analgesic _____

Column II

A. abnormal uterine bleeding caused by hormonal imbalance

B. severe behavior disturbances and anxiety

C. epilepsy

D. congestive heart failure and hypertension

E. epigastric discomfort

F. myalgia and neuralgia

G. anaphylactic shock

H. thrombosis and embolism

I. streptococcal pharyngitis

J. asthma

K. Complete the following terms based on definitions given.

1. agent that reduces fever: anti _____

2. agent that reduces itching: anti _____

3. habit-forming analgesic: _____ tic

4. two drugs cause an effect greater than the sum of each alone: syn _____

5. antibiotic derived from a red mold: _____ mycin

6. legal nonproprietary name of a drug: _____ name

7. factor in a patient's condition that prevents the use of a particular drug: contra _____

8. drug that produces an absence of sensation or feeling: an _____

L. Using the terms listed below, complete the following sentences.

ACE inhibitor   antiestrogen   diuretic
anesthetic   antihistamine   NSAID
anticonvulsant   antiviral   oral antidiabetic
antidepressant   bactericidal   SERM

1. Cephalosporins (such as cefuroxime and cefprozil) and penicillins are examples of a (an)

   _____ drug.

2. Advil (ibuprofen) is an example of a (an) _____.

3. Tegretol (carbamazepine) and phenytoin (Dilantin) are examples of a (an) _____
   drug.

4. Zovirax (acyclovir) and Crixivan (indinavir) are both types of a (an) _____
   drug.

5. Nolvadex (tamoxifen), used to treat estrogen receptor positive breast cancer in women, is an

   example of a (an) _____ drug.

6. Patients with high blood pressure may need Vasotec (enalapril) or Zestril (lisinopril). Both of these

   are examples of a (an) _____.

7. Glucophage (metformin) and rosiglitazone (Avandia) are two types of _____
   drugs.

8. Evista (raloxifene), used to treat osteoporosis in postmenopausal women, is an example of

   a selective estrogen receptor modulator or _____.

9. Elavil (amitriptyline) and fluoxetine (Prozac) are two types of a (an) _____
   drug.

10. If you have an allergy, your doctor may prescribe Allegra (fexofenadine), which is a (an)

    _____ drug.

11. Two agents that reduce the amount of fluid in the blood and thus lower blood pressure are Lasix

    (furosemide) and Aldactone (spironolactone). These are _____ drugs.

12. Xylocaine (lidocaine) and Pentothal (thiopental) are examples of a (an) _____
    drug.

M. Give the meanings of the following abbreviations.

1. NSAID _____   8. s̄ _____

2. p.r.n. _____   9. NPO _____

3. q.i.d. _____   10. p.c. _____

4. ad lib _____   11. b.i.d. _____

5. t.i.d. _____   12. q.h. _____

6. mg _____   13. p.o. _____

7. c̄ _____   14. q _____

N. Circle the term that best completes the meaning of the sentence.

1. After his heart attack, Bernie was supposed to take many drugs, including diuretics and a(an) **(progestin, laxative, anticoagulant)** to prevent blood clots.

2. Estelle was always anxious and had a hard time sleeping. Dr. Max felt that a mild **(antacid, anticonvulsant, tranquilizer)** would help her relax and concentrate on her work.

3. During chemotherapy Helen was very nauseated. Dr. Cohen prescribed an **(antihypertensive, antiemetic, antianginal)** to relieve her symptoms of queasy stomach.

4. The two antibiotics worked together and were therefore **(idiosyncratic, generic, synergistic)** in killing the bacteria in Susan's bloodstream.

5. The label warned that the drug might impair fine motor skills. It listed the **(side effects, antidote, pharmacodynamics)** of taking the sedative.

6. After receiving the results of Judy's sputum culture, her physician, an expert in **(endocrinology, cardiology, infectious disease)**, recommended Biaxin and other **(antihistamines, antibiotics, antidepressants)** to combat the mycobacterium avian complex disease in her **(heart, thyroid gland, lungs)**.

7. Our dog, Eli, has had seizures since he was hit by a car last year. The veterinarian currently prescribes phenobarbital, an **(anticoagulant, antinauseant, anticonvulsant)**, 45 mg b.i.d. **(every other day, twice a day, every evening)**.

8. To control his Type 1 **(heart disease, asthma, diabetes)**, David gives himself daily injections of **(oral drugs, insulin, aromatase inhibitors)**.

9. Many students who want to stay awake to study are taking **(stimulants, sedatives, tranquilizers)** containing **(Lithium, caffeine, butabarbital)**.

10. Shelly's wheezing, coughing, and shortness of breath when she is stressed and exposed to animal dander all pointed to a diagnosis of **(pneumonia, asthma, heart disease)**, which required treatment with steroids and **(antivirals, diuretics, bronchodilators)**.

XII. Answers to Exercises

A

1. chemotherapy
2. medicinal chemistry
3. molecular pharmacology
4. toxicology
5. pharmacodynamics
6. pharmacokinetics

B

1. toxicologist
2. antidote
3. Food and Drug Administration
4. trade (brand) name
5. chemical name
6. generic name
7. pharmacist
8. pharmacologist
9. Physicians' Desk Reference
10. United States Pharmacopeia

C

1. rectal
2. inhalation
3. sublingual
4. topical
5. parenteral
6. oral

D

1. within a vein
2. within a sheath (membranes around the spinal cord or brain)
3. an agent that works against infection
4. an agent that works against itching
5. a solution of particles (drug) in air (vapor or gas)
6. within a muscle
7. under the skin
8. within a cavity
9. physical and psychological dependence on a drug

E

1. G
2. F
3. B
4. A
5. H
6. D
7. E
8. C

F

1. synergism (potentiation)
2. additive action
3. tolerance
4. idiosyncrasy
5. antagonistic

G

1. an agent that inhibits or kills germ life (microorganisms)
2. an agent that relieves the symptoms of depression
3. an agent that blocks the action of histamine and relieves allergic symptoms
4. an agent that relieves pain
5. an agent that prevents blood clotting
6. an agent that reduces or eliminates sensation
7. an agent used to prevent diabetes mellitus
8. an agent (mildly hypnotic) that relaxes and calms nervousness
9. an agent that excites and promotes activity
10. a drug used to control anxiety and severe disturbances of behavior

H

1. H
2. F
3. C
4. E
5. B
6. A
7. D
8. G

I

1. drug that blocks the action of epinephrine at sites of receptors of heart muscles, blood vessels, and bronchial tubes (antihypertensive, antianginal, and antiarrhythmic)
2. a drug that produces male sexual characteristics
3. a hormone from the adrenal glands that reduces inflammation and raises blood sugar
4. a drug that blocks the entrance of calcium into heart muscle and blood vessel walls (antianginal, antiarrhythmic, and antihypertensive)
5. a hormone that produces female sexual characteristics
6. a drug that neutralizes acid in the stomach
7. a drug that relieves constipation
8. a drug that prevents nausea and vomiting
9. a drug that opens air passages
10. an agent that produces sleep
11. a drug that reduces the volume of blood and lowers blood pressure
12. a drug that reduces hypercholesterolemia

J

1. C
2. H
3. E
4. A
5. I
6. D
7. J
8. G
9. B
10. F

K

1. antipyretic
2. antipruritic
3. narcotic
4. synergism
5. erythromycin
6. generic
7. contraindication
8. anesthetic

L

1. bactericidal
2. NSAID
3. anticonvulsant
4. antiviral
5. antiestrogen
6. ACE inhibitor
7. oral antidiabetic for type 2 diabetes
8. SERM
9. antidepressant
10. antihistamine
11. diuretic
12. anesthetic

M

1. nonsteroidal anti-inflammatory drug
2. when requested
3. four times a day
4. freely as desired
5. three times a day
6. milligram
7. with
8. without
9. nothing by mouth
10. after meals
11. twice a day
12. every hour
13. by mouth
14. every

N

1. anticoagulant
2. tranquilizer
3. antiemetic
4. synergistic
5. side effects
6. infectious disease, antibiotics, lungs
7. anticonvulsant, twice a day
8. diabetes, insulin
9. stimulants, caffeine
10. asthma, bronchodilators

Answers to Practical Applications

Prescriptions
(A) 4
(B) 6
(C) 1
(D) 3
(E) 2
(F) 5

XIII. Pronunciation of Terms

Pronunciation Guide

ā as in āpe   ă as in ăpple
ē as in ēven   ĕ as in ĕvery
ī as in īce   ĭ as in ĭnterest
ō as in ōpen   ŏ as in pŏt
ū as in ūnit   ŭ as in ŭnder

To test your understanding of the terminology in this chapter, write the meaning of each term in the space provided. In addition, you may wish to cover the terms and write them by looking at your definitions. Make sure your spelling is correct. The page number after each term indicates where it is defined or used in the text so you can easily check your responses.

Term	Pronunciation	Meaning
ACE inhibitor (865)	ĀCE ĭn-HĬB-ĭ-tŏr	
addiction (863)	ă-DIK-shun	
additive action (863)	AD-ĭ-tĭv ĂK-shŭn	
aerosol (863)	Ā-ĕr-ō-sōl	
amphetamine (865)	ăm-FĔT-ă-mēn	
analgesic (865)	ăn-ăl-JĒ-zĭk	
anaphylaxis (863)	ăn-ă-fĭ-LĂK-sĭs	
androgen (865)	ĂN-drō-jĭn	
anesthesia (868)	ăn-ĕs-THĒ-zē-ă	
anesthetic (865)	ăn-ĕs-THĔ-tĭk	
angiotensin II receptor antagonist (865)	ăn-jē-ō-TĔN-sĭn II rē-SĔP-tŏr ăn-TĂG-ō-nĭst	
antacid (865)	ănt-ĂS-ĭd	
antagonistic action (863)	ăn-tă-gŏn-NĬS-tĭk ĂK-shŭn	
antiandrogen (865)	ăn-tē-ĂN-drō-jĕn	
antiarrhthymic (865)	ăn-tē-ā-RĬTH-mĭk	
antibiotic (865)	ăn-tĭ-bī-ŎT-ĭk	
anticoagulant (866)	ăn-tĭ-kō-ĂG-ū-lănt	
anticonvulsant (866)	ăn-tĭ-kŏn-VŬL-sănt	
antidepressant (866)	ăn-tĭ-dĕ-PRĔS-ănt	
antidiabetic (866)	ăn-tĭ-dī-ă-BĔT-ĭk	

antidiarrheal (866)	ăn-tĭ-dī-ă-RĒ-ăl	_____
antidote (863)	ĂN-tĭ-dōt	_____
antiemetic (866)	ăn-tĭ-ĕ-MĔ-tĭk	_____
antihistamine (866)	ăn-tĭ-HĬS-tă-mēn	_____
antinauseant (866)	ăn-tĭ-NAW-zē-ănt	_____
antiplatelet (866)	ăn-tĭ-PLĀT-lĕt	_____
antipruritic (869)	ăn-tĭ-prōō-RĬT-ĭk	_____
antipyretic (869)	ăn-tĭ-pĭ-RĔT-ĭk	_____
antiulcer (866)	ăn-tĭ-ŬL-ser	_____
antiviral (866)	ăn-tē-VĪ-răl	_____
aromatase inhibitor (866)	ă-RŌ-mă-tās ĭn-HĬB-ĭ-tŏr	_____
bactericidal (866)	băk-tē-rĭ-SĪ-dăl	_____
bacteriostatic (866)	băk-te-rē-ō-STĂ-tĭk	_____
beta-blocker (866)	BĀ-tă-BLŎK-er	_____
bronchodilator (868)	brŏng-kō-DĪ-lā-tĕr	_____
benzodiazepine (862)	bĕn-zō-dī-ĂZ-ĕ-pēn	_____
bisphosphonate (866)	bĭs-FŎS-fō-nāt	_____
brand name (863)	brănd nām	_____
caffeine (866)	kăf-ĒN	_____
calcium antagonist (866)	KĂL-sē-ŭm ăn-TĂ-gōn-ĭst	_____
cathartic (866)	kă-THĂR-tĭk	_____
chemical name (863)	KĔM-ĭ-kal nām	_____
chemotherapy (868)	kē-mō-THĔR-ă-pē	_____
contraindication (863)	kŏn-tră-ĭn-dĭ-KĀ-shŭn	_____
diuretic (867)	dī-ū-RĔT-ĭk	_____
emetic (867)	ĕ-MĔT-ĭk	_____
erythromycin (869)	ĕ-rīth-rō-MĪ-sĭn	_____
estrogen (867)	ĔS-trō-jŭn	_____

generic name (863)   jĕ-NĔR-ĭk nām   _____

glucocorticoid (867)   glōō-kō-KŌR-tĭ-koyd   _____

hypnotic (867)   hĭp-NŎT-ĭk   _____

hypodermic (868)   hī-pō-DĔR-mĭk   _____

iatrogenic (864)   ī-ăt-rō-JĔN-ĭk   _____

idiosyncrasy (864)   ĭd-ē-ō-SĬN-kră-sē   _____

inhalation (864)   ĭn-hă-LĀ-shŭn   _____

intrathecal (853)   ĭn-tră-THĒ-kăl   _____

laxative (867)   LĂK-să-tĭv   _____

medicinal chemistry (864) mĕ-DĬ-sĭ-năl KĔM-ĭs-trē _____

molecular   mō-LĔK-ū-lăr   _____
  pharmacology (864)   făr-mă-KŎL-ō-jē

narcotic (867)   năr-KŎT-ĭk   _____

parenteral (864)   pă-RĔN-tĕr-ăl   _____

pharmacist (864)   FĂR-mă-sĭst   _____

pharmacy (864)   FĂR-mă-sē   _____

pharmacodynamics (864)   făr-mă-kō-dī-NĂM-ĭks _____

pharmacokinetics (864)   făr-mă-kō-kĭ-NĔT-ĭks _____

pharmacologist (864)   făr-mă-KŎL-ō-gĭst   _____

pharmacology (864)   făr-mă-KŎL-ō-gē   _____

progestin (867)   prō-GĔS-tĭn   _____

purgative (867)   PŬR-gă-tĭv   _____

sedative (867)   SĔD-ă-tĭv   _____

SERM (867)   sĕrm   _____

stimulant (867)   STĬM-ū-lănt   _____

subcutaneous (868)   sŭb-KŪ-tā-nē-ŭs   _____

sublingual (864)   sŭb-LĬNG-wăl   _____

synergism (864)	SĬN-ĕr-jĭzm	_____
synergistic (870)	sĭn-ĕr-JĬS-tĭk	_____
syringe (865)	sĭ-RĬNJ	_____
thyroid hormone (867)	THĪ-royd HŎR-mōn	_____
tolerance (865)	TŎL-ĕr-ănz	_____
toxicity (865)	tŏk-SĬS-ĭ-tē	_____
toxicology (865)	tŏk-sĭ-KŎL-ō-jē	_____
tranquilizer (867)	TRĂN-kwĭ-lī-zĕr	_____
vasodilator (869)	văz-ō-DĪ-lā-tŏr	_____
vitamin (865)	VĪ-tă-mĭn	_____

XIV. Review Sheet

Write the meanings of the word parts in the spaces provided and test yourself. Check your answers with the information in the chapter or in the glossary (Medical Terms—English) at the back of the book.

COMBINING FORMS

Combining Form	Meaning	Combining Form	Meaning
aer/o		lingu/o	
alges/o		myc/o	
bronch/o		narc/o	
chem/o		or/o	
cras/o		pharmac/o	
cutane/o		prurit/o	
derm/o		pyret/o	
enter/o		thec/o	
erg/o		tox/o	
esthes/o		toxic/o	
hist/o		vas/o	
hypn/o		ven/o	
iatr/o		vit/o	

SUFFIXES

Suffix	Meaning	Suffix	Meaning
-amine		-in	
-dote		-phylaxis	
-genic		-sol	

PREFIXES

Prefix	Meaning	Prefix	Meaning
ana-		par-	
anti-		syn-	
contra-			

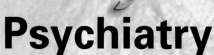

Psychiatry

This chapter is divided into the following sections

In this chapter you will

- Differentiate among a psychiatrist, a psychologist, and other mental health specialists.
- Learn of tests used by clinical psychologists to evaluate a patient's mental health and intelligence.
- Define terms that describe major psychiatric disorders.
- Identify terms that describe psychiatric symptoms.
- Compare different types of therapy for psychiatric disorders.
- Learn the categories and names of common psychiatric drugs.
- Define combining forms, suffixes, prefixes, and abbreviations related to psychiatry.
- Apply your new knowledge to understanding medical terms in their proper contexts, such as medical reports and records.

I. Introduction

You will find this chapter different from others in the book. Most psychiatric disorders are not readily explainable in terms of abnormalities in the structure or chemistry of an organ or tissue, as are other illnesses. In addition, the causes of mental disorders are complex and include significant psychological and social as well as chemical and structural elements. Our purpose here is to provide a simple outline and definitions of major psychiatric terms. For more extensive and detailed information, you may wish to consult the **Diagnostic and Statistical Manual of Mental Disorders: DSM-IV** (American Psychiatric Association, Washington, DC, 1994), as well as other textbooks of psychiatry.

Psychiatry (psych/o means mind, **iatr/o** means treatment) is the branch of medicine that deals with the diagnosis, treatment, and prevention of mental illness. It is a specialty of clinical medicine comparable to surgery, internal medicine, pediatrics, and obstetrics.

Psychiatrists complete the same medical training (4 years of medical school) as other physicians and receive an M.D. degree. Then they spend a varying number of years training in the methods and practice of **psychotherapy** (psychological techniques for treating mental disorders) and drug therapy. Psychiatrists can also take additional years of training to specialize in various aspects of psychiatry. **Child psychiatrists** specialize in the treatment of children; **forensic psychiatrists** specialize in the legal aspects of psychiatry, such as the determination of mental competence in criminal cases. **Psychoanalysts** complete 3 to 5 years of training in a special psychotherapeutic technique called **psychoanalysis** in which the patient freely relates her or his thoughts to the analyst, who does not interfere in the flow of thoughts.

A **psychologist** is a nonmedical person who is trained in methods of psychotherapy, analysis, and research and completes a master's or doctor of philosophy (Ph.D.) degree in a specific field of interest, such as **clinical** (patient-oriented) **psychology, experimental psychology,** or **social psychology** (focusing on social interaction and the ways the actions of others influence the behavior of the individual). A clinical psychologist, like a psychiatrist, can use various methods of psychotherapy to treat patients, but, unlike the psychiatrist, cannot prescribe drugs or electroconvulsive therapy. Other nonphysicians trained in the treatment of mental illness are licensed clinical social workers and psychiatric nurses.

Clinical psychologists are trained in the use of tests to evaluate various aspects of a patient's mental health and intelligence. Examples are **intelligence (I.Q.) tests** such as the **Wechsler Adult Intelligence Scale (WAIS)** and the **Stanford-Binet Intelligence Scale. Projective (personality) tests** are the **Rorschach technique** (inkblots, as shown in Fig. 22–1, are used to bring out associations) and the **Thematic Apperception Test (TAT),** in which pictures are used as stimuli for making up stories (Fig. 22–2). Both tests are especially revealing of personality structure. **Graphomotor projection tests** are the **Draw a Person Test,** in which the patient is asked to draw a body, and the **Bender-Gestalt Test,** in which the patient is asked to draw certain geometric designs. The Bender-Gestalt Test picks up deficits in mental processing and memory caused by brain damage. The **Minnesota Multiphasic Personality Inventory (MMPI)** contains true-false questions that reveal aspects of personality, such as sense of duty or responsibility, ability to relate to others, and dominance. This test is widely used as an objective measure of psychological disorders in adolescents and adults. A patient's responses to questions are compared with responses made by patients with diagnoses of schizophrenia, depression, and so on.

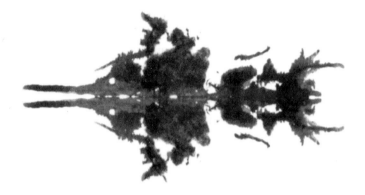

Figure 22-1

Inkblots like this one are presented on 10 cards in the Rorschach test. The patient describes images seen in the blot.

II. Psychiatric Clinical Symptoms

These terms describe abnormalities in behavior that are evident to an examining mental health professional. They will help you to understand Section III, Psychiatric Disorders.

amnesia   Loss of memory.

anxiety   Varying degrees of uneasiness, apprehension, or dread often accompanied by palpitations, tightness in the chest, breathlessness, and choking sensations.

apathy   Absence of emotions; lack of interest or emotional involvement.

autism   Severe lack of responsiveness to others, preoccupation with inner thoughts; withdrawal and retarded language development. (Auto- means self.)

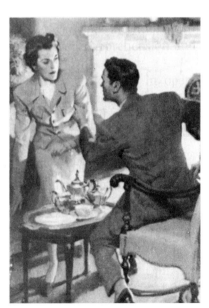

Figure 22-2

A sample picture from the **Thematic Apperception Test.** The patient is asked to tell the story that the picture illustrates. (From Gleitman H: Psychology, New York, WW Norton, 1991.)

therapy, there are fewer indications for electroconvulsive therapy, although it can be life saving when a rapid response is needed.

Drug Therapy

The following are categories of drugs used to treat psychiatric disorders. Figure 22–4 reviews these groups and lists specific drugs in each category.

- **Antianxiety and antipanic agents.** These drugs lessen anxiety, tension, and agitation, especially when they are associated with panic attacks. Examples are **benzodiazepines (BZDs),** which act as antianxiety agents, sedatives, or anticonvulsants (clonazepam). Benzodiazepines directly affect the brain to slow down the transmission of nerve impulses. Other antianxiety and antipanic agents are **selective serotonin reuptake inhibitors (SSRIs).** These agents prevent the reuptake of serotonin (a neurotransmitter) into nerve endings, allowing it to remain in the space surrounding the next nerve cell.
- **Antidepressants.** These drugs gradually reverse depressive symptoms and produce feelings of well-being. The basis of depression is thought to be an imbalance in the levels of neurotransmitters in the brain. Several groups of drugs are used as antidepressants. These include:
    1. **SSRIs (selective serotonin reuptake inhibitors)** such as fluoxetine (Prozac). They improve mood, mental alertness, physical activity, and sleep patterns.
    2. **Monoamine oxidase (MAO) inhibitors.** These drugs suppress an enzyme (monoamine oxidase) that normally degrades neurotransmitters. MAO inhibitors are not as widely prescribed as other antidepressants because serious cardiovascular and liver complications can occur with their use.
    3. **Tricyclic antidepressants.** These drugs contain three fused rings (tricyclic) in their chemical structure. They block the reuptake of neurotransmitters at nerve endings.
    4. **Atypical antidepressants.** These are antidepressants that do not fit in the previous categories.
- **Anti–obsessive-compulsive disorder (OCD) agents.** These drugs are prescribed to relieve the symptoms of obsessive-compulsive disorder. Tricyclic antidepressants and SSRIs are examples of these agents.
- **Antipsychotics (neuroleptics).** These drugs modify psychotic symptoms and behavior (neur/o = nerve, -leptic = taking hold). Examples are **phenothiazines,** which are tranquilizers that reduce the anxiety, tension, agitation, and aggressiveness associated with psychoses and modify psychotic symptoms such as delusions and hallucinations. Atypical drugs are examples of antipsychotics other than phenothiazines.
- An important side effect of taking neuroleptic drugs is **tardive dyskinesia** (tardive means late and dyskinesias are abnormal movements). This is a potentially irreversible condition marked by involuntary movements. Early detection is important.
- **Hypnotics.** These drugs are used to produce sleep (hypn/o = sleep) and relieve insomnia. Examples are sedatives and benzodiazepines.
- **Mood stabilizers.** These drugs treat the manic episodes of bipolar illness. **Lithium** (Eskalith, Lithane) is commonly used to reduce the levels of manic symptoms, such as rapid speech, hyperactive movements, grandiose ideas, poor judgment, aggressiveness, and hostility. It is also used as an adjunct in the treatment of depression. Lithium is a simple salt that is thought to stabilize nerve membranes. Anticonvulsant drugs are also used as mood stabilizers.
- **Stimulants.** These drugs **(amphetamines)** are prescribed for **attention-deficit hyperactivity disorder (ADHD)** in children. Common symptoms of ADHD are having a short attention span and being easily distracted, emotionally unstable, impulsive, and moderately to severely hyperactive.

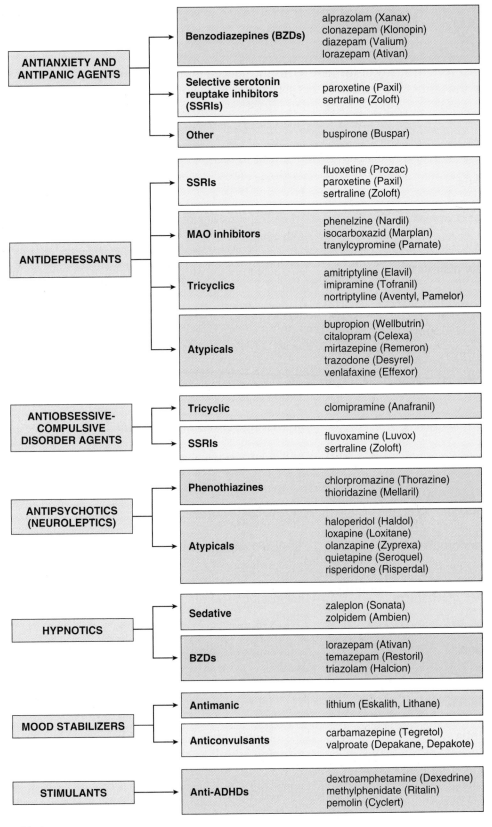

Figure 22–4

Psychiatric drug therapies and specific drugs.

V. Vocabulary

This list reviews many of the new terms introduced in the text. Short definitions reinforce your understanding of the terms. See Section XI of this chapter for help in pronouncing the more difficult terms.

General Terms, Symptoms, and Disorders

affect	The external expression of emotion, or emotional response.
amnesia	Loss of memory.
anorexia nervosa	An eating disorder of excessive dieting and refusal to maintain a normal body weight.
anxiety disorders	Characterized by unpleasant tension, distress, and avoidance behavior; examples are phobias, obsessive-compulsive disorder, and post-traumatic stress disorder.
apathy	Absence of emotions; lack of interest or emotional involvement.
autism	Severe lack of response to other people; withdrawal, inability to interact, and retarded language development.
bipolar disorder	Alternating periods of mania and depression.
bulimia nervosa	Eating disorder of binge eating followed by vomiting, purging, and depression.
compulsion	Uncontrollable urge to perform an act repeatedly.
conversion disorder	Physical symptom, with no organic basis, appearing as a result of anxiety and conflict.
defense mechanism	Unconscious technique a person uses to resolve or conceal conflicts and anxiety.
delirium	Confusion in thinking; faulty perceptions and irrational behavior. **Delirium tremens** is associated with alcohol withdrawal.
delusion	Fixed, false belief that cannot be changed by logical reasoning or evidence.
dementia	Loss of intellectual abilities with impairment of memory, judgment, and reasoning as well as changes in personality.
depression	Major mood disorder with chronic sadness, loss of energy, hopelessness, worry, and discouragement and, commonly, suicidal impulses and thoughts.
dissociative disorder	Chronic or sudden disturbance of memory, identity, or consciousness; dissociative identity disorder, amnesia, and fugue.

ego	Central coordinating branch of the personality.
fugue	Amnesia with flight from customary surroundings.
gender identity disorder	Strong and persistent cross-gender identification with the opposite sex.
hallucination	False sensory perception.
id	Major unconscious part of the personality; energy from instinctual drives and desires.
intelligence (I.Q.) test	A standardized test designed to determine mental age of an individual by measuring capacity to absorb information and solve problems.
labile	Unstable; undergoing rapid emotional change.
mania	Extreme excitement, hyperactivity, inflated self-esteem.
mood disorders	Prolonged emotion dominates a person's life; examples are bipolar and depressive disorders.
mutism	Nonreactive state; stupor.
obsessive-compulsive disorder	Anxiety disorder in which recurrent thoughts and repetitive acts dominate behavior.
paranoia	Delusions of persecution or grandeur or combinations of the two.
paraphilia	Recurrent intense sexual urge, fantasy, or behavior that involves unusual objects, activities, or situations.
personality disorders	Lifelong personality patterns marked by inflexibility and impairment of social functioning.
phobia	Irrational or disabling fear of an object or situation.
post-traumatic stress disorder	Anxiety-related symptoms appear following exposure to personal experience of a traumatic event.
projective (personality) test	Diagnostic, personality test that uses unstructured stimuli (inkblots, pictures, abstract patterns, incomplete sentences) to evoke responses that reflect aspects of an individual's personality.
psychiatrist	Physician with medical training in the diagnosis, prevention, and treatment of mental disorders. Examples are a **child psychiatrist** (diagnosing and treating children) and a **forensic psychiatrist** (specializing in legal aspects such as criminal responsibility, guardianship, and competence to stand trial). Forensic comes from the Latin, *forum,* meaning "public place."

psychologist	Individual (often a Ph.D.) specializing in mental processes and how the brain functions in health and disease. Areas of interest are **clinical psychology** (providing testing and counseling services to patients with mental and emotional disorders), **experimental psychology** (performing laboratory tests and experiments in a controlled environment to study mental processes), and **social psychology** (study of the effects of group membership on behavior and attitudes of individuals).
psychosis	Impairment of mental capacity to recognize reality, communicate, and relate to others.
reality testing	Ability to perceive fact from fantasy; severely impaired in psychoses.
repression	Defense mechanism by which unacceptable thoughts, feelings, and impulses are automatically pushed into the unconscious.
schizophrenia	Withdrawal from reality into an inner world of disorganized thinking and conflict.
sexual disorders	Disorders of paraphilias and sexual dysfunctions.
somatoform disorders	Having physical symptoms that cannot be explained by any actual physical disorder or other well-described mental disorder such as depression.
substance-related disorders	Regular overuse of psychoactive substances (alcohol, amphetamines, cannabis, cocaine, hallucinogens, opioids, and sedatives) that affect the central nervous system.
superego	Internalized conscience and moral part of the personality.

Therapy

amphetamines	Central nervous system stimulants that may be used to treat depression and attention-deficit hyperactivity disorder.
benzodiazepines	Drugs that lessen anxiety, tension, agitation and panic attacks.
cognitive behavior therapy	Conditioning (changing behavior patterns by training and repetition) is used to relieve anxiety and improve symptoms of illness.
electroconvulsive therapy	Electric current is used to produce convulsions in the treatment of depression. Modern techniques use anesthesia, so the convulsion is not observable.
family therapy	Treatment of an entire family to resolve and understand conflicts.
free association	Psychoanalytic technique in which the patient verbalizes, without censorship, the passing contents of his or her mind.
group therapy	Group of patients with similar problems gain insight into their personalities through discussion and interaction with each other.
hypnosis	Trance (state of altered consciousness) is used to increase the pace of psychotherapy.

insight-oriented therapy	Face-to-face discussion of life problems and associated feelings.
lithium	Medication used to treat the manic stage of manic-depressive illness.
neuroleptic drug	Any drug that favorably modifies psychotic symptoms. Examples are phenothiazines.
phenothiazines	Tranquilizers used to treat psychoses.
play therapy	Treatment in which a child, through use of toys in a playroom setting, expresses conflicts and feelings unable to be communicated in a direct manner.
psychoanalysis	Treatment that allows the patient to explore inner emotions and conflicts so as to understand and change current behavior.
psychodrama	Group therapy in which a patient expresses feelings by acting out roles with other patients.
psychopharmacology	Treatment of psychiatric disorders with drugs.
sedatives	Drugs that lessen anxiety.
supportive psychotherapy	Offering encouragement, support, and hope to patients facing difficult life transitions and events.
transference	Psychoanalytic process in which the patient relates to the therapist as he or she did to a prominent childhood figure.
tricyclic antidepressants	Drugs used to treat severe depression; three-ringed fused structure.

VI. Combining Forms, Suffixes, Prefixes, and Terminology

Write the meanings of the medical terms in the spaces provided.

Combining Forms			
Combining Form	Meaning	Terminology	Meaning
anxi/o	uneasy, anxious, distressed	anxiolytic _____ *This type of drug relieves anxiety.*	
hallucin/o	hallucination, to wander in the mind	hallucinogen _____ *A **hallucination** is a sensory perception in the absence of any external stimuli, and an **illusion** is an error in perception in which sensory stimuli are present but incorrectly interpreted.*	

hypn/o	sleep	hypnosis _____

The Greek god of sleep (Hypnos) put people to sleep by touching them with his magic wand or by fanning them with his dark wings.

iatr/o	treatment	psychiatrist _____
ment/o	mind	mental _____
neur/o	nerve	neurosis _____

A term formerly used to describe mental disorders in which symptoms are distressing but reality testing is intact.

phil/o	attraction to, love	paraphilia _____

para- means abnormal.

phren/o	mind	schizophrenia _____

schiz/o means split.

psych/o	mind	psychosis _____

Significant impairment of reality testing with symptoms such as delusions, hallucinations, and bizarre behavior.

psychopharmacology _____

psychotherapy _____

schiz/o	split	schizoid _____

Used to describe a mild form of schizophrenia or a withdrawn, introverted personality.

somat/o	body	psychosomatic _____

somatoform disorder _____

-form means resembling. Symptoms of these disorders resemble those of actual physical disease, but the origins are in the mind (psychogenic).

Suffixes

Suffix	Meaning	Terminology	Meaning
-genic	produced by	psychogenic _____	
-leptic	to seize hold of	neuroleptic drugs _____	
-mania	obsessive preoccupation	kleptomania _____	

klept/o means to steal.

pyromania _____

pyr/o means fire, heat.

-phobia   fear (irrational and often disabling)   agoraphobia _____

agora- means marketplace. Agoraphobics fear being left alone and feel anxious when away from familiar surroundings.

xenophobia _____

xen/o means stranger. Table 22–2 lists other phobias.

-phoria   feeling, bearing   euphoria _____

dysphoria _____

-thymia   mind   cyclothymia _____

cycl/o means circle, recurring. Alternating periods of hypomania and depression.

dysthymia _____

Depressed mood that is not as severe as major depression.

Table 22–2. PHOBIAS

Phobia	Medical Term
Air	Aerophobia
Animals	Zoophobia
Bees	Apiphobia, melissophobia
Blood or bleeding	Hematophobia, hemophobia
Books	Bibliophobia
Cats	Ailurophobia
Corpses	Necrophobia
Crossing a bridge	Gephyrophobia
Darkness	Nyctophobia, scotophobia
Death	Thanatophobia
Dogs	Cynophobia
Drugs	Pharmacophobia
Eating	Phagophobia
Enclosed places	Claustrophobia
Hair	Trichophobia, trichopathophobia
Heights	Acrophobia
Insects	Entomophobia
Light	Photophobia
Marriage	Gamophobia
Men	Androphobia
Needles	Belonephobia
Sexual intercourse	Coitophobia, cypridophobia
Sleep	Hypnophobia
Snakes	Ophidiophobia
Spiders	Arachnophobia
Traveling	Hodophobia
Vomiting	Emetophobia
Women	Gynephobia
Worms	Helminthophobia
Writing	Graphophobia

IX. Exercises

Remember to check your answers carefully with those given in Section X, Answers to Exercises.

A. Give the terms for the following definitions.

1. physician specializing in treating mental illness: _____

2. nonphysician trained in the treatment of mental illness: _____

3. therapist who practices psychoanalysis: _____

4. branch of psychiatry dealing with legal matters: _____ psychiatry

5. unconscious part of the personality: _____

6. conscious, coordinating part of the personality: _____

7. conscience or moral part of the personality: _____

8. the ability to perceive fact from fantasy: _____ testing

9. unconscious technique used to resolve or conceal conflicts and anxiety:

   mechanism _____

10. branch of psychology dealing with patient care: _____ psychology

B. Match the following psychiatric symptoms with their meanings as given below.

amnesia	compulsion	hallucination
anxiety	conversion	mania
apathy	delusion	mutism
autism	dissociation	obsession

1. a nonreactive state; stupor _____

2. state of excessive excitability; agitation _____

3. loss of memory _____

4. uncontrollable urge to perform an act repeatedly _____

5. persistent idea, emotion, or urge _____

6. feelings of apprehension, uneasiness, dread _____

7. uncomfortable feelings are separated from their real object and redirected toward a second object or

   behavior pattern _____

8. anxiety becomes a bodily symptom that has no organic basis _____

9. lack of responsiveness to others _____

10. absence of emotions _____

11. fixed false belief that cannot be changed by logical reasoning or evidence _____

12. false or unreal sensory perception _____

C. Give the meanings of the following terms.

1. dysphoria _____

2. euphoria _____

3. amnesia _____

4. paranoia _____

5. psychosis _____

6. neurosis _____

7. phobia _____

8. agoraphobia _____

9. labile _____

10. affect _____

D. Select from the following terms to complete the sentences below.

anxiety disorder   eating disorder   sexual disorder
delirium   mood disorder   somatoform disorder
dementia   personality disorder   substance-related disorder
dissociative disorder

1. Disturbance of memory and identity that hides the anxiety of unconscious conflicts

   is _____.

2. Troubled feelings, unpleasant tension, distress, and avoidance behavior describe a (an)

   _____.

3. An illness related to regular use of drugs and alcohol is a (an) _____.

4. Bulimia nervosa is an example of a (an) _____.

5. A disorder involving paraphilias is a (an) _____.

6. An illness marked by prolonged emotions (mania and depression) is a (an) _____.

7. A mental disorder in which physical symptoms cannot be explained by an actual physical disorder

   is a (an) _____.

8. A lifelong personality pattern that is inflexible and causes distress, conflict, and impairment of social

   functioning is a (an) _____.

9. Loss of intellectual abilities with impairment of memory, judgment, and reasoning is

   _____.

10. Confusion in thinking with faulty perceptions and irrational behavior is _____.

E. Give the meanings of the following terms.

1. obsessive-compulsive disorder _____

2. post-traumatic stress disorder _____

3. bipolar disorder _____

4. fugue _____

5. paranoia _____

6. amphetamines _____

7. cannabis _____

8. schizophrenia _____

9. sexual sadism _____

10. hypochondriasis _____

F. Match the general psychiatric disorder in column I with its example in column II. Write the letter of the answer in the space provided.

Column I

1. somatoform disorder _____

2. sexual disorder _____

3. anxiety disorder _____

4. mood disorder _____

5. substance-related disorder _____

6. schizophrenia _____

7. dissociative disorder _____

8. personality disorder _____

Column II

A. conversion disorder
B. cocaine abuse
C. phobia
D. catatonia
E. pedophilia
F. fugue
G. bipolar I and II
H. narcissism

G. Give the meanings of the following terms.

1. anorexia nervosa _____

2. bulimia nervosa _____

3. repression _____

4. dementia _____

5. hypomania _____

6. hallucinogen _____

7. opioids _____

8. cocaine _____

9. cyclothymic disorder _____

10. dysthymia _____

H

1. histrionic
2. antisocial
3. narcissistic
4. paranoid
5. schizoid
6. borderline

I

1. psychodrama
2. hypnosis
3. psychoanalysis
4. play therapy
5. behavioral therapy
6. sexual therapy
7. electroconvulsive therapy
8. psychopharmacology, or drug therapy
9. insight oriented therapy
10. supportive psychotherapy

J

1. xenophobia
2. kleptomania
3. MAO inhibitors
4. dysthymia
5. phenothiazines
6. agoraphobia
7. amphetamines
8. cyclothymia
9. pyromania
10. tricyclic antidepressants
11. benzodiazepines
12. lithium

K

1. mind
2. sleep
3. body
4. love, attraction to
5. treatment
6. split
7. obsessive preoccupation
8. fear
9. mind
10. to influence, turn
11. produced by
12. abnormal
13. deficient, less than, below
14. down

L

1. bipolar
2. Prozac
3. agoraphobia
4. delirium tremens
5. paranoid
6. tardive dyskinesia
7. panic attack
8. post-traumatic stress disorder
9. psychiatrist; bulimia nervosa; psychotherapy
10. SAD; hypomania

XI. Pronunciation of Terms

Pronunciation Guide

ā as in āpe   ă as in ăpple
ē as in ēven   ĕ as in ĕvery
ī as in īce   ĭ as in ĭnterest
ō as in ōpen   ŏ as in pŏt
ū as in ūnit   ŭ as in ŭnder

To test your understanding of the terminology in this chapter, write the meaning of each term in the space provided. In addition, you may wish to cover the terms and write them by looking at your definitions. Make sure your spelling is correct. The page number after each term indicates where it is defined or used in the text so you can easily check your responses.

Term	Pronunciation	Meaning
affect (902)	ĂF-fĕkt	_____
agoraphobia (907)	ăg-ŏ-ră-FŌ-bē-ă	_____
amnesia (902)	ăm-NĒ-zē-ă	_____
amphetamines (904)	ăm-FĔT-ă-mēnz	_____

anorexia nervosa (902)	ăn-ō-RĔK-sē-ă nĕr-VŌ-să	_____
antisocial personality (894)	ăn-tē-SŌ-shăl pĕr-sŏ-NĂL-ĭ-tē	_____
anxiety disorders (902)	ăng-ZĪ-ĕ-tē dĭs-ŎR-derz	_____
anxiolytic (905)	ăng-zī-ō-LĬT-ik	_____
apathy (902)	ĂP-ă-thē	_____
autism (902)	ĂW-tĭzm	_____
benzodiazepines (904)	bĕn-zō-dī-ĂZ-ĕ-pēnz	_____
bipolar disorder (902)	bī-PŌ-lăr dĭs-ŎR-dĕr	_____
borderline personality (894)	BŎR-dĕr-līn pĕr-sŏ-NĂL-ĭ-tē	_____
bulimia nervosa (902)	bū-LĒ-mē-ă nĕr-VŌ-să	_____
cannabis (897)	KĂ-nă-bis	_____
catatonic stupor (908)	kăt-ă-TŎN-ĭk STOO-pĕr	_____
claustrophobia (892)	klaws-trō-FŌ-bē-ă	_____
cognitive behavior therapy (904)	KŎG-nĭ-tĭv bē-HĀV-yŏr THĔR-ă-pē	_____
compulsion (902)	kŏm-PŬL-shŭn	_____
conversion disorder (902)	kŏn-VĔR-zhŭn dĭs-ŎR-dĕr	_____
cyclothymia (907)	sī-klō-THĪ-mē-ă	_____
defense mechanism (902)	dē-FĔNS mĕ-kăn-NĬ-zm	_____
delirium (902)	dĕ-LĬR-ē-ŭm	_____
delirium tremens (902)	dĕ-LĬR-ē-ŭm TRĒ-mĕnz	_____
delusion (902)	dĕ-LŪ-zhŭn	_____
dementia (902)	dē-MĔN-shē-ă	_____
depression (902)	dē-PRĔ-shŭn	_____
dissociative disorder (902)	dĭs-SŌ-shē-ă-tĭv dĭs-ŎR-der	_____
dysphoria (907)	dĭs-FŎR-ē-ă	_____
dysthymia (907)	dĭs-THĪ-mē-ă	_____
ego (903)	Ē-gō	_____

electroconvulsive therapy (904)	ē-lĕk-trō-kŏn-VŬL-sĭv THĔR-ă-pē	_____
euphoria (907)	ū-FŎR-ē-ă	_____
exhibitionism (895)	ĕk-sĭ-BĬSH-ŭ-nĭzm	_____
family therapy (904)	FĂM-ĭ-lē THĔR-ă-pē	_____
fetishism (895)	FĔT-ĭsh-ĭzm	_____
free association (904)	frē ă-sō-shē-Ā-shŭn	_____
fugue (903)	fūg	_____
gender-identity disorder (903)	GĔN-dĕr ī-DĔN-tĭ-te dĭs-ŎR-dĕr	_____
group therapy (904)	grōōp THĔR-ă-pē	_____
hallucination (903)	hă-lū-sĭ-NĀ-shŭn	_____
hallucinogen (905)	hă-LŪ-sĭ-nō-jĕn	_____
histrionic personality (894)	hĭs-trē-ŎN-ĭk pĕr-sŏn-ĂL-ĭ-tē	_____
hypnosis (904)	hĭp-NŌ-sĭs	_____
hypochondriasis (908)	hī-pō-kŏn-DRĪ-ă-sĭs	_____
hypomania (908)	hī-pō-MĀ-nē-ă	_____
id (903)	ĭd	_____
insight-oriented therapy (905)	ĬN-sīt ŎR-ē-ĕn-tĕd THĔR-ă-pē	_____
kleptomania (906)	klĕp-tō-MĀ-nē-ă	_____
labile (903)	LĀ-bĭl	_____
lithium (905)	LĬTH-ē-ŭm	_____
mania (903)	MĀ-nē-ă	_____
mental (906)	MĔN-tăl	_____
mood disorders (903)	MŌŌD dĭs-ŎR-dĕrz	_____
mutism (903)	MŪ-tĭzm	_____
narcissistic personality (894)	năr-sĭ-SĬS-tik pĕr-sĕ-NĂL-ĭ-tē	_____
neuroleptic drug (905)	nū-rō-LĔP-tik drŭg	_____

neurosis (906)	nū-RŌ-sĭs
obsession (890)	ŏb-SĔSH-ŭn
obsessive-compulsive disorder (903)	ŏb-SĔS-ĭv cŏm-PŬL-sĭv dĭs-ŎR-dĕr
opioid (897)	Ō-pē-ŏyd
paranoia (903)	păr-ă-NŎY-ă
paranoid personality (894)	PĂR-ă-nŏyd pĕr-sĕ-NĂL-ĭ-tē
paraphilia (903)	păr-ă-FĬL-ē-ă
pedophilia (895)	pē-dō-FĬL-ē-ă
personality disorders (903)	pĕr-sĕ-NĂL-ĭ-tē dĭs-ŎR-dĕrz
phenothiazines (905)	fē-nō-THĬ-ă-zēnz
phobia (903)	FŌ-bē-ă
play therapy (905)	plā THĔR-ă-pē
post-traumatic stress disorder (903)	pōst-trăw-MĂT-ĭk strĕs dĭs-ŎR-der
projective test (903)	prō-JĔK-tĭv tĕst
psychiatrist (903)	sī-KĪ-ă-trĭst
psychiatry (888)	sī-KĪ-ă-trē
psychoanalysis (905)	sī-kō-ă-NĂL-ĭ-sĭs
psychodrama (905)	sī-kō-DRĂ-mă
psychogenic (906)	sī-kō-JĔN-ĭk
psychologist (904)	sī-KŌL-ō-jĭst
psychopharmacology (905)	sī-kō-făr-mă-KŎL-ō-jē
psychosis (904)	sī-KŌ-sĭs
psychosomatic (906)	sī-kō-sō-MĂT-ĭk
psychotherapy (906)	sī-kō-THĔR-ă-pē
pyromania (907)	pī-rō-MĀ-nē-ă
reality testing (904)	rē-ĂL-ĭ-tē TĔS-tĭng
repression (904)	rē-PRĔ-shŭn

schizoid
  personality (906)   SKĬZ-ŏyd or SKĬT-sŏyd
     pĕr-sĕ-NĂL-ĭ-tē   _____

schizophrenia (904)   skĭz-ō-FRĒ-nē-ă or
     skĭt-sō-FRĒ-nē-ă   _____

sedatives (905)   SĔD-ă-tĭvz   _____

sexual disorders (904)   SĔX-ū-ăl dĭs-ŎR-dĕrz   _____

sexual masochism (895)   SĔX-ū-ăl MĂS-ō-kĭzm   _____

sexual sadism (895)   SĔX-ŭ-ăl SĀ-dĭzm   _____

somatoform disorders (904)   sō-MĂT-ō-fŏrm dĭs-ŎR-dĕrz   _____

superego (904)   sū-pĕr-Ē-gō   _____

supportive therapy (905)   sū-PŎR-tiv THĔR-ă-pē   _____

tolerance (896)   TŎL-ĕr-ănz   _____

transference (905)   trăns-FŬR-ĕns   _____

transvestic fetishism (895)   trăns-VĔS-tĭk FĔT-ĭsh-ĭzm   _____

tricyclic
  antidepressants (905)   trī-SĬK-lĭk
     ăn-tĭ-dĕ-PRĔ-săntz   _____

voyeurism (895)   VŎY-yĕr-ĭzm   _____

xenophobia (907)   zĕn-ō-FŌ-bē-ă   _____

XII. Review Sheet

Write the meanings of the word parts in the spaces provided and test yourself. Check your answers with the information in the chapter or in the glossary (Medical Terms—English) at the back of the book.

COMBINING FORMS

Combining Form	Meaning	Combining Form	Meaning
anxi/o	_____	phil/o	_____
cycl/o	_____	phren/o	_____
hallucin/o	_____	psych/o	_____
hypn/o	_____	pyr/o	_____
iatr/o	_____	schiz/o	_____
klept/o	_____	somat/o	_____
ment/o	_____	ton/o	_____
neur/o	_____	xen/o	_____

SUFFIXES

Suffix	Meaning	Suffix	Meaning
-form	_____	-pathy	_____
-genic	_____	-phobia	_____
-kinesia	_____	-phoria	_____
-leptic	_____	-somnia	_____
-mania	_____	-thymia	_____
-oid	_____	-tropic	_____

PREFIXES

Prefix	Meaning	Prefix	Meaning
a-, an-	_____	dys-	_____
agora-	_____	hypo-	_____
cata-	_____	para-	_____

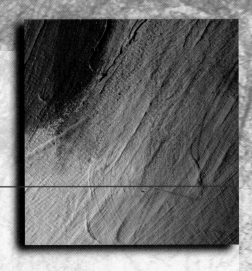

Glossary

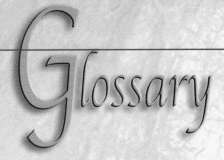

Medical Word Parts—English

Combining Form, Suffix or Prefix	Meaning	Combining Form, Suffix or Prefix	Meaning
a-, an-	no; not; without	-agra	excessive pain
ab-	away from	-al	pertaining to
abdomin/o	abdomen	alb/o	white
-ac	pertaining to	albin/o	white
acanth/o	spiny; thorny	albumin/o	albumin (protein)
acetabul/o	acetabulum (hip socket)	alges/o	sensitivity to pain
acous/o	hearing	-algesia	sensitivity to pain
acr/o	extremities; top; extreme point	-algia	pain
acromi/o	acromion (extension of shoulder bone)	all/o	other
		alveol/o	alveolus; air sac; small sac
actin/o	light	ambly/o	dim; dull
acu/o	sharp; severe; sudden	-amine	nitrogen compound
-acusis	hearing	amni/o	amnion (sac surrounding the embryo)
ad-	toward		
aden/o	gland	amyl/o	starch
adenoid/o	adenoids	an/o	anus
adip/o	fat	-an	pertaining to
adren/o	adrenal gland	ana-	up; apart; backward; again, anew
adrenal/o	adrenal gland	andr/o	male
aer/o	air	aneurysm/o	aneurysm (widened blood vessel)
af-	toward	angi/o	vessel (blood)
agglutin/o	clumping; sticking together	anis/o	unequal
-agon	to assemble, gather	ankyl/o	stiff
agora-	marketplace	ante-	before; forward

Combining Form, Suffix or Prefix	Meaning	Combining Form, Suffix or Prefix	Meaning
anter/o	front	**blephar/o**	eyelid
anthrac/o	coal	**bol/o**	cast; throw
anthr/o	antrum of the stomach	**brachi/o**	arm
anti-	against	**brachy-**	short
anxi/o	uneasy; anxious	**brady-**	slow
aort/o	aorta (largest artery)	**bronch/o**	bronchial tube
-apheresis	removal	**bronchi/o**	bronchial tube
aphth/o	ulcer	**bronchiol/o**	bronchiole
apo-	off, away	**bucc/o**	cheek
aponeur/o	aponeurosis (type of tendon)	**bunion/o**	bunion
append/o	appendix	**burs/o**	bursa (sac of fluid near joints)
appendic/o	appendix	**byssin/o**	cotton dust
aque/o	water		
-ar	pertaining to		
-arche	beginning	**cac/o**	bad
arter/o	artery	**calc/o**	calcium
arteri/o	artery	**calcane/o**	calcaneus (heel bone)
arteriol/o	arteriole (small artery)	**calci/o**	calcium
arthr/o	joint	**cali/o**	calyx
-arthria	articulate (speak distinctly)	**calic/o**	calyx
articul/o	joint	**capillar/o**	capillary (tiniest blood vessel)
-ary	pertaining to	**capn/o**	carbon dioxide
asbest/o	asbestos	**-capnia**	carbon dioxide
-ase	enzyme	**carcin/o**	cancerous; cancer
-asthenia	lack of strength	**cardi/o**	heart
atel/o	incomplete	**carp/o**	wrist bones (carpals)
ather/o	plaque (fatty substance)	**cata-**	down
-ation	process; condition	**caud/o**	tail; lower part of body
atri/o	atrium (upper heart chamber)	**caus/o**	burn; burning
audi/o	hearing	**cauter/o**	heat; burn
audit/o	hearing	**cec/o**	cecum (first part of the colon)
aur/o	ear	**-cele**	hernia
auricul/o	ear	**celi/o**	belly; abdomen
auto-	self, own	**-centesis**	surgical puncture to remove fluid
axill/o	armpit	**cephal/o**	head
azot/o	urea; nitrogen	**cerebell/o**	cerebellum (posterior part of the brain)
		cerebr/o	cerebrum (largest part of the brain)
bacill/o	bacilli (bacteria)	**cerumin/o**	cerumen
bacteri/o	bacteria	**cervic/o**	neck; cervix (neck of uterus)
balan/o	glans penis	**-chalasia**	relaxation
bar/o	pressure; weight	**-chalasis**	relaxation
bartholin/o	Bartholin glands	**cheil/o**	lip
bas/o	base; opposite of acid	**chem/o**	drug; chemical
bi-	two	**-chezia**	defecation; elimination of wastes
bi/o	life	**chir/o**	hand
bil/i	bile; gall	**chlor/o**	green
bilirubin/o	bilirubin	**chlorhydr/o**	hydrochloric acid
-blast	embryonic; immature	**chol/e**	bile; gall
-blastoma	immature tumor (cells)	**cholangi/o**	bile vessel

Combining Form, Suffix or Prefix	Meaning	Combining Form, Suffix or Prefix	Meaning
cholecyst/o	gallbladder	**-crit**	to separate
choledoch/o	common bile duct	**cry/o**	cold
cholesterol/o	cholesterol	**crypt/o**	hidden
chondr/o	cartilage	**culd/o**	cul-de-sac
chore/o	dance	**-cusis**	hearing
chori/o	chorion (outermost membrane of the fetus)	**cutane/o**	skin
		cyan/o	blue
chorion/o	chorion	**cycl/o**	ciliary body of eye; cycle; circle
choroid/o	choroid layer of eye	**-cyesis**	pregnancy
chrom/o	color	**cyst/o**	urinary bladder; cyst; sac of fluid
chron/o	time	**cyt/o**	cell
chym/o	to pour	**-cyte**	cell
cib/o	meal	**-cytosis**	condition of cells; slight increase in numbers
-cide	killing		
-cidal	pertaining to killing		
cine/o	movement		
cirrh/o	orange-yellow	**dacry/o**	tear
cis/o	to cut	**dacryoaden/o**	tear gland
-clasis	to break	**dacryocyst/o**	tear sac; lacrimal sac
-clast	to break	**dactyl/o**	fingers; toes
claustr/o	enclosed space	**de-**	lack of; down; less; removal of
clavicul/o	clavicle (collar bone)	**dem/o**	people
-clysis	irrigation; washing	**dent/i**	tooth
coagul/o	coagulation (clotting)	**derm/o**	skin
-coccus (-cocci, pl.)	berry-shaped bacterium	**-derma**	skin
		dermat/o	skin
coccyg/o	coccyx (tailbone)	**desicc/o**	drying
cochle/o	cochlea (inner part of ear)	**-desis**	to bind, tie together
col/o	colon (large intestine)	**dia-**	complete; through
coll/a	glue	**diaphor/o**	sweat
colon/o	colon (large intestine)	**-dilation**	widening; stretching; expanding
colp/o	vagina	**dipl/o**	double
comat/o	deep sleep	**dips/o**	thirst
comi/o	to care for	**dist/o**	far; distant
con-	together, with	**dors/o**	back (of body)
coni/o	dust	**dorsi-**	back
conjunctiv/o	conjunctiva (lines the eyelids)	**-dote**	to give
-constriction	narrowing	**-drome**	to run
contra-	against; opposite	**duct/o**	to lead, carry
cor/o	pupil	**duoden/o**	duodenum
core/o	pupil	**dur/o**	dura mater
corne/o	cornea	**-dynia**	pain
coron/o	heart	**dys-**	bad; painful; difficult; abnormal
corpor/o	body		
cortic/o	cortex, outer region		
cost/o	rib	**-eal**	pertaining to
crani/o	skull	**ec-**	out; outside
cras/o	mixture; temperament	**echo-**	reflected sound
crin/o	secrete	**-ectasia**	stretching; dilation; expansion
-crine	secrete; separate	**-ectasis**	stretching; dilation; expansion

Combining Form, Suffix or Prefix	Meaning	Combining Form, Suffix or Prefix	Meaning
ecto-	out; outside	-fication	process of making
-ectomy	removal; excision; resection	-fida	split
-edema	swelling	flex/o	to bend
-elasma	flat plate	fluor/o	luminous
electr/o	electricity	follicul/o	follicle; small sac
em-	in	-form	resembling; in the shape of
-ema	condition	fung/i	fungus; mushroom
-emesis	vomiting	furc/o	forking; branching
-emia	blood condition	-fusion	to pour; to come together
-emic	pertaining to blood condition		
emmetr/o	in due measure		
en-	in; within	galact/o	milk
encephal/o	brain	ganglion/o	ganglion; collection of nerve cell bodies
endo-	in; within		
enter/o	intestines (usually small intestine)	gastr/o	stomach
eosin/o	red; rosy; dawn-colored	-gen	producing; forming
epi-	above; upon; on	-genesis	producing; forming
epididym/o	epididymis	-genic	produced by or in
epiglott/o	epiglottis	ger/o	old age
episi/o	vulva (external female genitalia)	gest/o	pregnancy
epitheli/o	skin; epithelium	gester/o	pregnancy
equin/o	horse	gingiv/o	gum
-er	one who	glauc/o	gray
erg/o	work	gli/o	glue; neuroglial tissue (supportive tissue of nervous system)
erythem/o	flushed; redness		
erythr/o	red	-globin	protein
-esis	condition	-globulin	protein
eso-	inward	glomerul/o	glomerulus
esophag/o	esophagus	gloss/o	tongue
esthes/o	nervous sensation (feeling)	gluc/o	glucose; sugar
esthesi/o	nervous sensation	glyc/o	glucose; sugar
-esthesia	nervous sensation	glycogen/o	glycogen; animal starch
estr/o	female	glycos/o	glucose; sugar
ethm/o	sieve	gnos/o	knowledge
eti/o	cause	gon/o	seed
eu-	good; normal	gonad/o	sex glands
-eurysm	widening	goni/o	angle
ex-	out; away from	-grade	to go
exanthemat/o	rash	-gram	record
exo-	out; away from	granul/o	granule(s)
extra-	outside	-graph	instrument for recording
		-graphy	process of recording
		gravid/o	pregnancy
faci/o	face	-gravida	pregnant woman
fasci/o	fascia (membrane supporting muscles)	gynec/o	woman; female
femor/o	femur (thigh bone)		
-ferent	to carry		
fibr/o	fiber	hallucin/o	hallucination
fibros/o	fibrous connective tissue	hem/o	blood
fibul/o	fibula	hemat/o	blood

Combining Form, Suffix or Prefix	Meaning	Combining Form, Suffix or Prefix	Meaning
hemi-	half	**ischi/o**	ischium (part of hip bone)
hemoglobin/o	hemoglobin	**-ism**	process; condition
hepat/o	liver	**-ist**	specialist
herni/o	hernia	**-itis**	inflammation
-hexia	habit	**-ium**	structure; tissue
hidr/o	sweat		
hist/o	tissue		
histi/o	tissue	**jaund/o**	yellow
home/o	sameness; unchanging; constant	**jejun/o**	jejunum
hormon/o	hormone		
humer/o	humerus (upper arm bone)		
hydr/o	water	**kal/i**	potassium
hyper-	above; excessive	**kary/o**	nucleus
hypn/o	sleep	**kerat/o**	horny, hard; cornea
hypo-	deficient; below; under; less than normal	**kern-**	nucleus (collection of nerve cells in the brain)
hypophys/o	pituitary gland	**ket/o**	ketones; acetones
hyster/o	uterus; womb	**keton/o**	ketones; acetones
		kines/o	movement
		kinesi/o	movement
-ia	condition	**-kinesia**	movement
-iac	pertaining to	**-kinesis**	movement
-iasis	abnormal condition	**klept/o**	to steal
iatr/o	physician; treatment	**kyph/o**	humpback
-ic	pertaining to		
-ical	pertaining to		
ichthy/o	dry; scaly	**labi/o**	lip
-icle	small	**lacrim/o**	tear; tear duct; lacrimal duct
idi/o	unknown; individual; distinct	**lact/o**	milk
ile/o	ileum	**lamin/o**	lamina (part of vertebral arch)
ili/o	ilium	**lapar/o**	abdominal wall; abdomen
immun/o	immune; protection; safe	**-lapse**	to slide, fall, sag
in-	in; into; not	**laryng/o**	larynx (voice box)
-in, -ine	a substance	**later/o**	side
-ine	pertaining to	**leiomy/o**	smooth (visceral) muscle
infra-	below; inferior to; beneath	**-lemma**	sheath, covering
inguin/o	groin	**-lepsy**	seizure
insulin/o	insulin (pancreatic hormone)	**lept/o**	thin, slender
inter-	between	**-leptic**	to seize, take hold of
intra-	within; into	**leth/o**	death
iod/o	iodine	**leuk/o**	white
ion/o	ion; to wander	**lex/o**	word; phrase
-ion	process	**-lexia**	word; phrase
-ior	pertaining to	**ligament/o**	ligament
ipsi-	same	**lingu/o**	tongue
ir-	in	**lip/o**	fat; lipid
ir/o	iris (colored portion of eye)	**-listhesis**	slipping
irid/o	iris (colored portion of eye)	**lith/o**	stone; calculus
is/o	same; equal	**-lithiasis**	condition of stones
isch/o	to hold back; back	**-lithotomy**	incision (for removal) of a stone

Combining Form, Suffix or Prefix	Meaning	Combining Form, Suffix or Prefix	Meaning
lob/o	lobe	**-mission**	to send
log/o	study of	**mon/o**	one; single
-logy	study of	**morph/o**	shape; form
lord/o	curve; swayback	**mort/o**	death
-lucent	to shine	**-mortem**	death
lumb/o	lower back; loin	**-motor**	movement
lute/o	yellow	**muc/o**	mucus
lux/o	to slide	**mucos/o**	mucous membrane (mucosa)
lymph/o	lymph	**multi-**	many
lymphaden/o	lymph gland (node)	**mut/a**	genetic change
lymphangi/o	lymph vessel	**mutagen/o**	causing genetic change
-lysis	breakdown; separation; destruction; loosening	**my/o**	muscle
		myc/o	fungus
-lytic	to reduce, destroy; separate; breakdown	**mydr/o**	wide
		myel/o	spinal cord; bone marrow
		myocardi/o	myocardium (heart muscle)
		myom/o	muscle tumor
macro-	large	**myos/o**	muscle
mal-	bad	**myring/o**	tympanic membrane (eardrum)
-malacia	softening	**myx/o**	mucus
malleol/o	malleolus		
mamm/o	breast		
mandibul/o	mandible (lower jaw bone)	**narc/o**	numbness; stupor; sleep
-mania	obsessive preoccupation	**nas/o**	nose
mast/o	breast	**nat/i**	birth
mastoid/o	mastoid process (behind the ear)	**natr/o**	sodium
maxill/o	maxilla (upper jaw bone)	**necr/o**	death
meat/o	meatus (opening)	**nect/o**	to bind, tie, connect
medi/o	middle	**neo-**	new
mediastin/o	mediastinum	**nephr/o**	kidney
medull/o	medulla (inner section); middle; soft, marrow	**neur/o**	nerve
		neutr/o	neither; neutral; neutrophil
mega-	large	**nid/o**	nest
-megaly	enlargement	**noct/i**	night
melan/o	black	**norm/o**	rule; order
men/o	menses; menstruation	**nos/o**	disease
mening/o	meninges (membranes covering the spinal cord and brain)	**nucle/o**	nucleus
		nulli-	none
meningi/o	meninges	**nyct/o**	night
ment/o	mind; chin		
meso-	middle		
meta-	change; beyond	**obstetr/o**	midwife
metacarp/o	metacarpals (hand bones)	**ocul/o**	eye
metatars/o	metatarsals (foot bones)	**odont/o**	tooth
-meter	measure	**odyn/o**	pain
metr/o	uterus (womb); measure	**-oid**	resembling
metri/o	uterus (womb)	**-ole**	little; small
mi/o	smaller; less	**olecran/o**	olecranon (elbow)
micro-	small	**olig/o**	scanty
-mimetic	mimic; copy	**om/o**	shoulder

Combining Form, Suffix or Prefix	Meaning	Combining Form, Suffix or Prefix	Meaning
-oma	tumor; mass; fluid collection	**parathyroid/o**	parathyroid glands
omphal/o	umbilicus (navel)	**-paresis**	slight paralysis
onc/o	tumor	**-pareunia**	sexual intercourse
-one	hormone	**-partum**	birth; labor
onych/o	nail (of fingers or toes)	**patell/a**	patella
o/o	egg	**patell/o**	patella
oophor/o	ovary	**path/o**	disease
-opaque	obscure	**-pathy**	disease; emotion
ophthalm/o	eye	**pector/o**	chest
-opia	vision	**ped/o**	child; foot
-opsia	vision	**pelv/i**	pelvic bone; hip
-opsy	view of	**pend/o**	to hang
opt/o	eye; vision	**-penia**	deficiency
optic/o	eye; vision	**-pepsia**	digestion
-or	one who	**per-**	through
or/o	mouth	**peri-**	surrounding
orch/o	testis	**perine/o**	perineum
orchi/o	testis	**peritone/o**	peritoneum
orchid/o	testis	**perone/o**	fibula
-orexia	appetite	**-pexy**	fixation; to put in place
orth/o	straight	**phac/o**	lens of eye
-ose	full of; pertaining to; sugar	**phag/o**	eat; swallow
-osis	condition, usually abnormal	**-phage**	eat; swallow
-osmia	smell	**-phagia**	eating; swallowing
ossicul/o	ossicle (small bone)	**phak/o**	lens of eye
oste/o	bone	**phalang/o**	phalanges (fingers and toes)
-ostosis	condition of bone	**phall/o**	penis
ot/o	ear	**pharmac/o**	drug
-otia	ear condition	**pharmaceut/o**	drug
-ous	pertaining to	**pharyng/o**	throat (pharynx)
ov/o	egg	**phas/o**	speech
ovari/o	ovary	**-phasia**	speech
ovul/o	egg	**phe/o**	dusky; dark
ox/o	oxygen	**-pheresis**	removal
-oxia	oxygen	**phil/o**	like; love; attraction to
oxy-	swift; sharp; acid	**-phil**	attraction for
oxysm/o	sudden	**-philia**	attraction for
		phim/o	muzzle
		phleb/o	vein
pachy-	heavy; thick	**phob/o**	fear
palat/o	palate (roof of the mouth)	**-phobia**	fear
palpebr/o	eyelid	**phon/o**	voice; sound
pan-	all	**-phonia**	voice; sound
pancreat/o	pancreas	**-phor/o**	to bear
papill/o	nipple-like; optic disc (disk)	**-phoresis**	carrying; transmission
par-	other than; abnormal	**-phoria**	to bear, carry; feeling (mental state)
para-	near; beside; abnormal; apart from; along the side of	**phot/o**	light
		phren/o	diaphragm; mind
-para	to bear, bring forth (live births)	**-phthisis**	wasting away
-parous	to bear, bring forth	**-phylaxis**	protection

Combining Form, Suffix or Prefix	Meaning	Combining Form, Suffix or Prefix	Meaning
physi/o	nature; function	-ptysis	spitting
-physis	to grow	pub/o	pubis (anterior part of hip bone)
phyt/o	plant	pulmon/o	lung
-phyte	plant	pupill/o	pupil (dark center of the eye)
pil/o	hair	purul/o	pus
pineal/o	pineal gland	py/o	pus
pituitar/o	pituitary gland	pyel/o	renal pelvis
-plakia	plaque	pylor/o	pylorus; pyloric sphincter
plant/o	sole of the foot	pyr/o	fever; fire
plas/o	development; formation	pyret/o	fever
-plasia	development; formation; growth	pyrex/o	fever
-plasm	formation		
-plastic	pertaining to formation		
-plasty	surgical repair	quadri-	four
ple/o	more; many		
-plegia	paralysis; palsy		
-plegic	paralysis; palsy	rachi/o	spinal column; vertebrae
pleur/o	pleura	radi/o	x-rays; radioactivity; radius (lateral lower arm bone)
plex/o	plexus; network (of nerves)		
-pnea	breathing	radicul/o	nerve root
pneum/o	lung; air; gas	re-	back; again; backward
pneumon/o	lung; air; gas	rect/o	rectum
pod/o	foot	ren/o	kidney
-poiesis	formation	reticul/o	network
-poietin	substance that forms	retin/o	retina
poikil/o	varied; irregular	retro-	behind; back; backward
pol/o	extreme	rhabdomy/o	striated (skeletal) muscle
polio-	gray matter (of brain or spinal cord)	rheumat/o	watery flow
poly-	many; much	rhin/o	nose
polyp/o	polyp; small growth	rhytid/o	wrinkle
pont/o	pons (a part of the brain)	roentgen/o	x-rays
-porosis	condition of pores (spaces)	-rrhage	bursting forth (of blood)
post-	after; behind	-rrhagia	bursting forth (of blood)
poster/o	back (of body); behind	-rrhaphy	suture
-prandial	meal	-rrhea	flow; discharge
-praxia	action	-rrhexis	rupture
pre-	before; in front of	rrhythm/o	rhythm
presby/o	old age		
primi-	first		
pro-	before; forward	sacr/o	sacrum
proct/o	anus and rectum	salping/o	fallopian tube; auditory (eustachian) tube
pros-	before; forward		
prostat/o	prostate gland	-salpinx	fallopian tube; oviduct
prot/o	first	sarc/o	flesh (connective tissue)
prote/o	protein	scapul/o	scapula; shoulder blade
proxim/o	near	-schisis	to split
prurit/o	itching	schiz/o	split
pseudo-	false	scint/i	spark
psych/o	mind	scirrh/o	hard
-ptosis	droop; sag; prolapse; fall	scler/o	sclera (white of eye)

Combining Form, Suffix or Prefix	Meaning
-sclerosis	hardening
scoli/o	crooked; bent
-scope	instrument for visual examination
-scopy	visual examination
scot/o	darkness
seb/o	sebum
sebace/o	sebum
sect/o	to cut
semi-	half
semin/i	semen; seed
seps/o	infection
sial/o	saliva
sialaden/o	salivary gland
sider/o	iron
sigmoid/o	sigmoid colon
silic/o	glass
sinus/o	sinus
-sis	state of; condition
-sol	solution
somat/o	body
-some	body
somn/o	sleep
-somnia	sleep
son/o	sound
-spadia	to tear, cut
-spasm	sudden contraction of muscles
sperm/o	spermatozoa; sperm cells
spermat/o	spermatozoa; sperm cells
sphen/o	wedge; sphenoid bone
spher/o	globe-shaped; round
sphygm/o	pulse
-sphyxia	pulse
splanchn/o	viscera (internal organs)
spin/o	spine (backbone)
spir/o	to breathe
splen/o	spleen
spondyl/o	vertebra (backbone)
squam/o	scale
-stalsis	contraction
staped/o	stapes (middle ear bone)
staphyl/o	clusters; uvula
-stasis	to stop; control; place
-static	pertaining to stopping; controlling
steat/o	fat, sebum
-stenosis	tightening; stricture
ster/o	solid structure; steroid
stere/o	solid; three-dimensional
stern/o	sternum (breastbone)
steth/o	chest
-sthenia	strength

Combining Form, Suffix or Prefix	Meaning
-stitial	to set; pertaining to standing or positioned
stomat/o	mouth
-stomia	condition of the mouth
-stomy	new opening (to form a mouth)
strept/o	twisted chains
styl/o	pole or stake
sub-	under; below
submaxill/o	mandible (lower jaw bone)
-suppression	to stop
supra-	above, upper
sym-	together; with
syn-	together; with
syncop/o	to cut off, cut short; faint
syndesm/o	ligament
synov/o	synovia; synovial membrane; sheath around a tendon
syring/o	tube
tachy-	fast
tars/o	tarsus; hindfoot or ankle (7 bones between the foot and the leg)
tax/o	order; coordination
tel/o	complete
tele/o	distant
ten/o	tendon
tendin/o	tendon
-tension	pressure
terat/o	monster; malformed fetus
test/o	testis (testicle)
tetra-	four
thalam/o	thalamus
thalass/o	sea
the/o	put; place
thec/o	sheath
thel/o	nipple
therapeut/o	treatment
-therapy	treatment
therm/o	heat
thorac/o	chest
-thorax	chest; pleural cavity
thromb/o	clot
thym/o	thymus gland
-thymia	mind (condition of)
-thymic	pertaining to mind
thyr/o	thyroid gland; shield
thyroid/o	thyroid gland
tibi/o	tibia (shin bone)
-tic	pertaining to

Combining Form, Suffix or Prefix	Meaning	Combining Form, Suffix or Prefix	Meaning
toc/o	labor; birth	**uve/o**	uvea, vascular layer of eye (iris, choroid, ciliary body)
-tocia	labor; birth (condition of)		
-tocin	labor; birth (a substance for)	**uvul/o**	uvula
tom/o	to cut		
-tome	instrument to cut		
-tomy	process of cutting	**vag/o**	vagus nerve
ton/o	tension	**vagin/o**	vagina
tone/o	to stretch	**valv/o**	valve
tonsill/o	tonsil	**valvul/o**	valve
top/o	place; position; location	**varic/o**	varicose veins
tox/o	poison	**vas/o**	vessel; duct; vas deferens
toxic/o	poison	**vascul/o**	vessel (blood)
trache/o	trachea (windpipe)	**ven/o; ven/i**	vein
trans-	across; through	**vener/o**	venereal (sexual contact)
-tresia	opening	**ventr/o**	belly side of body
tri-	three	**ventricul/o**	ventricle (of heart or brain)
trich/o	hair	**venul/o**	venule (small vein)
trigon/o	trigone (area within the bladder)	**-verse**	to turn
-tripsy	to crush	**-version**	to turn
troph/o	nourishment; development	**vertebr/o**	vertebra (backbone)
-trophy	nourishment; development	**vesic/o**	urinary bladder
-tropia	to turn	**vesicul/o**	seminal vesicle
-tropic	turning	**vestibul/o**	vestibule of the inner ear
-tropin	stimulate; act on	**viscer/o**	internal organs
tympan/o	tympanic membrane (eardrum); middle ear	**vit/o**	life
		vitr/o	vitreous body (of the eye)
-type	classification; picture	**vitre/o**	glass
		viv/o	life
		vol/o	to roll
-ule	little; small	**vulv/o**	vulva (female external genitalia)
uln/o	ulna (medial lower arm bone)		
ultra-	beyond; excess		
-um	structure; tissue; thing	**xanth/o**	yellow
umbilic/o	umbilicus (navel)	**xen/o**	stranger
ungu/o	nail	**xer/o**	dry
uni-	one	**xiph/o**	sword
ur/o	urine; urinary tract		
ureter/o	ureter		
urethr/o	urethra	**-y**	condition; process
-uria	urination; condition of urine		
urin/o	urine		
-us	structure; thing	**zo/o**	animal life
uter/o	uterus (womb)		

English—Medical Word Parts

Meaning	Combining Form, Suffix or Prefix	Meaning	Combining Form, Suffix or Prefix
abdomen	abdomin/o (use with -al, -centesis)	apart	ana-
		apart from	para-
	celi/o (use with -ac)	appendix	append/o (use with -ectomy)
	lapar/o (use with -scope, -scopy, -tomy)		appendic/o (use with -itis)
		appetite	-orexia
abdominal wall	lapar/o	arm	brachi/o
abnormal	dys-	arm bone, lower, lateral	radi/o
	par-	arm bone, lower, medial	uln/o
	para-	arm bone, upper	humer/o
abnormal condition	-iasis	armpit	axill/o
	-osis	arteriole	arteriol/o
above	epi-	artery	arter/o
	hyper-		arteri/o
	supra-	articulate	-arthria
acetabulum	acetabul/o	(speak distinctly)	
acetones	ket/o	asbestos	asbest/o
	keton/o	assemble	-agon
acid	oxy-	atrium	atri/o
acromion	acromi/o	attraction for	-phil
across	trans-		-philia
action	-praxia	attraction to	phil/o
act on	-tropin	auditory tube	salping/o
adrenal glands	adren/o	away from	ab-
	adrenal/o		apo-
after	post-		ex-
again	ana-, re-		exo-
against	anti-		
	contra-		
air	aer/o	back	re-
	pneum/o		retro-
	pneumon/o	back, lower	lumb/o
air sac	alveol/o	back portion of body	dorsi-
albumin	albumin/o		dors/o
all	pan-		poster/o
along the side of	para-	backbone	spin/o (use with -al)
alveolus	alveol/o		spondyl/o (use with -itis, -listhesis, -osis, -pathy)
anew	ana-		
amnion	amni/o		vertebr/o (use with -al)
aneurysm	aneurysm/o	backward	ana-
angle	goni/o		retro-
animal life	zo/o	bacteria	bacteri/o
animal starch	glycogen/o	bacterium (berry-shaped)	-coccus (-cocci, pl.)
ankle	tars/o	bacilli (rod-shaped bacteria)	bacill/o
antrum (of stomach)	antr/o		
anus	an/o	bad	cac/o
anus and rectum	proct/o		dys-
anxiety	anxi/o		mal-

Meaning	Combining Form, Suffix or Prefix	Meaning	Combining Form, Suffix or Prefix
barrier	claustr/o	**blood condition**	-emia
base (not acidic)	bas/o		-emic
bear (to)	-para	**blood vessel**	angi/o (use with -ectomy,
	-parous		-genesis, -gram, -graphy,
	-phoria		-oma, -plasty, -spasm)
	phor/o		vas/o (use with -constriction,
before	ante-		-dilation, -motor)
	pre-		vascul/o (use with -ar, -itis)
	pro-	**blue**	cyan/o
	pros-	**body**	corpor/o
beginning	-arche		somat/o
behind	post-		-some
	poster/o	**bone**	oste/o
	retro-	**bone condition**	-ostosis
belly	celi/o	**bone marrow**	myel/o
belly side of body	ventr/o	**brain**	encephal/o
below, beneath	hypo-		cerebr/o
	infra-	**branching**	furc/o
	sub-	**break**	-clasis
bend (to)	flex/o		-clast
bent	scoli/o	**breakdown**	-lysis
beside	para-	**breast**	mamm/o (use with
between	inter-		-ary, -gram, -graphy,
beyond	hyper-		-plasty)
	meta-		mast/o (use with
	ultra-		-algia, -dynia, -ectomy,
bile	bil/i		-itis)
	chol/e	**breastbone**	stern/o
bile vessel	cholangi/o	**breathe**	spir/o
bilirubin	bilirubin/o	**breathing**	-pnea
bind	-desis	**bring forth**	-para
	nect/o		-parous
birth	nat/i	**bronchial tube (bronchus)**	bronch/o
	-partum		bronchi/o
	toc/o	**bronchiole**	bronchiol/o
	-tocia	**bunion**	bunion/o
birth (substance for)	-tocin	**burn**	caus/o
births (live)	-para		cauter/o
black	anthrac/o, melan/o	**bursa**	burs/o
bladder (urinary)	cyst/o (use with -ic, -itis,	**bursting forth (of blood)**	-rrhage
	-cele, -gram, -scopy,		-rrhagia
	-stomy, -tomy)		
	vesic/o (use with -al)		
blood	hem/o (use with -dialysis,	**calcaneus**	calcane/o
	-globin, -lysis, -philia,	**calcium**	calc/o
	-ptysis, -rrhage, -stasis,		calci/o
	-stat)	**calculus**	lith/o
	hemat/o (use with -crit,	**calyx**	cali/o
	-emesis, -logist, -logy,		calic/o
	-oma, -poiesis, -uria)	**cancerous**	carcin/o

Meaning	Combining Form, Suffix or Prefix	Meaning	Combining Form, Suffix or Prefix
capillary	capillar/o	come together	-fusion
carbon dioxide	capn/o	common bile duct	choledoch/o
	-capnia	complete	dia-
care for (to)	comi/o		tel/o
carry	duct/o	condition	-ation
	-ferent		-ema
	-phoria		-esis
carrying	-phoresis		-ia
cartilage	chondr/o		-ism
cast; throw	bol/o		-sis
cause	eti/o		-y
cecum	cec/o	condition, abnormal	-iasis
cell	cyt/o		-osis
	-cyte	connect	nect/o
cells, condition of	-cytosis	connective tissue	sarc/o
cerebellum	cerebell/o	constant	home/o
cerebrum	cerebr/o	control	-stasis, -stat
cerumen	cerumin/o	contraction	-stalsis
cervix	cervic/o	contraction of muscles, sudden	-spasm
change	meta-		
cheek	bucc/o	coordination	tax/o
chemical	chem/o	copy	-mimetic
chest	pector/o	cornea (of the eye)	corne/o
	steth/o		kerat/o
	thorac/o	cortex	cortic/o
	-thorax	cotton dust	byssin/o
child	ped/o	crooked	scoli/o
chin	ment/o	crush (to)	-tripsy
cholesterol	cholesterol/o	curve	lord/o
chorion	chori/o	cut	cis/o
	chorion/o		sect/o, -section
choroid layer (of the eye)	choroid/o		tom/o
ciliary body (of the eye)	cycl/o	cut off	syncop/o
circle or cycle	cycl/o	cutting, process of	-tomy
clavicle (collar bone)	clavicul/o	cycle	cycl/o
clot	thromb/o	cyst (sac of fluid)	cyst/o
clumping	agglutin/o		
clusters	staphyl/o		
coagulation	coagul/o	dance	chore/o
coal dust	anthrac/o	dark	phe/o
coccyx	coccyg/o	darkness	scot/o
cochlea	cochle/o	dawn-colored	eosin/o
cold	cry/o	death	leth/o
collar bone	clavicul/o		mort/o, -mortem
colon	col/o (use with -ectomy, -itis, -pexy, -stomy)		necr/o
	colon/o (use with -ic, -pathy, -scope, -scopy)	defecation	-chezia
		deficiency	-penia
		deficient	hypo-
color	chrom/o	destroy	-lytic

Meaning	Combining Form, Suffix or Prefix	Meaning	Combining Form, Suffix or Prefix
destruction	-lysis	egg cell	o/o
development	plas/o		ov/o
	-plasia		ovul/o
	troph/o	elbow	olecran/o
	-trophy	electricity	electr/o
diaphragm	phren/o	elimination of wastes	-chezia
difficult	dys-	embryonic	-blast
digestion	-pepsia	enlargement	-megaly
dilation	-ectasia	enzyme	-ase
	-ectasis	epididymis	epididym/o
dim	ambly/o	epiglottis	epiglott/o
discharge	-rrhea	equal	is/o
disease	nos/o	esophagus	esophag/o
	path/o	eustachian tube	salping/o
	-pathy	excess	ultra-
distant	dist/o	excessive	hyper-
	tele/o	excision	-ectomy
distinct	idi/o	expansion	-ectasia
double	dipl/o		-ectasis
down	cata-	extreme	pol/o
	de-	extreme point	acr/o
droop	-ptosis	extremities	acr/o
drug	chem/o	eye	ocul/o (use with -ar, -facial, -motor)
	pharmac/o		
	pharmaceut/o		ophthalm/o (use with -ia, -ic, -logist, -logy, -pathy, -plasty, -plegia, -scope, -scopy)
dry	ichthy/o		
	xer/o		
drying	desicc/o		opt/o (use with -ic, -metrist)
duct	vas/o		optic/o (use with -al, -ian)
dull	ambly/o	eyelid	blephar/o (use with -chalasis, -itis, -plasty, -plegia, -ptosis, -tomy)
duodenum	duoden/o		
dura mater	dur/o		
dusky	phe/o		
dust	coni/o		palpebr/o (use with -al)
ear	aur/o (use with -al, -icle)	face	faci/o
	auricul/o (use with -ar)	faint	syncop/o
	ot/o (use with -algia, -ic, -itis, -logy, -mycosis, -rrhea, -sclerosis, -scope, -scopy)	fall	-ptosis
		fallopian tube	salping/o
			-salpinx
		false	pseudo-
ear (condition of)	-otia	far	dist/o
eardrum	myring/o (use with -ectomy, -itis, -tomy)	fascia	fasci/o
		fast	tachy-
	tympan/o (use with, -ic, -metry, -plasty)	fat	adip/o (use with -ose, -osis)
			lip/o (use with -ase, -cyte, -genesis, -oid, -oma)
eat	phag/o		
	-phage		steat/o (use with -oma, -rrhea)
eating	-phagia		

Meaning	Combining Form, Suffix or Prefix	Meaning	Combining Form, Suffix or Prefix
fear	phob/o	gas	pneum/o
	-phobia		pneumon/o
feeling	esthesi/o	gather	-agon
	-phoria	genetic change	mut/a
female	estr/o (use with -gen, -genic)		mutagen/o
	gynec/o (use with -logist,	give (to)	-dote
	-logy, -mastia)	given (what is)	-dote
femur	femor/o	gland	aden/o
fever	pyr/o	glans penis	balan/o
	pyret/o	glass	silic/o
	pyrex/o		vitre/o
fiber	fibr/o	globe-shaped	spher/o
fibrous connective tissue	fibros/o	glomerulus	glomerul/o
fibula	fibul/o (use with -ar)	glucose	gluc/o
	perone/o (use with -al)		glyc/o
finger and toe bones	phalang/o		glycos/o
fingers	dactyl/o	glue	coll/a
fire	pyr/o		gli/o
first	prot/o	glycogen	glycogen/o
fixation	-pexy	go (to)	-grade
flat plate	-elasma	good	eu-
flesh	sarc/o	granule(s)	granul/o
flow	-rrhea	gray	glauc/o
fluid collection	-oma	gray matter	poli/o
flushed	erythem/o	green	chlor/o
foot	pod/o	groin	inguin/o
foot bones	metatars/o	grow	-physis
forking	furc/o	growth	-plasia
form	morph/o	gum	gingiv/o
formation	plas/o		
	-plasia		
	-plasm	habit	-hexia
	-poiesis	hair	pil/o
forming	-genesis		trich/o
forward	ante-, pro-, pros-	half	hemi-
four	quadri-		semi-
front	anter/o	hallucination	hallucin/o
full of	-ose	hand	chir/o
fungus	fung/i (use with -cide, -oid,	hand bones	metacarp/o
	-ous, -stasis)	hang (to)	pend/o
	myc/o (use with -logist,	hard	kerat/o
	-logy, -osis, -tic)		scirrh/o
		hardening	-sclerosis
		head	cephal/o
gall	bil/i (use with -ary)	hearing	acous/o
	chol/e (use with -lithiasis)		audi/o
gallbladder	cholecyst/o		audit/o
ganglion	gangli/o		-acusis
	ganglion/o		-cusis

Meaning	Combining Form, Suffix or Prefix	Meaning	Combining Form, Suffix or Prefix
heart	cardi/o (use with -ac, -graphy, -logy, -logist, -megaly, -pathy, -vascular)	intestine, large	col/o
		intestine, small	enter/o
		iodine	iod/o
	coron/o (use with -ary)	ion	ion/o
heart muscle	myocardi/o	iris	ir/o
heat	cauter/o		irid/o
	therm/o	iron	sider/o
heavy	pachy-	irregular	poikil/o
heel bone	calcane/o	irrigation	-clysis
hemoglobin	hemoglobin/o	ischium	ischi/o
hernia	-cele	itching	prurit/o
	herni/o		
hidden	crypt/o		
hip	pelv/i	jaw, lower	mandibul/o
hold back	isch/o		submaxill/o
hormone	hormon/o	jaw, upper	maxill/o
	-one	joint	arthr/o
horny	kerat/o		articul/o
horse	equin/o		
humerus	humer/o		
humpback	kyph/o	ketones	ket/o
hydrochloric acid	chlorhydr/o		keton/o
		kidney	nephr/o (use with -algia, -ectomy, -ic, -itis, -lith, -megaly, -oma, -osis, -pathy, -ptosis, -sclerosis, -stomy, -tomy)
ileum	ile/o		
ilium	ili/o		
immature	-blast		ren/o (use with -al, -gram, -vascular)
immature tumor (cells)	-blastoma		
immune	immun/o		
in, into, within	em-	killing	-cidal
	en-		-cide
	endo-	knowledge	gnos/o
	in-, intra-		
	ir-		
in due measure	emmetr/o	labor	-partum
in front of	pre-		toc/o
incomplete	atel/o		-tocia
increase in numbers (blood cells)	-cytosis	labor (substance for)	-tocin
		lack of	de-
individual	idi/o	lack of strength	-asthenia
infection	seps/o	lacrimal duct	dacry/o
inferior to	infra-		lacrim/o
inflammation	-itis	lacrimal sac	dacryocyst/o
instrument for recording	-graph	lamina	lamin/o
instrument for visual examination	-scope	large	macro-
			mega-
instrument to cut	-tome	larynx	laryng/o
insulin	insulin/o	lead	duct/o
internal organs	splanchn/o, viscer/o	lens of eye	phac/o
			phak/o

Meaning	Combining Form, Suffix or Prefix	Meaning	Combining Form, Suffix or Prefix
less	de-	**meatus**	meat/o
	mi/o	**mediastinum**	mediastin/o
less than normal	hypo-	**medulla oblongata**	medull/o
life	bi/o	**meninges**	mening/o
	vit/o		meningi/o
	viv/o	**menstruation; menses**	men/o
ligament	ligament/o	**metacarpals**	metacarp/o
	syndesm/o	**metatarsals**	metatars/o
like	phil/o	**middle**	medi/o
lip	cheil/o		medull/o
	labi/o		meso-
lipid	lip/o	**middle ear**	tympan/o
little	-ole	**midwife**	obstetr/o
	-ule	**milk**	galact/o
liver	hepat/o		lact/o
lobe	lob/o	**mimic**	-mimetic
location	top/o	**mind**	ment/o
loin	lumb/o		phren/o
loosening	-lysis		psych/o
love	phil/o		-thymia
luminous	fluor/o		-thymic
lung	pneum/o (use with -coccus, -coniosis, -thorax)	**mixture**	cras/o
		monster	terat/o
	pneumon/o (use with -ectomy, -ia, -ic, -itis, -lysis)	**more**	ple/o
		mouth	or/o (use with -al)
			stomat/o (use with -itis)
	pulmon/o (use with -ary)		-stomia
lymph	lymph/o	**movement**	cine/o
lymph gland	lymphaden/o		kines/o
lymph vessel	lymphangi/o		kinesi/o
			-kinesia
			-kinesis
make (to)	-fication		-motor
male	andr/o	**much**	poly-
malformed fetus	terat/o	**mucous membrane**	mucos/o
malleolus	malleol/o	**mucus**	muc/o
mandible	mandibul/o		myx/o
	submaxill/o	**muscle**	muscul/o (use with -ar, -skeletal)
many	multi-		my/o (use with -algia, -ectomy, -oma, -neural, -pathy, -rrhaphy, -therapy)
	ple/o		
	poly-		
marketplace	agora-		
marrow	medull/o		myos/o (use with -in, -itis)
mass	-oma		
mastoid process	mastoid/o	**muscle, heart**	myocardi/o
maxilla	maxill/o	**muscle, smooth (visceral)**	leiomy/o
meal	cib/o	**muscle, striated (skeletal)**	rhabdomy/o
	-prandial	**muscle tumor**	myom/o
measure	-meter	**muzzle**	phim/o
	metr/o		

Meaning	Combining Form, Suffix or Prefix	Meaning	Combining Form, Suffix or Prefix
nail	onych/o	one	mon/o
	ungu/o		mono-
narrowing	-constriction		uni-
	-stenosis	one's own	aut/o
nature	physi/o		auto-
navel	omphal/o	one who	-er
	umbilic/o		-or
near	para-	opening	-tresia
	proxim/o	opening (new)	-stomy
neck	cervic/o	opposite	contra-
neither	neutr/o	optic disc (disk)	papill/o
nerve	neur/o	orange-yellow	cirrh/o
nerve root	radicul/o	order	norm/o
nest	nid/o		tax/o
new	neo-	organs, internal	viscer/o
network	reticul/o	ossicle	ossicul/o
network of nerves	plex/o	other	all/o
neutral	neutr/o	other than	par-
neutrophil	neutr/o	out, outside	ec-
night	nocti/i		ex-
	nyct/o		exo-
nipple	thel/o		extra-
nipple-like	papill/o	outer region	cortic/o
nitrogen	azot/o	ovary	oophor/o (use with -itis, -ectomy, -pexy)
nitrogen compound	-amine		ovari/o (use with -an)
no, not	a-	oxygen	ox/o
	an-		-oxia
none	nulli-		
normal	eu-		
nose	nas/o (use with -al)		
	rhin/o (use with -itis, -rrhea, -plasty)	pain	-algia
			-dynia
nourishment	troph/o		odyn/o
	-trophy	pain, excessive	-agra
nucleus	kary/o	pain, sensitivity to	-algesia
	nucle/o		algesi/o
nucleus (collection of nerve cells in the brain)	kern-	painful	dys-
		palate	palat/o
numbness	narc/o	palsy	-plegia
			-plegic
		pancreas	pancreat/o
obscure	-opaque	paralysis	-plegia
obsessive preoccupation	-mania		-plegic
off	apo-	paralysis, slight	-paresis
old age	ger/o	patella	patell/a (use with -pexy)
	presby/o		patell/o (use with -ar, -ectomy, -femoral)
olecranon (elbow)	olecran/o		
on	epi-		

Meaning	Combining Form, Suffix or Prefix	Meaning	Combining Form, Suffix or Prefix
pelvic bone, pelvis	pelv/i	**pregnancy**	-cyesis
	pelv/o		gest/o
penis	balan/o		gester/o
	phall/o		gravid/o
people	dem/o		-gravida
perineum	perine/o	**pressure**	bar/o
peritoneum	peritone/o		-tension
pertaining to	-ac (cardiac)	**process**	-ation
	-al (inguinal)		-ion
	-an (ovarian)		-ism
	-ar (palmar)		-y
	-ary (papillary)	**produced by or in**	-genic
	-eal (pharyngeal)	**producing**	-gen
	-iac (hypochondriac)		-genesis
	-ic (nucleic)	**prolapse**	-ptosis
	-ical (neurological)	**prostate gland**	prostat/o
	-ine (equine)	**protection**	immun/o
	-ior (superior)		-phylaxis
	-ose (adipose)	**protein**	-globin
	-ous (mucous)		-globulin
	-tic (necrotic)		prote/o
phalanges	phalang/o	**pubis**	pub/o
pharynx (throat)	pharyng/o	**pulse**	sphygm/o
phrase	-lexia		-sphyxia
physician	iatr/o	**puncture to remove fluid**	-centesis
pineal gland	pineal/o	**pupil**	cor/o
pituitary gland	hypophys/o		core/o
	pituit/o		pupill/o
	pituitar/o	**pus**	py/o, purul/o
place	-stasis	**put**	the/o
	the/o	**put in place**	-pexy
	top/o	**pyloric sphincter, pylorus**	pylor/o
plant	phyt/o		
	-phyte		
plaque	ather/o	**radioactivity**	radi/o
	-plakia	**radius (lower arm bone)**	radi/o
pleura	pleur/o	**rapid**	oxy-
pleural cavity	-thorax	**rash**	exanthemat/o
plexus	plex/o	**rays**	radi/o
poison	tox/o	**record**	-gram
	toxic/o	**recording, process of**	-graphy
pole	styl/o	**rectum**	rect/o
polyp	polyp/o	**recurring**	cycl/o
pons	pont/o	**red**	eosin/o
pores (condition of)	-porosis		erythr/o
position	top/o	**redness**	erythem/o
potassium	kal/i		erythemat/o
pour	chym/o	**reduce**	-lytic
	-fusion	**relaxation**	-chalasia, -chalasis

Meaning	Combining Form, Suffix or Prefix	Meaning	Combining Form, Suffix or Prefix
removal	-apheresis	separation	-lysis
	-ectomy	set (to)	-stitial
	-pheresis	severe	acu/o
renal pelvis	pyel/o	sex glands	gonad/o
repair	-plasty	sexual intercourse	-pareunia
resembling	-form	shape	-form
	-oid		morph/o
retina	retin/o	sharp	acu/o
rib	cost/o		oxy-
roll (to)	vol/o	sheath	thec/o
rosy	eosin/o	shield	thyr/o
round	spher/o	shin bone	tibi/o
rule	norm/o	shine	-lucent
run	-drome	short	brachy-
rupture	-rrhexis	shoulder	om/o
		side	later/o
		sieve	ethm/o
sac, small	alveol/o	sigmoid colon	sigmoid/o
	follicul/o	single	mon/o
sac of fluid	cyst/o	sinus	sinus/o
sacrum	sacr/o	skin	cutane/o (use with -ous)
safe	immun/o		derm/o (use with -al)
sag (to)	-ptosis		-derma (use with erythr/o, leuk/o)
saliva	sial/o		
salivary gland	sialaden/o		dermat/o (use with -itis, -logist, -logy, -osis)
same	ipsi-		
	is/o		epitheli/o (use with -al, -lysis, -oid, -oma, -um)
sameness	home/o		
scaly	ichthy/o		
scanty	olig/o	skull	crani/o
sclera	scler/o	sleep	hypn/o
scrotum	scrot/o		somn/o
sea	thalass/o		-somnia
sebum	seb/o	sleep (deep)	comat/o
	sebace/o	slender	lept/o
	steat/o	slide (to)	-lapse
secrete	crin/o		lux/o
	-crine	slipping	-listhesis
seed	gon/o	slow	brady-
	semin/i	small	-icle
seizure	-lepsy		micro-
seize (to); take hold of	-leptic		-ole
self	aut/o		-ule
	auto-	small intestine	enter/o
semen	semin/i	smaller	mi/o
seminal vesicle	vesicul/o	smell	-osmia
send (to)	-mission	sodium	natr/o
sensation (nervous)	-esthesia	soft	medull/o
separate	-crine	softening	-malacia
	-lytic	sole (of the foot)	plant/o

Meaning	Combining Form, Suffix or Prefix	Meaning	Combining Form, Suffix or Prefix
solution	-sol	substance	-in
sound	echo-		-ine
	phon/o	substance that forms	-poietin
	-phonia	sudden	acu/o
	son/o		oxysm/o
spark	scint/i	sugar	gluc/o
specialist	-ist		glyc/o
speech	phas/o		glycos/o
	-phasia		-ose
sperm cells	sperm/o	surgical repair	-plasty
(spermatozoa)	spermat/o	surrounding	peri-
spinal column	rachi/o	suture	-rrhaphy
spinal cord	myel/o	swallow	phag/o
spinal column (spine)	spin/o	swallowing	-phagia
	rachi/o	swayback	lord/o
	vertebr/o	sweat	diaphor/o (use with -esis)
spiny	acanth/o		hidr/o (use with -osis)
spitting	-ptysis	swift	oxy-
spleen	splen/o	sword	xiph/o
split	-fida	synovia (fluid)	synov/o
	schiz/o	synovial membrane	synov/o
split (to)	-schisis		
stake (pole)	styl/o		
stapes	staped/o	tail	caud/o
starch	amyl/o	tailbone	coccyg/o
state of	-sis	tear	dacry/o (use with -genic, -rrhea)
steal	klept/o		
sternum	stern/o		lacrim/o (use with -al, -ation)
steroid	ster/o		
sticking together	agglutin/o	tear (to cut)	-spadia
stiff	ankyl/o	tear gland	dacryoaden/o
stimulate	-tropin	tear sac	dacryocyst/o
stomach	gastr/o	temperament	cras/o
stone	lith/o	tendon	ten/o
stop	-suppression		tend/o
stopping	-stasis		tendin/o
	-static	tension	ton/o
straight	orth/o	testis	orch/o (use with -itis)
stranger	xen/o		orchi/o (use with -algia, -dynia, -ectomy, -pathy, -pexy, -tomy)
strength	-sthenia		
stretch	tone/o		
stretching	-ectasia		orchid/o (use with -ectomy, -pexy, -plasty, -ptosis, -tomy)
	-ectasis		
stricture	-stenosis		
structure	-ium		test/o (use with -sterone)
	-um, -us	thick	pachy-
structure, solid	ster/o	thigh bone	femor/o
study of	log/o	thin	lept/o
	-logy	thing	-um
stupor	narc/o		-us

Meaning	Combining Form, Suffix or Prefix	Meaning	Combining Form, Suffix or Prefix
thirst	dips/o	**ulcer**	aphth/o
thorny	acanth/o	**ulna**	uln/o
three	tri-	**umbilicus, navel**	omphal/o (use with -cele,
throat	pharyng/o		-ectomy, -rrhagia,
through	dia-		-rrhexis)
	per-		umbilic/o (use with -al)
	trans-	**unchanging**	home/o
throw (to)	bol/o	**under**	hypo-
thymus gland	thym/o	**unequal**	anis/o
thyroid gland	thyr/o	**unknown**	idi/o
	thyroid/o	**up**	ana-
tibia	tibi/o	**upon**	epi-
tie	nect/o	**urea**	azot/o
tie together	-desis	**ureter**	ureter/o
tightening	-stenosis	**urethra**	urethr/o
time	chron/o	**urinary bladder**	cyst/o (use with cele,
tissue	hist/o		-ectomy, -itis, -pexy,
	histi/o		-plasty, -plegia, -scope,
	-ium		-scopy, -stomy, -tomy)
	-um		vesic/o (use with -al)
toes	dactyl/o	**urinary tract**	ur/o
together	con-	**urination**	-uria
	sym-	**urine**	ur/o-uria
	syn-		urin/o
tongue	gloss/o (use with -al, -dynia,	**uterus**	hyster/o (use with -ectomy,
	-plasty, -plegia, -rrhaphy,		-graphy, -gram, -tomy)
	-spasm, -tomy)		metr/o (use with -rrhagia,
	lingu/o (use with -al)		-rrhea, -rrhexis)
tonsil	tonsill/o		metri/o (use with -osis)
tooth	dent/i		uter/o (use with -ine)
	odont/o	**uvea**	uve/o
top	acr/o	**uvula**	uvul/o (use with -ar, -itis,
toward	ad-		-ptosis)
	af-		staphyl/o (use with -ectomy,
trachea	trache/o		-plasty, -tomy)
transmission	-phoresis		
treatment	iatr/o		
	therapeut/o	**vagina**	colp/o (use with -pexy,
	-therapy		-plasty, -scope, -scopy,
trigone	trigon/o		-tomy)
tube	syring/o		vagin/o (use with -al, -itis)
tumor	-oma	**vagus nerve**	vag/o
	onc/o	**valve**	valv/o
turn	-tropia		valvul/o
	-verse	**varicose veins**	varic/o
	-version	**varied**	poikil/o
turning	-tropic	**vas deferens**	vas/o
twisted chains	strept/o	**vein**	phleb/o (use with -ectomy,
two	bi-		-itis, -tomy)
tympanic membrane	myring/o		ven/o (use with -ous, -gram)
	tympan/o		ven/i (use with -puncture)

Meaning	Combining Form, Suffix or Prefix	Meaning	Combining Form, Suffix or Prefix
vein, small	venul/o	**watery flow**	rheumat/o
venereal	vener/o	**wedge**	sphen/o
ventricle	ventricul/o	**weight**	bar/o
vertebra	rachi/o (use with -itis, -tomy)	**white**	alb/o
			albin/o
	spondyl/o (use with -itis, -listhesis, -osis, -pathy)		leuk/o
		wide	mydr/o
	vertebr/o (use with -al)	**widening**	-dilation
vessel	angi/o (use with -ectomy, -genesis, -gram, -graphy, -oma, -plasty, -spasm)		-ectasia
			-ectasis
			-eurysm
	vas/o (use with -constriction, -dilation, -motor)	**windpipe**	trache/o
		with	con-
	vascul/o (-ar, -itis)		sym-
view of	-opsy		syn-
viscera	splanchn/o	**within**	en-
vision	-opia		endo-
	-opsia		intra-
	opt/o	**woman**	gynec/o
	optic/o	**womb**	hyster/o
visual examination	-scopy		metr/o
vitreous body	vitr/o		metri/o
voice	phon/o		uter/o
	-phonia	**word**	-lexia
voice box	laryng/o	**work**	erg/o
vomiting	-emesis	**wrinkle**	rhytid/o
vulva	episi/o (use with -tomy)	**wrist bone**	carp/o
	vulv/o (use with -ar)		
		x-rays	radi/o
wander	ion/o		
washing	-clysis		
wasting away	-phthisis	**yellow**	lute/o
water	aque/o		jaund/o
	hydr/o		xanth/o

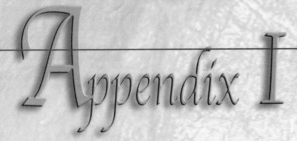

Appendix I

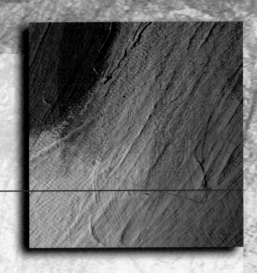

Plurals

The rules commonly used to form plurals of medical terms are as follows:

1. For words ending in **a**, retain the **a** and add **e**:
Examples:

Singular	Plural
vertebra	vertebrae
bursa	bursae
bulla	bullae

2. For words ending in **is**, drop the **is** and add **es**:
Examples:

Singular	Plural
anastomosis	anastomoses
metastasis	metastases
epiphysis	epiphyses
prosthesis	prostheses
pubis	pubes

3. For words ending in **ix** and **ex**, drop the **ix** or **ex** and add **ices**:
Examples:

Singular	Plural
apex	apices
varix	varices

4. For words ending in **on**, drop the **on** and add **a**:
Examples:

Singular	Plural
ganglion	ganglia
spermatozoon	spermatozoa

5. For words ending in **um**, drop the **um** and add **a**:
Examples:

Singular	Plural
bacterium	bacteria
diverticulum	diverticula
ovum	ova

6. For words ending in **us**, drop the **us** and add **i**:
Examples:

Singular	Plural
calculus	calculi
bronchus	bronchi
nucleus	nuclei

   Two exceptions to this rule are viruses and sinuses.

7. Examples of other plural changes are:

Singular	Plural
foramen	foramina
iris	irides
femur	femora
anomaly	anomalies
biopsy	biopsies
adenoma	adenomata

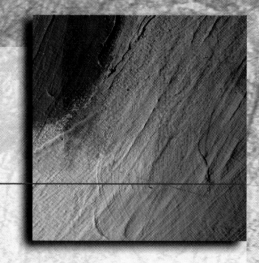

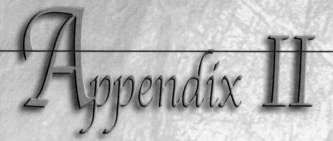

Appendix II

Abbreviations, Acronyms, and Symbols

Abbreviations

Many of these abbreviations may appear with or without periods and with either a capital or a lowercase first letter.

@	at
ā	before
A, B, AB, O	blood types; may have subscript numbers
ABCD	asymmetry, border, color, diameter (description of skin cancer lesions)
A2 or A$_2$	aortic valve closure (heart sound)
AAA	abdominal aortic aneurysm
AAL	anterior axillary line
AB/ab	abortion
Ab	antibody
abd	abdomen; abduction
ABGs	arterial blood gases
a.c.	before meals *(ante cibum)*
AC joint	acromioclavicular joint
ACE	angiotensin-converting enzyme (ACE inhibitors are used to treat hypertension)
ACh	acetylcholine (neurotransmitter)
ACL	anterior cruciate ligament (of knee)
ACS	acute coronary syndromes
ACTH	adrenocorticotropic hormone (secreted by the anterior pituitary gland)
AD	right ear *(auris dextra);* Alzheimer disease
ADD	attention deficit disorder
add	adduction

ADH	antidiuretic hormone; vasopressin (secreted by the posterior pituitary gland)
ADHD	attention-deficit hyperactivity disorder
ADL	activities of daily living
ADT	admission, discharge, transfer
ad lib.	as desired
AF	atrial fibrillation
AFB	acid-fast bacillus (bacilli); TB organism
AFO	ankle foot orthosis (device for stabilization)
AFP	alpha-fetoprotein
Ag	silver
AHF	antihemophilic factor (coagulation factor XIII)
AIDS	acquired immune deficiency syndrome
AIHA	autoimmune hemolytic anemia
AKA	above-knee amputation
alb	albumin (protein)
alk phos	alkaline phosphatase (elevated in liver disease)
ALL	acute lymphocytic leukemia
ALS	amyotrophic lateral sclerosis (Lou Gehrig disease)
ALT	alanine aminotransferase (elevated in liver and heart disease); formerly SGPT

a.m. or AM	in the morning or before noon
AMA	against medical advice; American Medical Association
Amb	ambulate, ambulatory (walking)
AMD	age-related macular degeneration
AMI	acute myocardial infarction
AML	acute myelocytic (myelogenous) leukemia
ANA	antinuclear antibody
ANC	absolute neutrophil count
AP or A/P	anteroposterior
A&P	auscultation and percussion
APC	acetylsalicylic acid (aspirin), phenacetin, and caffeine
aq.	water *(aqua);* aqueous
ARDS	adult respiratory distress syndrome
AROM	active range of motion
AS	left ear *(auris sinistra);* aortic stenosis
ASA	acetylsalicylic acid (aspirin)
ASD	atrial septal defect
ASHD	arteriosclerotic heart disease
AST	aspartate aminotransferase (elevated in liver and heart disease); formerly SGOT
AU	each ear, both ears *(auris uterque)*
Au	gold
AV	arteriovenous; atrioventricular
AVM	arteriovenous malformation
AVR	aortic valve replacement
A&W	alive and well
Ba	barium
BAL	bronchioalveolar lavage
bands	banded neutrophils
baso	basophils
BBB	bundle branch block
BC	bone conduction
B cells	lymphocytes produced in the bone marrow
BE	barium enema
b.i.d.	twice a day *(bis in die)*
BKA	below-knee amputation
BM	bowel movement
BMR	basal metabolic rate
BMT	bone marrow transplant
BP or B/P	blood pressure
BPH	benign prostatic hyperplasia (hypertrophy)
BRBPR	bright red blood per rectum; hematochezia
BSE	breast self-examination
BSO	bilateral salpingo-oophorectomy
BSP	bromsulphalein (dye used in liver function test; its retention is indicative of liver damage or disease)
BT	bleeding time
BUN	blood urea nitrogen
Bx, bx	biopsy

C	Carbon; calorie
°C	Celsius, centigrade (temperature scale)
c̄	with *(cum)*
C1, C2	first, second cervical vertebra
Ca	calcium
CA	cancer; carcinoma; cardiac arrest; chronological age
CABG	coronary artery bypass graft (surgery)
CAD	coronary artery disease
CAO	chronic airway obstruction
CAPD	continuous ambulatory peritoneal dialysis
cap	capsule
Cath	catheter; catheterization
CAT	computerized axial tomography
CBC	complete blood (cell) count
CBT	cognitive behavior therapy
CC	chief complaint
cc	cubic centimeter (same as ml; 1/1000 liter)
CCU	coronary care unit; critical care unit
CDC	Centers for Disease Control and Prevention
CDH	congenital dislocated hip
CEA	carcinoembryonic antigen
cf.	compare
CF	cystic fibrosis; complement fixation
cGy	centigray (one hundredth of a gray; a rad)
CHD	coronary heart disease; chronic heart disease
chemo	chemotherapy
CHF	congestive heart failure
chol	cholesterol
chr	chronic
μCi	microcurie
CIN	cervical intraepithelial neoplasia
CIS	carcinoma *in situ*
CK	creatine kinase
CKD	chronic kidney disease
Cl	chlorine
CLD	chronic liver disease
CLL	chronic lymphocytic leukemia
cm	centimeter (1/100 meter)
CMA	certified medical assistant
CMG	cystometrogram
CML	chronic myelogenous leukemia
CMV	cytomegalovirus
CNS	central nervous system
Co	cobalt
c/o	complains of
CO	carbon monoxide; cardiac output
CO_2	carbon dioxide
COD	condition on discharge
COPD	chronic obstructive pulmonary disease
CP	cerebral palsy; chest pain
CPA	costophrenic angle
CPAP	continuous positive airway pressure
CPD	cephalopelvic disproportion

CPR	cardiopulmonary resuscitation
CR	complete response; cardiorespiratory
CRF	chronic renal failure
C-section	cesarean section
C&S	culture and sensitivity
CSF	cerebrospinal fluid; colony-stimulating factor
C-spine	cervical spine films
ct.	count
CTA	clear to auscultation
CTS	carpal tunnel syndrome
CT	computed tomography (x-ray images in a cross-sectional view)
Cu	copper
CVA	cerebrovascular accident; costovertebral angle
CVP	central venous pressure
CVS	cardiovascular system; chorionic villus sampling
c/w	compare with; consistent with
CX (CXR)	chest x-ray
Cx	cervix
cysto	cystoscopy
D/C	discontinue; discharge
D&C	dilatation (dilation) and curettage
DCIS	ductal carcinoma *in situ*
DD	discharge diagnosis; differential diagnosis
Decub.	decubitus (lying down)
Derm.	dermatology
DES	diethylstilbestrol; diffuse esophageal spasm
DI	diabetes insipidus; diagnostic imaging
DIC	disseminated intravascular coagulation
DICOM	digital image communication in medicine
diff.	differential count (white blood cells)
DIG	digoxin; digitalis
dL, dl	deciliter (1/10 liter)
DLco	diffusion capacity of the lung for carbon monoxide
DLE	discoid lupus erythematosus
DM	diabetes mellitus
DNA	deoxyribonucleic acid
DNR	do not resuscitate
D.O.	Doctor of Osteopathy
DOA	dead on arrival
DOB	date of birth
DOE	dyspnea on exertion
DPI	dry powder inhaler
DPT	diphtheria, pertussis, tetanus (vaccine)
DRE	digital rectal exam
DRG	diagnosis-related group

DSA	digital subtraction angiography
DSM	Diagnostic and Statistical Manual of Mental Disorders
DT	delirium tremens (caused by alcohol withdrawal)
DTR	deep tendon reflexes
DUB	dysfunctional uterine bleeding
DVT	deep venous thrombosis
D/W	dextrose and water
Dx	diagnosis
EBV	Epstein-Barr virus
ECC	endocervical curettage; extracorporeal circulation
ECF	extended-care facility
ECG	electrocardiogram
ECHO	echocardiography
ECMO	extracorporeal membrane oxygenation
ECT	electroconvulsive therapy
ED	emergency department
EDC	estimated date of confinement
EEG	electroencephalogram
EENT	eyes, ears, nose, and throat
EGD	esophagogastroduodenoscopy
EKG	electrocardiogram
ELISA	enzyme-linked immunosorbent assay (AIDS test)
EM	electron microscope
EMB	endometrial biopsy
EMG	electromyogram
EMT	emergency medical technician
ENT	ear, nose, and throat
EOM	extraocular movement; extraocular muscles
eos.	eosinophil (type of white blood cell)
EPO	erythropoietin
ER	emergency room; estrogen receptor
ERCP	endoscopic retrograde cholangiopancreatography
ERT	estrogen replacement therapy
ESR	erythrocyte sedimentation rate
ESRD	end-stage renal disease
ESWL	extracorporeal shock wave lithotripsy
ETOH	ethyl alcohol
ETT	exercise tolerance test
F or °F	Fahrenheit
FACP	Fellow, American College of Physicians
FACS	Fellow, American College of Surgeons
FB	fingerbreadth; foreign body
FBS	fasting blood sugar
FDA	Food and Drug Administration

Fe	iron
FEF	forced expiratory flow
FEV$_1$	forced expiratory volume in first second
FH	family history
FHR	fetal heart rate
FROM	full range of movement/motion
FSH	follicle-stimulating hormone
F/u	follow-up
5-FU	5-fluorouracil (chemotherapy drug)
FUO	fever of undetermined origin
Fx	fracture
μg	microgram (one-millionth of a gram)
G	gravida (pregnant)
g, gm	gram
g/dL	gram per deciliter
Ga	gallium
GABA	gamma-aminobutyric acid (neurotransmitter)
GB	gallbladder
GBS	gallbladder series (x-rays)
GC	gonorrhea
G-CSF	granulocyte colony-stimulating factor
GERD	gastroesophageal reflux disease
GFR	glomerular filtration rate
GH	growth hormone
GI	gastrointestinal
G$_6$PD	glucose-6-phosphate dehydrogenase (enzyme missing in inherited red blood cell disorder)
GP	general practitioner
GM-CSF	granulocyte macrophage colony-stimulating factor
Grav. 1, 2, 3	first, second, third pregnancy
GTT	glucose tolerance test
gtt	drop (*gutta*), drops (*guttae*)
GU	genitourinary
Gy	gray (unit of radiation and equal to 100 rad)
GYN or gyn	gynecology
H	hydrogen
h., hr	hour
H2 blocker	H2 (histamine)-receptor antagonist (inhibitor of gastric acid secretion)
HAART	highly active antiretroviral therapy (for AIDS)
Hb; hgb	hemoglobin
HbA1C	glycosylated hemoglobin test (for diabetes)
HBV	hepatitis B virus
HCG (hCG)	human chorionic gonadotropin
HCl	hydrochloric acid
HCO$_3$	bicarbonate

Hct (HCT)	hematocrit
HCV	hepatitis C virus
HCVD	hypertensive cardiovascular disease
HD	hemodialysis (artificial kidney machine)
HDL	high-density lipoprotein
He	helium
HEENT	head, eyes, ears, nose, and throat
Hg	mercury
H&H	hematocrit and hemoglobin (rbc tests)
HIPAA	Health Insurance Portability and Accountability Act (of 1996)
HIV	human immunodeficiency virus
HLA	histocompatibility locus antigen (identifies cells as "self")
h/o	history of
H$_2$O	water
H&P	history and physical
HPF; hpf	high-power field (microscope)
HPI	history of present illness
HPV	human papillomavirus
HRT	hormone replacement therapy
h.s.	at bedtime (*hora somni*)
HSG	hysterosalpingography
HSV	herpes simplex virus
ht	height
HTN	hypertension (high blood pressure)
Hx	history
I	iodine
^{131}I	radioactive isotope of iodine
IBD	inflammatory bowel disease
ICD	implantable cardioverter/defibrillator
ICP	intracranial pressure
ICSH	interstitial cell-stimulating hormone
ICU	intensive care unit
I&D	incision and drainage
ID	infectious disease
IgA, IgD, IgE, IgG, IgM	immunoglobulins
IHD	ischemic heart disease
IHSS	idiopathic hypertrophic subaortic stenosis
IL1-15	interleukins
IM	intramuscular; infectious mononucleosis
inf.	infusion; inferior
INH	isoniazid (drug used to treat tuberculosis)
inj.	injection
I&O	intake and output (measurement of patient's fluids)
IOL	intraocular lens (implant)
IOP	intraocular pressure
IPPB	intermittent positive pressure breathing
I.Q.	intelligence quotient

ITP	idiopathic thrombocytopenic purpura
IUD	intrauterine device
IUP	intrauterine pregnancy
IV or I.V.	intravenous (injection)
IVP	intravenous pyelogram
K	potassium
kg	kilogram (1000 grams)
KJ	knee jerk
KS	Kaposi sarcoma
KUB	kidneys, ureters, bladder (x-ray exam)
μl	microliter (one-millionth of a liter)
L, l	liter; left; lower
L1, L2	first, second lumbar vertebra
LA	left atrium
LAD	left anterior descending (coronary artery)
lat	lateral
LB	large bowel
LBBB	left bundle branch block (heart block)
LD	lethal dose
LDH	lactate dehydrogenase
LDL	low-density lipoprotein (high levels associated with heart disease)
L-dopa	levodopa (used to treat Parkinson disease)
L.E.	lupus erythematosus
LEEP	loop electrocautery excision procedure
LES	lower esophageal sphincter
LFT	liver function test
LH	luteinizing hormone
LLL	left lower lobe (lung)
LLQ	left lower quadrant (abdomen)
LMP	last menstrual period
LMWH	low-molecular-weight heparin
LOC	loss of consciousness
LOS	length of stay
LP	lumbar puncture
lpf	low-power field (microscope)
LPN	licensed practical nurse
LS	lumbosacral spine
LSD	lysergic acid diethylamide
LSK	liver, spleen, and kidneys
LTB	laryngotracheal bronchitis (croup)
LTC	long-term care
LTH	luteotropic hormone (prolactin)
LUL	left upper lobe (lung)
LUQ	left upper quadrant (abdomen)
LV	left ventricle
LVAD	left ventricular assist device
L&W	living and well
lymphs	lymphocytes
lytes	electrolytes

MA	mental age
MAC	monitored anesthesia care
MAI	*Mycobacterium avium intracellulare*
MAOI	monoamine oxidase inhibitor (antidepressant drug)
MBD	minimal brain dysfunction
mcg	microgram
MCH	mean corpuscular hemoglobin (average amount in each red blood cell)
MCHC	mean corpuscular hemoglobin concentration (average concentration in a single red cell)
mCi	millicurie
μCi	microcurie
MCP	metacarpophalangeal joint
MCV	mean corpuscular volume (average size of a single red blood cell)
M.D.	Doctor of Medicine
MDI	metered-dose inhaler
MDR	minimum daily requirement
MED	minimum effective dose
mEq	milliequivalent
mEq/L	milliequivalent per liter (measurement of the concentration of a solution)
mets	metastases
MG	myasthenia gravis
Mg	magnesium
mg	milligram (1/1000 gram)
mg/cc	milligram per cubic centimeter
mg/dl	milligram per deciliter
μg	microgram (one-millionth of a gram)
MH	marital history; mental health
MI	myocardial infarction; mitral insufficiency
mL, ml	milliliter (1/1000 liter)
mm	millimeter (1/1000 meter; 0.039 inch)
mmHg	millimeters of mercury
MMPI	Minnesota Multiphasic Personality Inventory
MMR	measles-mumps-rubella (vaccine)
MMT	manual muscle testing
mμ	millimicron (1/1000 micron; a micron is 10^{-3} mm)
μm	micrometer (one-millionth of a meter)
MOAB	monoclonal antibody
monos	monocytes (white blood cells)
MR	mitral regurgitation; magnetic resonance
MRA	magnetic resonance angiogram
MRI	magnetic resonance imaging
mRNA	messenger RNA
MS	multiple sclerosis; mitral stenosis
MSL	midsternal line
MTX	methotrexate
MUGA	multiple-gated acquisition scan (of heart)
multip	multipara; multiparous
MVP	mitral valve prolapse

N	nitrogen
NA	not applicable
Na	sodium
NB	newborn
NBS	normal bowel or breath sounds
ND	normal delivery; normal development
NED	no evidence of disease
neg.	negative
NG tube	nasogastric tube
NHL	non-Hodgkin lymphoma
NICU	neonatal intensive care unit
NKA	no known allergies
NK cells	natural killer cells
NKDA	no known drug allergies
n.p.o.	nothing by mouth (*non per os*)
NSAID	nonsteroidal anti-inflammatory drug
NSR	normal sinus rhythm (of heart)
NTP	normal temperature and pressure

O, or O_2	oxygen
OA	osteoarthritis
OB/GYN	obstetrics and gynecology
OCPs	oral contraceptive pills
O.D.	Doctor of Optometry
OD	right eye (*oculus dexter*); overdose
OR	operating room
ORIF	open reduction internal fixation
ORTH; Ortho.	orthopedics
OS	left eye (*oculus sinister*)
os	opening; bone
O.T.	occupational therapy
OU	each eye (*oculus uterque*); both eyes
oz.	ounce

P	phosphorus; posterior; pressure; pulse; pupil
p̄	after
P2 or P_2	pulmonary valve closure (heart sound)
PA	pulmonary artery; posteroanterior
P-A	posteroanterior
P&A	percussion and auscultation
PAC	premature atrial contraction
PACS	picture archival communications system
$PaCO_2$, pCO_2	partial pressure of carbon dioxide in blood
palp.	palpable; palpation
PALS	pediatric advanced life support
PaO_2, pO_2	partial pressure of oxygen in blood
Pap smear	Papanicolaou smear (cells from cervix and vagina)

Para 1, 2, 3	unipara, bipara, tripara (number of viable births)
p.c.	after meals (*post cibum*)
PCA	patient controlled anesthesia
PCI	percutaneous coronary interventions
PCP	*Pneumocystis carinii* pneumonia; phencyclidine (hallucinogen)
PCR	polymerase chain reaction (process allows making copies of genes)
PD	peritoneal dialysis
PDA	patent ductus arteriosus
PDR	Physicians' Desk Reference
PE	physical examination; pulmonary embolism
PEEP	positive end-expiratory pressure
PEG	percutaneous endoscopic gastrostomy (a feeding tube)
PEJ	percutaneous endoscopic jejunostomy (a feeding tube)
per os	by mouth
PERRLA	pupils equal, round, react to light and accommodation
PET	positron emission tomography
PE tube	ventilating tube for eardrum
PFT	pulmonary function test
PG	prostaglandin
PH	past history
pH	hydrogen ion concentration (alkalinity and acidity measurement)
PI	present illness
PID	pelvic inflammatory disease
PIP	proximal interphalangeal joint
PKU	phenylketonuria
PM or p.m.	afternoon (post meridian)
PMH	past medical history
PMN	polymorphonuclear leukocyte
PMS	premenstrual syndrome
PND	paroxysmal nocturnal dyspnea
p/o	postoperative
p.o.	by mouth (*per os*)
poly	polymorphonuclear leukocyte
postop	postoperative (after surgery)
PPBS	postprandial blood sugar
PPD	purified protein derivative (test for tuberculosis)
preop	preoperative
prep	prepare for
PR	partial response
primip	primipara
PRL	prolactin
p.r.n.	as required (*pro re nata*)
procto	proctoscopy
prot.	protocol

Pro. time	prothrombin time (test of blood clotting)	**RLL**	right lower lobe (lung)
PSA	prostate-specific antigen	**RLQ**	right lower quadrant (abdomen)
pt.	patient	**RML**	right middle lobe (lung)
PT	prothrombin time; physical therapy	**RNA**	ribonucleic acid
PTA	prior to admission (to hospital)	**R/O**	rule out
PTC	percutaneous transhepatic cholangiography	**ROM**	range of motion
PTCA	percutaneous transluminal coronary angioplasty	**ROS**	review of systems
		RRR	regular rate and rhythm (of the heart)
PTH	parathyroid hormone	**RT**	right; radiation therapy
PTHC	percutaneous transhepatic cholangiography	**RUL**	right upper lobe (lung)
		RUQ	right upper quadrant (abdomen)
PTSD	post-traumatic stress disorder	**RV**	right ventricle
PTT	partial thromboplastin time (test of blood clotting)	**Rx**	treatment; therapy; prescription

Pro. time prothrombin time (test of blood clotting)
PSA prostate-specific antigen
pt. patient
PT prothrombin time; physical therapy
PTA prior to admission (to hospital)
PTC percutaneous transhepatic cholangiography
PTCA percutaneous transluminal coronary angioplasty
PTH parathyroid hormone
PTHC percutaneous transhepatic cholangiography
PTSD post-traumatic stress disorder
PTT partial thromboplastin time (test of blood clotting)
PU pregnancy urine
PUVA therapy psoralen ultraviolet A (treatment for psoriasis)
PVC premature ventricular contraction
PVD peripheral vascular disease
PWB partial weight bearing
Px prognosis

q every (*quaque*)
qAM every morning
q.d. every day (*quaque die*)
q.h. every hour (*quaque hora*)
q.2h. every 2 hours
q.i.d. four times daily (*quater in die*)
qns quantity not sufficient
qPM every evening
QRS wave complex in an electrocardiographic study
q.s. as much as suffices (*quantum sufficit*)
qt quart

R respiration; right
RA rheumatoid arthritis; right atrium
Ra radium
rad radiation absorbed dose
RBBB right bundle branch block
RBC, rbc red blood count (cell)
R.D.D.A. recommended daily dietary allowance
RDS respiratory distress syndrome
REM rapid eye movement
RF rheumatoid factor
Rh (factor) rhesus (monkey) factor in blood
RhoGAM drug to prevent Rh factor reaction in Rh-negative women
RIA radioimmunoassay (minute quantities are measured)

RLL right lower lobe (lung)
RLQ right lower quadrant (abdomen)
RML right middle lobe (lung)
RNA ribonucleic acid
R/O rule out
ROM range of motion
ROS review of systems
RRR regular rate and rhythm (of the heart)
RT right; radiation therapy
RUL right upper lobe (lung)
RUQ right upper quadrant (abdomen)
RV right ventricle
Rx treatment; therapy; prescription

s̄ without (*sine*)
S1, S2 first, second sacral vertebra
S-A node sinoatrial node (pacemaker of heart)
SAD seasonal affective disorder
SARS severe acute respiratory syndrome
SBE subacute bacterial endocarditis
SBFT small bowel follow-through (x-rays of small intestine)
SC, subcut subcutaneous
sed. rate sedimentation rate (rate of erythrocyte sedimentation)
segs segmented neutrophils; polys
SERM selective estrogen receptor modulator
SGOT (AST) serum glutamic-oxaloacetic transaminase
SGPT (ALT) serum glutamic-pyruvic transaminase
SIADH syndrome of inappropriate antidiuretic hormone
SIDS sudden infant death syndrome
sig. let it be labeled
SL sublingual
SLE systemic lupus erythematosus
SMAC automated analytical device for testing blood
SMA 12 twelve blood chemistries
SOAP subjective, objective, assessment, and plan (used for patient notes)
SOB shortness of breath
s.o.s. if necessary (*si opus sit*)
S/P status post (previous disease condition)
SPECT single-photon emission computed tomography
sp. gr. specific gravity
S/S signs and symptoms
SSCP substernal chest pain
SSRI selective serotonin reuptake inhibitor (antidepressant)

Staph.	staphylococci (berry-shaped bacteria in clusters)
stat.	immediately *(statim)*
STH	somatotropin (growth hormone)
STI	sexually transmitted infection
Strep.	streptococci (berry-shaped bacteria in twisted chains)
sc	subcutaneous
SVC	superior vena cava
SVD	spontaneous vaginal delivery
Sx	signs and symptoms
Sz	seizure

T	temperature; time
T tube	tube placed in biliary tract for drainage
T1, T2	first, second thoracic vertebra
T$_3$	triiodothyronine test
T$_4$	thyroxine test
TA	therapeutic abortion
T&A	tonsillectomy and adenoidectomy
TAB	therapeutic abortion
TAH	total abdominal hysterectomy
TAT	Thematic Apperception Test
TB	tuberculosis
Tc	technetium
T cells	lymphocytes produced in the thymus gland
TEE	transesophageal echocardiogram
TENS	transcutaneous electrical nerve stimulation
TFT	thyroid function test
TIA	transient ischemic attack
t.i.d.	three times daily *(ter in die)*
TLC	total lung capacity
TM	tympanic membrane
TMJ	temporomandibular joint
TNM	tumor, nodes, and metastases
tPA	tissue plasminogen activator
TPN	total parenteral nutrition
TPR	temperature, pulse, and respiration
TRUS	transrectal ultrasound
TSH	thyroid-stimulating hormone
TSS	toxic shock syndrome
TUR, TURP	transurethral resection of the prostate
TVH	total vaginal hysterectomy
Tx	treatment

U	unit
UA	urinalysis
UAO	upper airway obstruction
UC	uterine contractions
UE	upper extremity
UGI	upper gastrointestinal
umb.	navel *(umbilicus)*
U/O	urinary output
URI	upper respiratory infection
U/S	ultrasound
UTI	urinary tract infection
UV	ultraviolet

VA	visual acuity
VATS	video-assisted thorascopy
VC	vital capacity (of lungs)
VCUG	voiding cystourethrogram
VDRL	test for syphilis (venereal disease research laboratory)
VEGF	vascular endothelial growth factor
VF	visual fields
vis à vis	as compared with; in relation to
V/Q scan	ventilation-perfusion scan
V/S	vital signs; versus
VSD	ventricular septal defect
VT	ventricular tachycardia (abnormal heart rhythm)
VTE	venous thromboembolism

WAIS	Wechsler Adult Intelligence Scale
WBC, wbc	white blood cell; white blood count
WDWN	well developed, well nourished
WISC	Wechsler Intelligence Scale for Children
WNL	within normal limits
wt	weight

XRT	radiation therapy

y/o, yrs	year(s) old

Acronyms

An acronym is the name for an abbreviation that forms a pronounceable word.

ACE (ace) angiotensin-converting enzyme
AIDS (ades) acquired immune deficiency syndrome
BUN (bun) blood, urea, nitrogen
CABG (cabbage) coronary artery bypass graft
CAT (cat) computerized axial tomography
CPAP (seepap) continuous positive airway pressure
ELISA (eliza) enzyme-linked immunosorbent assay
GERD (gerd) gastroesophageal reflux disease
HIPAA (hipa) Health Insurance Portability and Accountability Act of 1996
LASER (lazer) light amplification by stimulated emission of radiation
LASIK (lasik) laser *in situ* keratomileusis
LEEP (leep) loop electrocautery excision procedure
MICU (miku) medical intensive care unit
MUGA (mugah) multiple-gated acquisition (scan)
NSAID (nsayd) nonsteroidal anti-inflammatory drug
NICU (niku) neonatal intensive care unit
PACS (paks) picture archival communications system
PALS (pahlz) pediatric advanced life support
PEEP (peep) positive end expiratory pressure

PEG (peg) percutaneous endoscopic gastrostomy
PERRLA (perlah) pupils equal, round, reactive to light and accommodation
PET (pet) positron emission tomography
PICU (piku) pediatric intensive care unit
PIP (pip) proximal interphalangeal joint
PUVA (poovah) psoralen ultraviolet A
REM (rem) rapid eye movement
SAD (sad) seasonal affective disorder
SARS (sarz) severe acute respiratory syndrome
SERM (serm) selective estrogen receptor modulator
SIDS (sidz) sudden infant death syndrome
SMAC (smak) sequential multiple analyzer computer (blood testing)
SOAP (sop) subjective, objective, assessment, plan
SPECT (spekt) single-photon emission computed tomography
TENS (tenz) transcutaneous electrical nerve stimulation
TRUS (truhs) transrectal ultrasound
TURP (turp) transurethral resection of the prostate
VATS (vahtz) video-assisted thorascopy

Symbols

=	equal	%	percent
≠	unequal	°	degree; hour
+	positive	:	ratio; "is to"
−	negative	±	plus or minus (either positive or negative)
↑	above, increase	′	foot
↓	below, decrease	″	inch
♀	female	∴	therefore
♂	male	@	at, each
→	to (in direction of)	c̄	with
>	is greater than	s̄	without
<	is less than	#	pound
1°	primary to	≅	approximately, about
2°	secondary to	Δ	change
ʒ	dram	p	short arm of a chromosome
℥	ounce	q	long arm of a chromosome

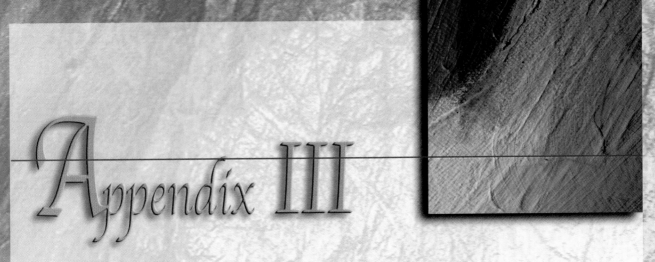

Appendix III

Normal Hematological Reference Values and Implications of Abnormal Results

The implications of abnormal results are major ones in each category. SI units are the International System of Units that are generally accepted for all scientific and technical uses. All laboratory values should be interpreted with caution since normal values differ widely among clinical laboratories.

cu mm = cubic millimeter (mm^3)
dL = deciliter (1/10 liter or 100 mL)
g = gram
L = liter
mg = milligram (1/1000 gram)
mL = milliliter
mEq = milliequivalent

mill = million
mm = millimeter (1/1000 meter)
mmol = millimole
thou = thousand
U = unit
μl = microliter
μmol = micromole (one-millionth of a mole)

Cell Counts

	Conventional Units	**SI Units**	**Implications**
Erythrocytes (RBC)			
Females	4.0–5.5 million/mm^3 or μl	4.0–5.5 $\times$ 10^{12}/L	*High* ◆ Polycythemia
Males	4.5–6.0 million/mm^3 or μl	4.5–6.0 $\times$ 10^{12}/L	◆ Dehydration
			Low ◆ Iron deficiency anemia
			◆ Blood loss
Leukocytes (WBC)			
Total	5000–10,000/mm^3 or μl	5.0–10.0 $\times$ 10^9/L	*High* ◆ Bacterial infection
			◆ Leukemia
Differential	%		◆ Eosinophils high in allergy
Neutrophils	54–62		*Low* ◆ Viral infection
Lymphocytes	20–40		◆ Aplastic anemia
Monocytes	3–7		◆ Chemotherapy
Eosinophils	1–3		
Basophils	0–1		
Platelets	150,000–350,000/mm^3 or μl	200–400 $\times$ 10^9/L	*High* ◆ Hemorrhage
			◆ Infections
			◆ Malignancy
			◆ Splenectomy
			Low ◆ Aplastic anemia
			◆ Chemotherapy
			◆ Hypersplenism

Coagulation Tests

	Conventional Units	**SI Units**	**Implications**
Bleeding time	2.75–8.0 min	2.7–8.0 min	*Prolonged* ◆ Aspirin ingestion
(template method)			◆ Low platelet count
Coagulation time	5–15 min	5–15 min	*Prolonged* ◆ Heparin therapy
Prothrombin time (PT)	12–14 sec	12–14 sec	*Prolonged* ◆ Vitamin K deficiency
			◆ Hepatic disease
			◆ Oral anticoagulant therapy

Red Blood Cell Tests

	Conventional Units	**SI Units**	**Implications**
Hematocrit (Hct)			
Females	37%–47%	0.37–0.47	*High* ◆ Polycythemia
Males	40%–54%	0.40–0.54	◆ Dehydration
			Low ◆ Loss of blood
			◆ Anemia
Hemoglobin (Hb, Hgb)			
Females	12.0–14.0 gm/dL	1.86–2.48 mmol/L	*High* ◆ Polycythemia
Males	14.0–16.0 gm/dL	2.17–2.79 mmol/L	◆ Dehydration
			Low ◆ Anemia
			◆ Blood loss

Serum Tests

	Conventional Units	SI Units	Implications
Alanine aminotransferase (ALT, SGPT)	5–30 U/L	5–30 U/L	*High* ♦ Hepatitis
Albumin	3.5–5.5 g/dl	35–55 g/L	*Low* ♦ Hepatic disease ♦ Malnutrition ♦ Nephritis and nephrosis
Alkaline phosphatase (ALP)	20–90 U/L	20–90 U/L	*High* ♦ Bone disease ♦ Hepatitis or tumor infiltration of liver ♦ Biliary obstruction
Aspartate aminotransferase (AST, SGOT)	10–30 U/L	10–30 U/L	*High* ♦ Hepatitis ♦ Cardiac and muscle injury

Bilirubin
    Total
    Neonates
	0.3–1.0 mg/dL
	1–12 mg/dL
		5.1–17 μmol/L
		17–205 μmol/L
			High ♦ Hemolysis
			♦ Neonatal hepatic immaturity
			♦ Cirrhosis
			♦ Biliary tract obstruction

Blood urea nitrogen (BUN)	10–20 mg/dL	3.6–7.1 mmol/L	*High* ♦ Renal disease ♦ Reduced renal blood flow ♦ Urinary tract obstruction *Low* ♦ Hepatic damage ♦ Malnutrition
Calcium	9.0–10.5 mg/dL	2.2–2.6 mmol/L	*High* ♦ Hyperparathyroidism ♦ Multiple myeloma ♦ Metastatic cancer *Low* ♦ Hypoparathyroidism ♦ Total parathyroidectomy

Cholesterol (desirable range)
    Total
    LDL cholesterol
    HDL cholesteol
	<200 mg/dL
	<130 mg/dL
	>60 mg/dL
		<5.2 mmol/L
		<3.36 mmol/L
		>1.55 mmol/L
			High ♦ High fat diet
			♦ Inherited hypercholesterolemia
			Low ♦ Starvation

Creatine kinase (CK)
    Females
    Males
	30–135 U/L
	55–170 U/L
		30–135 U/L
		55–170 U/L
			High ♦ Myocardial infarction
			♦ Muscle disease

Creatinine	<1.5 mg/dL	<133 μmol/L	*High* ♦ Renal disease
Glucose (fasting)	75–115 mg/dL	4.2–6.4 mmol/L	*High* ♦ Diabetes mellitus *Low* ♦ Hyperinsulinism ♦ Fasting ♦ Hypothyroidism ♦ Addison disease ♦ Pituitary insufficiency
Lactate dehydrogenase (LDH)	100–190 U/L	100–190 U/L	*High* ♦ Tissue necrosis ♦ Lymphomas ♦ Muscle disease
Phosphate ($-PO_4$)	3.0–4.5 mg/dL	1.0–1.5 mmol/L	*High* ♦ Renal failure ♦ Bone metastases ♦ Hypoparathyroidism *Low* ♦ Malnutrition ♦ Malabsorption ♦ Hyperparathyroidism

	Conventional Units	SI Units	Implications
Potassium (K)	3.5–5.0 mEq/L	3.5–5.0 mmol/L	*High* ♦ Burn victims ♦ Renal failure ♦ Diabetic ketoacidosis *Low* ♦ Cushing syndrome ♦ Loss of body fluids
Sodium (Na)	136–145 mEq/L	136–145 mmol/L	*High* ♦ Inadequate water intake ♦ Water loss in excess of sodium *Low* ♦ Adrenal insufficiency ♦ Inadequate sodium intake ♦ Excessive sodium loss
Thyroxine (T$_4$)	5–12 μg/dL	64–154 nmol/L	*High* ♦ Graves disease (hyperthyroidism) *Low* ♦ Hypothyroidism
Uric acid			
Females	2.5–8.0 mg/dL	150–480 μmol/L	*High* ♦ Gout
Males	1.5–6.0 mg/dL	90–360 μmol/L	♦ Leukemia

Appendix IV

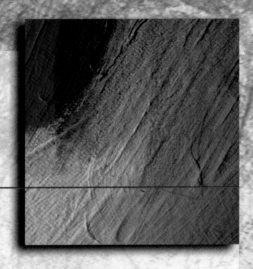

Drugs

This is an alphabetized list of drugs in Chapter 21 (tables) with brand name in parentheses and explanation of use (class or type).

Generic (Brand Name)	Explanation of Use
acarbose (Precose)	Antidiabetic/Type 2/alphaglucoside inhibitor
acetaminophen (Tylenol)	Analgesic/mild
acyclovir (Zovirax)	Antiviral
albuterol (Proventil)	Bronchodilator
alendronate (Fosamax)	Antiosteoporosis/bisphosphonate
alprazolam (Xanax)	Tranquilizer/minor/benzodiazepine
aluminum antacid (Rolaids)	GI/antacid
aluminum + magnesium antacid (Gaviscon)	GI/antacid
amiodarone (Cordarone)	Cardiovascular/antiarrhythmic
amlodipine (Norvasc)	Cardiovascular/calcium antagonist
amoxicillin trihydrate (Amoxil, Trimox)	Antibiotic/penicillin
amoxicillin + clavulanate (Augmentin)	Antibiotic/penicillin
anastrozole (Arimidex)	Endocrine/aromatase inhibitor
aspirin	Analgesic/mild: antiplatelet
atenolol (Tenormin)	Cardiovascular/beta-blocker
atorvastatin (Lipitor)	Cardiovascular/cholesterol-lowering
azithromycin (Zithromax)	Antibiotic/erythromycin class
beclomethasone (Vanceril)	Respiratory/steroid inhaler
buspirone (BuSpar)	Tranquilizer/minor
butabarbital (Butisol)	Sedative/hypnotic
caffeine	Stimulant
carbamazepine (Tegretol)	Anticonvulsant
cefprozil (Cefzil)	Antibiotic/cephalosporin
ceftazidine (Fortaz)	Antibiotic/cephalosporin

Generic (Brand Name)	Explanation of Use
cefuroxime axetil (Ceftin)	Antibiotic/cephalosporin
celecoxib (Celebrex)	Analgesic/NSAID
cephalexin (Keflex)	Antibiotic/cephalosporin
cetirizine (Zyrtec)	Antihistamine
chlorpheniramine maleate (Chor-Trimeton)	Antihistamine
chlorpromazine (Thorazine)	Tranquilizer/major/phenothiazine
cholestyramine (Questran)	Cardiovascular/cholesterol-lowering
cimetidine (Tagamet)	GI/antiulcer/anti-GERD
ciprofloxacin (Cipro)	Antibiotic/quinolone
cisapride (Propulsid)	GI/antiulcer/anti-GERD
clarithromycin (Biaxin)	Antibiotic/erythromycin class
codeine	Analgesic/narcotic
dextroamphetamine sulfate (Dexedrine)	Stimulant
diazepam (Valium)	Tranquilizer/minor/benzodiazepine
diclofenac (Voltaren)	Analgesic/NSAID
digoxin (Lanoxin)	Cardiovascular/anti-CHF
diltiazem (Cardizem CD)	Cardiovascular/calcium antagonist
diphenhydramine (Benadryl)	Antihistamine
diphenoxylate + atropine (Lomotil)	GI/antidiarrheal
doxycycline	Antibiotic/tetracycline
enalapril maleate (Vasotec)	Cardiovascular ACE inhibitor
enoxaparin sodium (Lovenox)	Anticoagulant
epinephrine	Bronchodilator
erythromycin (Ery-Tab)	Antibiotic/erythromycin
estrogen (Premarin, Prempro, Estradiol)	Endocrine/estrogen
ether	Anesthetic/general
extended insulin zinc suspension (Ultralente)	Antidiabetic/Type 1
famotidine (Pepcid)	GI/antiulcer/anti-GERD
felbamate (Felbatol)	Anticonvulsant
fexofenadine (Allegra)	Antihistamine
flecainide (Tambocor)	Cardiovascular/antiarrhythmic
fluconazole (Diflucan)	Antifungal
flunisolide (AeroBid)	Respiratory/steroid inhaler
fluoxymesterone (Halotestin)	Endocrine/androgen
flutamide (Eulexin)	Endocrine/antiandrogen
fluticasone propionate (Flovent)	Respiratory/steroid inhaler
fluvastatin (Lescol)	Cardiovascular/cholesterol-lowering
fulvestrant (Faslodex)	Endocrine/aromatase inhibitor
furosemide (Lasix)	Cardiovascular/diuretic
gabapentin (Neurontin)	Anticonvulsant
glipizide (Glucotrol XL)	Antidiabetic/Type 2/sulfonylurea
glyburide	Antidiabetic/Type 2/sulfonylurea
halothane (Fluothane)	Anesthetic/general
human insulin (Humalog)	Antidiabetic/Type 1
human insulin NPH (Humulin N)	Antidiabetic/Type 1
hydrochlorothiazide (Diuril)	Cardiovascular/diuretic
hydrocodone w/APAP	Analgesic/narcotic
hydromorphone (Dilaudid)	Analgesic/narcotic
ibuprofen (Motrin, Advil)	Analgesic/NSAID
indinavir (Crixivan)	Antiviral/protease inhibitor/anti-HIV
insulin zinc suspension (Lente)	Antidiabetic/Type 1
interferon Alfa-n1 (Wellferon)	Antiviral/anti-cancer drug
ipratropium bromide + albuterol (Atrovent)	Bronchodilator

Generic (Brand Name)	Explanation of Use
irbesartan (Avapro)	Cardiovascular/angiotensin II receptor antagonist
isoniazid or INH (Nydrazid)	Antitubercular
lamivudine (Epivir)	Antiviral/reverse transcriptase inhibitor/anti-HIV
lansoprazole (Prevacid)	GI/antiulcer/anti-GERD
letrozole (Femara)	Endocrine/aromatase inhibitor
levothyroxine (Levoxyl, Levothroid, Synthroid)	Endocrine/thyroid hormone
lidocaine (Xylocaine)	Anesthetic/local
lidocaine + prilocaine (EMLA)	Anesthetic/local
liothyronine (Cytomel)	Endocrine/thyroid hormone
liotrix (Thyrolar)	Endocrine/thyroid hormone
lisinopril (Prinivil, Zestril)	Cardiovascular/ACE inhibitor
lithium carbonate (Eskalith)	Tranquilizer/major
loperamide (Imodium)	GI/antidiarrheal
loratadine (Claritin)	Antihistamine
lorazepam (Ativan)	Tranquilizer/minor/benzodiazepine
losartan potassium (Cozaar)	Cardiovascular/angiotensin II receptor antagonist
lovastatin (Mevacor)	Cardiovascular/cholesterol-lowering
magnesium antacid (milk of magnesia)	GI/antacid
meclizine (Antivert)	Antihistamine
medroxyprogesterone acetate (Cycrin, Provera)	Endocrine/progestin
megestrol (Megace)	Endocrine/progestin
meperidine (Demerol)	Analgesic/narcotic
metaproterenol (Alupent)	Bronchodilator
metformin (Glucophage)	Antidiabetic/Type 2/biguanide
methylphenidate (Ritalin)	Stimulant
methylprednisolone (Medrol)	Respiratory/steroid IV or oral
methyltestosterone (Virilon)	Endocrine/androgen
metoclopramide (Reglan)	GI/antinauseant
metoprolol (Lopressor, Toprol-XL)	Cardiovascular/beta-blocker
miconazole (Monostat)	Antifungal
modafinil (Provigil)	Stimulant/sleep antagonist
montelukast (Singulair)	Respiratory/leukotriene modifier
nafcillin (Unipen)	Antibiotic/penicillin
naproxen (Naprosyn, Aleve)	Analgesic/NSAID
nifedipine (Adalat CC, Procardia)	Cardiovascular/calcium antagonist
nilutamide (Casodex)	Endocrine/antiandrogen
nitrofurantoin (Macrobid)	Antibiotic/sulfonamide
nitroglycerin	Cardiovascular/antianginal
nitrous oxide	Anesthetic/general
nystatin (Nilstat)	Antifungal
ofloxacin (Floxin)	Antibiotic/quinolone
olanzapine (Zyprexa)	Tranquilizer/major/antipsychotic
omeprazole (Prilosec)	GI/antiulcer/anti-GERD
ondansetron (Zofran)	GI/antinauseant
oxacillin (Bactocill)	Antibiotic/penicillin
oxycodone (Oxycontin)	Analgesic/narcotic
pamidronate disodium (Aredia)	Anti-osteoporosis/bisphosphonate
paregoric	GI/antidiarrheal
phenergan (Promethazine)	Antihistamine/antinauseant
phenobarbital	Sedative/hypnotic/anticonvulsant
phenytoin sodium (Dilantin)	Anticonvulsant
pioglitazone (Actos)	Antidiabetic/Type 2
pravastatin (Pravachol)	Cardiovascular/cholesterol-lowering